TEXTBOOK OF ANESTHESIA

VOLUME 2
CLINICAL APPLICATIONS, ADVANCED TECHNIQUES, AND CRITICAL CARE PERSPECTIVES

Dr Krunal Bhatt

ALLIED HEALTH PRESS

Textbook of Anesthesia

Volume 2: Clinical Applications, Advanced Techniques, and Critical Care Perspectives

Author: **Dr Krunal Bhatt**

Allied Health Press
4164 Lakeshore Road
Burlington ON L7L 1A4
Canada
www.alliedhealthpress.com
Email: orders@arclereducation.com

ISBN: 978-1-77956-786-4

ABOUT THE AUTHOR

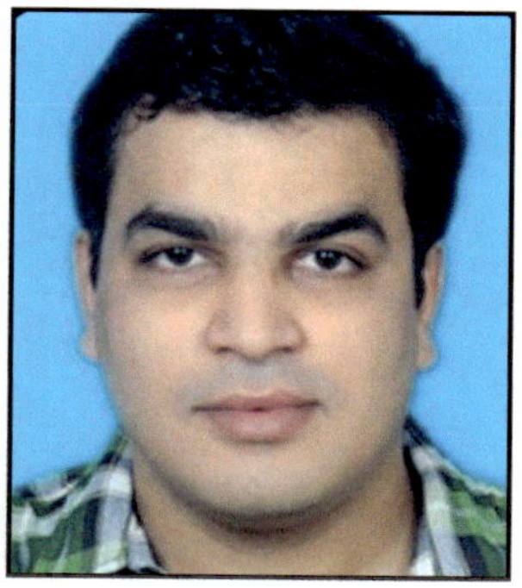

Dr Krunal Bhatt (1982) is presently working at Zydus hospital, Vadodara as a chief clinical intensivist and Anaesthesiologist for one year. He did his MBBS from Baroda Medical College. He has worked as a Medical Officer at various corporate hospitals in Vadodara (2006-2009). He joined Indian armed forces and posted to various locations during his tenure (2009-2018). He has served at Pune, Lucknow, Jodhpur, Jammu and Kashmir. He also has obtained Counter Insurgency ops medal and High Altitude serving medals for his serving tenure at line of control in Kashmir. He did his post-graduation in Anaesthesiology from AFMC, Pune, India in 2018. He is life member of Indian Medical Association, Indian Society of Anesthesiology, Indian Society of Critical Care Medicine, ad European Society of Anaesthesia.

Brief Table of Contents

Chapter Openers

A list of Chapter Outline is presented providing a brief Introduction to what will be covered in the chapter.

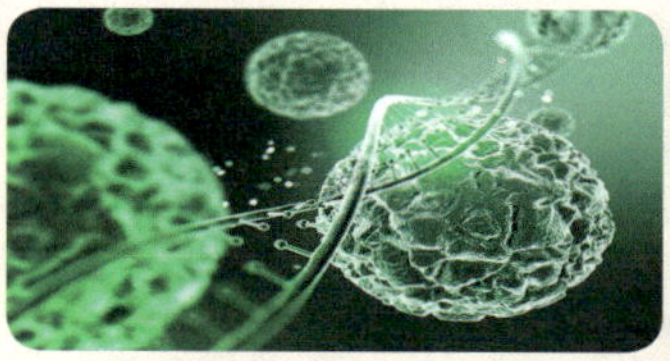

Introduction

Often referred to as the science of life, biology is a broad field of study aimed at comprehending the several kinds of life on Earth, from tiny creatures to sophisticated multicellular entities. Comprising several subfields, including molecular biology, ecology, and evolutionary biology, each of which advances our knowledge of living systems, this field clarifies the mechanisms controlling life events, including development, reproduction, and interaction with the surroundings, which is the central goal of biology. Moreover, biology fills in the void between the natural sciences and medicine by offering a necessary understanding of health, illness, and the interactions between organisms and their environments. Dealing with urgent global issues such as climate change, biodiversity loss, and new diseases depends on an awareness of these complex biological interactions, therefore highlighting the critical part biology plays in modern civilization. Fundamentally, biology explores and tests ideas about the living world using the scientific method. Through methodical observation and experimentation,

LEARNING OBJECTIVES

After studying this chapter, you will be able to:

1. Discuss the scientific method in biology;
2. Explain the cell theory;
3. Discuss the genetics and heredity;
4. Evolution and natural selection;
5. Focus on ecology and ecosystems;
6. Learn about human biology;
7. Evaluate the plant biology;
8. Explain the microbiology;
9. Focus on current trends in biology.

1.1. The Scientific Method in Biology

Learning Outcome

1. Describe the steps of the scientific method;
2. Focus on hypothesis formation;
3. Learn about experimental design.

Learning Outcomes

The beginning of each section of every chapter contains a set of Learning Outcomes that inform students of concepts they should understand. These outcomes help students understand what they should be able to do if they have mastered the material in that section.

Test Your Knowledge

Throughout each chapter, Test Your Knowledge cues you to note which topics have been covered and to self-test your understanding of the material presented.

Test Your Knowledge

1. Explain why correlation does not imply causation in scientific experiments.
2. How does the scientific method help reduce the influence of personal opinions in research?

Chapter Summary

The Summary Section appear at the end of each chapter and summarize main concepts covered throughout the chapter. These points provide key concepts in an engaging and meaningful way.

Summary

The investigation of biological principles highlights the importance of a comprehensive view of life by reflecting the intricate interactions that occur within living systems. The complexity of biology goes beyond individual species or systems, as this essay highlights; it also includes the interactions that mold ecosystems and affect biodiversity. Researchers can conduct in-depth analyses of metabolomic data using sophisticated technologies like MetaboAnalyst, which offer insights into the molecular mechanisms underlying these interactions. As demonstrated by the developments in MetaboAnalyst, for example, the integration of diverse omics data promotes a thorough understanding of metabolic pathways and helps identify important biological markers necessary for research on development and disease (Chong et al., 2018). Additionally, the phenomenon of ecological invasions is a key component of biological research and a vital field of study. The introduction of non-native species into unfamiliar habitats has significant ramifications and calls for multidisciplinary management strategies. Examining the origins and effects of these biological incursions, invasion science has become a crucial field that highlights the need to comprehend ecological dynamics and community interactions. As interest in biological invasions increases, new findings are emerging that put conventional ecological theories and practices to the test. The importance of incorporating various scientific viewpoints is shown by this developing discipline, which also highlights how invasive species shape ecosystems and advances our knowledge of ecological resilience (David et al., 2013). When taken as a whole, these discoveries from invasion science and metabolomics highlight the value of multidisciplinary biology research. Fostering cross-disciplinary collaboration and utilizing technological breakthroughs to improve our comprehension of intricate biological interactions are crucial as we look to the future of biological research. In addition to deepening our understanding of the complexities of life, this method lays the groundwork for tackling urgent environmental issues. Future studies can ensure the continued relevance of biology in a world that is constantly changing by acknowledging the interconnection of biological systems and opening the door to creative solutions that support sustainability and biodiversity conservation. We might imagine a thorough comprehension of life that serves both academia and society at large through ongoing investigation and integration of scientific knowledge.

Knowledge Assessment

The chapter includes material designed to review and reinforce each content. It includes Critical Thinking Questions to help test of your understanding of information presented in the chapter and Short answer Questions to review your understanding of the key concepts presented in the chapter.

Critical Thinking Questions

1. **Who is known as the "Father of Modern Biology"?**
   a. Aristotle
   b. Charles Darwin
   c. Gregor Mendel
   d. Louis Pasteur
2. **What is the basic unit of life?**
   a. Atom
   b. Molecule
   c. Cell
   d. Organism
3. **Which branch of biology studies the interaction of organisms with their environment?**
   a. Genetics
   b. Ecology
   c. Physiology
   d. Botany
4. **Which macromolecule is the main source of energy for living organisms?**
   a. Proteins
   b. Lipids
   c. Carbohydrates
   d. Nucleic acids
5. **DNA is primarily responsible for which function in living organisms?**
   a. Energy production
   b. Protein synthesis
   c. Storing genetic information
   d. Regulating body temperature

Short Answer Questions

1. What is biology, and why is it important to study biology?
2. What are the three main domains of life, and how are they different from one another?
3. Define homeostasis and give an example of how it works in living organisms.
4. What is the cell theory, and why is it fundamental to biology?
5. How do autotrophs and heterotrophs differ in the way they obtain energy?
6. What is the scientific method, and how is it applied in biological research?
7. Discuss how biology helps address global challenges such as climate change, disease, and food security.
8. Explain the levels of biological organization from the smallest unit to the largest. Provide examples at each level.
9. Describe the relationship between structure and function in biology, giving specific examples from cells or organs.
10. How has the discovery of genetics shaped our understanding of inheritance and variation among organisms?

Supplementary Materials

Key Terms: A list of key terms is given for quick reference

KEY TERMS FROM THIS CHAPTER

Annotation enrichment analysis
Cell theory
Ecosystems
Microbiology
Plant biology
Biological structure
Cellular structure
Genetics
Natural selection
Cell
Ecology
Human biology
Organism

Further Resources: Recommendations for additional readings, websites, and multimedia resources.

References

1. Argelaguet, R., Velten, B., Arnol, D., Dietrich, S., Zenz, T., Marioni, J. C., Buettner, F., et al. (2018). Multi-omics factor analysis—A framework for unsupervised integration of multi-omics data sets. *Molecular Systems Biology, 14*. https://doi.org/10.15252/msb.20178124.
2. Bacher, S., Blackburn, T. M., Essl, F., & Genovesi, P. (2017). *Socio-Economic Impact Classification of Alien Taxa (SEICAT)*. https://core.ac.uk/download/286567949.pdf (accessed on 8th March 2025).
3. Barnett, R., Brace, S., Cucchi, T., & Dobney, K. (2013). *Divergent Evolutionary Processes Associated with Colonization of Offshore Islands*. https://core.ac.uk/download/20664364.pdf (accessed on 8th March 2025).

Detailed Table of Contents

CHAPTER 8

CHAPTER 9

CHAPTER 10

CHAPTER 11

LIST OF FIGURES

PREFACE

Complex surgical procedures demand anesthesiology practitioners to be extremely clinically flexible, anatomically knowledgeable, and procedurally pre-planned. Every subspecialty—cardiothoracic, neurosurgery, obstetrics, or pediatrics—is associated with physiological, technical, and pharmacologic challenges. Anesthesia as a profession, therefore, evolves not merely based on generic principles but also based on specialized clinical expertise relevant to the operative milieu. Appreciation for these distinctions is imperative to deliver safety to the patient, success to the procedure, and optimum results in all fields of medicine.

Subspecialty anesthesia has arisen to prominence within the last several decades with the development of directed anesthetic techniques, modern monitoring techniques, and multidisciplinary collaboration. The role of the anesthesiologist in complex cases is more nuanced and based on operative positioning, intraoperative difficulty, patient comorbidities, and procedure-specific risk. In addition, the rising role of anesthesia outside of the traditional operating room—e.g., diagnostic suites and critical care areas—has expanded the range of expertise required on a daily basis.

Textbook of Anesthesia – Volume 2 is designed to meet the educational and clinical needs of higher learners and practitioners by addressing the specific needs of varied surgical and non-surgical specialties. Following the fundamental knowledge established in Volume 1, the present volume has a comprehensive focus on the application of anesthesia in a large range of specialties so that there is a better appreciation of issues related to procedure, patient variability, and modern-day therapeutic maneuvers.

Chapter 1 describes cardiothoracic anesthesia, covering areas of cardiopulmonary bypass management methods, myocardial protection methods, hemodynamic monitoring, and care after cardiac surgery in the cardiac surgical intensive care unit. Chapter 2 discusses anesthesia for neurosurgery, specifically cerebral physiology, positioning concerns, anesthetic goals in intracranial and spinal surgery, and neuroprotective measures.

Chapter 3 discusses obstetric anesthesia, the double concern of maternal and fetal safety, choices for labor analgesia, cesarean section anesthesia, and side effects such as hypotension and high spinal blockade. Chapter 4 discusses pediatric anesthesia, offering recommendations on age-related anatomy, pharmacokinetics, fluid therapy, and perioperative anxiolysis in children and infants. Chapter 5 discusses ENT and airway surgery anesthesia, such as airway-sharing procedures, tracheostomy, and laser safety during airway interventions.

Chapter 6 outlines anesthesia for renal and urologic surgery, with specific concerns regarding positioning, patient management in renal failure, and anesthetic aspects of transurethral procedures. Chapter 7 summarizes anesthesia for trauma and orthopedic surgery, both elective and emergent, and covers blood loss, regional blocks, and special cases in polytrauma patients.

Chapter 8 addresses anesthesia of liver and gastrointestinal surgery and addresses topics like coagulopathy, fluid shift, and hepatic drug metabolism. Chapter 9 addresses non-operating room anesthesia (NORA), with an emphasis on sedation and anesthesia delivery outside the operating room, such as in radiology, endoscopy, and interventional suites and equipment, and safety considerations pertinent to such sites.

Chapter 10 presents an overview of critical care and intensive care anesthesia, covering ventilatory support, hemodynamic stabilization, sedation in the intensive care unit, and ethical dilemmas in critically ill patients. Chapter 11 introduces the idea of chronic pain and palliative care, highlighting long-term pharmacologic management, interventional techniques, and quality-of-life enhancement strategies in terminal illness.

Chapter 12 concludes the book through recent advancements and evidence-based anesthetics, summarizing future technologies, guidelines, and findings that define contemporary anesthetic practice. Among these are point-of-care ultrasound, goal-directed therapy, perioperative medicine, and the impact of artificial intelligence on anesthesia.

It is written for anesthesia residents, senior trainees, and practicing anesthesiologists who wish to extend their skills in specialty-specific anesthesia. It is also useful for surgeons, critical care physicians, and allied postgraduate students who require a deeper appreciation of the anesthetic concerns relevant to their specialties.

ANESTHESIA FOR CARDIOTHORACIC SURGERY

1

LEARNING OBJECTIVES

After studying this chapter, you will be able to:

1. Discuss the types of anesthesia used in cardiothoracic surgery
2. Focus on preoperative assessment and preparation
3. Explain the anesthetic techniques and agents
4. Know monitoring during surgery
5. Understand postoperative care and management
6. Focus on advances in anesthesia for cardiothoracic surgery

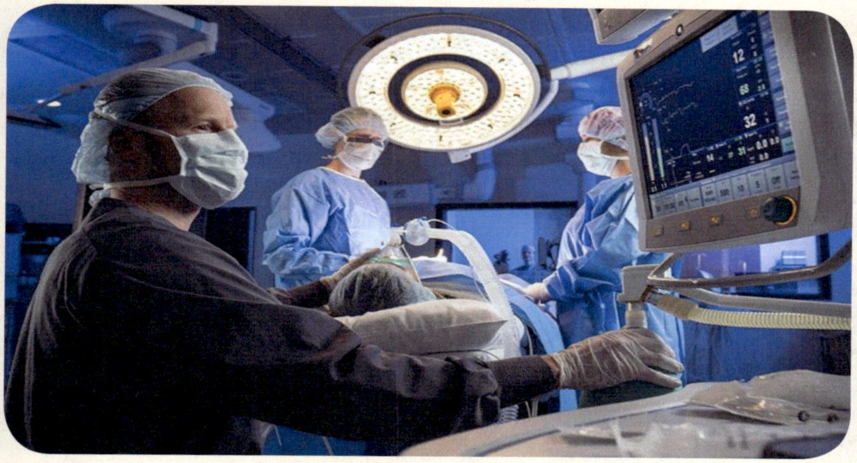

Introduction

In cardiothoracic surgery, anesthesia plays a key role in enabling complicated surgeries while ensuring patient safety and comfort. The subtle manipulation of the heart and lungs involved in cardiothoracic surgery requires a masterful expertise in anesthesia practice. Anesthesiologists must be acquainted with many anesthetic medications and monitoring equipment to condition the physiological reactions that occur during surgery. This initial perspective aims to highlight the wide-ranging impact that anesthetic choice has on surgical results, recovery from surgery, and the success of cardiothoracic interventions as a whole. With ever-advancing surgical techniques, particularly in the face of the greater popularity of minimally invasive surgeries, the regimens of anesthesia used must also adapt to counter the unique challenges of these newer surgical techniques. One of the more prevalent aspects of contemporary cardiothoracic surgery is the evolution of minimally invasive techniques, which have transformed patient care. As a result of technologies like robot-assisted surgeries, anesthesiologists are now faced with the challenges of new positioning, ventilation, and hemodynamic stability issues. As the surgical intervention landscape alters, it is more critical to explore how anesthesia practice must evolve in response to these developments. For example, while robotically assisted operations hold the potential for improved recovery and postoperative results, they also necessitate a sophisticated anesthesia strategy that optimizes patient exposure and reduces complications. Recent literature has outlined the importance of formulating strong protocols and team management to support such innovations, placing the intersection of surgical innovation and patient-anesthetic expertise as an area of future research priority (Lehr et al., 2016). Also, the establishment of minimally invasive mitral valve surgery is indicative of evolving standards for both anesthesiology and surgery. Not only do advances in less invasive procedures enhance patient recovery, but this progression is also aligned with present practices aimed at ensuring optimal surgical efficacy. Anesthesiologists are responsible for instituting best practices associated with such surgery that can differ significantly from what has been practiced historically. This dynamic practice environment of evolving methods, particularly that of mitral valve procedures, beckons serious attention to postoperative care and anesthetic aspects (Lehr et al., 2016). By integrating new technology with tried-and-true anesthetic maxims, health professionals are able to design an environment that not only prioritizes patient outcomes but also fosters continual professional development and dedication to optimal practices among the surgical and anesthetic teams (Figure 1.1).

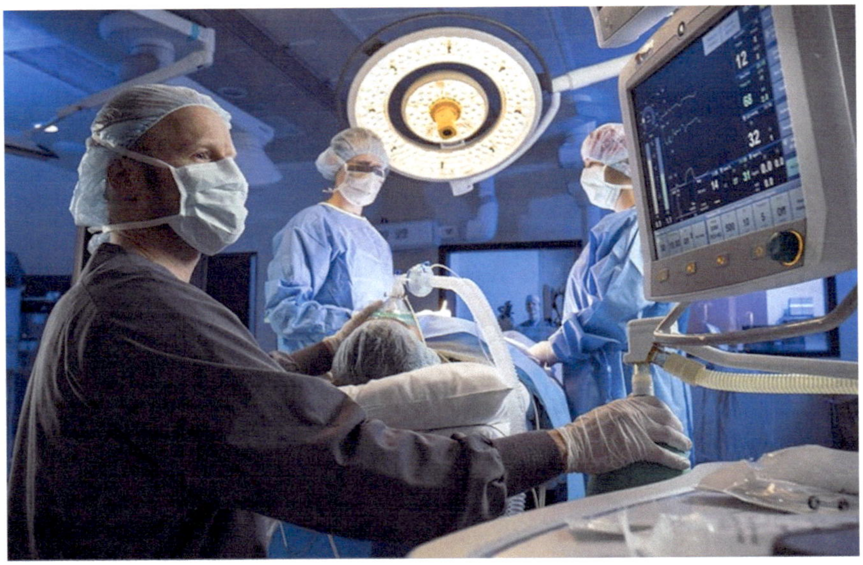

Figure 1.1. In the realm of cardiothoracic surgery, anesthesia plays a critical role in facilitating complex procedures.

Source: https://www.foxcitiesaha.com/wp-content/uploads/aha11.jpg.

Definition of Cardiothoracic Surgery

Cardiothoracic surgery is a branch of medicine that consists of surgical procedures on organs within the thorax, but with particular focus on the heart and the lungs. It combines cardiac and thoracic surgery practice because it treats conditions such as coronary artery disease, valvular heart disease, lung carcinoma, and congenital heart deformities. Similar to advancements in surgical techniques, cardiothoracic surgery has incorporated the use of minimally invasive techniques, giving patients shorter recovery times and fewer morbidity problems postoperatively. These procedures are technically demanding in that they require a lot of training and expertise, as they are generally very complicated surgeries that require in-depth knowledge of not only surgical techniques but also the disease pathophysiology being treated. Practitioners must then not only possess technical skills but also the skill of making the right decisions during the most adverse situations. Patient care throughout cardiothoracic surgery extends beyond the operating room, particularly regarding perioperative care and anesthesiology services. Anesthesia plays a vital role in patient safety and comfort during surgery, such that the surgeon can perform complex procedures without compromising physiological function. With the complications that are associated with such operations, anesthesiologists must carefully assess the cardiovascular status of their patients, mainly since patients having cardiac operations often have comorbidities. Furthermore, anesthesia regimens are planned not only to manage pain but also to optimize hemodynamic stability in operations. More advanced techniques, such as cardiopulmonary bypass, highly rely on anesthetic intervention to provide appropriate physiological parameters, and competence within the specialty is hence crucial for successful surgical outcome as well as enhanced patient recovery. Postoperative durations are still of greatest concern, with successful anesthesia management contributing to quicker recoveries as well as minimizing complications such as prolonged intensive care unit (ICU) stay. Studies also indicate that recovery time may be influenced by such variables as the complexity of the procedure and non-elective surgery. For instance, prolonged ICU stay has been associated with various patient-related factors, such as renal failure, in addition to the characteristics of surgery itself (Almashrafi et al., 2016). Likewise, in pediatric cardiothoracic surgery, the trend towards multimodal analgesia and regional anesthesia techniques has been shown to curtail opioid consumption and improve recovery time, and it is a credit to innovative practice in anesthetic management to optimize postoperative outcomes (Hall et al., 2024). Hence, the significance of anesthesia in cardiothoracic surgery cannot be overstated as its function plays an important role in the success of surgical interventions both in the short and long term (Figure 1.2).

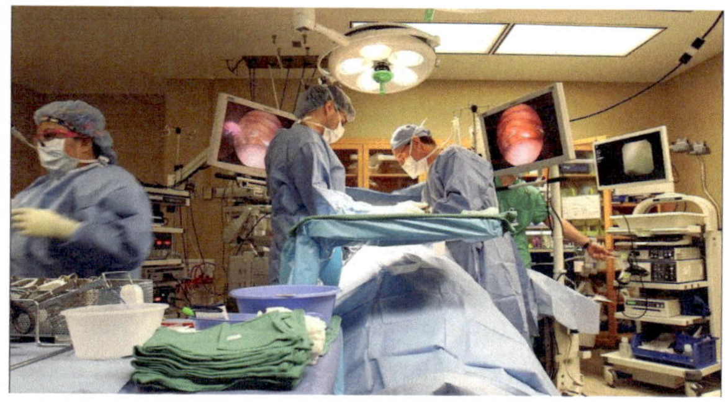

Figure 1.2. Cardiothoracic surgery represents a specialized domain within medicine that encompasses surgical procedures.

Source: https://i.ytimg.com/vi/qid-tK9I7uw/maxresdefault.jpg?sqp=-oaymwEmCIAKENAF8quKqQMa8AEB-AH-CYAC0AWKAgwIABABGHIgUigqMA8=&rs=AOn4CLDcdierdQGLsWqM8t7BWU4QytoKyw.

Importance of Anesthesia in Surgical Outcomes

The role of anesthesia within cardiothoracic surgery is pivotal, not only in the continuation of pain relief but also in optimizing overall surgical results. Anesthesia plays a key role in patient hemodynamics, enabling surgeons to operate with optimal conditions while minimizing stress responses. Anesthetists are equipped to tailor anesthetic plans to individual patient needs, especially in high-risk groups routinely met in cardiothoracic surgery. With techniques such as regional anesthesia, one can further minimize the body's burden from surgery, providing faster recovery and decreased hospital stays. Furthermore, contemporary anesthesia technology also makes direct observation of physiological parameters possible, allowing for instant control in anesthetic delivery. Hence, these technologies highlight the importance of anesthesia as they provide not just the necessary facilitation for advanced surgical techniques but also the tool for improving postoperative recovery indices significantly. Furthermore, the use of multimodal anesthesia techniques can lead to better postoperative pain management and less opioid consumption, which are highly desirable in cardiothoracic settings. With a combination of anesthetic agents and analgesics, anesthesiologists can optimize pain control while minimizing the risk of complications, such as respiratory depression or prolonged sedation, as much as possible. This kind of care is particularly helpful in heart and lung surgery, where steady respiratory and cardiovascular function should be preserved at all times. Implementation of intraoperative fluid management and temperature control policies also demonstrates how anesthesia maximizes surgical outcomes by preventing excessive complications in cardiac surgery. Ultimately, these represent an expression of a complete comprehension of patient safety and comfort, reinforcing the anesthetist's role as a critical member of the surgical team dedicated to improved patient outcomes. More and more literature highlights the interconnection between anesthetic care quality and long-term patient outcome after cardiothoracic surgery. Recent evidence shows that quality anesthesia not only influence short-term success of surgery but also has impacts on long-term recovery and survival. For instance, studies have found that inadequately controlled intraoperative blood pressure or inadequate analgesia may lead to perioperative complications, including myocardial infarction or extended mechanical ventilation, that complicate recovery and extend hospital stay. In such situations, anesthesiologists are not only tasked with ensuring procedural efficiency but also with safeguarding patients' long-term health outcomes. Besides, the identification of burnout predictors among cardiac anesthesiologists also identifies the challenge and value of this specialty, highlighting the need for continued professional development and concern. As such, respect for anesthesia's contribution to operating rooms comes with an appreciation of its decisive role in planning the course of patient recovery after intricate cardiothoracic interventions.

1.1. Types of Anesthesia Used in Cardiothoracic Surgery

Learning Outcome

1. General anesthesia
2. Regional anesthesia
3. Local anesthesia

For cardiothoracic surgery, anesthesia is a pivotal element with immediate implications for patient outcome and surgical success. The three primary forms of anesthesia employed in cardiothoracic practice are general anesthesia, regional anesthesia, and their combination, each specifically indicated for procedure requirements and patient condition. General anesthetic remains the cornerstone of most cardiothoracic surgery, with the assurance of total unconsciousness and muscle relaxation required for procedures such as coronary artery bypass grafting (CABG) and valve replacement. Regional anesthetic techniques, such as thoracic epidural and paravertebral blocks, have become increasingly popular in recent years. These modalities ensure effective pain relief and may hasten recovery, although less frequently used than general anesthetics. It is crucial that anesthesiologists understand the advantages and constraints of each type to determine the most appropriate technique for each patient with complex cardiac surgery. The choice of anesthesia in cardiothoracic surgery not only relies on the type of surgery but also greatly on the preoperative status of the patients. For instance, the occurrence of comorbidities like congestive heart disease, renal insufficiency, or obesity can affect the selection of an anesthetic method (Almashrafi et al., 2016). General anesthesia, although prevalent, poses a higher risk to the patient with compromised pulmonary or cardiac function. Regional anesthesia may, however, be a better choice for other patients, with pain control strategies suited to their clinical condition.

Furthermore, the anesthetic regimen must remain flexible and modify real-time assessment throughout surgery and the postoperative course to achieve optimal patient outcomes. With careful thought and individualized approaches, anesthesiologists can easily minimize anesthesia and surgical complications. In addition, advances in monitoring technology and anesthetic technique continually redefine the future of anesthesia for cardiothoracic surgery. Advanced perioperative monitoring devices enable anesthesiologists to maintain close control of hemodynamic variables during surgery, ultimately recording better outcomes. Studies suggest that improved scheduling and planning within the operating room, closely linked to anesthesia control, can reduce waiting times as well as increase operating efficiency (Belien et al., 2010). This not only optimizes surgical resources but also boosts patient satisfaction. With ongoing development in the field, ongoing investigation into how well newer anesthetic medications and delivery methods function has promise to further optimize safety profiles and recovery times. In short, the use of tailored anesthesia protocols based on both surgical and patient-specific variables remains the foundation for cardiothoracic surgical excellence (Figure 1.3).

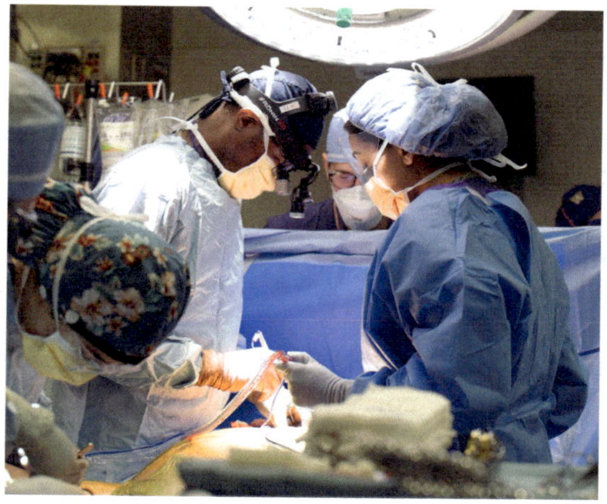

Figure 1.3. Types of anesthesia used in cardiothoracic surgery.

Source: https://anesthesiology.uw.edu/wp-content/uploads/2023/03/UWMC-CT-42-scaled.jpg.

1.1.1. General Anesthesia

General anesthesia application in cardiothoracic surgery is crucial to patient safety and effectiveness of operation. General anesthesia provides a level of controlled unconsciousness that allows surgeons to perform intricate procedures without causing pain or awareness to the patient. Intravenous or inhalational induction of anesthetic agents causes deep analgesia and muscle relaxation required for thoracic procedures. In addition, monitoring cardiovascular and respiratory function is essential in these operations due to the delicacy of thoracic procedures that produce significant physiological changes. These changes necessitate a tailored anesthetic approach based on patient-specific conditions like comorbidities, body habitus, and type of cardiac or thoracic surgery for maximum outcomes and minimization of morbidity. The pharmacological basis of general anesthesia is the intricacy of drug interactions and the subtle interplay between anesthetic depth and cardiovascular stability. Success in cardiothoracic surgery relies on the ability of the anesthesiologist to maintain hemodynamic stability and provide adequate cerebral perfusion. For example, hypnotic agents such as propofol or etomidate facilitate rapid induction of anesthesia but have different effects on cardiac output and blood pressure, with the need to make appropriate decisions depending on the patient background. Despite all advances made with anesthetics, intraoperative hypotension remains a nightmare. As the literature has outlined, brain function is very sensitive to having a good correlation between metabolic demand and regulation of cerebral blood flow, which emphasizes the task of anesthesiologists in regulating these parameters optimally (Claassen et al., 2021). Secondly, advanced monitoring equipment makes general anesthesia safer in complex surgeries. In cardiothoracic surgery, intraoperative transesophageal echocardiography, when coupled with current hemodynamic monitoring equipment, enables anesthesiologists to customize anesthesia care in real-time, making it possible for them to make anticipatory changes to avoid complications. Second, the use of protocols, including those used with extracorporeal membrane oxygenation (ECMO), serves as a reminder that having sophisticated systems to manage potential intraoperative complications in readiness is central to ensuring patient safety. The use of ECMO, while more common among pediatric patients undergoing cardiac procedures, is also suitable for adult cardiothoracic cases, particularly the case of high-risk cardiac arrest patients (Guerguerian et al., 2021). Such high-tech interventions complement the dynamic and multicentric nature of providing anesthesia in cardiothoracic surgery, where optimal outcomes rely on multidisciplinary collaboration and meticulous planning.

1.1.2. Regional Anesthesia

The use of regional anesthesia for cardiothoracic surgery presents a new way of managing postoperative pain, enhancing patient recovery, and minimizing opioid consumption. Techniques such as the erector spinae plane block (ESPB) have gained popularity in recent years because they are very effective for analgesia and can lower narcotic utilization following surgery. The ESPB preferentially blocks the sensory nerves of the thoracic spine with optimal analgesic effects while potentially minimizing the side effects of systemic opioids. This emphasis on regional blocks comes from the compelling evidence suggesting that insufficiently treated postoperative pain can enhance the risk for some complications, such as longer hospital stays and chronic pain syndromes, and undermine patient outcomes (Miller, 2023). Use of regional anesthesia techniques for cardiothoracic surgery entails recognition of the benefits and risks of each intervention. Multimodal analgesia is presently advised to optimize the patient's comfort and safety. This notwithstanding, the perceived dangers of neuraxial techniques, including the employment of epidurals, including hemorrhage and hemodynamic instability, have been a cause for caution (Miller, 2023). On the contrary, peripherally positioned nerve blocks like the ESPB offer a less invasive pathway with fewer complications, making it a suitable alternative for anesthesiologists. Efficacy studies establishing the validity of the ESPBs in varied surgery situations have shown growing interest among anesthesia providers, reflecting a trend towards the use of regional techniques in practice. Educational initiatives to educate anesthesia professionals on information about regional methods such as the ESPB can have a significant impact on standards of practice and patient care. Recent quality improvement projects have proved that formal instructional interventions can enhance providers' confidence in initiating these blocks, hence better outcomes within cardiothoracic surgery environments. Improvements in knowledge, attitudes and willingness to implement regional anesthesia methods are leading to an increasing understanding of their potential benefits. As practice under anesthesia changes, the inclusion of regional blocks in the standard procedure for cardiothoracic surgery not only paints a picture of a dedication to evidence-based practice but insists on the necessity for continuing education within the specialty, eventually working towards enhancing the quality of patient care (Figure 1.4).

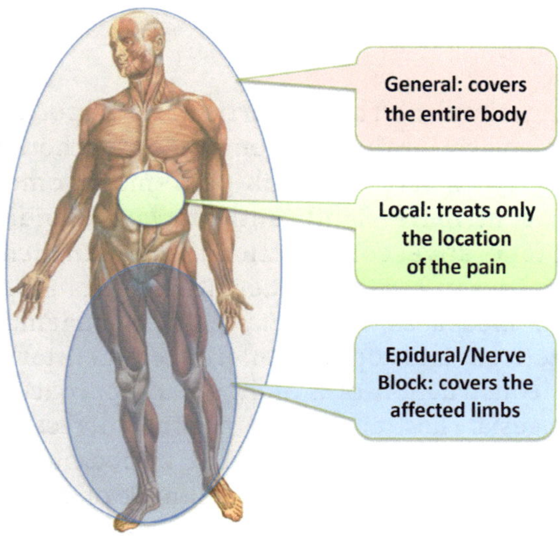

Figure 1.4. The use of regional anesthesia in cardiothoracic surgery.

Source: https://bcachemistry.wordpress.com/wp-content/uploads/2014/05/nerves1.png.

1.1.3. Local Anesthesia

The application of local anesthesia in cardiothoracic surgery is becoming a more vital aspect of perioperative pain management. Compared to general anesthesia, which typically implies complete sedation, local anesthesia enables partial pain relief with reduced potential for systemic complications. Not only does this technique lower the need for systemic opioids and related side effects, but it also leads to faster recovery. For instance, nerve blocks are also gaining popularity among the local anesthetic procedures to control pain without affecting overall consciousness, hence patients can remain alert and also participate more effectively in postoperative care. With advancements in agents and techniques, local anesthesia is increasingly being applied in cardiac and thoracic operations, improving overall patient outcomes while operating on perioperative pain efficiently. Recent studies indicate the advantages of integrating regional techniques with local anesthesia, which has been found to be effective in enhancing analgesia during cardiothoracic surgery. The application of technologies such as the erector spinae plane (ESP) block has introduced a new approach to initiating significant pain relief without being dependent on opioids to a large extent. These regional modes of anesthesia can be very beneficial in patients having complex thoracic procedures, wherein the outcome of recovery largely depends on pain management. These blocks not only limit postoperative pain but are also responsible for fewer respiratory disturbances, which can be of utmost importance in patients with a history of lung disease. The evidence indicates that when local anesthesia is combined with multimodal analgesia techniques, it leads to better patient satisfaction and final outcomes of the surgery, which needs further exploration and confirmation by randomized trials on larger groups (Cil et al., 2025).

In addition, synergistic use of imaging modalities and local anesthesia can enhance surgical precision and safety for the patient. Local anesthetics can be delivered by ultrasound and CT to target specific nerves or anatomical locations effectively, maximizing the drug delivery. This synergy is especially valuable in cardiothoracic surgery, where anatomical variability might interfere with traditional anesthetic methods. As operating teams utilize these advanced modalities, the convergence of imaging and anesthesia becomes apparent with the ultimate aim of creating a smooth interface that promotes the patient. The potential for improved outcomes and decreased adverse effects underscores the need for the coupling of local anesthesia with imaging technology, paving the way for future research in cardiothoracic anesthetic concepts (Almutairi et al., 2024).

Test Your Knowledge

1. Which type of anesthesia is most commonly used in cardiothoracic surgery?
2. What is the purpose of regional anesthesia in cardiothoracic procedures?

1.2. Preoperative Assessment and Preparation

Learning Outcome

1. Focus on Patient evaluation and medical history
2. Explain the Risk assessment and stratification
3. Understand Anesthetic plan development

In cardiothoracic surgery, preoperative assessment and preparation are critical elements that have a significant influence on patient outcomes. The evaluation is comprised of an in-depth examination of every patient's history, physical examination, and risk stratification in order to determine their suitability for surgery. In patients who are going to undergo surgery like mitral valve repair or replacement, careful assessment is employed to identify underlying comorbid disease and optimize the individual's physiological status before surgery. Also, collaborative decision-making by surgical and anesthetic teams is very important in formulating standardized guidelines for patient choice and surgical planning. By incorporating evidence-based recommendations, healthcare providers can enhance the effectiveness and safety of the perioperative process, which eventually translates to improved surgical results (Lehr et al., 2016). The anesthesiologist's function in the preoperative setting is more than being prepared for administering anesthesia; they are key to developing an individualized perioperative analgesic plan. This is particularly important, particularly for those patients on cardiothoracic surgery, where optimal pain management can contribute significantly toward avoiding postoperative complications and enhancing pathways of recovery. Anesthesiologists assess such measures as recent pain management practices and opioid tolerance, facilitating the construction of a multimodal approach to analgesia. These approaches not only correct pain in the immediate postoperative period but also strive to prevent the establishment of chronic versus acute pain, a risk especially pertinent among high-risk patient populations (Wenzel et al., 2016). Hence, the preoperative care team must collaborate in addressing expected pain management challenges to improve patient satisfaction and clinical outcomes. Preoperative preparation further entails patient education and psychological support, which are crucial in alleviating surgical anxiety. Patients commonly experience fear regarding their surgeries and potential consequences, and hence, clinicians must establish an open and supportive environment. Educational intervention can establish the surgical process, map out the role of anesthesia, and provide individualized assurances related to cardiothoracic surgery issues. Furthermore, rapport with patients allows for active patient involvement in preoperative processes, enabling them to make informed choices regarding their care. By covering both the physical and emotional bases of preoperative care, teams can maximize patients' general readiness for surgery and thus contribute positively to improved outcomes of surgery and improved recovery experiences (Figure 1.5).

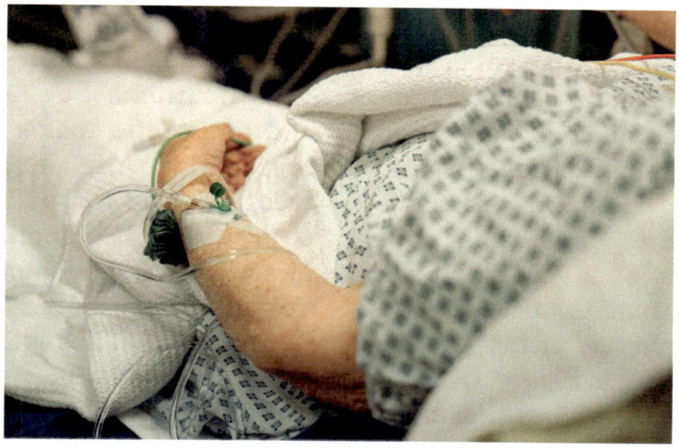

Figure 1.5. Preoperative assessment and preparation.

Source: https://www.nlg.nhs.uk/wp-content/uploads/2023/12/11072023_SGH_Theatres7-scaled.jpg.

1.2.1. Patient Evaluation and Medical History

Systematic patient evaluation and a comprehensive medical history are paramount in anesthesia for cardiothoracic surgery. The preoperative assessment allows anesthesiologists to identify prior medical conditions, current medications, and potential risk factors that may complicate the procedure. Cardiovascular disease, pulmonary disease, and diabetes significantly affect anesthesia management and patient outcomes. In addition, knowing the functional status of a patient, including any history of heart failure or arrhythmias, helps to form an individualized anesthetic plan. Successful perioperative management is reliant on such evaluations, as well as accurately predicting the patient's reaction to anesthesia, accurately and for the patient's anesthetic safety. Therefore, comprehensive history-taking not only facilitates effective preoperative planning but is also in accordance with best practice to optimize the surgical outcomes of patients for those procedures that are complex, like cardiothoracic operations, as outlined in recent guidelines for patient evaluation and selection for cardiac interventions (Lehr et al., 2016). Also important are specific preoperative determinants influencing postoperative recovery and length of stay in the cardiac intensive care unit (CICU). There are several factors that have been shown to correlate with extended recovery periods, which highlight the importance of careful preoperative evaluation. For example, factors such as the body mass index of the patients, comorbid conditions, and the complexity of the procedure are all critical in determining prognosis. A retrograde analysis of surgical patients concluded that combined coronary artery bypass grafting and valve surgery patients were at significantly greater likelihood of extended CICU stay (Almashrafi et al., 2016). Identifying these factors through an in-depth medical history is beneficial to anesthesiologists and surgical teams in risk stratification, allocation of resources, and postoperative care decision-making. Therefore, systems-based patient assessment directs not just anesthesiology care but overall surgical planning as well. Secondly, integration of evidence-based best practice into the patient evaluation process demonstrates a policy of extending surgical effectiveness and safety. Availability of protocols for routine measurement of anatomical and physiological parameters provides a means to identify high-risk patients and implement specific perioperative interventions. For patients under consideration of minimally invasive techniques, as highlighted by current expert recommendations, astute selection and planning demand extensive know-how of the patient's medical history and complications (Lehr et al., 2016). Such strategic evaluations translate to improved patient outcomes via lowered intraoperative risks and smooth postoperative recovery. Lastly, integration of a patient's history into anesthetic planning is one of the most important areas of clinical acumen and evidence-based practice overlap, providing a safer environment for patients who are undergoing cardiothoracic surgical interventions (Figure 1.6).

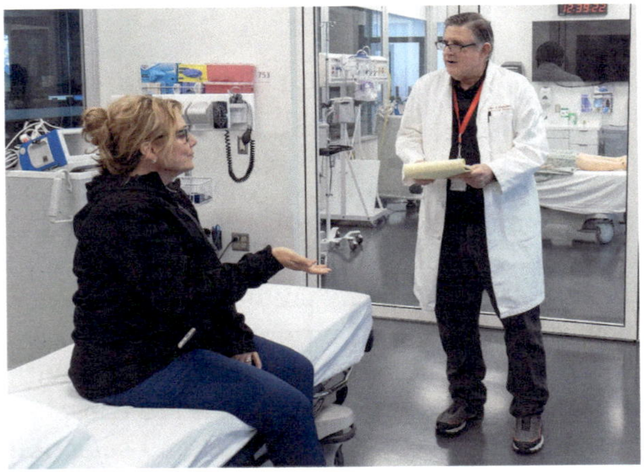

Figure 1.6. Patient evaluation and medical history.

Source: https://simzine.news/wp-content/uploads/2024/11/unnamed-2-2-scaled-e1732549335500.jpg.

1.2.2. Risk Assessment and Stratification

Risk assessment of cardiothoracic surgery patients is important to the attainment of ideal anesthesia care and successful postoperative results. It is an activity of evaluating a number of factors, including demographics, comorbid conditions, and the complexity of surgery. Risk stratification not only helps predict potential complications but also enables surgical and anesthetic teams to tailor interventions according to individual needs. For instance, recognition of the patients at heightened risk of prolonged postoperative hospitalization can direct preoperative counseling and postoperative utilization of resources, hence shaping recovery trajectories. Through the development of predictive models with preoperative data, institutions are able to improve patient management plans significantly, which ultimately enhances the quality of care offered in the CICU setting, as highlighted in studies targeting prolonged length of stay in cardiac surgery patients (Almashrafi et al., 2016). In addition to the traditional risk factors associated with cardiothoracic surgery, the elderly population is in special need of consideration in risk assessment and risk stratification. With the demographic shift in surgical patients and the rising proportion of patients older than 65 years being subjected to cardiac operations, an understanding of the impact of physiological changes with age on anesthetic management is essential. The perioperative risks are far higher in the elderly population due to the prevalence of comorbidities such as heart failure, renal failure, and cognitive impairment, all of which can increase surgical risk and make postoperative recovery more complex. Therefore, a thorough preoperative assessment of particular relevance to the patient's requirement for this age group is necessary to direct decision-making around surgical interventions (Birchenough, 2015). Understanding these aspects of risk stratification can lead to improved outcomes in this high-risk population. Ultimately, the inclusion of risk assessment and stratification in anesthesia planning for cardiothoracic surgery is an evolving process that can yield substantial dividends to patient care. With the use of predictive models that take into account many different variables from simple demographics to complex medical conditions, healthcare providers are better able to forecast complications and allocate resources more effectively. Moreover, constant updating of such risk assessment tools can improve their applicability and accuracy in line with advances in cardiothoracic surgery technology and perioperative care. As anesthesiology progresses, the shared focus on risk stratification will also grow in importance, influencing clinical pathways and dictating standards for quality improvement programs in cardiothoracic surgery (Almashrafi et al., 2016).

1.2.3. Anesthetic Plan Development

The development of an anesthetic strategy is one of the most important elements for enhancing patient protection and optimizing outcomes in cardiothoracic surgery. An entire anesthetic plan begins with a thorough preoperative assessment, which takes into account both the extent of surgery and the patient's individual physiological characteristics. Age, comorbidities, and cardiac function are some of the areas that must be thoroughly assessed to tailor the anesthetic method properly. For instance, patients with severe cardiovascular or pulmonary compromise may require a specially tailored anesthetic approach with emphasis on stable hemodynamics and adequate oxygenation. Moreover, the choice of anesthetic agents affects postoperative recovery, demanding balanced choice-making at planning time. This meticulous planning process then serves as the basis for a successful surgical procedure and postoperative recovery. Furthermore, understanding the specific surgical intervention directs anesthetic plan development. For cardiothoracic procedures such as minimally invasive mitral valve repair and replacement, an anesthetic plan must be compatible with hemodynamic barriers introduced by these techniques. Anesthesia, in more recent advances, has emphasized the importance of nonrobotic methods in minimizing trauma with good anesthesia.

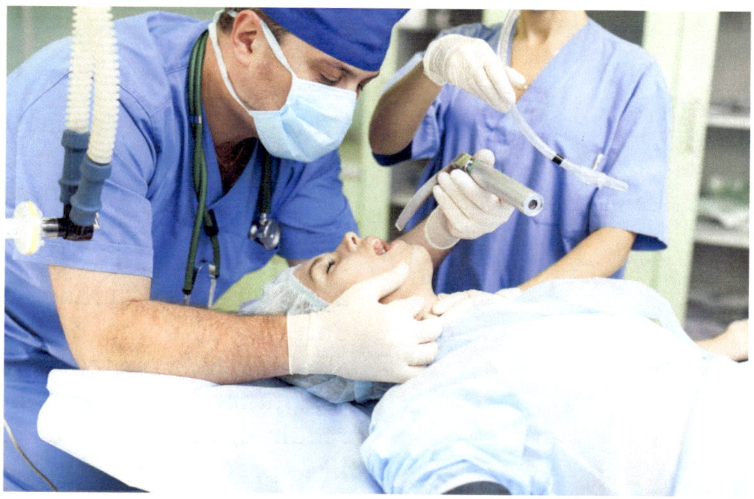

Figure 1.7. The development of an anesthetic plan is a critical component in enhancing patient safety.

Source: https://external-content.duckduckgo.com/iu/?u=http%3A%2F%2Fphotos.demandstudios.com%2Fgetty%2Farticle%2F99%2F128%2F489120943.jpg&f=1&nofb=1&ipt=be2e6f0404399fa66d044a88e41cee61262931fd9f417b9ebe8fa932f64abaec.

Anesthesiologists are obligated to adjust the plan to benefit from these newer surgical techniques while allowing smooth coordination between anesthetic care and surgery. As noted, current best practices for such cases involve not just preoperative planning but also uninterrupted intraoperative monitoring to respond early to any hemodynamic fluctuations throughout surgery (Lehr et al., 2016). This real-time adaptability accommodates favorable surgical results. Even postoperative care relies equally on the early establishment of the anesthetic plans. The strategy must incorporate interventions that lower postoperative complications such as pain, nausea, and respiratory complications, which are frequent among cardiothoracic patients. An effective anesthetic plan must consider multimodal analgesia techniques, minimizing opioid dependence and optimizing patient comfort. The ability to predict and handle postoperative complications can significantly optimize recovery pathways and decrease hospital lengths of stay. Notably, effective communication among the operating surgical team and the anesthetist is essential in this respect, ensuring continuity of care and addressing any emergent conditions likely to arise during the postoperative period. In most cases, a well-structured anesthetic plan is essential in ensuring patient safety, improving operating conditions for the surgeon, and ensuring successful recovery in cardiothoracic surgery (Department of Anesthesia, University of Iowa, 2011) (Figure 1.7).

Test Your Knowledge

1. What is the main purpose of preoperative assessment?
2. Why is patient preparation important before surgery?

1.3. Anesthetic Techniques and Agents

Learning Outcome

1. Understand Inhalational anesthetics
2. Focus on Intravenous anesthetics
3. Discuss the Neuromuscular blocking agents

In cardiothoracic surgery, the selection of the anesthetic techniques is crucial in enhancing the success of the patient and facilitating complex operations. General anesthetics are most frequently used for such operations, as it provides an even state of unconsciousness but allow rapid intubation and adequate ventilation. Utilization of complex anesthetic agents, such as intravenous agents and inhalational anesthetics, allows the maintenance of hemodynamic stability and modulation of pain response during surgery. Furthermore, the choice of agents like sevoflurane and propofol can not only regulate the depth of anesthesia but also influence postoperative recovery profiles. Adaptations of the anesthetic regimen will be required, depending on patient-specific items like preoperative cardiorespiratory health and comorbidities, which could complicate perioperative management. Combinations of multimodal anesthetic modalities can enhance analgesia with fewer side effects from opioid use. Regional anesthesia methods, including thoracic epidural analgesia or paravertebral block, have gained popularity in cardiothoracic practice since they can offer selective pain relief, enabling the patient to have more preserved respiratory function after surgery. The method has been most useful in cutting down the rate of respiratory complications, which is a major issue in thoracic surgery. In addition, a combination of local methods with common anesthesia may lead to more favorable outcomes, which in turn will allow for enhanced analgesia and reduced opioid requirements. As emphasized in current publications, inclusion of the methods has considerable effects on postoperative pain management, hence facilitating early mobilization and discharge for the patients, which is a key attribute of modern patient-oriented care in cardiothoracic surgery. The advent of neurophysiological monitoring with surgery is an exhilarating addition to anesthetic technology, particularly in high-risk surgery involving the nervous system.

Techniques such as intraoperative neurophysiological monitoring allow for real-time assessment of nerve function, thus minimizing the risk of neurologic complications with cardiac and thoracic surgery. The application of modalities such as somatosensory evoked potentials and electromyography gives the anesthesiologist a valuable complement to the evaluation of the functional integrity of key nervous structures during surgery. Such comprehensive multimodality monitoring, as controversial in the literature, represents a new dimension of safety and responsivity that permits more aggressive surgical practices when needed. By integrating this technology with effective anesthetic techniques, clinicians are able to create a patient-centric methodology that weighs operative efficiency and safety as priorities number one, making it possible to have a better prognosis in patients with complex interventions in the cardiothoracic department (Lehr et al., 2016; Singh et al., 2016) (Figure 1.8).

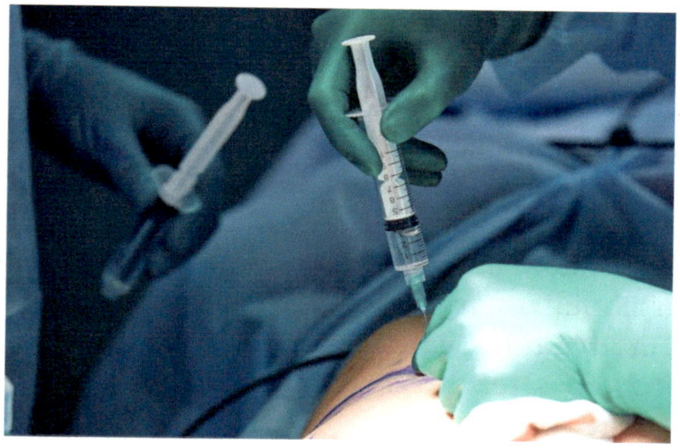

Figure 1.8. The selection of anesthetic techniques.

Source: https://philadelphiaanesthesiaservices.com/wp-content/uploads/2024/11/fieldblock.jpg.

1.3.1. Inhalational Anesthetics

Inhalational anesthetics are at the center of anesthesia control in cardiothoracic surgery, primarily due to their predictable pharmacokinetics and rapid adjustability. These anesthetics, such as sevoflurane and isoflurane, provide effective sedation and pain control, which is essential for patient comfort in lengthy and invasive procedures. Their ability to induce and maintain anesthesia with the potential to rapidly recover from it is ideally suited to the changing physiological needs typical in cardiothoracic settings. By design, such anesthetics permit an unbroken course through induction, maintenance, and recovery from anesthesia. Furthermore, their impact on hemodynamics is critical in that alterations of cardiovascular stability during surgery can be troublesome. Therefore, the choice of an anesthetic must take into account intraoperative control of the patient's cardiovascular condition to enhance outcomes. The unique demands of cardiothoracic surgery call for a thorough understanding of the interaction between cardiovascular physiology and inhalational anesthetics. Their administration should be closely observed as they have the potential to induce dose-dependent changes in heart rate and blood pressure, complicating intraoperative management. For example, certain inhalational agents produce vasodilation, thereby influencing systemic vascular resistance and cardiac output. This is most important in procedures involving cardiopulmonary bypass, wherein changes in hemodynamic values can end up affecting recovery after surgery and patient outcomes in general.

Anesthesiologists must be vigilant in regulating the depth of anesthesia provided by inhalational anesthetics, correlating their effects on hemodynamic stability and the loads imposed on the cardiovascular system by physiology throughout surgical intervention, especially taking into account the risks posed by such extensive surgery. Furthermore, the postoperative carryover from inhalational anesthetics not only impacts patient recovery but can also contribute to complications after the case, such as in the cardiothoracic patient. The choice of anesthetic influences not only intraoperative application but also the patient's postoperative course, particularly in patients who are at risk of developing complications like hemodynamic instability or respiratory depression.

This is relevant considering the fact that physiological changes induced by anesthesia and surgical interventions can complicate patterns of recovery. Effective management of the resulting effects is essential in averting postoperative care complications as well as providing adequate recovery. Hence, joint integration of inhalational anesthetics into the anesthetic strategy must also take into account intraoperative demand as well as potential postoperative outcomes, reiterating the demand for patient-specific anesthetic strategies in cardiothoracic surgery, precisely as noted in support of patient-specific models to enhance predictive power in surgical outcomes (Kaufmann & Kung, 2019) (Figure 1.9).

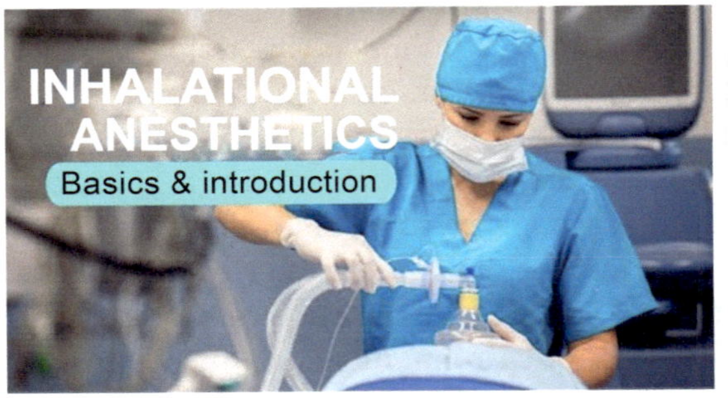

Figure 1.9. Inhalational anesthetics play a pivotal role in the management of anesthesia during cardiothoracic surgeries.

Source: https://external-content.duckduckgo.com/iu/?u=https%3A%2F%2Fi.ytimg.com%2Fvi%2FLAyjzEiajU4%2Fhqdefault.jpg&f=1&nofb=1&ipt=9b8cd54e19ec899ed6d988a2211b130ae894f15148223fc5f35ab6f51510b1e4.

1.3.2. Intravenous Anesthetics

Intravenous anesthetics occupy a central role in cardiothoracic surgery anesthesia induction, with deep impacts on the choice of anesthetic technique. These agents, e.g., propofol, etomidate, and thiopental, are favorites due to their rapid onset and ease of titration. Their pharmacokinetics are advantageous for rapid induction of anesthesia, enabling smooth transition to the operating phase, which is most critical in cardiothoracic surgery, where patient hemodynamics must be constantly monitored. In addition, intravenous anesthetics reduce the duration that patients are under anesthesia and thus can lower postoperative complications such as respiratory distress and enhance recovery times. This efficiency is critical in surgical specialties where time is of the essence and patients' stability needs to be maintained, and thus they form a vital part of the anesthetic arsenal for cardiothoracic procedures. Besides the quicker induction, the safety profile of intravenous anesthetics is another essential aspect that determines their application in cardiothoracic surgery. The titratable nature of such agents permits anesthesiologists to keep a close watch on the level of anesthesia and rapidly intervene in case of any hemodynamic variations. For example, there is emerging evidence that intravenous regional anesthesia (IVRA) can lead to shorter operation times and reduced postoperative analgesia requirements, as indicated in comparisons with standard practices (Kaufman & Kung, 2019).

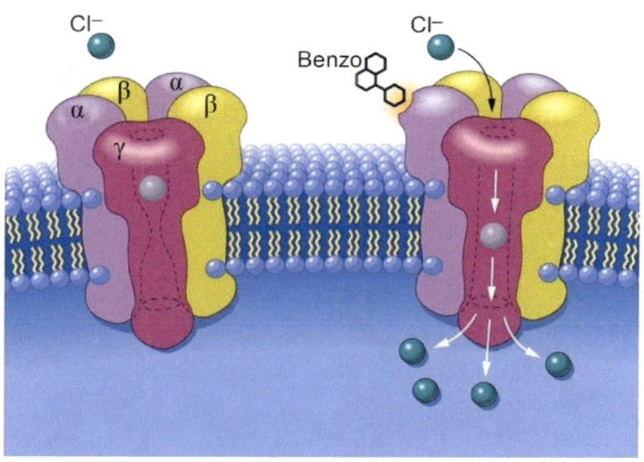

Figure 1.10. Intravenous anesthetics.

Source: https://www.nysora.com/wp-content/uploads/2022/06/8.8.jpg.

In this context, therefore, the use of intravenous anesthetics can enhance overall outcomes through decreased intraoperative complications coupled with effective pain control. This is a beneficial aspect for cardiothoracic patients, who often have complex medical histories that necessitate an expertly crafted anesthetic strategy. Secondly, intravenous anesthetics also facilitate postoperative multimodal analgesia consideration, which is most important in optimizing patient recovery. Rescue analgesics during procedures enhance pain control and may reduce the dependency on opioids post-procedure, thereby minimizing the risk of associated adverse side effects. To illustrate, studies have demonstrated the efficacy of intravenous anesthetics in combination with preoperative analgesia in proving their worth against intolerable perception of postoperative pain (Stasiowski et al., 2024). This paradigm of prevention has not only been effective in treating acute postoperative pain but has also reduced the incidence of chronic pain syndromes after surgery. Lastly, the wise selection and administration of intravenous anesthetics are paramount in achieving successful outcomes in cardiothoracic surgery, highlighting their key role in modern anesthetic practice (Figure 1.10).

1.3.3. Neuromuscular Blocking Agents

Neuromuscular blocking agents (NMBDs) are a necessary tool in the administration of anesthesia during cardiothoracic surgery, creating perfect conditions for surgery by inducing paralysis of the skeletal muscles. Paralysis gives the surgeon easier access to organs inside the thorax and significantly reduces the frequency of spontaneous muscle movement during delicate procedures. NMBDs such as succinylcholine and non-depolarizing drugs rocuronium, are critical for intubation and prolonged controlled ventilation. Appropriate paralysis also lessens the potential for complications from movement, which can jeopardize patient safety in a high-risk operation. In addition, the reversibility of these drugs allows anesthesiologists to modulate the depth and the duration of the neuromuscular blockade based on the requirements of surgery, thereby enhancing overall patient outcome in cardiothoracic operations. Effective communication between the surgical team and the anesthesiologist is very important during the administration of NMBAs in cardiothoracic surgery, particularly the dose and timing of administration of the agents. The anesthesiologist should effectively assess the status of patients for respiratory complications and neuromuscular diseases, which may affect drug efficacy and safety. For instance, patients with a history of pre-existing obstructive sleep apnea (OSA) have also been proven to be at risk of respiratory complications during the perioperative period due to synergistic effects of anesthesia and their disease, as reported in past literature (Diamond et al., 2019). Therefore, inclusion of methods such as neuromuscular monitoring is most critical in ensuring appropriate dosing and recovery monitoring. This vigil is useful in the personalization of NMBAs use, preventing residual paralysis, and enhancing patient safety during the recovery process. Moreover, innovations in advanced neuromuscular monitoring devices have enhanced NMBAs administration in cardiothoracic surgery significantly. These devices facilitate real-time monitoring of neuromuscular function, leading to precise titration of muscle relaxants and ensuring rapid recovery of neuromuscular function post-surgery. Techniques like the employment of train-of-four (TOF) and quantitative electromyography can accurately measure the extent of blockade and monitor recovery and preservation, with relevant information for the clinician. Advances in multimodal neuromonitoring have equipped AEs with the ability to promptly manage complications and navigate the intricacies surrounding the administration of NMBAs. Through these monitoring measures, risks of adverse events such as postoperative respiratory failure can be minimized, hence upholding the overall efficacy and safety of anesthesia in cardiothoracic surgery, as emphasized in the literature in regard to multimodal methods for patient monitoring during surgical interventions (Singh et al., 2016) (Figure 1.11).

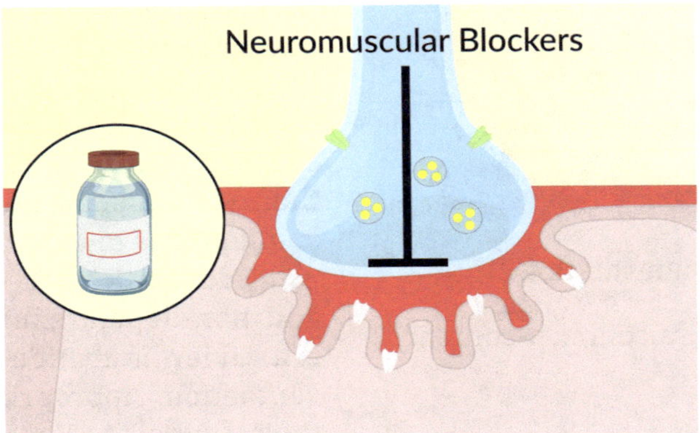

Figure 1.11. Neuromuscular blocking agents (NMBAs).

Source: https://external-content.duckduckgo.com/iu/?u=https%3A%2F%2Fcloudfront.jove.com%2Ffiles%2Fmedia%2Fscience-education%2Fscience-education-thumbs%2F14483.jpg&f=1&nofb=1&ipt=59a733a33480cb496df9f8f2d7bab5c5771191349e9d4d410cd5c8b5e949e4f6.

Test Your Knowledge

1. What is the main difference between inhalational anesthetics and intravenous anesthetics in terms of administration?
2. Give one example of an inhalational anesthetic and one example of an intravenous anesthetic.

1.4. Monitoring During Surgery

Learning Outcome

1. Explain the Vital signs and hemodynamic monitoring
2. Focus on Depth of anesthesia assessment
3. Discuss the Neuromuscular function monitoring

Surgical monitoring is a critical component of anesthesia care in cardiothoracic surgery. The procedures have a nature so complex that complex monitoring has to be used, such as hemodynamic values, oxygenation, and neuromuscular status. Continuous monitoring of vital parameters like heart rate, blood pressure, and oxygen saturation provides anesthesiologists with an opportunity to make real-time adjustments in anesthetic and supportive devices. This vigilant monitoring is required to recognize and manage intraoperative complications such as hypotension or hypoxemia, which can jeopardize patient outcomes. Advances in technology have also improved such monitoring functionalities, allowing for more sophisticated insight into patients' physiological status throughout the entire process of surgery, improving overall efficacy and safety of anesthesia management in cardiothoracic surgery. In recent years, the introduction of neuroelectrophysiological monitoring modalities has considerably enhanced the anesthetic practice for intricate operations, especially those involving the spine and thoracic cavity. Techniques such as somatosensory evoked potentials (SSEPs) and motor evoked potentials (MEPs) provide real-time information regarding neural pathway functional status during surgical manipulation. Not only do such modalities assist in the preservation of neurological integrity, but they also facilitate intraoperative decision-making. Optimization of neurophysiological monitoring has been shown to reduce intraoperative neurological complications, thereby ensuring patient safety and postoperative recovery (2025). Furthermore, individualized anesthesia strategies that make use of such high-level monitoring techniques will sufficiently prevent risk while streamlining anesthetic management and ensuring better surgical outcomes and patient satisfaction. Lung ultrasound monitoring of lung isolation in cardiothoracic surgery has also gained significance for its reliability and safety. Traditional methods, such as auscultation, have proved to be insensitive and nonspecific in identifying double-lumen tube placement endobronchial. Modern studies indicate lung ultrasound performs much better than auscultation, providing a more precise measure of ensuring proper ventilation and isolation of the lungs during one-lung ventilation procedures.

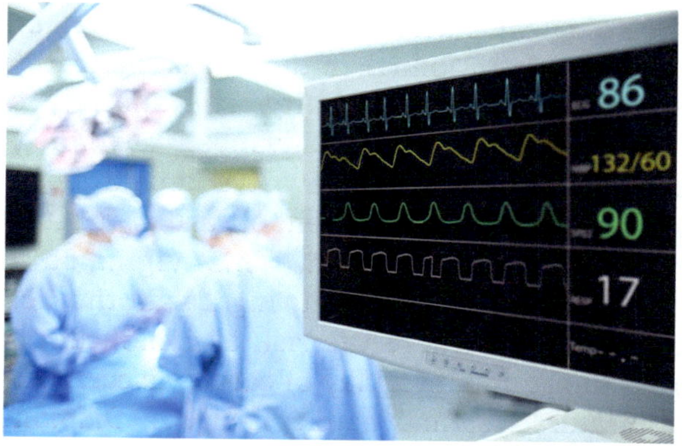

Figure 1.12. Monitoring during surgery is a critical component of anesthesia management in cardiothoracic procedures.

Source: https://external-content.duckduckgo.com/iu/?u=https%3A%2F%2Fphiladelphiaanesthesiaservices.com%2Fwp-content%2Fuploads%2F2022%2F09%2FarterialBPmonitoring.jpeg&f=1&nofb=1&ipt=71480697cc478f486320ecd61b30266d692eabc8f44fc2b1497beb46e625be78.

This more advanced monitoring is crucial since it allows anesthesiologists to provide optimal surgical access conditions while achieving adequate oxygenation. With advancing science, application of newer equipment such as ultrasound in routine monitoring procedures has good prospects of increasing the quality and safety of anesthesia control during cardiothoracic surgery (Agarwal et al., 2024) (Figure 1.12).

1.4.1. Vital Signs and Hemodynamic Monitoring

In the context of cardiothoracic surgery, maintaining ideal vital signs and hemodynamic parameters is crucial in order to guarantee patient safety and successful surgery. Access to ample knowledge of vital signs such as heart rate, blood pressure, and oxygen saturation and comprehensive hemodynamic monitoring allows anesthesiologists to deliver correct decision-making during surgery. These parameters allow for crucial monitors of the physiological status of a patient and enable timely intervention when there is an indication of hemodynamic instability. The subtlety of monitoring—employing advanced technology like invasive and non-invasive techniques—allows for timely assessment of cardiac function and systemic perfusion. This vigilance is particularly important during cardiothoracic interventions, where the risk of complications from the subtle interplay of cardiovascular and respiratory system dynamics is higher (Diamond et al., 2019). Cardiothoracic anesthesia inherently necessitates close monitoring of hemodynamic variables, given the great risk of perioperative cardiac complications. Blood pressure management is particularly important; hypotension or hypertension may precipitate adverse surgical outcomes or postoperative delay in recovery. Additionally, heart rate needs to be monitored to detect arrhythmias that can develop secondary to myocardial stress. Advanced hemodynamic monitoring techniques, such as the use of pulmonary artery catheters or echocardiography, provide information regarding ventricular performance and fluid status. Such techniques allow anesthesiologists to control fluid management, critical in avoiding events such as myocardial ischemia or cardiac arrest during and after surgery. The complexity of such cases calls for an interdisciplinary and multidisciplinary intervention to resolve all the variables impacting patient stability (Francesco et al., 2023). Furthermore, the use of hemodynamic monitoring and vital signs becomes necessary while treating patients suffering from underlying issues such as coronary artery disease or diabetes. For instance, multiple comorbid patients often require a tailored anesthetic practice considering their specific physiological problems.

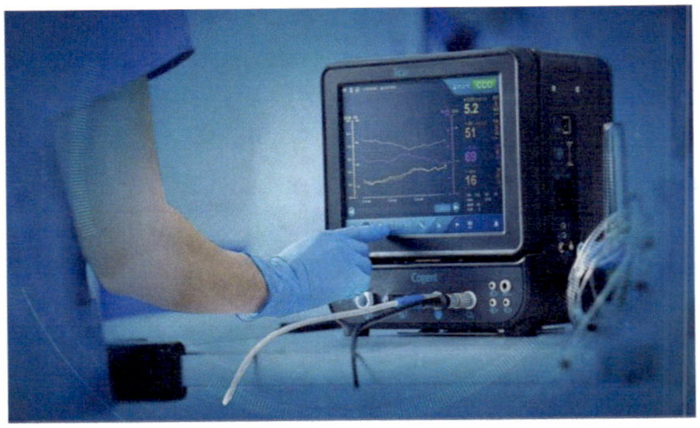

Figure 1.13. In the realm of cardiothoracic surgery, maintaining optimal vital signs and hemodynamic parameters is crucial for patient safety and surgical success.

Source: https://www.dicardiology.com/sites/default/files/styles/content_feed_large/public/field/image/Hemodynamic-Monitoring-Market-Website-New-e1659953386571.jpeg?itok=uVLihU7D.

Effective team communication, made possible through instantaneous hemodynamic feedback, allows anesthesiology protocols to be fine-tuned to meet the continuously evolving individual needs of each patient. With such a coordinated response, not only is the outcome of surgery enhanced, but postoperative complication risk is also minimized. Such interaction between watchful attention and responsive anesthetic management thus constitutes a cornerstone in ensuring patient safety as well as improving recovery processes among cardiothoracic surgery patients, underscoring the pivotal role of anesthesiology towards contemporary cardiac and thoracic interventions (Diamond et al., 2019) (Figure 1.13).

1.4.2. Depth of Anesthesia Assessment

Depth of anesthesia is an important factor in ensuring the safety and efficacy of anesthetic care, particularly in cardiothoracic surgery. This extremely technical surgical subspecialty creates unique challenges, with the requirement for tight anesthetic depth control to produce hemodynamic stability and optimal operating conditions. Patient physiology changes and the risk of cardiovascular compromise requires active monitoring to predict and prevent adverse events. Intraoperative anesthesia depth monitoring can be both subjective and objective, for example, clinical signs of anesthesia, hemodynamic considerations, and other newer technologies. The use of neuromonitoring, as made clear by contemporary literature, highlights the advantage of multimodality approaches in ventilating and titrating anesthesia depth, ensuring patient safety throughout the procedure. Hence, a complete understanding of these assessment tools is a necessary aspect for anesthesiologists in the context of cardiothoracic surgery. The use of multimodal monitoring techniques enables anesthesiologists to better navigate the intricacy of drug interactions and physiological effects. New advancements entail the use of neuromonitoring modalities, which can generate real-time feedback about the functional integrity of the nervous system while performing complex procedures. For instance, employing electroencephalography with somatosensory evoked potentials allows a more complete evaluation of the depth of anesthesia, aligning the administration of adequate analgesia with the prevention of awareness during anesthesia. While each modality is limited in some way, a multimodal approach takes advantage of the strengths of each method to enhance the overall measure of depth of anesthesia. This integrated philosophy is at the core of cardiothoracic surgery, in which anesthetic management is directly tied to patient outcome and emphasizes the necessity to integrate new monitoring technology into practice (Singh et al., 2016). Depth of anesthesia monitoring must also consider potential postoperative complications, like pulmonary edema, that have a significant impact on recovery and outcome in patients undergoing cardiothoracic surgery.

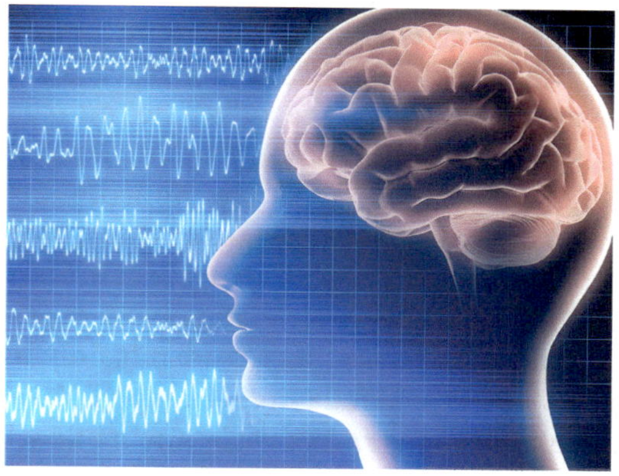

Figure 1.14. The assessment of depth of anesthesia.

Source: https://www.apsf.org/wp-content/uploads/newsletters/2019/3402/anesthesia-monitoring-featured.jpg.

The relationship between anesthetic depth and pulmonary function should be monitored cautiously perioperatively. Literature indicates that early diagnosis and intervention of complications like pulmonary edema can improve postoperative outcomes, which is why there is a need for timely diagnosis and management tools. Tools such as lung ultrasonography and transpulmonary thermodilution have proved to be effective modalities for the measurement of extravascular lung water and identification of high-risk patients. By their application in conjunction with depth of anesthesia monitoring, clinicians can more effectively optimize overall surgical care and patient safety (Assaad et al., 2018). Thus, critically evaluating anesthetic depth is not only fundamental to intraoperative care but also successful recovery for cardiothoracic surgery patients (Figure 1.14).

1.4.3. Neuromuscular Function Monitoring

The importance of monitoring neuromuscular function during cardiothoracic surgery cannot be overstressed, particularly in terms of patient safety and optimal postoperative outcomes. Neuromuscular blocking is commonly employed to facilitate intubation and improve surgical exposure, but its effect must be monitored carefully so that problems with residual paralysis can be prevented. Accurate neuromuscular function monitoring allows anesthesiologists to titrate neuromuscular drugs accurately as well as predict the return of muscle strength. Measuring neuromuscular transmission using technologies like electromyography (EMG) and acceleromyography offers real-time feedback on the adequacy of recovery and neuromuscular block, which is essential in a high-stakes setting like cardiothoracic surgery. Using these methods, postoperative complications like respiratory failure or the need for prolonged mechanical ventilation can be meaningfully reduced, illustrating the importance of continuous monitoring in patient safety. In addition to enhancing patient safety, neuromuscular function monitoring also offers a valuable means for assessing neuromuscular integrity in the operating room. In cardiothoracic surgery, and more specifically in complicated procedures of the heart and lungs, nervous system damage is a serious risk. With multimodal monitoring methods, as recent reports have emphasized, full safety evaluations of nervous system tissues can be provided, especially in procedures with delicate cranial and peripheral nerves. For example, intraoperative neurophysiological monitoring, through techniques such as transcranial electric motor evoked potentials and somatosensory evoked potentials, enables anesthesiologists to monitor the functional consistency of neural pathways on a constant basis throughout a procedure. Identification of neuromuscular dysfunction is a key to early intervention to prevent potential complications, and hence an overall safer operation (Singh et al., 2016).

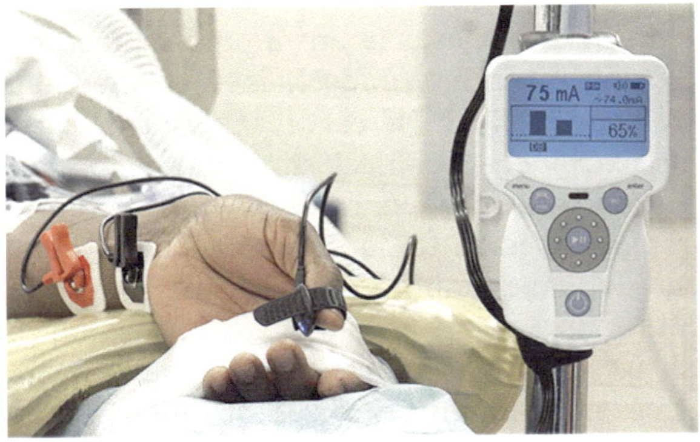

Figure 1.15. The importance of neuromuscular function monitoring.

Source: https://www.nejm.org/cms/10.1056/NEJMvcm1603741/asset/a6bcfab0-5aaa-4aee-9c54-559162f1e3b0/assets/images/large/nejmvcm1603741_f5.jpg.

Moreover, integration of continuous intraoperative neuromonitoring techniques is not merely measuring neuromuscular function but also has broader potential effects on surgical outcomes in advanced cardiothoracic surgery. Specifically, technological advancements in monitoring can facilitate early identification of positional brachial plexopathy, a risk factor in prolonged surgeries, particularly those involving arm positioning. As a number of case reports show, this monitoring has proven effective in identifying extensive amplitude loss of evoked potentials, compelling necessary positional adjustments to avert permanent nerve damage (Luginbuhl et al., 2012). By utilizing these techniques in cardiothoracic surgery, anesthesiologists are able not only to enhance the safety of the procedure but also to contribute to improving neurological outcomes, thereby confirming the essential importance of neuromuscular function monitoring to modern surgical practice (Figure 1.15).

Test Your Knowledge

1. Which vital signs are commonly monitored during surgery, and why is hemodynamic monitoring important?
2. What is neuromuscular function monitoring, and how does it help in assessing muscle relaxation during anesthesia?

1.5. Postoperative Care and Management

Learning Outcome

1. Discuss the Recovery from anesthesia
2 Explain the Pain management strategies
3 Focus on Complications and their management

Good postoperative management and care are crucial factors that will influence the overall result of the patient following cardiothoracic surgery. The postoperative course is often disturbed by complications such as low cardiac output, renal failure, and infection, which can have a profound impact on the recovery process. Observation is the most important thing, particularly within the first several hours following surgery, when patients are typically taken to the intensive care unit (ICU) for close monitoring and support. The fast-track model, intended to accelerate recovery and shorten hospital stays, requires meticulous planning and implementation. Research has indicated that following it deviates from this protocol can result in higher rates of readmission to the ICU, which are linked with adverse patient outcomes, including increased mortality and hospital length of stay, thus emphasizing the need for close observation at this juncture of recovery (Kiessling et al., 2013). Apart from physiological monitoring, postoperative care is an interdisciplinary process that weaves in anesthesia care, surgical follow-ups, and rehabilitation interventions. An instance is the introduction of physical therapy early on since this was shown to decrease recovery time through facilitated mobility and reducing the risk of postoperative complications like deep vein thrombosis and pulmonary embolism. Moreover, the anesthetic technique employed during surgery has a direct influence on postoperative pain management, and this is of critical significance for early mobilization. Individualized pain management should be initiated, with multimodal analgesia designed to optimize comfort while decreasing the use of opioids since such drugs have deleterious effects on respiratory function and recovery (Lehr et al., 2016). These combined strategies emphasize the importance of an integrated care model that will be able to manage the patient's complex needs following surgery. New technologies in minimally invasive techniques also call for a redefinition of postoperative care management. Improvements in nonrobotic and minimally invasive mitral valve replacement and repair, for instance, have seen shorter stays and reduced postoperative pain, revolutionizing traditional management practices. These developments necessitate modifying nursing and medical processes to enable the provision of new best practices pertaining to the specific physiological variations of less invasive procedures. Continuing education and in-service training for healthcare providers are needed to accommodate such evolving techniques and ensure postoperative care is in line with new evidence-based practices. Therefore, postoperative care in cardiothoracic surgery is not only focused on the handling of early postoperative needs but also emphasizes long-term patterns of recovery, which are vastly affected by advancements in surgical technology (Lehr et al., 2016).

1.5.1. Recovery From Anesthesia

Recovery from anesthesia, especially for cardiothoracic surgery, is a multidimensional process that prioritizes patient safety and comfort. The post-anesthetic phase is most important at the beginning, when patients move out of the influence of anesthesia and become fully conscious. Monitoring vital signs during this time is very important, as the signs may shift because of residual anesthetic drugs. The delivery of multimodal analgesia, where both regional and systemic drugs are given to alleviate pain, plays a central role in facilitating recovery. Not only does this method enhance patient comfort, but it also prevents the occurrence of complications arising from opioid addiction, making it imperative for overall pain management strategies to be employed in the recovery process after surgery. During the recovery of patients from anesthesia after cardiothoracic surgeries, the use of enhanced recovery after surgery (ERAS) protocols significantly influences their postoperative course. Prioritizing early mobilization and nutrition has been shown to result in faster recovery and discharge. In this system, postoperative pain management by interventions such as fascial plane blocks can maximize analgesia while having fewer systemic side effects. Evidence of the success of these measures attests to their suitability for optimizing the recovery process. Accordingly, a holistic technique combining zealous observation, best pain management practices, and mobilization provides a favorable setting for the patient, promoting not just recovery but overall well-being within the postoperative setting. The recovery process following surgery is, in addition, not just physical; psychological factors are of equal concern. Anxiety and distress post-cardiothoracic surgery can complicate recovery, and therefore, holistic interventions must be used that address physical and emotional needs. Non-pharmacological interventions like cognitive-behavioral therapy or patient education on the recovery process complement the entire experience by enhancing control and optimism. With such great stakes and risk levels riding on surgery in this specialized field, patient-centered practice, as indicated by Capuano et al. (2024), becomes a key to improving patient outcomes. All these practices work together to form a more streamlined recovery process, allowing for an improved transition from surgery to post-operative healing (Figure 1.16).

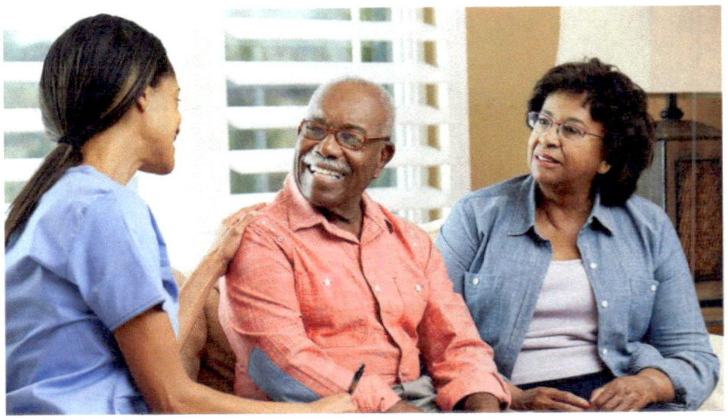

Figure 1.16. The recovery from anesthesia.

Source: https://medstarhealth-delivery.sitecorecontenthub.cloud/api/public/content/services%2FAnesthesia-Recovery-and-Going-Home?v=2dbec21d.

1.5.2. Pain Management Strategies

Effective pain management methods are at the forefront of the anesthesia world for cardiothoracic surgery, as they have a direct impact on patient outcomes and recovery.

Anesthesia administration is all about minimizing the pain of surgery without compromising patient safety. Techniques can include the use of regional anesthesia, which has gained popularity due to its perceived way of delivering localized relief from pain with less systemic drug exposure. It not only allows for pain management but also helps decrease opioid demand, thus lowering the risks of opioid dependency and side effects. In addition, multimodal analgesia with multiple pharmacologic agents such as the NSAIDs and local anesthetics can synergistically contribute to pain relief and offer a more comprehensive pain management approach that addresses many pain pathways and mechanisms, offering a definite advantage in the postoperative setting. The management of pain during the course of cardiothoracic procedures also entails the progressive application of non-pharmacologic therapies, which have increasingly been appreciated for their potential to complement standard practice. Techniques such as acupuncture, massage, and guided imagery are increasingly being used as adjunctive therapy to pharmacologic interventions in pain management schemes. Through these complementary approaches, medical professionals are in a position to address the various dimensions of pain, considering the psychological, emotional, and physiological factors that contribute to the patient's suffering. Research indicates that these steps lead to greater patient satisfaction and increased rates of recovery. In addition, integrating these non-pharmacological interventions with the overall pain management plan of cardiothoracic surgical patients can enable burnout problems in healthcare providers since greater patient outcomes are highly associated with reduced stress levels among caregivers in high-stress settings, as evidenced by studies of burnout among cardiac anesthesiologists (Sanfilippo et al., 2018). Lastly, evolving techniques in cardiothoracic surgery itself are also influencing pain management strategies. Minimally invasive surgical methods, such as robot-assisted surgery, have not only been encouraging in reducing tissue trauma but also significantly enhancing post-operative pain control (Lehr et al., 2016). Innovations achieved allow for less narcotic reliance during the post-surgical course and improve recovery at a faster rate, which is crucial in high-complexity cardiothoracic procedures. Pre-emptive optimization of the post-operative pain control approach relies on an understanding of the individual patient's requirements and response to the multiple modalities. By controlled assessment and tailoring of analgesic techniques, caregivers can offer patients total care encompassing immediate and long-term pain management and therefore strive for overall enhancement and quality of life for the patient following challenging surgery (Figure 1.17).

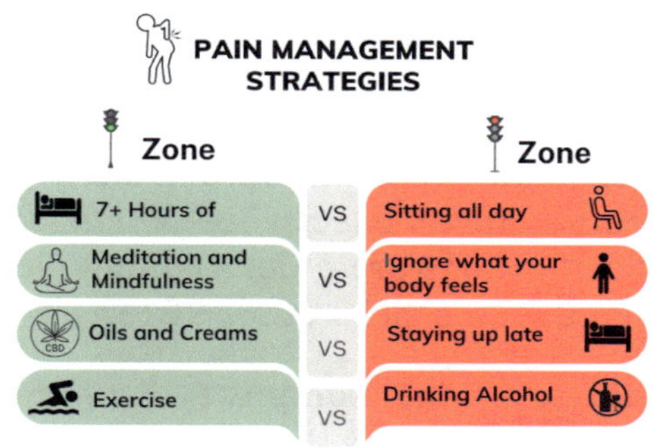

Figure 1.17. Pain management strategies.

Source: https://www.biaww.org/uploads/1/2/5/7/12574140/sessions-1-5-infographics1_orig.png.

1.5.3. Complications and Their Management

Management of complications during and following cardiothoracic surgery is a critical aspect of anesthetic management. Re-admission to the ICU following surgery is among the lingering issues, and it is an adverse indicator of patient prognosis. A review noted that roughly 36% of patients scheduled for fast-track care either could not be transferred to an intermediate care unit on the day of surgery or needed re-admission to the ICU following the first postoperative day, with mortality rates being a marker for this poor outcome. Risk predictors in this expedited protocol found include higher ASA and NYHA classifications and longer surgical times, all indicative of the necessity of meticulous preoperative analysis and planning (Kiessling et al., 2013). Sound care practices are not only needed to prevent these complications, but also the implementation of strict monitoring and intervention tactics to safeguard patient recuperation. Another severe complication often faced in cardiothoracic surgery is prolonged postoperative length of stay (LOS), particularly in the cardiac intensive care unit (CICU). Various factors converge to arrive at this outcome, among them the complexity of the procedure and the patient's conditions. For example, non-elective cases and congestive heart failure have been found to contribute considerably to longer LOS. Research indicates that approximately 30.5% of surgery patients experience prolonged LOS, and complications are a determining factor in this regard (Almashrafi et al., 2016).

Therefore, the complete awareness of individual patient risks allows anesthesiologists and surgical teams to optimize perioperative care accordingly, planning timely intervention in case of complications and optimizing the operations of available resources accordingly. Complication consequences are not solely confined to the immediate postoperative period; they can significantly affect long-term healing and global patient quality of life. The identification of risk factors for complications determines anesthetic management and enables the formation of a preventative plan for patient care. Studies have reported the utilization of predictive models that are based on a variety of preoperative variables and thus help to identify those patients who are at greater risk of complications such as prolonged CICU stay and re-admission (Almashrafi et al., 2016). These models support decision-making on resource allocation and tailoring the plans for patient management, thus improving surgical outcomes. Continued monitoring and refinement of anesthetic modalities and monitoring protocols will remain essential in their management, thereby ensuring maximally beneficial recovery profiles for patients undergoing cardiothoracic surgery.

Test Your Knowledge

1. What are the key components of postoperative care immediately after surgery?
2. Why is pain management important in postoperative patients, and what methods are commonly used?

1.6. Advances in Anesthesia for Cardiothoracic Surgery

Learning Outcome

1. Understand New anesthetic agents and techniques
2. Discuss the Technology in monitoring and safety
3. Learn about Research and future directions

The anesthetic care specialty for cardiothoracic procedures has witnessed tremendous advancements over the recent past, with enhanced patient safety and operation results. Of notable significance among such developments is the refining of anesthetic techniques, including the application of focused ultrasound to facilitate regional anesthetic placement. This modality also has enormous benefits with regard to real-time imaging, not only facilitating more effective nerve blocks but also minimizing risks associated with the employment of blind methods. Multimodal analgesia methods have also revolutionized pain control in the postoperative period, promoting reduced opioid consumption and improved recovery rates. By combining various analgesic agents, anesthesiologists are in a position to tailor pain control regimens to the unique requirements of each patient, thereby enabling greater ambulation and reduced length of stay, ultimately leading to better patient satisfaction and outcome (Department of Anesthesia, University of Iowa, 2011). Besides improved anesthetic techniques, the blending of technology has played a significant role in the administration of anesthesia in cardiothoracic surgery. The advent of sophisticated monitoring equipment has enabled real-time assessment of patients' cardiovascular and respiratory status during surgery. Such technologies are sophisticated hemodynamic monitoring through minimally invasive equipment that yields critical information on a patient's physiological status. Such advances not only allow anesthetists to respond to changes in patient condition on time but also provide information that can be used to make intraoperative decisions. On top of this, processing with machine learning algorithms will be capable of predicting patient outcomes based on historical data and therefore further optimizing the anesthetic approach on a case-by-case basis with improved safety and efficiency in patient care (Singh et al., 2016).

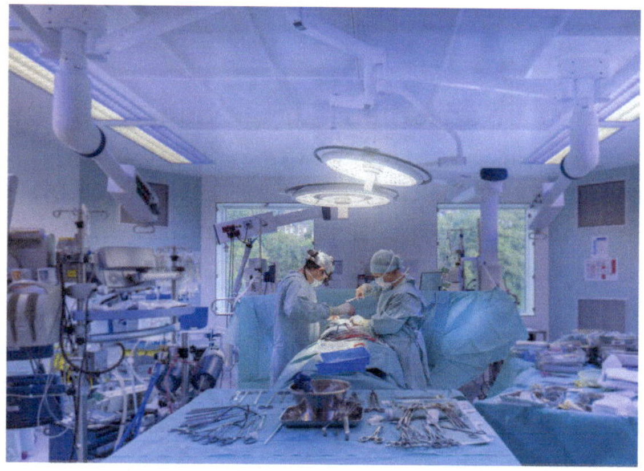

Figure 1.18. Advances in Anesthesia for Cardiothoracic Surgery.

Source: https://www.verywellhealth.com/thmb/6rr69Wz34ud5wlEvgN5ZHnGLnt4=/1500x0/filters:no_upscale():max_bytes(150000):strip_icc()/open_heart_surgery-14d3586d4c254057baae1f2256f8d404.jpg.

Another fascinating field of cardiothoracic anesthesia improvement is the intraoperative neurophysiological monitoring technique. With the advancements in neuromonitoring in high-risk procedures like heart and lung surgeries, multimodal strategies are increasingly in use. Through the use of synergies of neuromonitoring modalities like electroencephalography and somatosensory evoked potentials, anesthesiologists can offer real-time monitoring of neural circuits, making the patient safer. The multimodal strategy promotes the early detection of neural compromise during surgery and subsequent interventions earlier on, thereby preventing damage. With these technologies taking off, they have the potential to establish a new world where sophisticated neurophysiological monitoring can be integrated with ease into routine anesthetic practice in cardiothoracic surgery, pointing towards the critical intersection of technology and patient care (Singh et al., 2016) (Figure 1.18).

1.6.1. New Anesthetic Agents and Techniques

The area of anesthetic drugs and techniques is constantly evolving, particularly in cardiothoracic surgery. The introduction of new anesthetics such as remimazolam, which is a rapid-metabolizing benzodiazepine, is an interesting development. This agent offers precise control over the depth of sedation due to its fast onset and recovery time, making individualized anesthetic management possible that minimizes postoperative residual effects. Furthermore, multimodal analgesia methods are increasingly being added to enhance patient outcomes, reduce opioid consumption, and optimize pain management, which is a significant factor in patients presenting with complex surgical procedures. Such developments contribute to a more stable hemodynamic profile and allow for a quick recovery, which is of prime value in the cardiothoracic group often plagued by pre-existing comorbidities. Technological innovations, including regional anesthesia, have also shown promising results in enhancing patient care. Neuraxial blocks and other procedures are increasingly being applied together with general anesthesia in thoracic surgery to provide useful postoperative pain control. This combination reduces the doses required of systemic opioids, which in turn reduces side effects and complications associated with the administration of opioids. In addition, the use of ultrasound-guided regional anesthesia facilitates greater precision and efficiency of the nerve blocks, improving patient comfort as well as safety. For cardiothoracic surgical procedures, the synergistic application of these anesthetic techniques formulates a more integrated strategy in perioperative care to guarantee better patient outcomes and decreased hospital stay durations. The integration of intraoperative monitoring techniques has become essential in optimizing anesthetic administration and patient safety. Intraoperative neurophysiological monitoring during particularly complex surgery with vital structures can greatly enhance surgical safety. In endoscopic, endonasal skull base access, for instance, a multimodality monitoring approach that utilizes an array of techniques such as electroencephalography and somatosensory evoked potentials is used. It is not only feasible, but it also enhances the ability to assess at-risk neural structures' functional integrity in real time. These advancements are particular in cardiothoracic surgery, where safety in both intervention and anesthetic delivery is crucial in patients. They present the emphasis on crafting anesthetic practice, with efficiency and patient safety central to surgical care (Lehr et al., 2016; Singh et al., 2016).

1.6.2. Technology in Monitoring and Safety

In cardiothoracic surgery, the integration of advanced monitoring technologies has significantly enhanced patient safety and performance under anesthetic care. Live monitoring of critical parameters such as heart rate, blood pressure, and oxygen saturation is essential in assessing the condition of a patient. Advances have further extended the functionality of these systems to offer more sophisticated and integrated data acquisition. For example, the development of intravenous continuous glucose monitoring (ivCGM) systems has provided a promising alternative to glucose control in critically ill surgical patients. Besides ensuring timely adjustment of anesthetic protocols, this technology also helps to minimize the risk of hyperglycemic or hypoglycemic complications, which can be especially dangerous after surgery, as indicated in the study (Hochfellner et al., 2025). Another technical advancement involved in anesthetic safety in cardiothoracic surgery is the addition of neuroelectrophysiological monitoring. Such a technique gives instant feedback about neural function during surgery, and anesthesiologists can adjust their methods based on this, preventing nerve damage-related complications. Incorporation of such monitoring devices helps personalized management of anesthesia that reduces intraoperative risk and maximizes patient comfort. Besides, multimodal analgesia has gained widespread use as a technique involving multiple pain management modes to minimize the use of opioids, leading to fewer side effects while providing more effective pain control across recovery. Such advancements demonstrate the importance of using technology to enhance safety and optimize recovery in cardiothoracic anesthesia, as observed in Hochfellner et al. (2025).

While integration of modern monitoring and safety technology into anesthetic practice has held the greatest potential, ongoing challenges and refinements continue. The compromise between monitoring requirements and actual in-use equipment in the real world remains a crucial consideration, especially in high-stress operating theaters. Additionally, proper training of medical staff in the use of such advanced equipment remains critical to realizing their ultimate potential benefits. Continued research and development are needed to move existing systems forward and find new solutions that address the unique requirements of cardiothoracic surgery. Through a focus on implementing smart monitoring technologies and enhancing anesthetic protocols, healthcare providers can continue to push the level of care and provide patient safety throughout complicated cases, supporting the essential role of technology in anesthesia management in this field (Figure 1.19).

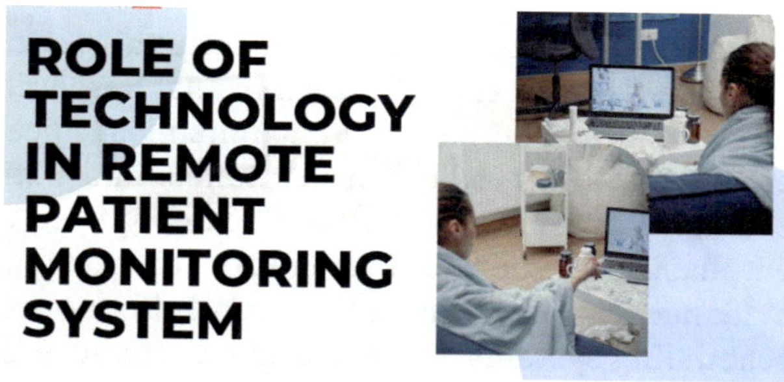

Figure 1.19. Technology in monitoring and safety.

Source: https://external-content.duckduckgo.com/iu/?u=https%3A%2F%2Fwww.aeologic.com%2Fblog%2Fwp-content%2Fuploads%2F2023%2F03%2FRemote-Patient-Monitoring-System-1180x664.jpg&f=1&nofb=1&ipt=3369acd4ed70293d288b3ae25d75186836bd2a67a87d5d0a3b0065793bc5c0e0.

1.6.3. Research and Future Directions

The history of anesthesia techniques in cardiothoracic surgery is an area that is rich in research potential, particularly with current advances in technology and techniques. Current evidence has demonstrated the impact of anesthetic management on patient outcomes such as length of stay and postoperative complications. Investigating the use of multimodal analgesia methods is a future horizon since it may not only enhance analgesia but also reduce opioid dependence, hence confining related complications. Future research increasingly targets individualization of anesthetic management strategies to the specific patient with regard to their own unique cardiovascular profile, which may serve to optimize efficacy and safety in surgical outcomes. Such tailored strategies may revolutionize practice in anesthesiology, necessitating ongoing exploration of factors related to the patient influencing anesthetic response and intraoperative overall performance (Black et al., 1981). With advancements in cardiac anesthesia, the emphasis on functional performance in operating rooms has been an issue of interest to researchers and clinicians. Research into operating room scheduling and planning is a fundamental component of maximizing surgical processes overall, as inefficiency can have adverse effects on both medical professionals and patients. A lot of contemporary literature provides an extensive overview of the methods employed to optimize scheduling efficiency, with findings that emphasize the merit of basing robust performance measures on operating procedures. By collating evidence from several studies, trends in this area become evident to highlight the call for adaptable scheduling systems that are capable of addressing the complexity of cardiothoracic procedures. In the future, anesthesiologists and surgery teams have to collaborate to lead research efforts focusing on delays and patient flow optimization using sophisticated scheduling techniques (Belien et al., 2010). Furthermore, research into new anesthetic agents and their application to cardiothoracic surgery is a new area of investigation. Advances in pharmacology have, within the recent past, generated interest in those agents that will offer an improved safety margin or outcomes during the perioperative period. The application of the newer anesthetics, if viewed with reference to specific patient groups—the elderly or those patients who have heavy comorbid loads—opens up opportunities for significant clinical benefits. Furthermore, technology integration, such as the use of real-time monitoring and data analysis, in anesthetic practice can help in more effective decision-making strategies, allowing for interventions on the spot in response to adverse events. Creating protocols that incorporate these innovations should be a focus of research in the future to improve patient safety and recovery in the complex scenario of cardiothoracic surgery. This translatability of clinical research into practice will find progress translate well into improved surgical outcomes (Black et al., 1981).

Test Your Knowledge

1. What are some recent technological advances that have improved anesthesia management in cardiothoracic surgery?
2. How have modern anesthetic techniques enhanced patient safety and recovery in cardiothoracic procedures?

SUMMARY

Finally, anesthesia in cardiothoracic surgery is critical in ensuring better patient outcomes and minimizing postoperative complications. Not only does anesthesia facilitate the surgery, but it also has a significant impact on patients' hemodynamic stability and recovery course. Appropriate anesthetic technique choice, general anesthesia or regional techniques, can minimize risks associated with surgery, especially in the elderly or comorbid patients. As seen from recent findings, newer techniques such as video-assisted aortic valve replacement offer hopeful results, balancing effectiveness against cost (Tripathiet al., 2011). The ability to achieve greater results with fewer invasive procedures expresses the evolving nature of anesthetic practice in cardiothoracic surgery. The management of postoperative complications, particularly acute kidney injury (AKI), also expresses the necessity of an evolutionary approach to anesthesia. Research has shown that the application of advanced analytical tools, such as machine learning, can be used to better inform the risk of postoperative AKI. Through enhanced predictive specificity regarding outcome in the patient, these models facilitate optimization of anesthetic care in each patient, which could enhance survival in the long term. The findings of the study reveal that postoperative AKI patients have significantly lower survival rates, thus validating the imperative for intensive monitoring and intervention actions in the perioperative setting (Choi et al., 2024). Ultimately, the practice of anesthesia for cardiothoracic surgery keeps progressing with advancing technologies and techniques that aim to improve patient care. The integration of evidence-based practice not only guides to enhance surgical outcomes but also emphasizes the role of anesthesia in a multidisciplinary treatment regimen. With the continued advancement of the discipline, research and education will be required to equip anesthesiologists with the knowledge needed to optimize both anesthesia techniques and perioperative care. By focusing on patient safety and evidence-based techniques, the goal of reducing morbidity and enhancing recovery during cardiothoracic surgery can be better achieved in the future.

Anesthesia management in cardiothoracic surgery is a complex and critical task that reflects well on patient results. The issues to highlight regarding anesthesiologists' challenges in cardiothoracic surgery are patient management with high-risk patients, who possess co-morbidities that complicate anesthesia administration. High levels of burnout among cardiac anesthesiologists have been found in a recent study, predominantly explained by the high-stress specialty. The respondents in the national survey indicated high emotional exhaustion and depersonalization, which points to the psychological stress of working on complicated cases under time pressure. Their resilience was, however, contrasted with a high sense of commitment to the profession because, despite the challenges, they could still exhibit a paradox where their self-satisfaction motivates them (Sanfilippo et al., 2018). In addition to the psychological stress, pain control management for patients undergoing cardiothoracic procedures is crucial. Effective postoperative pain relief not only enhances patient satisfaction but also reduces the risk of chronicity of acute pain. The opioid crisis, however, has made things so tricky that maintaining a balance between good control of pain and the risk of opioid complications is increasingly difficult. It is the responsibility of anesthesiologists to develop multimodal perioperative analgesic regimens that must begin preoperatively and extend into the postoperative period. This proactive approach attempts to minimize opioid dependence without compromising appropriate analgesia, particularly in opioid-dependent patients where higher doses can precipitate complications (Wenzel et al., 2016). Ultimately, the role of the anesthesiologist in cardiothoracic surgery underscores the need for specialized training and continuous evaluation of practice in this high-risk setting. Knowledge of the psychological implications of burnout, as well as effective pain management strategies are central to cultivating patient safety as well as anesthesiologist health. Emphasis on teamwork and communication of operating room staff also maximizes the collaboration model to improve surgery outcomes. With the development of the field, ongoing study and reciprocal sharing of best practice will be required in order to maximize anesthetic practice and address the specific issues that specialists in cardiothoracic settings face (Wenzel et al., 2016; Sanfilippo et al., 2018).

KEY TERMS FROM THIS CHAPTER

- Cardiac function
- Cardiothoracic operations
- Coronary artery bypass grafting (CABG)
- Erector spinae plane block (ESPB)
- Hemodynamic stability
- Intensive care unit (ICU)
- Potential complications
- Surgical efficacy
- Cardiac intensive care unit (CICU)
- Cardiothoracic surgery
- Erector spinae plane (ESP)
- Extracorporeal membrane oxygenation
- Influence postoperative
- Patient recovery
- Regional anesthesia
- Thorax

Critical Thinking Questions

1. **Which of the following is the most common induction agent used in cardiothoracic surgery?**
   a. Propofol
   b. Ketamine
   c. Thiopental
   d. Etomidate
2. **What is the primary goal of monitoring during cardiothoracic surgery?**
   a. Ensuring patient comfort
   b. Maintaining hemodynamic stability
   c. Monitoring for pain
   d. Enhancing surgical field visibility
3. **Which of the following is a key anesthetic consideration for cardiopulmonary bypass (CPB)?**
   a. Avoiding anticoagulation
   b. Managing hypothermia
   c. Increasing cardiac output
   d. Reducing systemic vascular resistance
4. **What is the primary purpose of transesophageal echocardiography (TEE) during cardiothoracic surgery?**
   a. Pain management
   b. Assessing cardiac function and structure
   c. Monitoring depth of anesthesia
   d. Preventing postoperative complications
5. **Which of the following drugs is commonly used for myocardial protection during cardiac surgery?**
   a. Lidocaine
   b. Nitroglycerin
   c. Adenosine
   d. Potassium chloride

Short Answer Questions

1. What are the primary anesthetic considerations for a patient undergoing cardiopulmonary bypass (CPB)?
2. What is the significance of mixed venous oxygen saturation (SvO_2) during cardiac surgery?
3. Define cardioplegia and its role in cardiac surgery.
4. Which monitoring techniques are essential during cardiac surgery?
5. How is hemodynamic stability maintained during off-pump coronary artery bypass (OPCAB)?
6. Discuss the role of antifibrinolytics during cardiac surgery.

Answer to Critical Thinking Questions

1. (a); 2. (b); 3. (b); 4. (b); 5. (d)

References

1. Agarwal, S., Verma, I., Sharma, J., & Dagar, N. (2024). Comparison of auscultation method versus lung ultrasound technique to evaluate the accuracy of positioning of left double lumen tube in patients undergoing cardiothoracic surgery. *Indonesian Journal of Anesthesiology and Reanimation*. https://www.semanticscholar.org/paper/54eea9663633949b05ff5a63a7cdd9abd4365973 (accessed on 28th June 2025).
2. Lehr, E. J., Guy, T. S., Smith, R. L., Grossi, E. A., Shemin, R. J., Rodriguez, E., Ailawadi, G., Agnihotri, A. K., Fayers, T. M., Hargrove, W. C., Hummel, B. W., Khan, J. H., Malaisrie, S. C., Mehall, J. R., Murphy, D. A., Ryan, W. H., Salemi, A., Segurola, R. J., Jr, Smith, J. M., Wolfe, J. A., ... Lewis, C. T. (2016). Minimally Invasive Mitral Valve Surgery III: Training and Robotic-Assisted Approaches. *Innovations (Philadelphia, Pa.)*, *11*(4), 260–267. https://doi.org/10.1097/IMI.0000000000000299(accessed on 28th June 2025).
3. Almashrafi, A., Alsabti, H., Mukaddirov, M., Balan, B., & Aylin, P. (2016). Factors associated with prolonged length of stay following cardiac surgery in a major referral hospital in Oman: a retrospective observational study. *BMJ open*, *6*(6), e010764. https://doi.org/10.1136/bmjopen-2015-010764(accessed on 28th June 2025).
4. Almutairi, A. H., Alshammas, N., Sulaiman, N., Aljehani, B. A., Al.Jarie, A., Alshehri, M., Alonazi, A. A., et al. (2024). Comprehensive review of radiological imaging techniques and anesthesia support in surgery. *Journal of Eco Humanism*. https://www.semanticscholar.org/paper/09e81e110c9e5f2122cdca886354f4011ad4155a (accessed on 28th June 2025).
5. Kaufmann J, Kung E. Factors Affecting Cardiovascular Physiology in Cardiothoracic Surgery: Implications for Lumped-Parameter Modeling. *Front Surg*. 2019;6:62. Published 2019 Nov 5. doi:10.3389/fsurg.2019.00062(accessed on 28th June 2025).
6. Sanfilippo, F., Noto, A., Palumbo, G. J., Ippolito, M., Gagliardone, M., Scarlata, M., Bignami, E., Sangalli, F., Cattaneo, S., Blangetti, I., Scolletta, S., Locatelli, A., Tritapepe, L., Lorini, F. L., & Arcadipane, A. (2018). Burnout in Cardiac Anesthesiologists: Results From a National Survey in Italy. *Journal of cardiothoracic and vascular anesthesia*, *32*(6), 2459–2466. https://doi.org/10.1053/j.jvca.2018.05.016(accessed on 28th June 2025).
7. Assaad, S., Kratzert, W. B., Shelley, B., Friedman, M. B., & Perrino, A., Jr (2018). Assessment of Pulmonary Edema: Principles and Practice. *Journal of cardiothoracic and vascular anesthesia*, *32*(2), 901–914. https://doi.org/10.1053/j.jvca.2017.08.028pdf (accessed on 28th June 2025).
8. Wenzel, J. T., Schwenk, E. S., Baratta, J. L., & Viscusi, E. R. (2016). Managing Opioid-Tolerant Patients in the Perioperative Surgical Home. *Anesthesiology clinics*, *34*(2), 287–301. https://doi.org/10.1016/j.anclin.2016.01.005(accessed on 28th June 2025).
9. Belien, J., Cardoen, B., & Demeulemeester, E. (2010). Operating room planning and scheduling: A literature review. https://core.ac.uk/download/pdf/6347245.pdf (accessed on 28th June 2025).
10. Bhardwaj, A., Deep, A., Chadha, A., & Kumar, Y. (2025). Advances in pain management in oral surgery. *Journal of Academy of Dental Education*. https://www.semanticscholar.org/paper/71c2a4b841ea69e235c3da0d26da94a929829d53 (accessed on 28th June 2025).

11. Kiessling, A. H., Huneke, P., Reyher, C., Bingold, T., Zierer, A., & Moritz, A. (2013). Risk factor analysis for fast track protocol failure. *Journal of cardiothoracic surgery, 8*, 47. https://doi.org/10.1186/1749-8090-8-47(accessed on 28th June 2025).

12. Birchenough, S. J. (2015). Assessment of the preoperative assessment: A case study. https://core.ac.uk/download/146517522.pdf (accessed on 28th June 2025).

13. Capuano, P., Sepolvere, G., Toscano, A., Scimia, P., Silvetti, S., Tedesco, M., Gentili, L., et al. (2024). Fascial plane blocks for cardiothoracic surgery: A narrative review. *Journal of Anesthesia, Analgesia and Critical Care, 4*. https://www.semanticscholar.org/paper/74308aab8ce04162f712172b40312549dcfe7a6a (accessed on 28th June 2025).

14. Choi, B. Y., Choi, W., Min, J., Chung, B. H., Koh, E. S., Hong, S., Ban, T. H., et al. (2024). Predicting long-term mortality of patients with postoperative acute kidney injury following noncardiac general anesthesia surgery using machine learning. *Kidney Research and Clinical Practice*. https://www.semanticscholar.org/paper/315eb58635c5e297dcc549f516ca9f128f501261 (accessed on 28th June 2025).

15. Cil, H., & Buren, M. A. (2025). The role of methadone and regional anesthesia in the management of patients undergoing complex spinal surgery. *Current Anesthesiology Reports*. https://www.semanticscholar.org/paper/6758b1d2ed51a30f93c929737916d54c864dd77f (accessed on 28th June 2025).

16. Claassen, J. A. H. R., Thijssen, D. H. J., Panerai, R. B., & Faraci, F. M. (2021). Regulation of cerebral blood flow in humans: Physiology and clinical implications of autoregulation. *Physiological Reviews, 101*, 1487–1559. https://doi.org/10.1152/physrev.00022.2020 (accessed on 28th June 2025).

17. Luginbuhl, A., Schwartz, D. M., Sestokas, A. K., Cognetti, D., & Pribitkin, E. (2012). Detection of evolving injury to the brachial plexus during transaxillary robotic thyroidectomy. *The Laryngoscope, 122*(1), 110–115. https://doi.org/10.1002/lary.22429(accessed on 28th June 2025).

18. Di Francesco, M., Magunia, H., Örgel, A., Tatagiba, M., Radwan, M., & Adib, S. (2023). Case report: Interdisciplinary treatment of complex C1/C2 fractures in a patient with concomitant three-vessel coronary artery disease requiring bypass surgery. *Frontiers in Surgery, 10*. https://www.semanticscholar.org/paper/073ad3a20941a8cc0b2c33c1799ada06dbd388c2 (accessed on 28th June 2025).

19. Diamond, B., Guerrier, G., Holliman, C., Marrero, D., et al. (2019). A quality improvement project to determine the incidence and prevalence of obstructive sleep apnea, best practice anesthesia guidelines, and the incidence of perioperative cardiac and respiratory complications after the implementation of the STOP-BANG questionnaire. https://core.ac.uk/download/301296636.pdf (accessed on 28th June 2025).

20. Singh, H., Vogel, R. W., Lober, R. M., Doan, A. T., Matsumoto, C. I., Kenning, T. J., & Evans, J. J. (2016). Intraoperative Neurophysiological Monitoring for Endoscopic Endonasal Approaches to the Skull Base: A Technical Guide. *Scientifica, 2016*, 1751245. https://doi.org/10.1155/2016/1751245(accessed on 28th June 2025).

21. Guerguerian, A. M., Sano, M., Todd, M., Honjo, O., Alexander, P., & Raman, L. (2021). Pediatric extracorporeal cardiopulmonary resuscitation ELSO guidelines. *ASAIO Journal, 67*, 229–237. https://doi.org/10.1097/mat.0000000000001345 (accessed on 28th June 2025).

22. Hall, M. (2024). Final scholarly project: Implementation guidelines of ultrasound-guided regional anesthesia in pediatric cardiac surgical patients. https://core.ac.uk/download/616421822.pdf (accessed on 28th June 2025).

23. Hochfellner, D., Poettler, T., Schoerghuber, M., Lukic, E., Yates, A., Keeling, I., Zimpfer, D., et al. (2025). Accuracy and safety of a novel intravenous continuous glucose monitoring system in patients admitted to a cardiothoracic ICU: A pilot trial. *Journal of Diabetes Science and Technology*. https://www.semanticscholar.org/paper/507ffeb917c8e4cbff9a4d30246ab81441295372 (accessed on 28th June 2025).

24. Kaufmann J, Kung E. Factors Affecting Cardiovascular Physiology in Cardiothoracic Surgery: Implications for Lumped-Parameter Modeling. *Front Surg*. 2019;6:62. Published 2019 Nov 5. doi:10.3389/fsurg.2019.00062(accessed on 28th June 2025).

25. Lopes, E. C. R., César, C. A., de Mello, M. A. A., Perez, G. B., Maya, P. A. H., Benfatti, R. A., Benfatti, A. F. C., et al. (2025). Display poster abstracts. *Innovations, 20*, 97S–130S. https://www.semanticscholar.org/paper/78d9ba128445a3ee1cebe864fc0354ae4a774f01 (accessed on 28th June 2025).

26. Miller, A. B., et al. (2023). A quality improvement project: Erector spinae plane blocks for patients undergoing cardiothoracic surgery. https://core.ac.uk/download/622984241.pdf (accessed on 28th June 2025).

27. Novikova, A. I., Lyubushkin, V. E., Studenikina, A. V., Albotova, D. K., Bakhmeteva, P. I., Torchinova, D. A., Chkareuli, D. N., et al. (2024). The role of anesthesiology in modern cardiac surgery: Overview of key techniques and issues. *Cardiometry*. https://www.semanticscholar.org/paper/e9ca845a8de28a31fca089396b62598feac4a104 (accessed on 28th June 2025).

28. Tripathi RS, Blum JM, Papadimos TJ, Rosenberg AL. A bibliometric search of citation classics in anesthesiology. *BMC Anesthesiol*. 2011;11:24. Published 2011 Dec 12. doi:10.1186/1471-2253-11-24(accessed on 28th June 2025).

29. Stasiowski, M., Lyssek-Boroń, A., Krysik, K., Majer, D., Zmarzły, N., & Grabarek, B. (2024). Evaluating the efficacy of pre-emptive peribulbar blocks with different local anesthetics or paracetamol using the adequacy of anesthesia guidance for vitreoretinal surgeries: A preliminary report. *Biomedicines, 12*. https://www.semanticscholar.org/paper/bc13c17805db43615fefd40d54b84d4412d4a76e (accessed on 28th June 2025).

ANESTHESIA FOR NEUROSURGERY

2

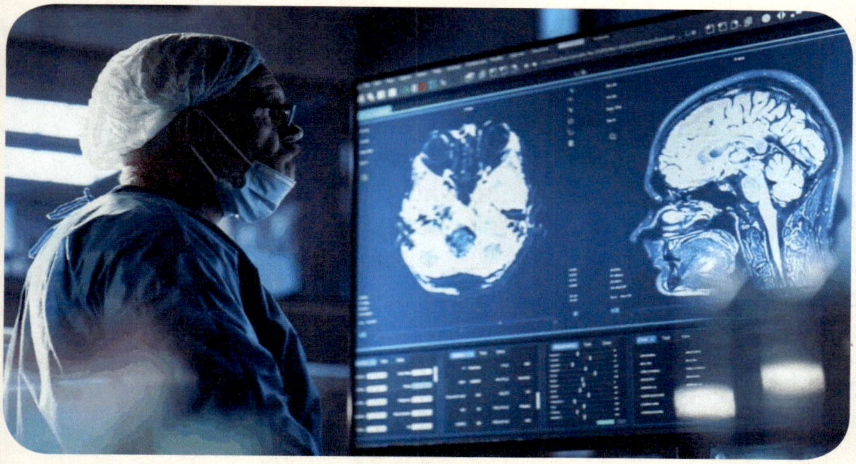

LEARNING OBJECTIVES

After studying this chapter, you will be able to:

1. Discuss the types of anesthesia used in neurosurgery
2. Focus on preoperative assessment
3. Explain the anesthetic techniques in neurosurgery
4. Know the challenges in anesthesia for neurosurgery
5. Understand postoperative care
6. Evaluate advances in anesthetic practices

Introduction

The highly advanced interaction between anesthesia and neurosurgery is a critical pillar of modern medicine. Because neurosurgical procedures often involve highly advanced manipulations of the central nervous system, ideal anesthetic management is of the utmost significance. Anesthesia not only matters for patient comfort and postoperative results but also has critical implications for intraoperative neurophysiological monitoring, which is needed to confirm neural protection in advanced surgical therapy. The use of a variety of monitoring techniques in neurosurgery, as detailed in more recent reports, indicates the potential of multimodal monitoring to contribute to real-time measurement of neurological function. This becomes relevant in complex operations, particularly endoscopic and endonasal surgery, where there is always a chance of damaging vital structures (Singh et al., 2016). Anesthetic techniques thus must be modified to fit the surgical procedure and specific neurological pathology unique to each operation. Besides the technical issues of anesthesia in neurosurgery, there is also a general argument about access to such basic services globally. Low- and middle-income countries (LMIC) have tremendous inequities in neurosurgical care, which can have a significant impact on the prognosis of the patient. Many of these patients with conditions such as epilepsy—potentially curable through functional neurosurgical therapy—are still out of the reach of optimal surgical therapy. The cost factors incurred in the introduction of sophisticated anesthetic and surgical techniques in these regions pose a monumental challenge (Fezeu et al., 2018). With the world discovering such inequities, a collaborative approach is necessary to create context-adjusted interventions that provide equitable access to neurosurgical care and anesthesia. Partnerships between HIC and LMIC can create opportunities for collaborative endeavors that attempt to bridge these disparities and improve surgical results in the world. The contribution of research and innovation in anesthetic science for neurosurgery cannot be overstated. Advances in pharmacologic agents and monitoring technology continue to advance anesthetic management, introducing increased safety and effectiveness to neurosurgical procedures. Technologies such as the availability of short-acting anesthetics and sophisticated neuromonitoring equipment allow clinicians to tailor anesthesia plans to a patient's unique needs and to specific surgery objectives. Moreover, understanding the neuroanatomical and physiological ramifications of these technologies is a precondition for anesthesiologists. As the specialty progresses, ongoing education and training in surgical and anesthetic techniques will be necessary for neuroanesthesiologists to be current and open to novel challenges and opportunities presented in the operating room. The interaction of these factors ultimately underscores the necessity of an integrating, global approach to anesthetic management of neurosurgery, where patient safety and operative success are ultimate objectives (Figure 2.1).

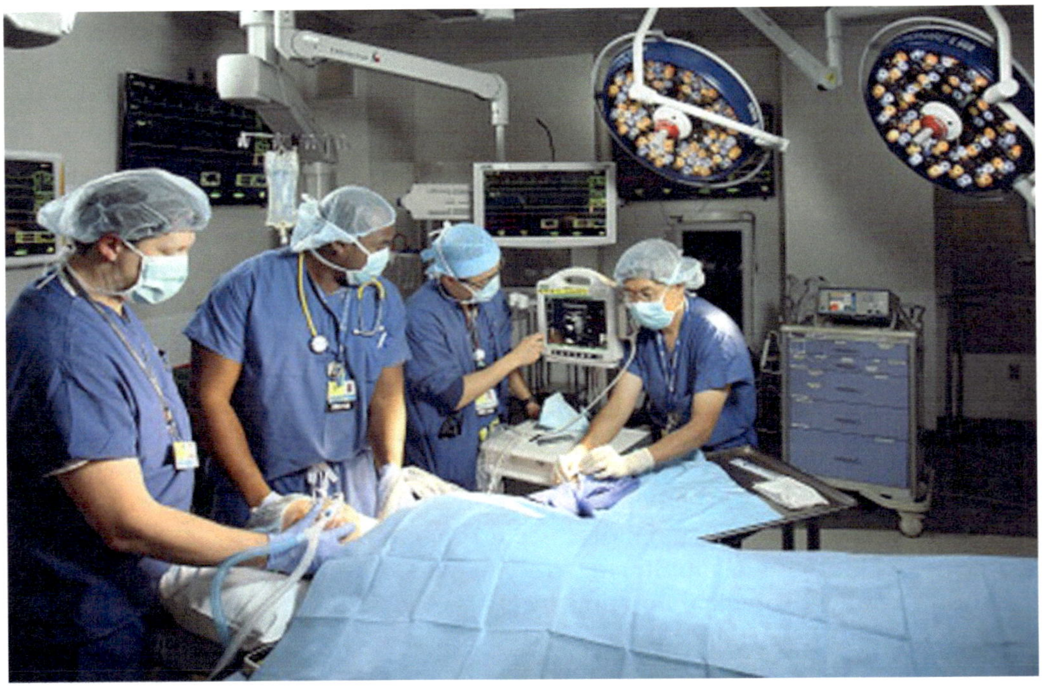

Figure 2.1. Neurosurgical anesthesia.

Source: https://anesthesiology.hopkinsmedicine.org/wp-content/uploads/2022/04/Neurosurgical-Anesthesia-Fellowship.jpg.

Definition of Anesthesia

Anesthesia is a clinical art employed to create a reversible loss of sensation or consciousness in the course of offering surgical procedures without exposing the patient to pain. This method is greatly necessary in neurosurgery, where precision is greatly desired and even the slightest movement of the patient can compromise the success of surgery. Anesthesia can be categorized into various types, including general anesthesia, which renders a patient completely unconscious, and regional or local anesthesia, which prevents sensory nerves in the body from functioning. Depending on the type of surgery to be performed, the patient's condition, and the nature of neurological procedures to be conducted, the kind of anesthesia typically administered is decided. Neurosurgical procedures, such as the removal of tumors or clipping of aneurysms, require careful planning to ensure that the anesthetic methods used ensure maximum safety and efficiency in a bid to avoid any risk associated with the patient's nervous system function. The complexity of carrying out neurosurgery requires a complete understanding of anesthesia's definition and application, particularly in the case of brain surgery. One of the distinctive characteristics of anesthesia is that, in addition to being analgesic, it is also amnesic and hence reduces the psychological distress of invasive procedures. When undergoing neurosurgery, the anesthetic management must tip towards proper sedation with careful monitoring of the patient's neurological condition during surgery. For instance, surgical techniques such as awake craniotomies allow surgeons to talk with patients during the procedure, ensuring that major brain functions are not compromised. Such nuances illustrate the evolving role of anesthesia as a way of assuring patient safety while enabling advanced surgical techniques, such as MRI-guided deep brain stimulation and focused ultrasound treatments, that have the potential to significantly enhance surgical precision (Eljamel et al., 2014). Furthermore, the definition of "anesthesia" has been extended beyond mere sedation to encompass the sophisticated monitoring and support required with intricate operations. Efficacious anesthesia in neurosurgery is not solely a matter of pharmacologic agents but also a function of technical innovation in monitoring cerebral function and vital signs. All of these components interact synergistically to create an environment conducive to optimal results. Here, anesthesiologists play a vital role, using their expertise to tailor anesthetic approaches considering the individual anatomical and physiological characteristics of patients. As science in the field of neurosurgery advances, the function of anesthesia also involves new customs and techniques to provide optimized anesthetic effectiveness and patient safety while aiming to capture the interacting equilibrium between anesthesia and neurological health (Hopayian et al., 2010) (Figure 2.2).

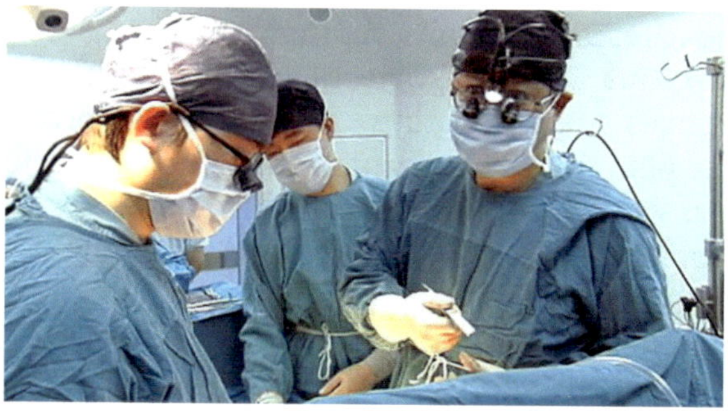

Figure 2.2. Anesthesia is a specialized medical technique.

Source: https://cdn.britannica.com/39/179539-138-7619C468/Discussion-medicine-focus-use-Chinese-anesthetic-surgery.jpg?w=800&h=450&c=crop.

Importance of Anesthesia in Neurosurgery

The role of anesthesia in neurosurgery cannot be overstated since it is a critical component in establishing patient and surgical safety.

Neurosurgical procedures constitute much like delicate manipulation of the brain and the surrounding tissues, which not only requires effective pain relief but also a precise tuning of a patient's physiological parameters. Anesthesia enables neurosurgeons to perform intricate operations by inducing unconsciousness and relaxing muscles, which can give better access to the point of operation. Additionally, the selectivity of most anesthetic agents allows for the preservation of hemodynamic stability, circumventing trends in heart rate and blood pressure during an operation. Stability is very important as even slight changes may lead to adverse outcomes. Thus, careful anesthetic management enables the intricate demands of neurosurgery while managing positioning complications and surgical duration-related concerns. Moreover, the influence of anesthesia on postoperative recovery for patients undergoing neurosurgery is great. Pain relief following craniotomy, for instance, has been augmented by reports indicating that effective anesthesia not only brings suffering to a stop, but also supports quicker recovery and reduces hospital stays. Research has proven that pain following craniotomy is accompanied by a variety of symptoms, such as nausea and fluctuations in blood pressure, which also complicate recovery (Guilkey et al., 2016). Anesthesiologists, therefore, play a significant role in the administration of multimodal analgesia protocols that efficiently minimize such complications, thereby improving overall patient outcomes. The parallel with advanced anesthetic techniques, e.g., regional anesthesia and nerve blocks, further emphasizes the importance of tailored anesthetic approaches to neurosurgery. Not only do these techniques enhance postoperative pain control, but they also decrease the risk of opioid addiction during the postoperative period. Moreover, anesthetic problems have a definitive role in the single event of worldwide health crises, such as the COVID-19 pandemic. The inherent risks of transmission of viruses in upper aerodigestive tract procedures necessitate safety protocols among healthcare workers (Givi et al., 2020). In neurosurgery, with potential aerosol-generating procedures, anesthesia staff must adopt additional measures, including proper personal protective interventions and ventilation policies. These additional measures are important to safeguard patients as well as healthcare workers while maintaining necessary surgical services. Therefore, the role of anesthesia is not merely the delivery of drugs; it is a comprehensive approach towards providing patient safety, handling complications, and cross-disciplinary practice in the face of evolving health challenges.

2.1. Types of Anesthesia Used in Neurosurgery

Learning Outcome

1. General anesthesia
2. Regional anesthesia
3. Local anesthesia

The application of anesthesia in neurosurgery is crucial not just for pain relief in patients but also for precision while undertaking operations on the brain. General anesthesia is frequently applied in various neurosurgical procedures to anesthetize patients to sleep and make them insensitive to intricate operations. Deep sedation, muscle relaxation, and analgesia are realized with this type of anesthesia and are required to perform delicate operations, such as tumor removal or cranial operations. Further, it allows for invasive monitoring of vital signs, which ensures optimal response to changing physiological patterns that can occur during neurosurgery. Through advancements in anesthetic medications, general anesthesia can now be safely administered, with complications minimized and the desired depth of sedation for the complex nature of neurosurgical procedures ensured. Aside from overall anesthesia, regional anesthesia is also significant in neurosurgery, particularly in the context of some procedures such as peripheral nerve blocks or spinal anesthesia. Techniques like the administration of epidural or spinal anesthesia may provide targeted analgesia for lower limb surgery or some intracranial surgery. Not only does it reduce the need for systemic opioids, but the risk of respiratory complications of general anesthesia is reduced as well. Also, regional anesthetic techniques have the advantage of preserving patients' ability to respond to verbal command, which is useful in neurosurgical cases where neuronal function must be monitored intraoperatively. Hence, the appropriate use of regional anesthesia combined with sedation techniques provides a dimensional concept, enhancing neurosurgical outcomes.

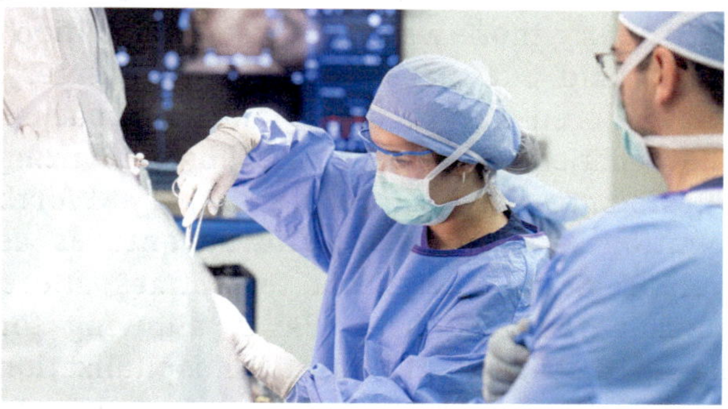

Figure 2.3. The application of anesthesia in neurosurgery.

Source: https://www.barrowneuro.org/wp-content/uploads/20240221-BNI-Neurosurgery-Parkinsons-DBS-Procedure-0018-2000x1125.jpg.

New techniques in anesthesia, such as monitored anesthesia care (MAC) and neuromonitoring in conjunction with anesthetic technique, demonstrate the range of techniques that can be applied to neurosurgical procedures. MAC offers a combination of sedation and local anesthesia to allow for patient awareness and comfort. This is particularly useful in procedures such as awake craniotomies, in which continuous neurological monitoring is essential. Furthermore, the merging of intraoperative imaging and monitored techniques, such as MRI-guided deep brain stimulation, mirrors the evolving nature of anesthetic application in neurosurgery (Eljamel et al., 2014; Benet et al., 2015). As these modalities advance, blending various forms of anesthesia ensures enhanced safety and efficacy of neurosurgical interventions, ultimately resulting in enhanced surgical outcomes and patient care (Figure 2.3).

2.1.1. General Anesthesia

General anesthesia is a critical element of neurosurgery, which delivers a reversible, controllable plane of unconsciousness necessary to perform intimate surgical manipulations on the brain and spinal cord. Under general anesthesia, the neurosurgeon is able to perform accurate dissections and manipulations with little patient movement, necessary to prevent intraoperative damage. Ensuring that patients are fully unresponsive to surgical stimuli also protects neurological function, particularly when surgery is being done in sensitive areas of the brain. The anesthetic agents themselves, propofol and inhalational anesthetics, are selected for their rapid onset and recovery of action to ensure patient safety and comfort and optimal surgical conditions. In neurosurgical cases, some things must be addressed regarding the pharmacokinetics and pharmacodynamics of drugs employed for anesthesia. For example, the choice of drugs can be based on potential effect on cerebrospinal fluid dynamics as well as intracranial tension. Drugs like nitrous oxide, which have cerebral vascular effects in addition to other recognition, are excluded on grounds of suspected intracranial tension rise. Besides, neuromuscular blockers are typically administered to achieve maximum muscle relaxation and enable precise dissection during surgery. Monitoring techniques are also employed by anesthesiologists to ensure ongoing assessment of cerebral perfusion and oxygenation levels during surgery to avert postoperative syndromes like postoperative cognitive dysfunction, especially dreaded in the elderly. Additionally, the effects of general anesthesia are not limited to the surgical operation itself but also reach the overall recovery process of patients undergoing neurosurgery. Neurotoxicity due to anesthesia is also of interest, as evidence is presented that there may be a relationship between specific anesthetic drugs and cognitive impairment, especially in susceptible patients. While risk due to such complications could be mitigated with the employment of advanced monitoring and tailored anesthetic protocols, more research is required to evaluate the long-term effects of general anesthesia in neurosurgical interventions. With the evolving field, collaboration among neurosurgeons and neuroanesthetists becomes essential to optimize perioperative practice so that general anesthesia benefits are maximized and side effects are kept to a minimum for the ultimate goal of optimizing patient outcomes within the challenging context of anesthetic management of neurosurgery (Figure 2.4).

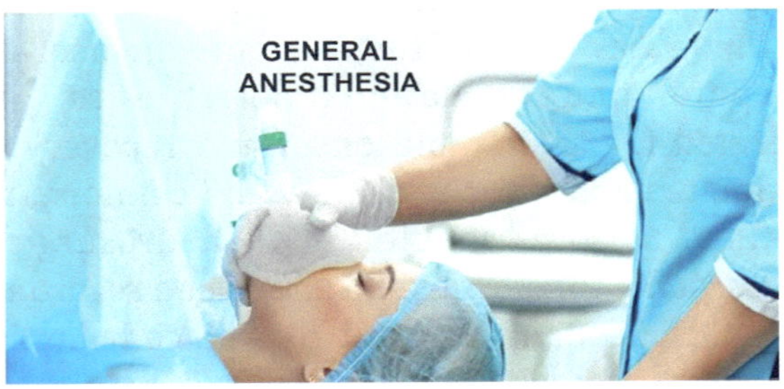

Figure 2.4. General anesthesia plays a crucial role in neurosurgery.

Source: https://img.icliniq.com/article/general-anesthesia-2141.webp.

2.1.2. Regional Anesthesia

Regional anesthesia is key to neurosurgical interventions, especially if one takes into consideration the delicate needs of spinal and brain surgeries. By focusing on specific nerve structures, regional anesthesia makes pain management easier while also potentially minimizing the use of systemic analgesics, which can be unwanted in nature. Its application in lumbar surgery has been found to have advantages compared to general anesthesia, including fewer postoperative complications and shorter operative time. For instance, recent studies indicate that spinal anesthesia can lead to significantly reduced operative times and decreased blood loss, and also adhere to improved patient outcomes and resource utilization (Pierce et al., 2017). This approach not only boosts the overall efficiency of surgical interventions but also facilitates a smoother process of recovery in patients undergoing extensive neurosurgical interventions. In addition, regional anesthesia provides a viable solution for patients with specific contraindications to general anesthesia, particularly those with pre-existing conditions that would put them at risk during surgery. The tailored nature of regional approaches allows patient-focused treatment by minimizing physiological stress during surgery. Worth mentioning are the logistic advantages as well; regional anesthesia techniques afford quicker recovery from PACU, allowing for earlier discharge and shorter hospitalization periods (Pierce et al., 2017). Both these are contributing to higher patient satisfaction along with economic benefits to healthcare systems, which increasingly consider the cost-effectiveness of various anesthetic approaches in neurosurgery. However, while the benefits of regional anesthesia are immense, its use in low- and middle-income countries (LMIC) illustrates one of the most significant challenges to global neurosurgical practice. Limited access to advanced anesthetic techniques and equipment could potentially restrict the use of regional anesthesia in these countries despite prevalent conditions necessitating neurosurgical intervention. There is an imbalance in access to effective and safe surgical care, and with increased visibility for functional neurosurgical techniques, closing this disparity needs to be a priority. Joint efforts between low- and high-income countries can help spread regional anesthesia practices and ensure that innovations in neurosurgical care are accessed equitably across the range of healthcare contexts.

2.1.3. Local Anesthesia

Loco-regional anesthesia is a key component of neurosurgical practice, transforming the surgical experience for the patient as well as the surgeon. The ability to selectively anesthetize specific areas while the patient remains awake and alert is particularly valuable in operations where patient feedback in real-time is crucial. Awake craniotomies, for instance, wherein surgeons operate near essential brain functions, can benefit the most from local anesthesia. This technique not only enables the expression of patients' feelings during the operation but also enhances the accuracy of tumor resections and other procedures. These modalities are critical because they illustrate the need to balance effective pain control with neurological function preservation—a primary concern in neurosurgical treatment. The physiological actions of local anesthesia in neurosurgery extend beyond the transient relief of pain. Studies of the functional structure of the brain, particularly in reference to local anesthetic action, reveal sophisticated dynamics in cortical regions. Experiments using current imaging techniques such as functional magnetic resonance imaging (fMRI) and electrocorticography (ECoG) demonstrate the manner in which local anesthetic activity can interact with and modify the brain's resting state networks. It is worth understanding these interactions since they provide insights into the brain's adaptive capability, especially for surgery on traumatized or ill tissue. By preserving some neurophysiological functions and minimizing pain, local anesthesia has been discovered to possibly influence recovery courses following neurosurgical operations and making light of the complex interplay between anesthesia and cortical physiology under operative circumstances (Bandt et al., 2017).

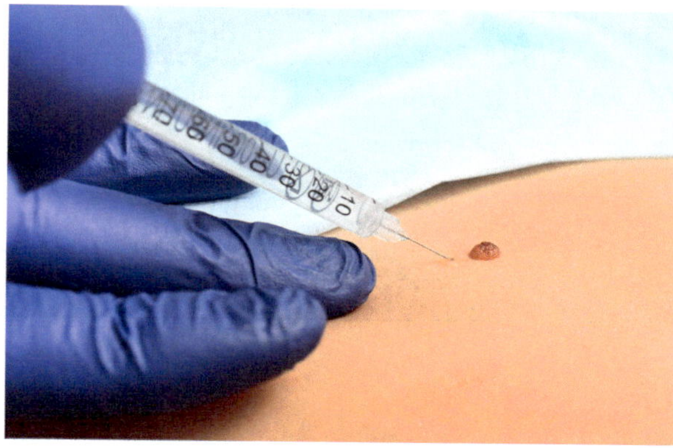

Figure 2.5. Local anesthesia serves a pivotal role.

Source: https://www.verywellhealth.com/thmb/OBM5z6-W9C0GVNtf_plkBIGdwTo=/3190x2125/filters:no_upscale():max_bytes(150000):strip_icc()/local_anesthesia_mole-b56769a7261945d2ba813c91f24767e2.jpg.

Secondly, the neurosurgical application of local anesthesia is founded on an interactive process among multidisciplinary teams, as the concept of skinning the cat theory suggests. Such an environment provokes ongoing dialogue among basic scientists and clinicians aimed at improving decision-making within the surgical field. Accordingly, local anesthesia is more than a procedure; it is a strategic component of an ongoing academic and clinical discussion aimed at enhancing patient outcomes. The integration of decision analysis and algorithmic thinking allows practitioners to customize anesthetic techniques based on unique patient needs and surgical conditions. By facilitating an interdisciplinary understanding of how local anesthesia is best utilized, the discipline continues to advance in efficiency and safety. This collaborative work ultimately enhances surgical performance with reduced risks associated with anesthesia, justifying its absolute value in contemporary neurosurgery (Lorenz et al., 1989) (Figure 2.5).

Test Your Knowledge

1. What are the main types of anesthesia commonly used in neurosurgery?
2. Why is total intravenous anesthesia (TIVA) often preferred in certain neurosurgical procedures?

2.2. Preoperative Assessment

Learning Outcome

1. Patient medical history
2. Neurological evaluation
3. Anesthetic risk assessment

One of the key components of quality anesthetic care in neurosurgical patients is strict preoperative assessment that systematically screens a patient's history, physical condition, and specific surgical needs. Preoperative assessment is vital in discovering any underlying conditions that can complicate surgery or anesthesia. In neurosurgery, if patients come to the hospital with complications of their neurological diseases, a proper history of previous surgeries, comorbidities, and current medicative management can have a huge impact on anesthetic choices and outcomes. The preoperative evaluation is not just to reduce risks but also to render the overall medical status of patients optimal before surgery. An integrated plan makes sure that anesthesiologists and surgical teams work together in close collaboration, thereby ensuring that their plans are coordinated with expected complications of the neurosurgical procedure (Pierce et al., 2017). Furthermore, within the preoperative assessment, there are certain neuromonitoring considerations that are specific to neurosurgery. Functional integrity of important neural pathways might become essential when the procedure is for the brain or spinal cord; thus, the anesthetic plan should take into account these issues. With this in mind, intraoperative neurophysiologic monitoring, as described by the current literature, focuses on its safety and applicability within the framework of endoscopic, endonasal skull base surgery. With the employment of diverse monitoring modalities, such as electroencephalography and somatosensory evoked potentials, anesthesiologists play a dynamic role in the preservation of neurologic function during the duration of surgery. These preoperative assessments ensure that anesthesia plans are specially tailored to both the procedure and each individual patient's specific needs, creating an environment for optimal intraoperative safety (Singh et al., 2016).

Finally, the value of preoperative assessments extends to postoperative care and potential complications. Postoperative complications such as neurological impairment or respiratory issues are risks for neurosurgical patients and need a specialized intervention for postoperative care. The information gained in the preoperative assessment controls the whole perioperative path, modulating recovery mechanisms and potential interventions. For instance, the cardiovascular stability of a patient, determined in this stage, may decide whether an ordinary recovery process can be taken or whether intensified monitoring and support are required. This progressive perspective later emphasizes the importance of proper preoperative assessment in preventing complications and obtaining maximum benefit in patients undergoing complex neurosurgical procedures (Pierce et al., 2017) (Figure 2.6).

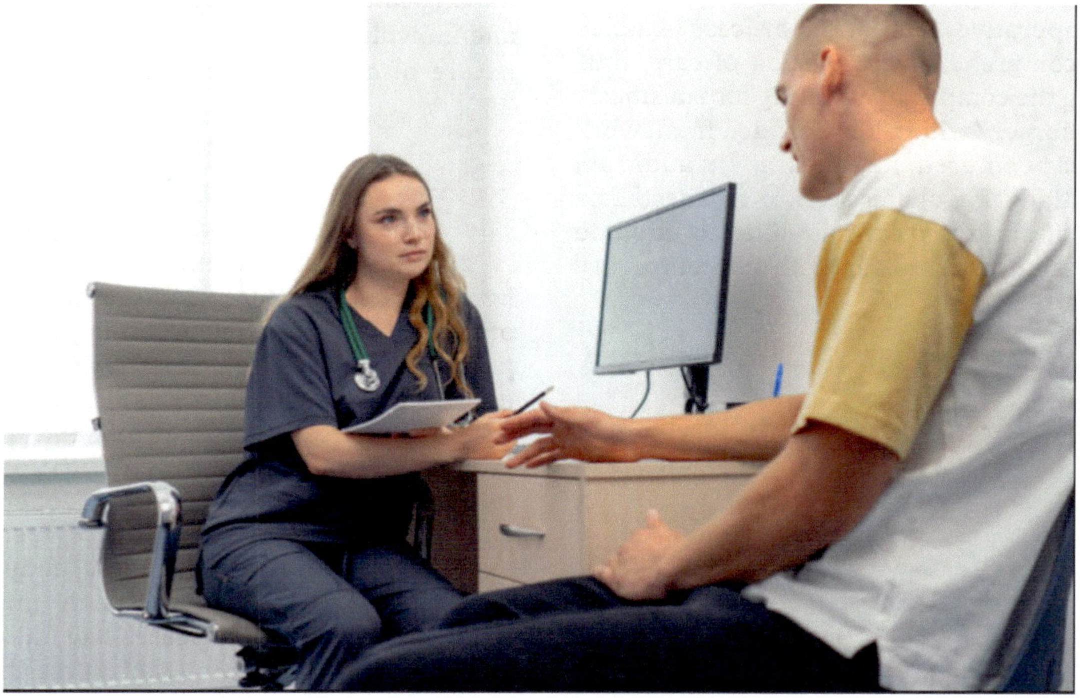

Figure 2.6. The rigorous preoperative assessment.

Source: https://www.nysora.com/wp-content/uploads/2025/01/preoperative-assessment-690x460.jpg.

2.2.1. Patient Medical History

Careful patient medical history is a corner stone in neurosurgical anesthesia practice, which determines anesthetic care and also surgical outcomes. Past medical conditions, operations, and drug use must be diligently noted and examined for signs of potential complications and altered anesthetic plans accordingly. For instance, patients with chronic pulmonary diseases react differently to anesthetic medications such that the choice of medication and routes of administration should be adjusted accordingly. In addition, a detailed review of the patient's neurological exam, history of brain surgery, or neurological disorder may alert the anesthesiology team of specific risks and allow them to take precautionary measures to prevent complications as outlined by the relevant literature, supported by strong evidence (Givi et al., 2020). This foundational knowledge not only optimizes postoperative results but also optimizes overall safety in neurosurgery. The intricacies of patient medical history extend beyond physiologic factors into the psychological and social realms of treatment. Psychological evaluation can reveal hidden anxiety disorders or intellectual disabilities that would complicate the perioperative course. Identification of such factors enables anesthesiologists to better address the unique needs of each patient, with interventions such as anxiolytic drugs or implementation of regional anesthesia techniques less psychologically invasive.

Furthermore, social determinants of health like support systems and living conditions significantly impact patient compliance and recovery. Taking such factors into account in the preoperative evaluation process enables a more comprehensive provision of care, thus reflecting the complexity of caring for anesthesia in neurosurgery within an expanded framework of patient-centered healthcare. In addition, the function of evolving science in anesthesia recommendations reminds one to include patient medical histories with contemporary methods.

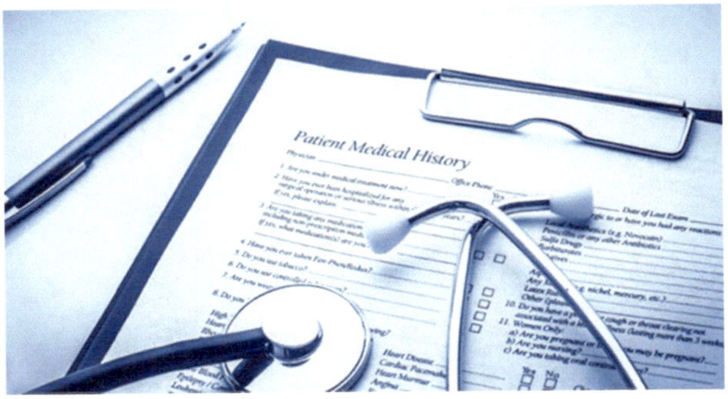

Figure 2.7. A comprehensive patient medical history.

Source: https://1.bp.blogspot.com/-IgdvjWaP7sA/XW-WrZKJgvI/AAAAAAAADIU/RhEpnr-HWm4T9rsg38_9Sak-Atu5jFV-wCLcBGAs/s1600/Importance%2Bof%2BThorough%2 BCommunication%2Bon%2BPatient%2BHistory.jpg.

While better neuromonitoring technologies, as described in recent literature for their ability and safety in use during neurosurgery, are emerging, anesthesiologists must also consider how a patient's past could affect how they interpret such monitoring. For instance, some neurological diseases could affect baseline neurophysiological responses, making intraoperative nervous system integrity assessments challenging (Singh et al., 2016). For this reason, knowledge of a patient's medical history, in addition to real-time monitor data, enables the anesthesia team to react quickly to possible complications, thus improving surgical effectiveness and patient safety. This moving interplay between history, technology, and individualized care represents the complex nature of anesthesia in neurosurgery (Figure 2.7).

2.2.2. Neurological Evaluation

The process of neurological assessment is extremely significant in anesthesia for neurosurgery because it offers an evaluation of the patient's baseline neurological function preoperatively. Such evaluations involve diversified assessments such as history taking, physical examination, and imaging studies. Through the identification of a patient's neurological status preoperatively, anesthesiologists are capable of identifying expected complications that may arise intraoperatively. This is especially important in the management of diseases like intracranial hypertension, where intracranial pressure (ICP) changes can have a colossal impact on patient outcome. For instance, ICP monitoring during anesthesia provides valuable information regarding cerebral perfusion and risks of head-up position, which allows for evidence-based anesthetic management strategies and surgical planning, as noted in the findings of Sturges et al. (2019). Other than standard neurological assessment, advanced techniques such as multilobar electrocorticography (mEcoG) have significant roles to play in neurological assessment during neurosurgery. mEcoG provides real-time cortical-level monitoring of brain activity with greater sensitivity to ischemic alterations than scalp EEG. This is of critical significance when aneurysm surgery causes temporary clipping that alters blood flow. The correlation of mEcoG findings with postoperative outcome underscores the significance of precise monitoring to adequately inform anesthetic management and surgical intervention. Interestingly, the emergence of abnormal trends on mEcoG has been associated with neurological dysfunction, thereby justifying the incorporation of this modality as a component of comprehensive neurological evaluations in the perioperative interval, as explicated in a study using mEcoG data from (Dehdashti et al., 2018). Furthermore, neurological evaluations after surgery are of paramount importance for assessing the efficacy of surgical techniques and anesthetic techniques in neurosurgery. Monitoring in real time postoperatively allows detection of emergent neurological changes, which can direct the need for acute interventions or patient management modifications. The pathologic importance of this examination is underscored by studies correlating persistent abnormalities noted on mEcoG with adverse outcomes, such as increased neurological deficit and imaging hypodensity. By encompassing thorough preoperative and perioperative neurological examinations, clinicians can optimize patient safety and enhance outcomes following neurosurgery. Lastly, the application of such evaluation strategies coupled with proper anesthetic care proves beyond doubt an extreme passion to improve patient care in the distinctive field of neurosurgery (Figure 2.8).

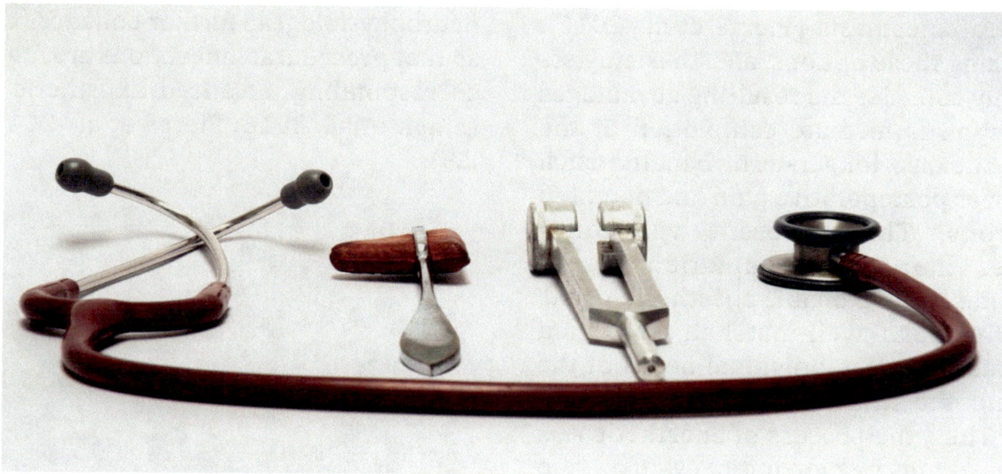

Figure 2.8. The process of neurological evaluation.

Source: https://external-content.duckduckgo.com/iu/?u=https%3A%2F%2Fnursingcecentral.com%2Fwp-content%2Fuploads%2F2022%2F06%2FBlog-Image-Banner-10-5.jpg&f=1&nofb=1&ipt=e58055c833d8cf9f5d99012f3c24f901890e16e66af2684b62ae28bbb9fa5c81.

2.2.3. Anesthetic Risk Assessment

In neurosurgery, anesthetic risk assessment is a critical component that dictates patient management as well as the surgical plan. Anesthetic risk assessment involves a thorough evaluation of patient factors, surgical complexity, and the likelihood of anesthesia-related complications. Underlying systemic diseases, neurological status, and some proposed operations are the critical components. By carefully evaluating these factors, anesthesiologists can tailor anesthetic methods to minimize risk and enhance outcomes. The addition of options such as intraoperative neurophysiological monitoring can provide immediate assessment of nervous system function during surgery, thereby making the procedure considerably safer. The literature increasingly supports the efficacy of multimodal monitoring techniques that offer assessment of the integrity of essential neural structures, particularly in high-complexity neurosurgical procedures where the risk of complication is greater (Singh et al., 2016). This dynamic risk assessment procedure ultimately leads to enhanced patient safety in addition to improved surgical procedures. Apart from the intrinsic complexities of the neurosurgical environment, the selection between other anesthetic methods can also affect the procedural risks involved with them. Anesthetic procedures, specifically general anesthesia vs. regional anesthesia, have varying implications on patient outcomes during neurosurgical procedures. Spinal anesthesia has been found in recent studies to result in briefer operative times and better postoperative recovery rates, though most procedures are still under general anesthesia (Pierce et al., 2017). When weighing these options, anesthesiologists need not only consider the resulting advantages and risks upon immediate completion of the procedure but also longer-term benefits such as control over postoperative pain and potential complications. This inherent variability necessitates thorough examination of the prevailing literature to enable anesthesiologists to optimally make well-matched, informed decisions based on the individual needs of the patients and the individual demands of the procedure. Thus, the process of anesthetic risk assessment extends beyond initial evaluation to include continuous monitoring and adjustment of anesthetic strategy throughout the surgical process. Last, anesthetic risk evaluation is the pillar in successful execution of neurosurgical operations. By combining in-depth evaluations of patient variables, surgical intricacies, and anesthetic modalities, health professionals are suitably positioned to manage the intricate world of anesthetic complications in neurosurgery. Ongoing advancement in monitoring technologies allows for sophisticated precision in risk estimates, allowing for a customized strategy focused on patient safety. Also, cumulative data obtained from previous research will continue to influence the best practices of anesthetic care. With the evolving science, ongoing research will be essential in optimizing risk assessment protocols and anesthetic practice to aid patient outcomes for neurosurgical patients. Ongoing liaison between anesthesiologists, surgeons, and neurophysiologists further enhances the process so that procedural innovations are matched with corresponding advanced anesthetic strategies (Singh et al., 2016; Pierce et al., 2017) (Figure 2.9).

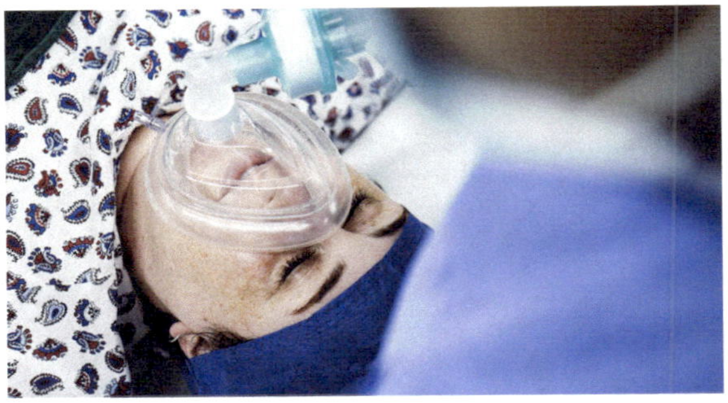

Figure 2.9. The evaluation of anesthetic risk.

Source: https://post.medicalnewstoday.com/wp-content/uploads/sites/3/2021/11/general_anesthesia_GettyImages910493382_Header-1024x575.jpg.

Test Your Knowledge

1. What information is gathered during a preoperative assessment?
2. How does preoperative assessment help reduce surgical risks?

2.3. Anesthetic Techniques in Neurosurgery

Learning Outcome

1. Induction methods
2. Maintenance of anesthesia
3. Monitoring during surgery

Choice of anesthetic techniques in neurosurgery has been a major determinant of optimizing patient results and procedural safety. Techniques such as total intravenous anesthesia (TIVA) and volatile anesthetics are extremely controversial when it comes to their efficacy in maintaining hemodynamic stability and providing adequate cerebral protection. TIVA, a favorite due to its recovery time and low post-operative nausea, is more appropriate for regulating the depth of anesthesia, such as in cases of surgery where neurological function needs to be closely monitored. Volatile anesthetics, on the other hand, can be neuroprotective, potentially preserving cerebral blood flow and metabolism. Intraoperative monitor integration would also serve to strengthen the anesthetic plan since it allows for real-time cerebral function monitoring, which is a vital aspect in maneuvering around sensitive structures within complex neurosurgical procedures. Multimodal intraoperative neurophysiologic monitoring has proven to increase the accuracy and safety of neurosurgical procedures in contemporary neurosurgery. A variety of techniques, including electroencephalography, somatosensory evoked potentials, and transcranial motor evoked potentials, provide surgeons with valuable information regarding the functional integrity of nervous tissue. Monitoring technologies such as these allow for early detection of potential neurological compromise and prompt intervention. These monitoring modalities have been found, according to recent literature, to be optimally integrated into anesthetic practices in order to ensure optimal results in procedures such as endoscopic, endonasal skull base surgery. The use of such advanced monitoring techniques not only improves patient safety but also makes the possibility of intensive management strategies available after the treatment of complex pathologies, thus emphasizing the importance of anesthetic techniques in neurosurgical settings (Singh et al., 2016). Secondly, the utilization of functional neurosurgery techniques reflects the disparities in the utilization of anesthetic techniques between different regions of the world.

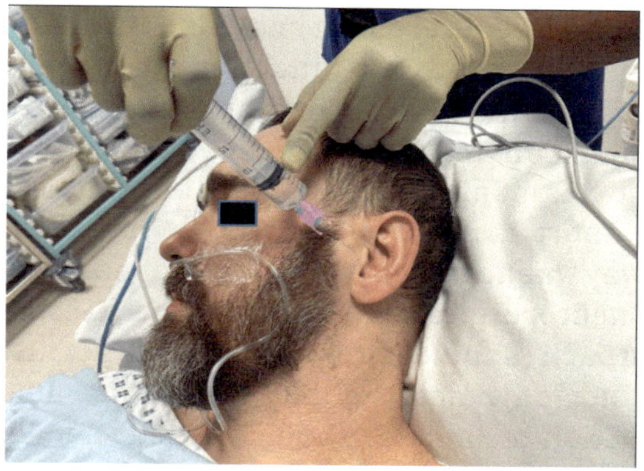

Figure 2.10. The choice of anesthetic techniques in neurosurgery.

Source: https://resources.wfsahq.org/wp-content/uploads/480_image_5.png.

While high-income countries (HIC) tend to have relatively universal access to cutting-edge neurosurgical care, low- and middle-income countries (LMIC) typically are limited by cost and resource factors. Greater access to anesthetic techniques in these countries can play a significant role in the management of diseases like epilepsy that are sensitive to functional surgery. Recent literature establishes that despite a large portion of the population in LMIC lacking access to safe surgical care, there is demand for functional neurosurgery (Fezeu et al., 2018). Institutional partnership between

HIC and LMIC can facilitate knowledge transfer and the adaptation of effective anesthetic practices appropriate to local conditions. These partnerships have promise for increasing surgical access and outcomes, highlighting the importance of augmenting anesthetic techniques in neurosurgery globally (Figure 2.10).

2.3.1. Induction Methods

The selection of appropriate induction methods of anesthesia in neurosurgery is critical because it instantly influences the success of the patients and the overall safety of the procedure. Intravenous or inhalational drugs employed for induction are typically directed towards ensuring rapid and effortless progression to unconsciousness. Propofol is most commonly used due to its onset of action and short half-life, which allows for efficient airway management and hemodynamics. In the neurosurgical environment, the anesthetic approach should prefer cerebral perfusion and hemodynamic stability; the choice among induction techniques should be determined by the patient's particular needs, e.g., pre-existing neurologic disease and hemodynamic status. The combination of general anesthesia with regional techniques, e.g., scalp block, may result in dramatic benefits. Scalp blocks, done after induction of general anesthesia, have been able to efficiently prevent hemodynamic variations that are normally encountered in craniotomy procedures, in harmony with the best results in neurosurgery (Tonković et al., 2015). Coordination of various anesthesia induction methods with neurophysiologic monitoring also has the promise of providing robust information on the functional integrity of neurological tissues during surgery. The incorporation of multimodal neuromonitoring systems allows anesthetists to assess real-time changes in neurologic function during the induction of anesthesia. Some of the methods used to enhance traditional anesthesia methods include electroencephalography and somatosensory evoked potentials, which improve sensitivity to the effect of anesthesia on vital neural pathways. For instance, in endoscopic skull base procedures, employing these monitoring techniques will help in assessing the impact of anesthesia induction on the cranial nerves and cerebral cortex. With the inclusion of these monitoring techniques, the anesthesiology team can dynamically modify induction protocols to promote greater safety, in addition to appropriate management of complications resulting from the anesthesia used (Singh et al., 2016). Finally, the emphasis on patient-specific induction methods in neurosurgery is a reflection of growing recognition of the diversity of patient populations and needs within the specialty. Anesthesia must be tailored not only to the character of the surgical procedure and the specific anatomical problem, but to the individual patient's special hemodynamic and neurologic status.

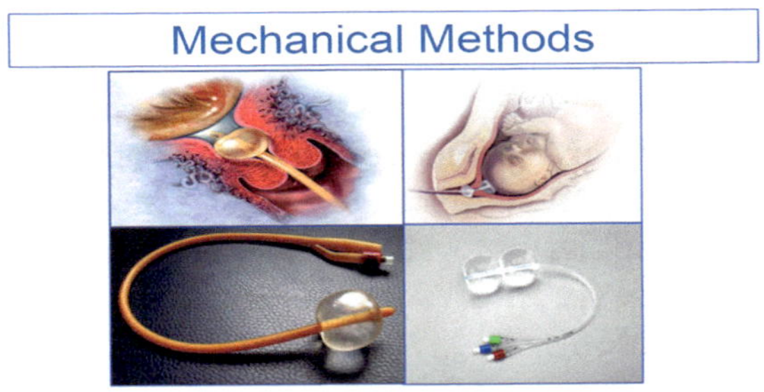

Figure 2.11. The selection of appropriate induction methods for anesthesia in neurosurgery.

Source: https://ars.els-cdn.com/content/image/1-s2.0-S0002937823000819-mmc4.jpg.

Methods that provide hemodynamic stability, such as general anesthesia with regional blocks, may significantly improve patient outcomes by reducing the risks of intraoperative complications. Monitoring of hemodynamic parameters following induction allows for prompt correction of any deviation and enhanced stability during surgery by the anesthesia practitioners. Lastly, ongoing developments in induction methods demonstrate an evolving context with new approaches centering on patient safety and procedural success in neurosurgical practice (Tonković et al., 2015) (Figure 2.11).

2.3.2. Maintenance of Anesthesia

In neurosurgery, anesthesia support is a critical component to ensure patient safety and surgical success. Maintenance of anesthesia refers to the administration of anesthetic drugs in a manner that offers adequate analgesia and unconsciousness with hemodynamic stability. During long-duration neurosurgical procedures, the anesthesiologist must observe the patient constantly and alter the anesthesia plan based on the physiological status of the patient and the requirements of the surgical team. Such flexibility is particularly valuable in neurosurgery, where small alterations in brain perfusion can have disastrous implications. The use of real-time monitoring techniques, such as bispectral index (BIS) monitoring, evaluates the depth of anesthesia, allowing for prompt modification to optimize patient comfort and surgical conditions. In addition, the use of advanced neuromonitoring techniques in neurosurgical cases has the potential to enhance the safety and efficacy of the maintenance of anesthesia. The application of multimodality neuromonitoring, including modalities such as electroencephalography and somatosensory evoked potentials, is to allow for a complete assessment of susceptible neural structures. For instance, during endonasal procedures to the skull base, monitoring cerebral cortex and cranial nerve viability is important to prevent intraoperative damage. Such monitoring enables the surgical team and anesthesiologist to make informed decisions about anesthesia maintenance, enabling them to more aggressively but safely treat complex brain tumors. The success of this multimodality protocol underscores the importance of mutual awareness during neurosurgical anesthesia maintenance in unifying the integration of real-time information into clinical care (Singh et al., 2016). Further, the use of transcranial Doppler (TCD) in combination with routine anesthesia monitoring could improve cerebral hemodynamic assessment during procedures with a significant impact on brain perfusion. TCD's ability to detect cerebral circulation arrest is informative, especially when working with brain death or life-threatening surgeries. Research has demonstrated that adding procedures such as insonation of the extracranial internal carotid artery (ICA) to TCD raises its sensitivity and thus enables deeper investigation of intracranial blood flow. These ancillary monitoring modalities are particularly useful in neurosurgical contexts when optimal cerebral perfusion is crucial. By utilizing TCD as a component in the plan of anesthesia maintenance, anesthesiologists are able to ensure greater precision in managing the critical balance between drug effect and neurological status, ultimately resulting in better outcomes for patients during and after surgery (Conti et al., 2006).

2.3.3. Monitoring During Surgery

The role of monitoring in surgery extends beyond the provision of general physiological stability; it is also critical to the anticipation and management of complications that may arise in neurosurgical cases. Care intraoperatively is centered on continuous monitoring of vital signs, including heart rate, blood pressure, and oxygen saturation, which allow anesthesiologists to detect variations from baseline and make suitable interventions. In neurosurgery, however, such attention is even crucial because cerebral perfusion must be closely monitored in case neurological damage is to be prevented. Moreover, advances in technology have led to specialized monitoring tools, like the analgesia nociception index, which give details about a patient's pain response so that interventions can be made accordingly (Kamath, 2023). This level of monitoring enhances patient safety as well as the more efficient management of pain during the surgical process. In neurosurgical settings, the intensity of the procedures necessitates a multidimensional strategy for monitoring. The modified park bench position used in certain surgeries poses special challenges, particularly in cardiovascular stability management and access to the airway. Anesthesiologists must plan the administration of anesthesia carefully, involving both invasive and non-invasive monitoring techniques to keep the patient's physiological state stable throughout the surgery (Wanda et al., 2024).

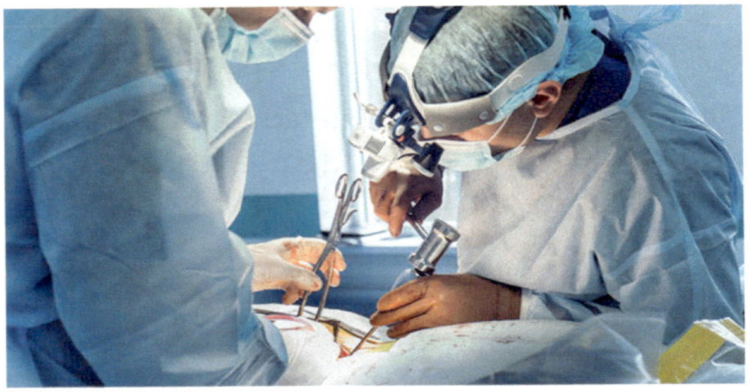

Figure 2.12. The role of monitoring during surgery.

Source: https://www.rwkgoodman.com/wp-content/uploads/2024/01/Spinal-surgery.jpg.

Arterial lines permit real-time blood pressure, whereas central venous catheters can provide information on fluid status as well as cardiac function. Monitoring of neuromuscular function also helps assess the effectiveness of neuromuscular blockade. This comprehensive monitoring strategy not only aids in real-time intraoperative decision-making but also forms the cornerstone for effective postoperative recovery and pain management. Integrating advanced monitoring techniques in neurosurgery proves to be valuable not just for short-term patient outcomes but also for subsequent recovery trajectories. Postoperatively, patients are usually managed in intensive care units in which constant evaluation of neurological status and vital parameters is crucial. The findings of research indicate a high incidence rate of postoperative pain, highlighting the seriousness of adequate analgesia protocols (Kamath, 2023). Effective communication and coordination between the surgical and anesthetic teams ensures that any occurred complication can be addressed with urgency. Furthermore, use of multimodal analgesia, possibly with the use of non-opioids along with traditional opioids, has been shown to maximize surgical recovery and minimize possible opioid side effects. Lastly, restrictive monitoring practices intra-operatively and post-operatively are a testament to an emphasis on patient safety and recovery within the rigorous field of neurosurgery (Figure 2.12).

Test Your Knowledge

1. Which type of anesthesia is commonly used in neurosurgery?
2. Why is careful control of intracranial pressure important during anesthesia?

2.4. Challenges in Anesthesia for Neurosurgery

Learning Outcome

1. Patient positioning
2. Management of intracranial pressure
3 Potential for neurological complications

Anesthesia administration in neurosurgery presents a range of specialty issues demanding greater acuity and competence on the part of anesthesiologists. One of the key concerns is the physiological impact of neuroanesthesia on cerebral perfusion and metabolism. Anesthetics possess a potential impact on intracranial pressure (ICP) that can nullify cerebral blood flow and brain oxygen supply. This is particularly crucial in brain tumor or trauma surgery, in which stable cerebral perfusion pressure should be ensured to prevent secondary brain injury. Anesthesiologists must therefore be proficient in the use of controlled hypotension or judicious fluid management strategies to ensure stability during surgery, but respond easily to real intraoperative variations in patient condition. Furthermore, the multidisciplinary nature of neurosurgical procedures makes anesthesia management that much more daunting. Collaborative work between neurosurgeons and anesthesiologists is essential, as variation in surgical technique can significantly influence anesthetic technique. For instance, differences in surgical technique during intraoperative neurophysiological monitoring require consideration in the choice of anesthetics to avoid interference with evoked potentials. The evolution of high-technology neurosurgical techniques, such as functional neurosurgery, also increases the need for a tailored anesthetic approach (Fezeu et al., 2018). With these procedures growing more common, especially in low- and middle-income nations (LMIC), the challenge to balance efficacy and safety is even greater due to limited access to advanced monitoring and anesthesia facilities. The global scope of medical emergencies, such as the COVID-19 pandemic, has also presented novel challenges for anesthesiology in neurosurgery. Anesthesiologists come into contact with greater concentrations of infectious agents, and on this account, strict safety protocols need to be maintained in order to protect both patients and staff. With the advent of the pandemic, the degree of anesthesia management complexity has dramatically increased due to the necessity of greater infection control measures (Givi et al., 2020). Such a shift has pushed healthcare systems to rapidly adapt, reinforcing the importance of effective communication and anesthetic and inter-surgical collaboration. Therefore, addressing these evolving needs is through ongoing learning and collaboration to ensure that the quality of care provided to neurosurgery patients is maintained during these unprecedented times.

2.4.1. Patient Positioning

Proper patient positioning is extremely critical in neurosurgery, not only because it enhances surgical exposure but also because it works considerably towards ensuring patient safety during surgery. Surgical exposures vary and therefore specific positioning techniques must be used to allow for optimal visualization and ease of handling of neural structures. For instance, in craniotomies, the head is normally immobilized in a position to allow access to the cranial cavity with minimal movement, thus reducing the risk of nerve injury. This precise fixation allows for the proper creation of a stable field for the surgeon and thus the accuracy of interventions. Moreover, patient position can influence intracranial dynamics, and therefore adjustments should be made based on how ICP and cerebrospinal fluid flow are affected during surgery. Hemodynamic stability is also critical when it comes to patient position for neurosurgical procedures. Changes in the position of the head can lead to changes in cerebral perfusion of blood to the brain, which influences neural tissue perfusion and oxygenation. Techniques such as the Trendelenburg position, where the body is placed in supine with a tilt with the legs in elevation, can be utilized to counteract hypotension but must be balanced against the risk of increased ICP. The positioning also causes complications such as pressure sores or nerve injury, particularly where stability for more than a prolonged period is required. An intimate understanding of these principles is to the advantage of surgical teams and anesthesiologists when selecting the optimal positioning strategy to provide maximum surgical outcomes and patient safety. Intraoperative neurophysiological monitoring is particularly beneficial in the context of patient positioning.

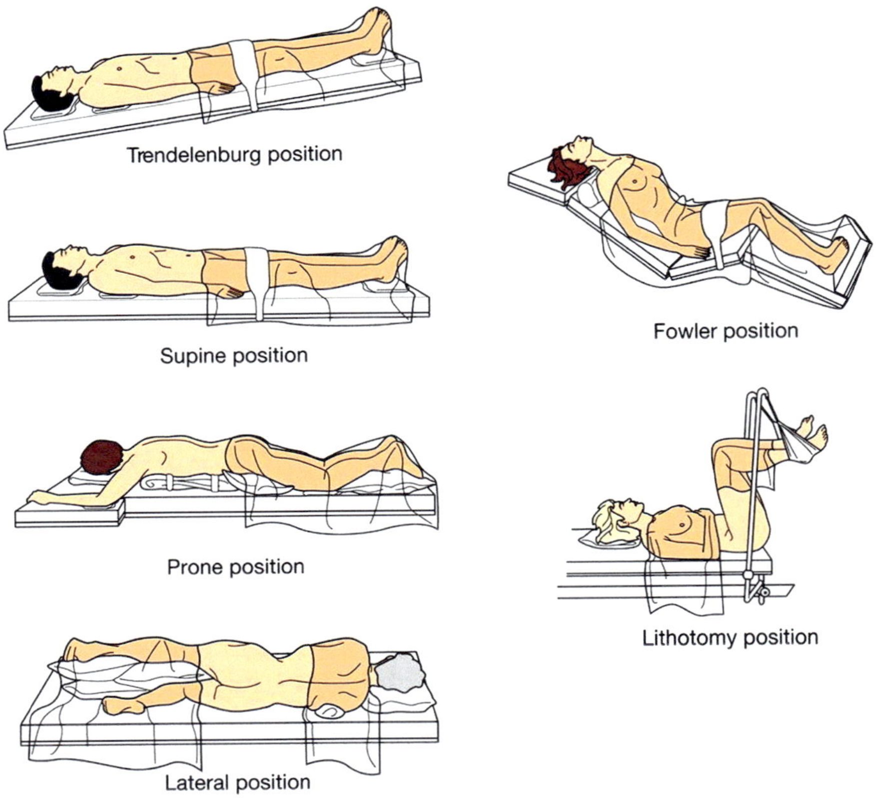

Figure 2.13. The administration of anesthesia in neurosurgery presents a range of unique challenges.

Source: https://blog.georgiaemsacademy.com/wp-content/uploads/2020/09/1073774_550144461709322_942723524_o.jpg.

Multimodal monitoring techniques provide real-time feedback regarding the functional status of neural anatomy during surgery, enhancing the capability of the surgeons to respond to intraoperative changes on the basis of positioning. This skill is especially critical in endonasal approaches to the skull base, where exposure is limited by anatomical complexity and proximity to sensitive neurologic structures. As studies show, application of total neuromonitoring approaches allows for safer management of high-risk cases by facilitating prompt interventions upon detection of abnormalities, thereby providing better patient outcomes and avoiding the risk of postoperative positioning-related complications (Singh et al., 2016). Enhancing patient positioning along with neurophysiological monitoring finally depicts the intricate interface between anesthesia management and surgical technique in neurosurgery (Figure 2.13).

2.4.2. Management of Intracranial Pressure

ICP management is a crucial aspect of anesthesiology in neurosurgery, particularly because it directly impacts the result of surgery and patient safety. Because intracranial hypertension can significantly impair cerebral perfusion, monitoring and control of ICP with caution are critical during surgery. Anesthesia professionals are obligated to employ various techniques to maintain ICP within normal limits. These techniques usually include careful fluid management, induction of mild respiratory alkalosis by hyperventilation, and pharmacologic interventions such as administration of osmotic agents.

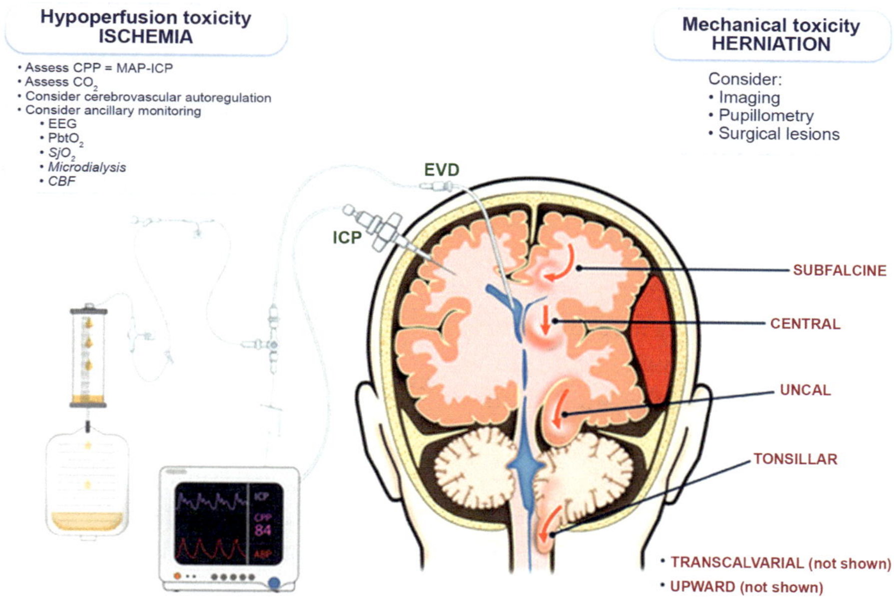

Figure 2.14. The management of intracranial pressure (ICP).

Source: https://media.springernature.com/lw685/springer-static/image/art%3A10.1007%2Fs00134-022-06786-y/MediaObjects/134_2022_6786_Fig1_HTML.png.

Effective management of ICP not only helps to guard against brain dysfunction but also enhances visualization of the surgical site, thereby facilitating the surgery for the surgeons and ultimately optimizing prognostic results for patients who are undergoing neurosurgical procedures. The value of monitoring intracranial pressure during anesthesia is confirmed by numerous studies that provide evidence of the safety and feasibility of monitoring ICP using microsensor technology. In one study, intraparenchymal transducers made continuous, real-time intracranial pressure monitoring possible without significantly impacting measurements regardless of where the transducer was placed, although side effects were more prominent with intraparenchymal placements. The results emphasize the importance of simplifying ICP measurement techniques within the operating room environment. By using protocols for therapeutic response to variations in ICP, anesthesiologists are capable of enhancing patient outcomes. Placement of the subdural sensor appears to have specific advantages, thus guiding anesthesia providers on the management of ICP during neurosurgery (Sturges et al., 2019). Multimodal neuromonitoring is a key aspect in the management of ICP in high-level neurosurgical interventions as well. It is a technique that integrates various forms of monitoring, i.e., electroencephalography and somatosensory evoked potentials, which allow for real-time assessment of nervous system integrity. In endoscopic, endonasal surgery, multimodal monitoring comes in handy to conduct comprehensive evaluations of such crucial neurological structures as the cerebral cortex and cranial nerves. Utilization of such an extensive method enhances the security of the surgical procedure, facilitates appropriate interventions within an appropriate time when an abnormal ICP value is detected, and presents a model for gentle and aggressive tumor manipulation. The addition of these monitoring techniques during the process of anesthesia, therefore, reinforces the complete effectiveness and safety of neurosurgical practice (Singh et al., 2016) (Figure 2.14).

2.4.3. Potential for Neurological Complications

Regarding the neurological complications of neurosurgical procedures, the anesthetic technique employed plays a critical role. Particularly, spinal anesthesia (SA) has been weighed in terms of advantages and disadvantages compared to general anesthesia. Evidence indicates that SA can result in less operative time, decreased blood loss, and reduced total hospital stay for patients who have undergone lumbar procedures such as diskectomy and laminectomy. Nevertheless, the threat of adverse neurological outcomes is an issue of primary significance. As far as one research discovered just one case of spinal hematoma within the SA group, an event that healed without any long-term sequelae, it still reiterates the intrinsic risks of spinal approaches in neurosurgery, even though this sample lacked complications such as paraparesis and post-dural puncture headache (Pierce et al., 2017). An accurate appreciation of the risk of neurological complications, thus, plays an important role in planning the appropriate anesthetic approach. An additional factor in the assessment of neurological complications is where neurosurgery is being performed. Availability of safe surgery in LMIC is a significant challenge, resulting in a higher burden of neurological conditions potentially amenable to neurosurgical intervention. Poor resources, nonetheless, limit the application of functional neurosurgery that may, in turn, lead to untreatable diseases that would otherwise be managed well. According to the literature, surgically amenable disease morbidity is underreported in these regions, and therefore, equality in treatment access is also hindered (Fezeu et al., 2018). Increased understanding of such gaps can result in targeted efforts toward the establishment of improved surgical infrastructure and anesthetic care, minimizing the risk of neurosurgical complications. Such efforts, combined with HIC, may enhance outcomes and reduce neurological complications in LMIC patients. Moreover, the selection of an anesthetic approach should also consider the individual condition of the patient since various comorbid conditions might predispose to neurological complications. For example, those patients with pre-existing neurological deficits or requiring complex neurosurgical interventions can develop exaggerated sensitivity to the side effects of anesthesia. Such a well-thought-out anesthetic plan then has to be multidisciplinary in character with thorough preoperative assessment and postoperative monitoring for the identification of any prodromal signs of complications. An aggressive strategy of this sort can significantly reduce the risk associated with different anesthetic modalities. With evolving neurosurgical methods, continuous research on the effectiveness of various anesthetic drugs and techniques will be of critical value in the improvement of patient safety and best results, thereby helping solve the persistent issue of neurological complications of anesthesia in neurosurgery (Figure 2.15).

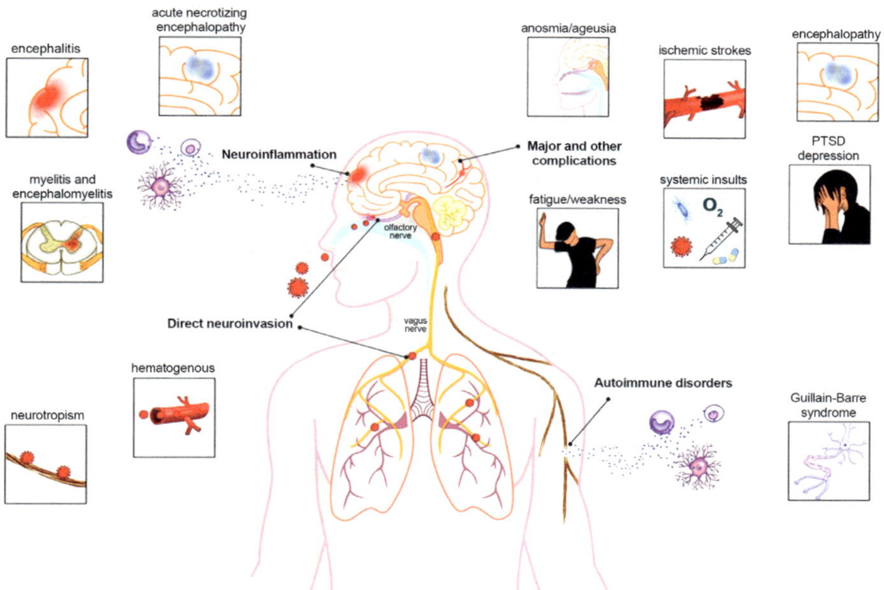

Figure 2.15. Potential for neurological complications.

Source: https://media.springernature.com/lw685/springer-static/image/art%3A10.1007%2Fs00134-021-06439-6/MediaObjects/134_2021_6439_Fig1_HTML.png.

Test Your Knowledge

1. What is a major challenge in maintaining brain stability during neurosurgery?
2. Why is monitoring vital functions critical in neurosurgical anesthesia?

2.5. Postoperative Care

Learning Outcome

1. Recovery from anesthesia
2. Pain management strategies
3. Monitoring for complications

The significance of postoperative care in neurosurgery can perhaps be overstated, since it is of critical significance to patient recovery and general outcomes of surgery. Postoperative patients who underwent procedures involving anesthesia, particularly neurosurgery, need to be watched closely to avoid potential complications such as respiratory distress, infection, and neurological impairment. Ideal care at this stage consists of extensive assessments that monitor vital functions and neurological status and ensure that these changes are intervened upon promptly. The choice between spinal and general anesthesia has been shown to affect recovery-related metrics, including postoperative nausea and pain scores. For instance, spinal anesthesia has been associated with reduced operative times and hospital stays and demonstrated its potency in managing postoperative care effectively (Pierce et al., 2017). Additionally, patient-specific postoperative plans can enhance patient comfort and aid quicker rehabilitation, ultimately saving the healthcare system. In neurosurgical environments, postoperative management is increasingly informed by the most up-to-date developments in the delivery of anesthesia, showing an active cross-talk between surgical technique and recuperation algorithms. As a case in point, new studies define the advantage of spinal anesthesia, which not only reduces surgery time but also enables minimization of the requirement for extensive observation in the post-anesthesia care unit (PACU) (Pierce et al., 2017). Sophisticated monitoring techniques, such as real-time neuromonitoring, enable clinicians to identify complications early in the game, meaning timely interventions. No one role is larger, either, than that of multidisciplinary teams, with anesthesiologists, nurses, and physiotherapists collaborating to create personalized postoperative treatment plans. By sharing their expertise, they optimize patient outcomes and ensure complications such as urinary retention or postoperative headache are minimized, thus enabling a smooth recovery process. In addition, the necessity of an integrative strategy for postoperative care is emphasized in low- and middle-income countries (LMIC), where there are unique challenges in this respect. In spite of high incidence rates of conditions that are appropriate for functional neurosurgical interventions in these nations, few resources have the tendency to generate disparities in the provision of care, with detrimental impacts on patients' outcomes.

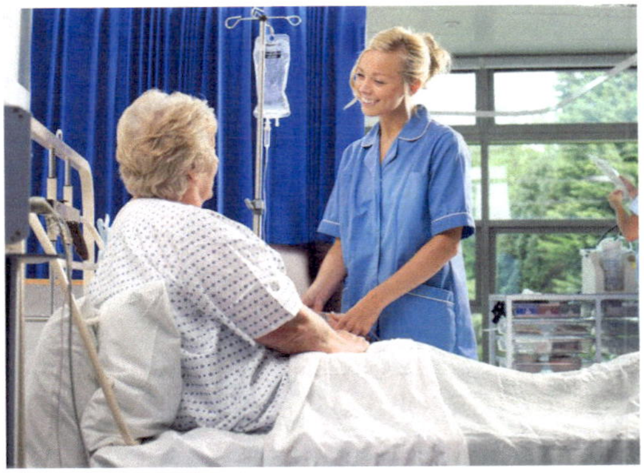

Figure 2.16. The significance of postoperative care in neurosurgery.

Source: https://media.post.rvohealth.io/wp-content/uploads/2020/08/postoperative-care_thumb.jpg.

Effective postoperative policies in LMIC must consider not just the surgical and anesthetic methods but also system factors such as access to follow-up and rehabilitation care. The setting up of international collaboration and awareness about such inequalities can result in activities that can promote postoperative care policies. Certain strategies, such as community aid, education, and resource, are essential in addressing the individual needs of these groups. With continued advancements in neurosurgery, the need for equitable and inclusive postoperative care remains an underpinning to improving surgical efficiency globally (Figure 2.16).

2.5.1. Recovery from Anesthesia

Recovery from anesthesia is a critical component of the perioperative process, particularly with neurosurgery in consideration, wherein patient stability and mental status are the prime considerations. Different techniques of anesthesia, such as general anesthesia and spinal anesthesia, can have significant impacts on recovery outcomes. For instance, studies have suggested that spinal anesthesia can lead to decreased operative time and improved recovery results, including less total hospital stay and decreased postoperative pain levels. Interestingly enough, though spinal anesthesia has such positive attributes as reduced blood loss and minimal complications, there is an awareness to address the variation among patients, which will have a significant impact on recovery experiences (Pierce et al., 2017). Such assessments are critical to optimize patient management practices to enable neurosurgical patients to recover well and safely. Recovery from anesthesia involves both early postoperative care and subsequent recovery markers. Early recovery typically occurs in the PACU, where patients remain under close observation for untoward effects or complications. Studies have indicated that recovery from spinal anesthesia also has prolonged PACU stays, which can be attributed to the need for longer monitoring after the procedure (Pierce et al., 2017). It should also be considered in evaluating recovery, not only time for consciousness or motor function return but also the degree to which patients are able to return to work and cognitive function. Anesthesia protocols also play an important role in these recovery stages, affecting such outcomes as postoperative nausea and general satisfaction with the surgical experience. Anesthetic technique comparisons underscore the importance of individually directed care measures in neurosurgical recovery. Debates regarding the superiority of inhalational versus intravenous anesthesia continue to linger, but the roles that these choices play in recovery outcomes are becoming a concern. Factors like the quality and speed of reawakening and postoperative adverse events are well-researched, but increasingly, new evidence also highlights the importance of long-term morbidity and patient satisfaction after surgery. It follows that the focus should be placed on holistic measures that cater not just to the short-term recovery but also to the long-term effects of anesthesia decisions on the quality of life of a patient. This multi-faceted approach is crucial in maximizing patient outcomes during the sensitive recovery period following neurosurgical procedures (Figure 2.17).

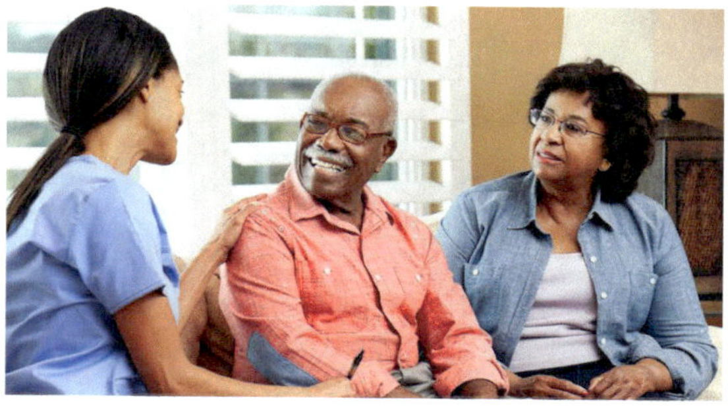

Figure 2.17. The recovery from anesthesia.

Source: https://medstarhealth-delivery.sitecorecontenthub.cloud/api/public/content/services%2FAnesthesia-Recovery-and-Going-Home?v=2dbec21d.

2.5.2. Pain Management Strategies

The most effective pain management methods are integral components of neurosurgical anesthesia as they directly influence recovery and postoperative results. Postoperative pain severity can be affected to a large extent by the method of anesthesia employed; i.e., spinal anesthesia (SA) has been associated with reduced operative time, blood loss, and hospital stay in comparison to general anesthesia in lumbar procedures. Moreover, studies have indicated that SA can lead to lower frequencies of postoperative complications such as urinary retention and nausea, which further benefits the patient experience in the PACU (Pierce et al., 2017).

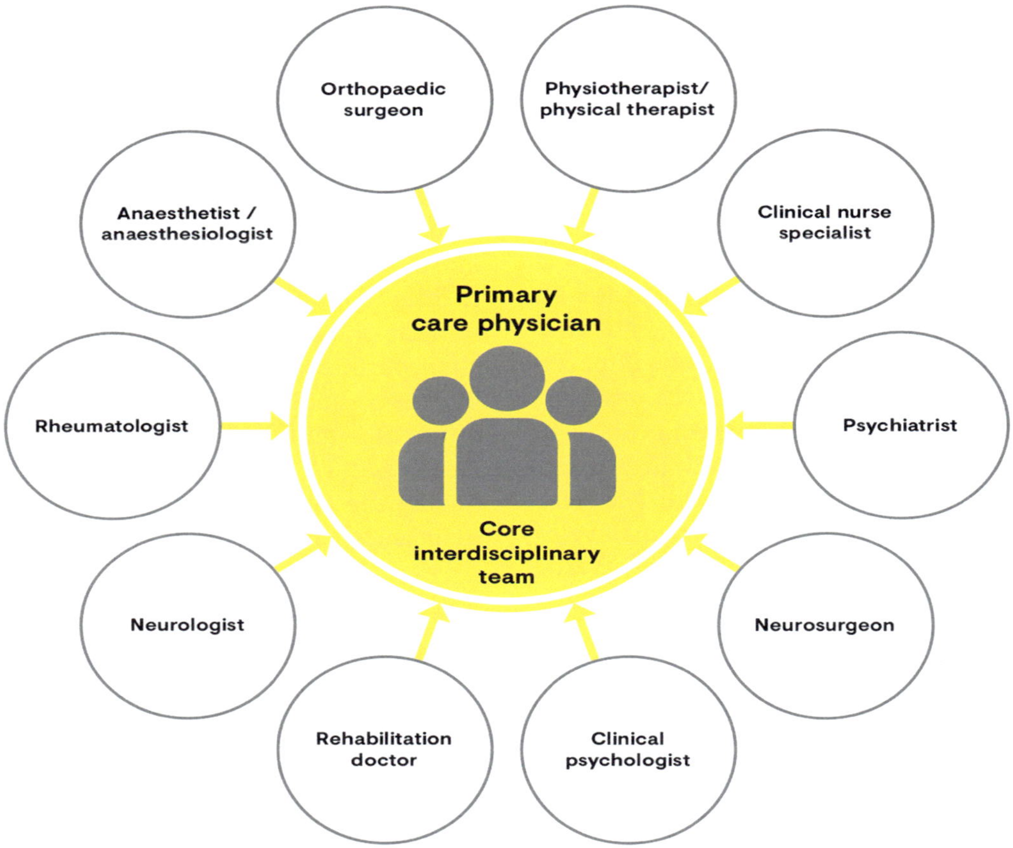

Figure 2.18. The pain management strategies.

Source: https://www.grunenthal.com/-/media/projects/change-pain/pain-basics/en/p-basics4.png?rev=298f0a5efd7d43619c14681a87869d99&hash=A25EDCF1FBCA61BCE019CA0B8C84C195.

Thus, the use of SA in appropriate neurosurgical procedures not only helps to alleviate pain quickly but also makes the entire process of management in the perioperative period easier, thereby enhancing surgical efficiency and patient satisfaction. Outside of the choice of anesthetic technique, multimodal analgesia is an important pain management technique in neurosurgical patients. By the use of several analgesic drugs—e.g., non-steroidal anti-inflammatory drugs (NSAIDs), acetaminophen, and regional blocks—the practitioner can reduce opioid dependence, with resultant reduction in side effects. Combined effect upon several pain pathways optimizes analgesic effect while reducing total drug dosages required for effective pain relief. Besides, studies have indicated early intervention with multimodal analgesia has been linked to improved recovery profiles, reduced hospital stays, and high patient satisfaction, particularly in cases of neurosurgery where pain management has a direct impact on neurological function (Fezeu et al., 2018). Emphasis on multimodal strategies offers a robust paradigm for handling the complex pain needs of neurosurgical patients. Furthermore, effective neurosurgical pain management also demands individualized approaches tailored to the specific demands of every patient. Factors related to the type of neurosurgery, the patient's past medical history, and potential comorbidities are all factors to be considered when formulating an integrated pain management policy. The application of high-technology techniques such as PCA or regional anesthesia may provide better pain control and allow for early mobilization. Empirical data are available to confirm that improved pain management leads to fewer complications, shorter length of stay, and greater overall satisfaction with care (Pierce et al., 2017). Eventually, an accurate understanding of such factors enables anesthesiologists and surgeons to develop individualized pain management plans that optimize the effectiveness of anesthesia in neurosurgical settings to the advantage of both patient and healthcare systems (Figure 2.18).

2.5.3. Monitoring for Complications

The multifaceted relationship between anesthesia and neurosurgery necessitates vigilant monitoring for complications in the perioperative period. Monitoring for complications is a prophylactic measure intended to guarantee patient outcomes in central nervous system procedures. The delicacy of neural structures necessitates that the risk of adverse events, such as elevated intracranial pressure (ICP) or loss of neurophysiological function, warrants constant monitoring. For instance, established protocols involving microsensor transducers in the measurement of ICP have demonstrated their effectiveness in providing real-time data on intracranial dynamics and thus allowing for timely interventions whenever necessary. Monitoring strategies enhance clinical decision-making against anticipated complications, ultimately improving patient safety and recovery. Further, persistent monitoring of hemodynamic stability throughout the procedure is significant in the prevention of secondary injury due to underperfusion of the brain. Another central aspect of monitoring for neurosurgery is the incorporation of intraoperative neurophysiological tests. These tests are significant for instances where the functional integrity of significant neural structures at risk should be assessed. Techniques such as electroencephalography and somatosensory evoked potentials are also extremely useful in the intraoperative monitoring of nervous system function in real time, allowing the surgeon and anesthesiologist to identify developing complications just as they are starting to occur intraoperatively. The multimodality approach not only increases the scope of monitoring but also its usefulness by combining several technologies for a comprehensive evaluation of neurological conditions. Through the combination of these modalities, the clinical team can rapidly identify changes that are indicative of impending complications and therefore take immediate remedial action that can minimize the risk of injury to critical neural pathways, as documented in recent literature on the subject (Singh et al., 2016). Beyond direct neurological monitoring, watchfulness for observation of systemic responses to anesthesia and surgery also plays a role, as these too can precipitate complications. Neurosurgical anesthesia generally employs agents with an effect upon cerebral perfusion and general physiology. Continuous monitoring of parameters such as heart rate, blood pressure, and oxygen saturation is essential to detect early indicators of an impending adverse reaction. Alteration from baseline readings may signal the onset of an emerging complication requiring immediate treatment. For instance, arterial pressure alterations influence cerebral perfusion, making stable hemodynamics during surgeries a requirement. Comprehensive monitoring not only attends to intracranial pathology, but systemic homeostasis is also maintained, reducing postoperative complications and enhancing the quality of patient management generally in neurosurgical procedures (Sturges et al., 2019).

Test Your Knowledge

1. What is the primary goal of postoperative care?
2. Why is pain management important after surgery?

2.6. Advances in Anesthetic Practices

Learning Outcome

1. New anesthetic agents
2. Technology in monitoring
3. Enhanced recovery protocols

The recent developments in anesthetic practice have significantly enhanced patient management in neurosurgical procedures. One of the breakthroughs is the increasing use of spinal anesthesia for selected operations, particularly lumbar spine stabilization. It was demonstrated that spinal anesthesia is a satisfactory substitute for general anesthesia in carefully selected high-risk patients to provide cardiovascular stability without adverse effects such as hypotension and bradycardia. Very systematic research involving 497 patients established the effectiveness of spinal anesthesia, obtained with subarachnoid block utilizing appropriate dosages of bupivacaine and adjuvant medication, in such a manner that there was no incidence of significant intraoperative complications and it facilitated quicker recovery time. This switch to spinal anesthesia in neurosurgery reflects a broader pattern of employing more focused and less invasive anesthesia techniques, eventually leading to better patient outcomes and safety in complex procedures (Erbaş et al., 2015). With progress in local anesthesia techniques, multimodal analgesia has emerged as a critical advancement in anesthetic care in neurosurgery. Through the blending of various analgesic drugs, i.e., dexmedetomidine before induction, experts can considerably reduce the need for opioid analgesics during the perioperative period. One of the recent projects aimed at anesthesia providers' training for dexmedetomidine found a considerable increase in its expected use, which was found to alter clinical practice in the direction of opioid-sparing techniques. Not only does this approach decrease risks associated with opioid use, such as dependence and respiratory depression, but it also enhances patients' satisfaction by ensuring improved pain management (Nilsson, 2024). Thus, the inclusion of multimodal analgesia in anesthetic regimens for neurosurgery is a preventive step to optimize perioperative management. Moreover, advancements in monitoring and anesthesia delivery technology have been the key driving force in determining practices for neurosurgery. With the advent of high-tech monitoring, it has become possible for anesthesiologists to obtain instant feedback regarding a patient's physiological status and intervene in a timely fashion when needed. In addition, improvements in computer-controlled anesthesia delivery systems enable precise delivery of medication according to the patient's requirements. This improvement leads to a reduced rate of complications and improved overall success of the surgery. Improved monitoring techniques also enable early detection of potential problems, for example, fluctuation in blood pressure or oxygen saturation, thus making the surgical procedure safer. With the progress of anesthesia practices through these technologies, the focus is on attaining optimal patient safety as well as a smooth and optimized surgical procedure in neurosurgical procedures (Figure 2.19).

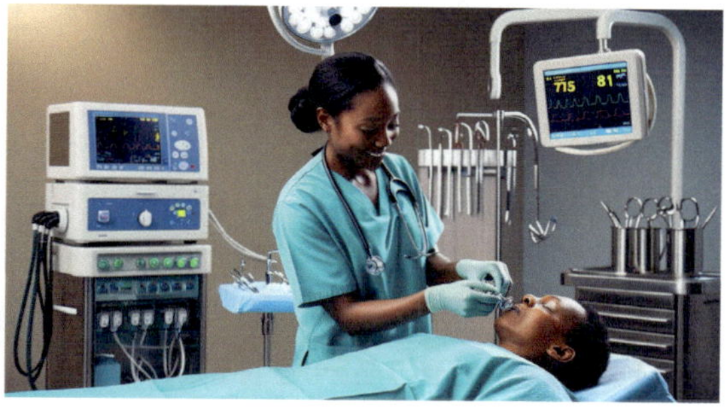

Figure 2.19. Recent advancements in anesthetic practices.

Source: https://www.ines.ac.rw/media/faculties/Anestesia.jpg.

2.6.1. New Anesthetic Agents

The evolution of anesthetic drugs has far-reaching implications on neurosurgery, influencing intraoperative management as well as postoperative outcomes. The older drugs have paved the way for new techniques that promise a better future of safety and efficacy. Among the new developments, ultra-short-acting intravenous anesthetics are increasingly being employed with the benefits of rapid onset and rapid recovery. These agents decrease the risk of prolonged anesthesia, especially in neurosurgical situations where patient responsiveness can influence the success of surgery. Multimodal analgesia is also now being integrated into anesthetic practice to reduce opioid use and its associated side effects. With the use of agents that provide superior quality anesthesia and recovery, neurosurgeons are able to create the optimal surgical result, thereby again reflecting on the necessity of continued research and development of anesthetic methods. In addition to the creation of intravenous anesthetics, inhalational agents have been formulated as well, with significant revisions to enhance their profile in neurosurgery. These inhalational drugs have also been contrasted with intravenous drugs of late in studies using several key endpoints such as induction quality, hemodynamic stability, and postoperative recovery parameters. Interestingly, the newer inhalational drugs offer a safer profile, reducing the incidence of postoperative nausea and vomiting, which complicates recovery. Secondly, the economic studies of these anesthetics are now going beyond the initial drug costs to encompass hospital efficiency and patient outcomes.

Findings show not only that newer inhalation agents improve patient satisfaction but also that they can decrease postoperative recovery time, hence contributing to increased overall hospital throughput (Sneyd & Holmes, 2011). The effects of new anesthetic agents extend beyond recovery in patients to touch intraoperative monitoring, particularly in neurosurgery. The addition of advanced monitoring techniques made possible through the employment of modern anesthetic agents allows cerebral and neuromuscular function to be assessed in real-time. This is particularly relevant in operations on the sensitive structures of the central nervous system. Current literature now focuses on the multimodal technique of neuromonitoring, and the employment of technologies such as electromyography and transcranial stimulation yields more specific information regarding neurophysiological status intraoperatively (Singh et al., 2016). Therefore, with advances in these agents and monitoring technologies, neurosurgeons can safely navigate intricate topographies in surgery, and there is a decrease in complication rates along with improved patient outcomes in the long term (Figure 2.20).

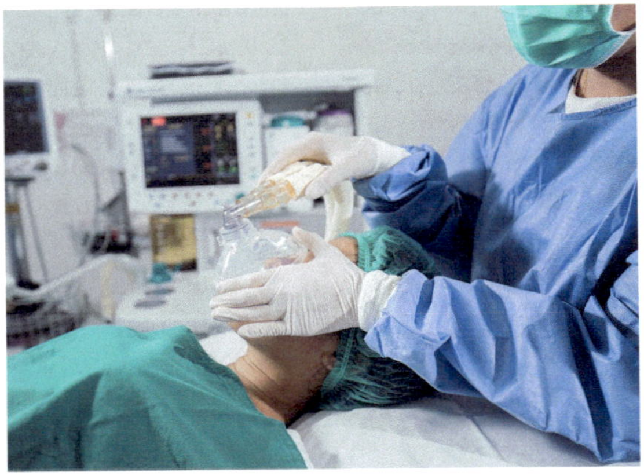

Figure 2.20. The evolution of anesthetic agents.

Source: https://images-cdn.welcomesoftware.com/Zz02NGZkOWRmMDUwZDkxMWVkOTBhZWRlODhjZWY2OTFkOQ==/doctors-were-anesthetize.jpg.

2.6.2. Technology in Monitoring

The use of advanced technology in monitoring has become essential in the neurosurgical field, particularly with anesthesia management and patient safety. Technology, such as built-in physiological monitoring systems, allows for real-time analysis of vital signs, ICP, and breath mechanics in neurosurgery. These systems enable anesthesiologists to evaluate variations in patient conditions promptly and hence make more informed decisions regarding ventilation and fluid management. For instance, the use of standardized ventilatory settings can enhance patient outcomes, but interinstitutional practice variation can lead to variations in care, influencing overall survival rates (Robba et al., 2025). Therefore, the adoption of cutting-edge monitoring tools not only enhances intraoperative management accuracy but also allows for a more considered approach in tailoring anesthetic interventions to suit the specific needs of individual patients. Moreover, multimodal neuromonitoring has been identified as an ideal practice in the management of severe traumatic brain injury (TBI), which is a prevalent observation in neurosurgical practice. ICP monitors in relation to cerebral perfusion pressure provide critical information that dictates anesthetic management and surgical strategies. Though plenty of data are generated through such monitoring procedures, the challenge is how to translate such data into guidelines. Still, the literature has presented the lack of robust evidence for specific therapies or intervention protocols to adequately control ICP, indicating a critical need for professional agreement. Together, there is a need to establish comprehensive guidelines based on expert consensus and current evidence, thus ultimately leading to improved patient outcomes after and during neurosurgical procedures (Iaccarino et al., 2021). Finally, with anesthesiology continuing to expand, new technology will continue to redefine neurosurgical monitoring procedures. For instance, wireless and portable monitoring devices could make it more convenient and provide real-time streams of data in a non-invasive procedure, which might reduce complications caused by the traditional process. In addition, artificial intelligence (AI) has the ability to review vast amounts of physiological information to predict adverse occurrences or detect unanticipated patient status changes. Such prediction capability could be the solution for maximizing anesthetic technology and techniques. As the setting of neurosurgical anesthesia becomes more progressive through these technologies, it is imperative to regularly update and refine protocols in order to ensure the best possible care. This commitment to innovation will ultimately enhance patient outcomes and safety in the challenging specialty of neurosurgical anesthesia (Figure 2.21).

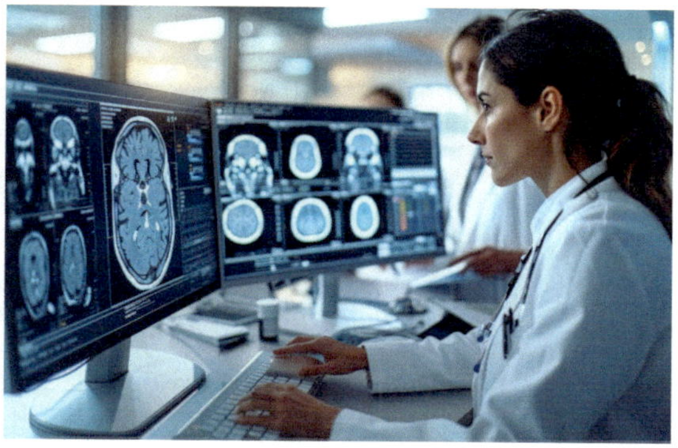

Figure 2.21. The integration of advanced technology in monitoring.

Source: https://www.chitkara.edu.in/wp-content/uploads/2025/01/mrit-desk-1.jpg.

2.6.3. Enhanced Recovery Protocols

It has been an example of strategic design to optimize patient recovery results in numerous fields of surgery, even neurosurgery. The pathways are designed to lessen the physiological and psychological stressors of surgical procedures, thereby making the recovery process more effective. With the addition of a multidisciplinary process of anesthesiologists, surgeons, nurses, and nutritionists, improved recovery pathways attempt to standardize preoperative, intraoperative, and postoperative care. This includes techniques like optimization of analgesia protocols and minimization of opioid consumption, which not only reduce pain but also avoid postoperative complications from occurring. Early mobilization and adequate fluid administration also enhance recovery, which results in reduced stay in the hospital and improved patient satisfaction, rendering such protocols highly applicable to neurosurgical patients who are known to have complicated recovery profiles. The use of enhanced recovery protocols is particularly important when nutritional needs in neurosurgical patients are being met. Malnutrition has been demonstrated to significantly escalate the risk of postoperative morbidity and extended hospitalization, warranting the use of preoperative optimization of nutrition. An example includes a specific perioperative nutrition pathway that was instituted for elective spinal fusion patients in the context of a neurosurgery office practice, emphasizing the integration of nutritional evaluation as a part of routine surgical practice. These channels are designed to identify at-risk patients for malnutrition and stimulate early nutrition treatment, for example, the intravenous administration of supplemental fluids like Ensure. Although early outcomes with these programs can report no statistically significant decrease in hospitalization stay, they identify areas for improvement, i.e., for adequate nutrition assessments that are designed specifically for the neurosurgical patient, especially the comorbid patient. Besides, better recovery pathways contribute to maximizing the overall surgery experience and outcomes by systematically addressing postoperative care issues. This involves very important factors such as patient education, psychological care, and timely rehabilitation services, which have a tendency to significantly affect recovery patterns among neurosurgery patients. For example, establishing protocols involving pre- and postoperative psychological testing can be utilized to determine at-risk patients for neurocognitive impairments, with individualized interventions being directed towards cognitive recovery. More so, establishing ongoing feedback loops in such protocols enables one to continuously improve based on patient outcomes and staff experience. With the evolution of neurosurgery, integration of more effective recovery protocols has become the solution to not only improve clinical outcomes but also manage healthcare costs for extended hospital stay and postsurgical complications, as underscored in evidence on surgical costs and the importance of effective care pathways (McKay, 2019).

Test Your Knowledge

1. What is one recent advancement in anesthetic practices?
2. How do new anesthetic techniques improve patient safety?

Summary

The crossover of anesthetic management and neurosurgical intervention demands vigilance of detail. Not only is anesthesia important for patient comfort, but it is also important for the best surgical conditions and results. The success of this synergy is enhanced when one considers the unique challenges posed by varying neurosurgical procedures. For instance, while standard protocols can be applied to straightforward surgeries, complex interventions entail a profound understanding of neurophysiological principles and the potential impact of anesthetics on cerebral function. Establishing synergy between the anesthesiologist and the neurosurgical team has the potential to enhance patient safety and procedure outcome, highlighting the shared responsibility in achieving best practices of care. Also, the varying availability of neurosurgery facilities across the globe, particularly among HIC and LMIC, requires an urgent imperative for more collaborative action. The vast disparity reported in the availability of functional neurosurgery techniques in LMIC speaks volumes about an important gap that must be urgently addressed. It is essential that activities for increasing access to safe surgical procedures, such as in HIC, are developed and put in place in LMIC contexts. This could involve partnerships that generate financial and technical support, providing a system where effective neurosurgical techniques can be applied more widely. Recognition of world disparities also serves to encourage research and development of guidelines that are appropriate to local epidemiological needs, thus enabling patients to receive treatment that is proper and timely. Finally, as improvements in neurosurgical technique and anesthetics continue to keep abreast of advances, ongoing research and clinical trials are necessary to establish the safety and efficacy of new modalities. Application of microsensor technologies for intracranial monitoring illustrates the possibility of enhanced monitoring capacity, yet there are still limitations, particularly in terms of determining optimal device location and prevention of negative consequences. Continuous examination of practice, in conjunction with fact-based recommendations, will shape best practices for anesthetic care for various neurosurgical conditions. With the advancement of the discipline, a focus on patient outcomes regarding the complexities of anesthesia will be crucial in achieving excellence in neurosurgical practice and closing the gaps that continue to exist globally.

Anesthetic delivery in neurosurgery is a complex and sensitive process that entails extensive preclusion of the unique physiological needs of neurological surgery. Most prominent among them is the maintenance of cerebral perfusion and prevention of intraoperative damage. Diligent selection of anesthetic drugs must be done to prevent the decrement of cerebral blood flow or the rise of intracranial pressure (ICP). This concern with neuroprotection is crucial, particularly in procedures involving delicate structures like the brain or spinal cord, where even perfusion variation can result in serious postoperative neurological deterioration. Techniques like controlled hypotension may also be used for enhancing surgical visibility, although these strategies need to be balanced against the risk of compromising cerebral perfusion, hence making it critical that monitoring during the procedure should be done with utmost care. Neuroendoscopic procedures, particularly for conditions such as colloid cysts, have seen pioneering advancements. The introduction of technologies such as the Nd:YAG laser guidance is a testament to where the field of anesthesia intersects with better neurosurgical outcomes. Studies that have looked into such procedures indicated that those patients who underwent stereotactic neuroendoscopy experienced tremendous clinical improvement following the procedure with minimal complications and rapid recuperation. Most notably, reversible morbidities alone were reported, including transient diabetes insipidus, which emphasizes the necessity of global perioperative management. These findings introduce the critical function of merging anesthetic management with contemporary surgical technologies to provide the best patient outcomes, while underlining the central significance of the selection of appropriate anesthetic techniques allowing for successful procedures (Pinto et al., 2009). Furthermore, the use of endovascular techniques in the treatment of intracranial aneurysms has totally changed the practice of neuroanesthesia. Utilization of self-expanding stents for the management of wide-necked aneurysms is not only a reflection of surgical ingenuity but also evidence of the role anesthesiology has played in advancing patient safety and procedural success. These minimally invasive interventions can be performed safely with anesthesia, and there is little risk of complications if technical success rates and excellent long-term results are indicative, as noted. A multimodal anesthetic regimen that encourages hemodynamic stability and avoids neurological risk is central to the excellent results achieved with these interventions. With such advancements in the neurosurgery branch, as the field continues to expand, ongoing research and emphasis on anesthetic optimization are essential (Vannucci, 2012).

KEY TERMS FROM THIS CHAPTER

- Amnesia
- Electrocorticography (ECoG)
- High-income countries (HIC)
- Neuroanesthesiologists
- Neurosurgery
- Patient care
- Pharmacodynamics
- Post-anesthesia care unit (PACU)
- Anesthetic
- Functional magnetic resonance imaging
- Monitored anesthesia care (MAC)
- Neuromonitoring
- Optimal anesthetic management
- Patient-centered care
- Pharmacokinetics

Critical Thinking Questions

1. **Which of the following is not a common effect of volatile anesthetics on intracranial pressure (ICP)?**
   a. Increase in cerebral blood flow (CBF)
   b. Decrease in cerebral metabolic rate (CMR)
   c. Decrease in cerebrospinal fluid (CSF) production
   d. Increase in ICP
2. **Which agent is preferred for rapid reduction of intracranial pressure?**
   a. Mannitol
   b. Furosemide
   c. Dexamethasone
   d. Propofol
3. **The most critical parameter to monitor during neurosurgery is:**
   a. Central venous pressure (CVP)
   b. Intracranial pressure (ICP)
   c. Mean arterial pressure (MAP)
   d. Cerebral perfusion pressure (CPP)
4. **Which positioning complication is most associated with neurosurgery in the sitting position?**
   a. Venous air embolism (VAE)
   b. Hypotension
   c. Hypertension
   d. Pulmonary edema
5. **What is the primary effect of hyperventilation during neurosurgery?**
   a. Decreased cerebral blood flow (CBF)
   b. Increased cerebral metabolic rate (CMR)
   c. Increased intracranial pressure (ICP)
   d. Decreased oxygen delivery

Short Answer Questions

1. Define the Monroe-Kellie Doctrine.
2. What is the role of hyperventilation during neurosurgical procedures?
3. How is cerebral perfusion pressure (CPP) calculated, and why is it important?
4. Describe the role of mannitol in neurosurgical anesthesia.
5. What are the considerations for patient positioning in neurosurgery, such as the prone or sitting position?

Answer to Critical Thinking Questions

1. (c); 2. (a); 3. (d); 4. (a); 5. (a)

References

1. Benet, A., Plata-Bello, J., Abla, A. A., Acevedo-Bolton, G., Saloner, D., & Lawton, M. T. (2015). Implantation of 3D-Printed Patient-Specific Aneurysm Models into Cadaveric Specimens: A New Training Paradigm to Allow for Improvements in Cerebrovascular Surgery and Research. *BioMed research international, 2015*, 939387. https://doi.org/10.1155/2015/939387(accessed on 28th June 2025).

2. Robba, C., Giardiello, D., Almondo, C., Asehnoune, K., Badenes, R., Cinotti, R., Elhadi, M., Graziano, F., Helbok, R., Jiang, L., Chen, W., Laffey, J. G., Messina, A., Putensen, C., Schultz, M. J., Wahlster, S., Rebora, P., Galimberti, S., Taccone, F. S., Citerio, G., ... VENTIBRAIN study group (2025). Ventilation practices in acute brain injured patients and association with outcomes: the VENTIBRAIN multicenter observational study. *Intensive care medicine*, *51*(2), 318–331. https://doi.org/10.1007/s00134-025-07808-1 (accessed on 28th June 2025).

3. Mangus, D. B., Huang, L., Applegate, P. M., Gatling, J. W., Zhang, J., & Applegate, R. L., 2nd (2014). A systematic review of neuroprotective strategies after cardiac arrest: from bench to bedside (Part I - Protection via specific pathways). *Medical gas research*, *4*, 9. https://doi.org/10.1186/2045-9912-4-9(accessed on 28th June 2025).

4. Pierce, J. T., Kositratna, G., Attiah, M. A., Kallan, M. J., Koenigsberg, R., Syre, P., Wyler, D., Marcotte, P. J., Kofke, W. A., & Welch, W. C. (2017). Efficiency of spinal anesthesia versus general anesthesia for lumbar spinal surgery: a retrospective analysis of 544 patients. *Local and regional anesthesia*, *10*, 91–98. https://doi.org/10.2147/LRA.S141233(accessed on 28th June 2025).

5. Bandt, S. K., Roland, J. L., Pahwa, M., Hacker, C. D., et al. (2017). The impact of high-grade glial neoplasms on human cortical electrophysiology. https://core.ac.uk/download/212869036.pdf (accessed on 28th June 2025).

6. Eljamel, S., Volovick, A., Saliev, T., Eisma, R., & Melzer, A. (2014). Evaluation of Thiel cadaveric model for MRI-guided stereotactic procedures in neurosurgery. *Surgical neurology international*, *5*(Suppl 8), S404–S409. https://doi.org/10.4103/2152-7806.140199(accessed on 28th June 2025).

7. Erbaş, Y. C., Erdoğan, E., Bengisun, Z. K., Pusat, S., et al. (2015). *Dejeneratif spondilolistezis, spinal stenoz, lomber kompresyon fraktürü olan yüksek riskli hastalarda spinal anestezi ile posterior lomber stabilizasyon cerrahisi.* https://core.ac.uk/download/492892134.pdf (accessed on 28th June 2025).

8. Iaccarino, C., Lippa, L., Munari, M., Castioni, C. A., Robba, C., Caricato, A., Pompucci, A., Signoretti, S., Zona, G., Rasulo, F. A., & Traumatic Brain Injury Section of the Italian Society of Neurosurgery (SINch) and the Neuroanesthesia and Neurocritical Care Study Group of the Italian Society of Anesthesia, Analgesia, Resuscitation and Intensive Care (SIAARTI) (2021). Management of intracranial hypertension following traumatic brain injury: a best clinical practice adoption proposal for intracranial pressure monitoring and decompressive craniectomy. Joint statements by the Traumatic Brain Injury Section of the Italian Society of Neurosurgery (SINch) and the Neuroanesthesia and Neurocritical Care Study Group of the Italian Society of Anesthesia, Analgesia, Resuscitation and Intensive Care (SIAARTI). *Journal of neurosurgical sciences*, *65*(3), 219–238. https://doi.org/10.23736/S0390-5616.21.05383-2(accessed on 28th June 2025).

9. Guilkey RE, Von Ah D, Carpenter JS, Stone C, Draucker CB. Integrative review: postcraniotomy pain in the brain tumour patient. *J Adv Nurs*. 2016;72(6):1221-1235. doi:10.1111/jan.12890(accessed on 28th June 2025).

10. Hopayian, K., Song, F., Riera, R., & Sambandan, S. (2010). The clinical features of the piriformis syndrome: a systematic review. *European spine journal : official publication of the European Spine Society, the European Spinal Deformity Society, and the European Section of the Cervical Spine Research Society*, *19*(12), 2095–2109. https://doi.org/10.1007/s00586-010-1504-9(accessed on 28th June 2025).

11. Pinto, F. C., Chavantes, M. C., Fonoff, E. T., & Teixeira, M. J. (2009). Treatment of colloid cysts of the third ventricle through neuroendoscopic Nd: YAG laser stereotaxis. *Arquivos de neuro-psiquiatria*, *67*(4), 1082–1087. https://doi.org/10.1590/s0004-282x2009000600023(accessed on 28th June 2025).

12. Givi, B., Schiff, B. A., Chinn, S. B., Clayburgh, D., Iyer, N. G., Jalisi, S., Moore, M. G., Nathan, C. A., Orloff, L. A., O'Neill, J. P., Parker, N., Zender, C., Morris, L. G. T., & Davies, L. (2020). Safety Recommendations for Evaluation and Surgery of the Head and Neck During the COVID-19 Pandemic. *JAMA otolaryngology-- head & neck surgery*, *146*(6), 579–584. https://doi.org/10.1001/jamaoto.2020.0780 (accessed on 28th June 2025).

13. Conti, A., Aaslid, R., Alkire, B., Aoki, N., Bedforth, N., Boisseau, N., et al. (2006). Cerebral hemodynamic changes during propofol-remifentanil or sevoflurane anesthesia: Transcranial Doppler study under bispectral index monitoring. https://core.ac.uk/download/53221344.pdf (accessed on 28th June 2025).

14. Dehdashti, A. R., Pralong, E., Debatisse, D., & Regli, L. (2006). Multilobar electrocorticography monitoring during intracranial aneurysm surgery. *Neurocritical care*, *4*(3), 215–222. https://doi.org/10.1385/NCC:4:3:215(accessed on 28th June 2025).

15. Sturges, B. K., Dickinson, P. J., Tripp, L. D., Udaltsova, I., & LeCouteur, R. A. (2019). Intracranial pressure monitoring in normal dogs using subdural and intraparenchymal miniature strain-gauge transducers. *Journal of veterinary internal medicine*, *33*(2), 708–716. https://doi.org/10.1111/jvim.15333(accessed on 28th June 2025).

16. Singh, H., Vogel, R. W., Lober, R. M., Doan, A. T., Matsumoto, C. I., Kenning, T. J., & Evans, J. J. (2016). Intraoperative Neurophysiological Monitoring for Endoscopic Endonasal Approaches to the Skull Base: A Technical Guide. *Scientifica*, *2016*, 1751245. https://doi.org/10.1155/2016/1751245(accessed on 28th June 2025).

17. Fezeu F, Ramesh A, Melmer PD, Moosa S, Larson PS, Henderson F Jr. Challenges and Solutions for Functional Neurosurgery in Developing Countries. *Cureus*. 2018;10(9):e3314. Published 2018 Sep 17. doi:10.7759/cureus.3314(accessed on 28th June 2025).

18. Sneyd, J. R., & Holmes, K. A. (2011). Inhalational or total intravenous anaesthesia: is total intravenous anaesthesia useful and are there economic benefits?. *Current opinion in anaesthesiology*, *24*(2), 182–187. https://doi.org/10.1097/ACO.0b013e328343f3ac(accessed on 28th June 2025).

19. Kamath, S. (2023). Assessment and management of perioperative pain in neurosurgical patients. https://core.ac.uk/download/593035646.pdf (accessed on 28th June 2025).

20. Lorenz, W., & Rothmund, M. (1989). Theoretical surgery: A new specialty in operative medicine. https://core.ac.uk/download/11550720.pdf (accessed on 28th June 2025).

21. McKay, A. J. (2019). Nutrition and neurosurgery: Designing a perioperative pathway for elective spine fusion patients. https://core.ac.uk/download/220125581.pdf (accessed on 28th June 2025).

22. Nilsson, A. (2024). Reducing perioperative opioid use through utilization of dexmedetomidine prior to induction: Provider education. https://core.ac.uk/download/604145967.pdf (accessed on 28th June 2025).

23. Wanda, A. ., Suarjaya, I. P. P. ., Widnyana, M. G. ., Sutawan, I. K. J. ., & Ryalino, C. . (2024). ANESTHESIA MANAGEMENT IN MODIFIED PARK BENCH POSITION IN NEUROSURGERY : A CASE REPORT. *PREPOTIF : JURNAL KESEHATAN MASYARAKAT*, *8*(2), 3679–3687. https://doi.org/10.31004/prepotif.v8i2.31222 (accessed on 28th June 2025).

24. Tonković, D., Lozić, M., Sekulić, A., Bandić Pavlović, D., Perić, M., Martinović, P., Baronica, R., et al. (2015). Scalp block for hemodynamic stability during neurosurgery. PERIODICUM BIOLOGORUM UDC 57:61 VOL. 117, No 2, 247–250, 2015. https://core.ac.uk/download/33282685.pdf (accessed on 28th June 2025).

25. Vannucci, S. (2012). Stent-assisted reconstructive endovascular repair of intracranial aneurysms: Long-term clinical and angiographic follow-up. https://core.ac.uk/download/14704130.pdf (accessed on 28th June 2025).

OBSTETRIC ANESTHESIA

3

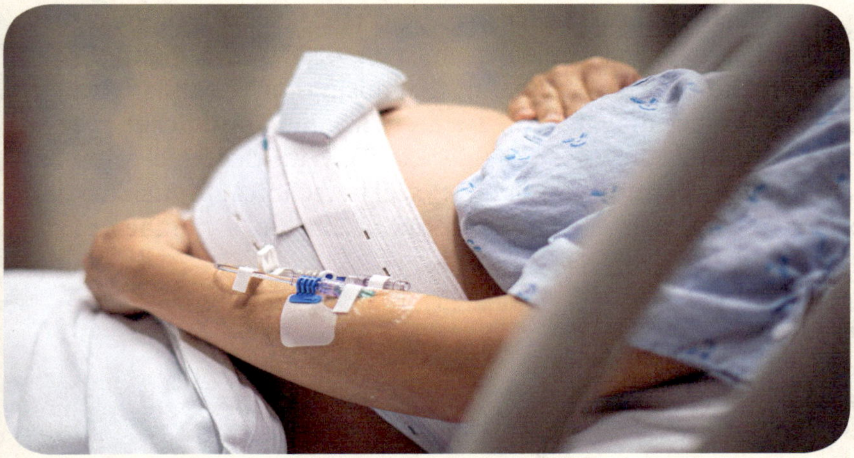

LEARNING OBJECTIVES

After studying this chapter, you will be able to:

1. Discuss the types of anesthesia used in obstetrics
2. Describe the indications for obstetric anesthesia
3. Explain the benefits of obstetric anesthesia
4. Focus on risks and complications
5. Discuss the role of anesthesiologists in obstetric care
6. Know current trends and innovations in obstetric anesthesia

Introduction

Obstetric anesthesia is the specialty in the spotlight of contemporary maternity care, symbolizing both the delicacy of pain relief and the imperative for the safeguarding of maternal and neonatal health during labor and delivery. As the journey to motherhood encompasses countless physical and emotional obstacles, effective anesthesia becomes vital. Not only does obstetric anesthesia alleviate the pain, but it also enhances the birthing process in general, which brings relief to otherwise be a painful and stressful experience. In this regard, obstetric anesthesia professionals have to work in a world of techniques—epidurals, spinal blocks, and so on—each with its own benefits and risks. The evolution of anesthetic history has transformed the childbirth experience with the ability for the mother to exercise her desired pain-relief options, showing a more advanced attitude towards patient-centered care. Despite the progress in obstetric anesthesia, challenges still persist, such as the deployment of best practices in varying birthing conditions. Skin-to-skin contact, for instance, is increasingly supported for its benefits both to mothers and babies, such as bonding and facilitating breastfeeding. However, the practices have largely been underutilized in cesarean birth. A trial of an educational intervention for operating room staff is representative of the potential barriers to the use of skin-to-skin contact within these environments. This inequality underscores the need for enhanced training and sensitization of medical professionals about the advantages of incorporating anesthetic procedures into mother and neonate care protocols to ensure that optimal outcomes are realized regardless of delivery mode (Loebig, 2020). In addressing such problems, the practice can enhance not only pain control measures but also integrative care approaches. In addition, the global health inequities setting adds an extra layer of obstetric anesthesia complexity. Where there is a setting such as Bihar, India, an integral quality improvement program to enhance the skills of providers in managing obstetric complications yielded promising results. Focusing on postpartum hemorrhage (PPH) and intrapartum asphyxia, programs such as these address critical issues that complicate childbirth. Mentoring and training of healthcare professionals in such environments highlight the importance of equipping providers with the necessary skills in diagnosing and dealing with complications effectively. Increased rates of correct diagnosis in such environments indicate the promise of enhanced maternal and neonatal health outcomes (Loebig, 2020). With the developing branch of obstetric anesthesia, it is essential that practitioners not only excel in technical proficiency but also engage with broader discussions regarding systemic concerns arising in a number of different healthcare environments (Figure 3.1).

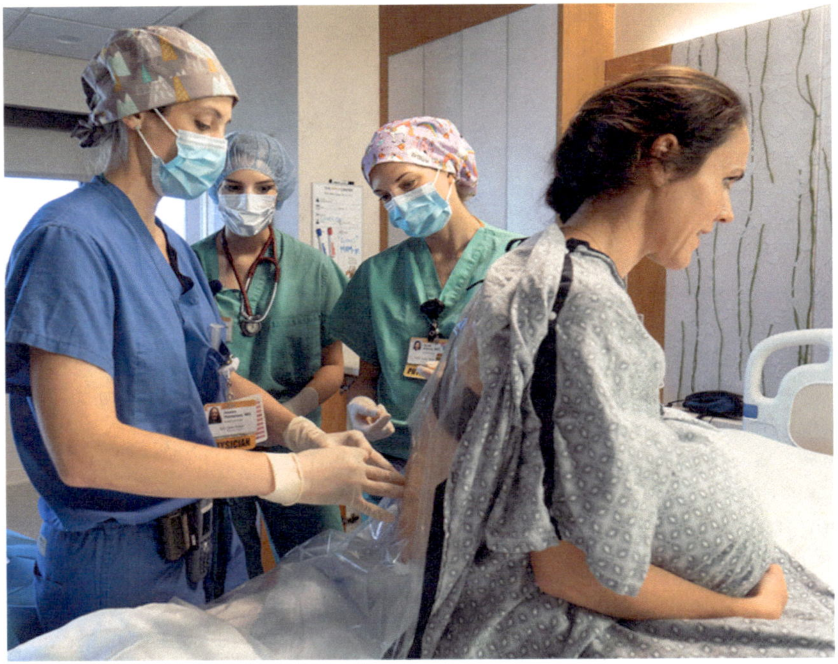

Figure 3.1. Obstetrical anesthesia rotation – anesthesiology.

Source: https://cdn.atriumhealth.org/-/media/wakeforest/school/images/page-content/education-and-training/residencies-and-fellowships/anesthesiology-residency/anes-res-curr-obstetric-anes-2.jpg?h=646&w=800&rev=bb7f85fe3be34686a8fb139f2b0e4690&hash=F3AADFADB2C2ADF98E0BA7582FA45282.

Definition of Obstetric Anesthesia

Obstetric anesthesia is a specialty of anesthesia that involves pain relief and comfort in the perinatal period, i.e., labor, delivery, and the first few hours postpartum. The primary goal of obstetric anesthesia is to ensure the mother's comfort and safety while facilitating the baby's delivery. It encompasses various techniques, such as epidural anesthesia, spinal anesthesia, and general anesthesia, each selected based on the patient's medical status and mode of delivery. Familiarity with the nuances of these techniques is essential since they are specific pharmacological therapies and technique maneuvers that require training and knowledge. The ultimate goal is pain reduction with the greatest safety, thereby promoting healthy birth experiences for both the mother and the baby, demonstrating the importance of specialist skills in this branch of medicine. Epidural anesthesia has been the most extensively utilized technique in obstetric anesthesia, particularly for relief of labor pain. This method involves the insertion of a catheter into the epidural space within the spine to facilitate the continuous delivery of anesthetic drugs. The significance of this method is that it can provide effective pain relief while the mobility and active contribution to the process of labor by the mothers are maintained. Besides, it can be tailored to the individual's needs, with the dose and drug form depending on the response of the patient. Administration of epidural anesthesia must also involve adequate assessment of contraindications and complications to ensure maternal and fetal safety during labor. Therefore, selection and application of epidural anesthesia are pivotal in maximizing the obstetric process. Other than epidural techniques, spinal anesthesia is also frequently employed during cesareans, characterized by speed of onset of profound analgesia as well as effective pain management. Spinal anesthesia involves the injection of anesthetic agents directly into the cerebrospinal fluid to produce immediate analgesia below the level of injection. The strategic accuracy of spinal anesthesia renders it extremely appropriate for surgical interventions with instant action. However, it is important to consider patient-specific factors, such as differences in anatomy and disease, which may affect the success of the procedure and also any associated risk. The complications of spinal anesthesia represent the complexity of obstetric anesthesia, highlighting the importance of careful preoperative assessment and informed consent to ensure safe and effective management of mothers and their offspring. Thus, obstetric anesthesia is an active component of current-day obstetric practice, and one needs to have comprehensive knowledge of various techniques and their use in varied conditions (Loebig, 2020).

Importance in Maternal and Fetal Health

The priority of fetal and maternal well-being during pregnancy cannot be overemphasized, as it is the foundation of the mother's and child's general health. In obstetric anesthesia, a compromise has to be achieved between ensuring that interventions that are undertaken do not jeopardize fetal viability while simultaneously acknowledging the mother's pain and comfort. This sensitive balancing act includes an advanced understanding of anesthetic technologies and their potential effects on uteroplacental perfusion. As in the case of emergencies like surgical interventions during pregnancy, such as trauma, the success of the anesthetic management can even be extremely crucial to both fetal and maternal outcomes. Cooperation between obstetricians, anesthesiologists, and surgical teams is necessary in realizing the intricate nature of difficulties posed by such cases, ultimately maintaining the importance of holistic care for the mother. In addition, threats of maternal complications such as amniotic fluid embolism (AFE) underscore the urgent necessity of increased monitoring and rapid action in obstetric anesthesia. AFE is especially difficult with an unpreventable onset and high maternal morbidity and mortality, further calling for multimodal therapy. The cooperation among healthcare professionals can initiate early diagnosis and intervention, which can save the mother and child from disastrous results. Through the promotion of publicity of such complications and cross-talk about the best practices, the healthcare facilities can enhance their preparedness for such events. Continuing education and research remain necessary in identifying effective measures of diagnosis and treatment, thus more and more are recording the importance of optimal maternal and fetal health in obstetric care.

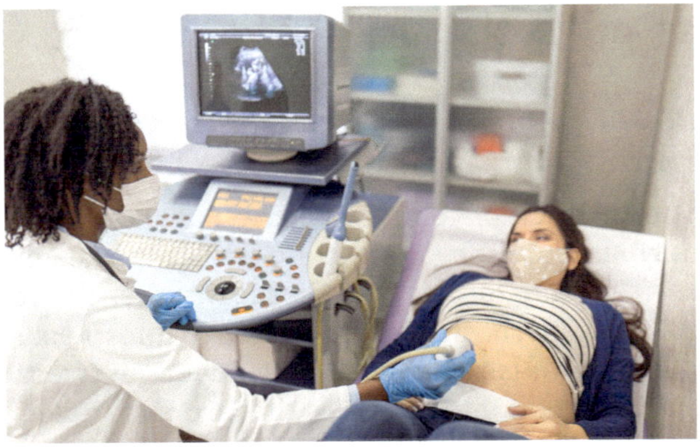

Figure 3.2. The significance of maternal and fetal health during pregnancy cannot be overstated.

Source: https://www.cedars-sinai.org/content/dam/cedars-sinai/blog/2021/3/perinatologists-in-pregnancy.jpg.

Furthermore, integration of technological advancements into maternal-fetal monitoring has enormously improved the capacity to evaluate and respond to changes in fetal health under anesthetic care. Equipment such as continuous fetal heart rate monitoring allows for real-time measurement, greatly increasing timely intervention that can prevent fetal distress. This technology is particularly crucial during surgery when maternal positioning can hinder uteroplacental perfusion, where close observation is required. As illustrated in case reports, harmonious coordination can ensure that both the surgical procedure and anesthetic process have the optimal safety protocol for mother and fetus. As a whole, these factors summarize the importance of obstetric anesthesia to fetal and maternal health to reinforce the need for close attention by all those who have responsibility for the antenatal and perinatal periods (Figure 3.2).

Historical Development of Obstetric Anesthesia

The history of obstetric anesthesia has been marked by landmark developments that have redefined the nature of child birth. Pain in labor in ancient periods was largely managed through non-pharmacological interventions. Traditional birth attendants and midwives employed diverse techniques, from herbal medicine to soothing rituals, to minimize pain. When anesthesia was discovered in the 19th Century, obstetric care evolved, with methods like ether and chloroform applied in labor. These initial drugs were groundbreaking, providing mothers with unparalleled ease and changing the social culture around giving birth. This revolution created increasing demand for anesthetic options in obstetric practice, which paved the way for future advances and the creation of safer and more effective anesthetic procedures. With advancement in the field of obstetric anesthesia in the 20th century, improved and specialized techniques were formulated, particularly following the discovery of regional anesthesia. Spinal and epidural blocks were made to become favored for their effectiveness, allowing the woman to remain awake and take an active role in the birth process with pain control. Increased understanding of drug action and interaction with pregnancy physiology was important for these improvements. The unique alterations involved with pregnancy, such as edema and altered respiratory function, posed new challenges to safe use of anesthesia. Data from previous practice informed these advancements, with a focus on individualized approaches to adapt to parturients' needs, which ultimately maximized fetal and maternal safety during the process of birth (Habek et al., 2023). Over the last few years, the integration of ultrasound technology into obstetric anesthesia has also maximized needle placement procedures, with tremendous advancements in outcomes, particularly for obese parturients. Historically, anatomical landmark identification challenges in these types of patients presented challenges to effective regional anesthetic practice. However, current surveys indicate that most certified registered nurse anesthetists (CRNAs) have incorporated ultrasound into their spinal and epidural practice, enjoying its role in enhancing precision and safety (Loebig, 2020).

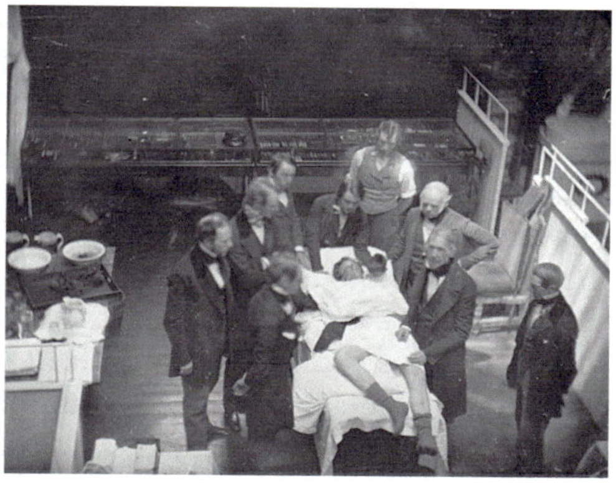

Figure 3.3. The historical development of obstetric anesthesia.

Source: https://upload.wikimedia.org/wikipedia/commons/thumb/4/4b/Southworth_%26_Hawes_-_First_etherized_operation_%28re-enactment%29.jpg/500px-Southworth_%26_Hawes_-_First_etherized_operation_%28re-enactment%29.jpg.

Despite this, barriers such as limited training and access to ultrasound machines persist. Further research must be conducted to bridge the differences and continue with the progress in obstetric anesthesia, emphasizing not just the historical background of these developments but also the probable future improvements to increase maternal care and overall health outcomes of childbirth (Figure 3.3).

3.1. Types of Anesthesia Used in Obstetrics

Learning Outcome

1. Epidural anesthesia
2. Spinal anesthesia
3. General anesthesia

The practice of obstetric anesthesia encompasses various techniques intended to enhance maternal relaxation and fetal security during labor and delivery. Epidural and spinal anesthesia are the most common types, both capable of alleviating pain while leaving the mother alert and aware. Epidural anesthesia is the administration of an anesthetic drug into the epidural space of the lumbar region, resulting in reduced sensation below the waist. Not only does it ease labor pain, but it also enables the patient to participate actively in the birth process. Spinal anesthesia, on the other hand, is one anesthetic injection into cerebrospinal fluid with a rapid onset and profound anesthesia, widely used in cesarean sections. These procedures are illustrative of how obstetric anesthesia innovation weighs both medical effectiveness and maternal control equally. General anesthesia, though less common in obstetrics, is still a useful option under some conditions, especially when rapid intervention is needed. This technique is defined by the complete unconsciousness of the patient and is typically reserved for emergent cesarean deliveries or for contraindications to regional anesthesia. General anesthesia is also accompanied by a careful balancing of both maternal and fetal risks, including potential respiratory complications and the effect of anesthetic agents on the neonate. Moreover, current evidence suggests increased emphasis on minimizing exposure to general anesthesia where feasible, particularly in light of its associations with adverse neonatal consequences. Thus, obstetric choice of anesthesia is based on a balanced assessment of the clinical scenario, potential risks, and maternal desire and promotes collaborative decision-making. In addition to these primary methods of anesthesia, there are several adjunctive techniques that might play significant roles in the management of obstetric pain. Nitrous oxide, for example, is a very popular choice among women who desire less invasive pain relief during labor. Nitrous oxide is an inhalational anesthetic that can be used very effectively to provide analgesia with the added advantage of preserving maternal control over its use.

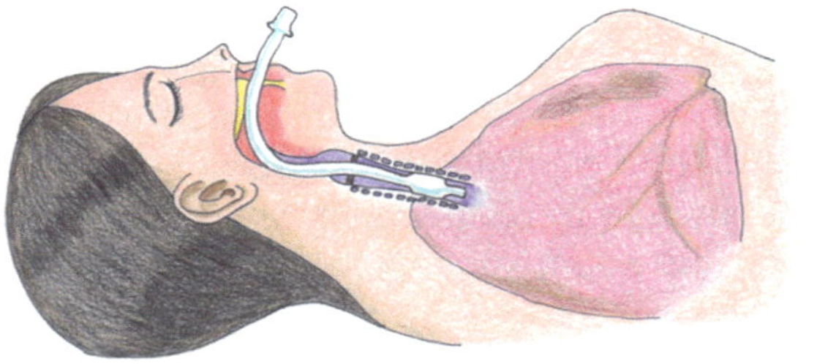

Figure 3.4. The realm of obstetric anesthesia encompasses a range of techniques.

Source: https://obgyn.com.my/wp-content/uploads/2020/07/endotracheal-tube-ETT-final-border.png.

Local anesthesia, on the other hand, can be utilized for perineal repair after delivery to provide comfort for required procedures without the use of more profound regional blocks. These diverse anesthetic strategies served to demonstrate the value of patient-centered obstetric care, ensuring both safety and comfort for the mother as well as positively improving the birthing experience. As the discipline evolves, incorporation of evidence-based practices in obstetric anesthesia will be critical in maximizing outcomes for both the mother and infant, a quest fostered by continued research and clinical evidence (Vanhaesebrouck et al., 2010; Guenther et al., 2012) (Figure 3.4).

3.1.1. Epidural Anesthesia

Epidural anesthesia is now a standard of pain relief in labor and delivery, and it has brought much relief to parturient with minimal systemic side effects compared to other analgesia. Administration involves injecting anesthetics into the epidural space, which breaks the transmission of pain impulses from the cervix and uterus. Its use has been linked to a decrease in the perception of pain during contractions, thereby enhancing the overall process of childbirth. Epidural anesthesia is particularly noted for its effectiveness in providing pain relief while making the mother aware and active in the process of birth, thus contributing to maternal satisfaction and instilling a supportive environment for the mother and child. Though it has numerous advantages, administration of epidural anesthesia is not risk-free either. One such area of concern is the risk of infectious complications, although these are statistically rare. Systematic review estimates the overall rate of infectious complications following central neuraxial blocks, including epidurals, at approximately 9 per 100,000 blocks, with central nervous system infections far lower. Specifically, the obstetric cohort shows a significantly lower incidence of these complications, underscoring the relative safety of epidural anesthesia in the context of control. The implications of these data underscore the importance of careful procedural technique and infection control measures, essential for guaranteeing the health of both mother and neonate during labor. Further, careful examination of outcomes of epidural anesthesia holds nuanced implications for maternal and neonatal health. Evidence indicates that, while epidural use can be associated with prolongation of labor and is associated with increased rates of instrumental delivery, overall maternal morbidity is low. Comparative studies in women who are undergoing vaginal delivery indicate that there are no differences between women who have and do not have epidural anesthesia concerning neonatal morbidity. Interestingly, the Greentop guideline does acknowledge the lack of extensive evidence in relation to the use of epidural anesthesia in specific cases, such as breech delivery, and insists on further research. On that account, while epidurals are an effective method of pain relief, additional research into their impact on diverse delivery conditions is essential (Allert et al., 2023; Selvamani et al., 2024) (Figure 3.5).

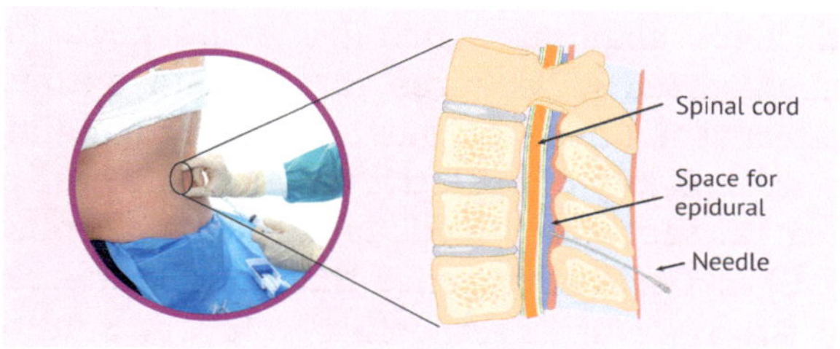

Figure 3.5. Epidural anesthesia.

Source: https://www.invitra.com/en/wp-content/uploads/2014/07/epidural-anesthesia-labor.jpg.

3.1.2. Spinal Anesthesia

Spinal anesthesia is a pillar in the practice of obstetric anesthesia and a vehicle to accomplish successful and safe cesarean delivery. Spinal anesthesia refers to the delivery of anesthetic medication into the subarachnoid space, characterized by rapid onset and widespread sensory and motor blockade. The study found the main advantage of spinal anesthesia lies in its possible provision of adequate pain relief with surgery without rendering the mother unconscious and the ability to actively participate in the birth process. Choice of anesthetic medications such as bupivacaine or ropivacaine, along with adjunct medications such as opioids, is key to achieving optimal analgesia and preventing side effects. As this method is now common practice in elective cesarean section, anesthesiologists must be aware of the subtleties of its application for protecting both mother and fetus. Amongst the complications associated with the use of spinal anesthesia, one must note particularly hypotension, which is increasingly secondary to sympathetic blockade and vasodilation. This condition can have critical complications in both mother and child and thus, preventive measures are essential. Recent research has focused on the prophylactic use of vasopressors such as metaraminol to avoid the incidence of hypotensive events during and after spinal anesthesia. Results showed that the efficacy of metaraminol in the prevention of hypotensive events is dose-dependent, with ED50 and ED90 at 0.64 μg/kg/min and 2.00 μg/kg/min, respectively. Such findings emphasize the need for personalized vasopressor regimens that can effectively prevent spinal anesthesia-induced hypotension and attain superior maternal hemodynamic stability and neonatal outcomes in cesarean sections (Xiao et al., 2021).

In addition, technological improvements in intraoperative monitoring have caught up to track hemodynamic alterations after the administration of a spinal anesthetic. The perfusion index (PI), as an invisible monitor, has emerged as a valuable tool to predict impending hypotension. Several studies have documented a broad range of rapid increases in PI among parturient developing acute hypotension, which indicates that it can serve as an early warning symptom for anesthesiologists. This allows for timely intervention by vasopressors or fluid boluses and thereby reduces maternal morbidity from hypotension complications. With the evolution of methods and surveillance protocols, focus continues to be placed upon patient safety and outcomes from cesarean delivery, establishing spinal anesthesia as a pillar of obstetric anesthesia (Mallawaarachchi et al., 2020) (Figure 3.6).

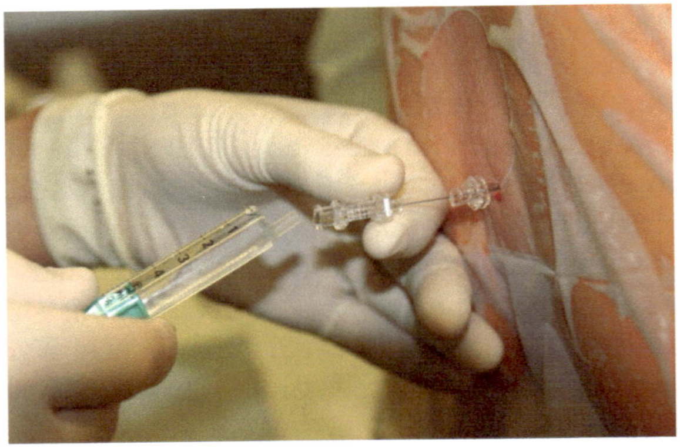

Figure 3.6. Spinal anesthesia.

Source: https://upload.wikimedia.org/wikipedia/commons/e/e5/Liquor_bei_Spinalanaesthesie.JPG.

3.1.3. General Anesthesia

General anesthesia also plays a significant role in obstetric anesthesia, particularly in cesarean section, wherein it may be needed to ensure the safety and comfort of the patient. General anesthesia places the patient in a reversible state of unconsciousness and, therefore, medical professionals can perform their surgical procedures without any awareness or sensation of pain on the part of the patient. General anesthesia is also used judiciously in chosen situations, particularly when there is an emergent necessity for delivery. Nevertheless, it must be managed and monitored appropriately due to potential risk to both mother and infant. The anesthesiologist's skill plays a significant role in minimizing such risks through the evaluation of the patient's medical history, preoperative assessments, and guaranteeing evidence-based care for the application of making the most secure environment possible in the process. The application of general anesthesia as compared to regional techniques, such as neuraxial blockade, remains a significant consideration in the management of obstetric patients. In cases of severe preeclampsia or in the urgency of cesarean delivery, general anesthesia can be used when time considerations are a factor in the application of neuraxial techniques. It has been demonstrated through research that there is inconsistency in patient management practice patterns, particularly in those with preeclampsia, where there is disagreement among anesthesiologists regarding adequate hemostatic conditions for the placement of neuraxial blockade (Sultan & Butwick, 2013). All these challenges bring out the need for standardized procedures to maintain optimal maternal and neonatal outcomes when handling the complexity of obstetric cases. In the case of cesarean sections, immediate skin-to-skin contact (SSC) is a critical practice that can be affected by the type of anesthesia employed. Studies show that patients under general anesthesia are likely to miss SSC opportunities as compared to women who experience vaginal deliveries or cesareans under regional anesthesia (Balatero, 2018). Obstetric nurses see multiple barriers to facilitating SSC after cesarean surgery despite the complete realization of its vast benefits in terms of maternal-infant bonding. The findings by healthcare providers illustrate the necessity of enhancing perioperative practice to enhance the maternal and neonatal experiences after surgery. Integration of these into common anesthetic practice guarantees that even during operative procedures, the benefits of maintaining significant rituals of bonding are not overlooked.

Test Your Knowledge

1. What are the common types of anesthesia used during labor and cesarean section?
2. When is regional anesthesia preferred over general anesthesia in obstetric patients?

3.2. Indications for Obstetric Anesthesia

Learning Outcome

1. Pain management during labor
2. Surgical interventions such as cesarean sections
3. Special considerations for high-risk pregnancies

In obstetric anesthesia, the indication for use covers a broad area of clinical conditions calling for pain management during labor and delivery. The primary indication remains giving analgesia to women in labor with the general aim of pain relief and facilitation of the childbirth process. Modern techniques such as epidural and spinal anesthesia have facilitated labor pain management so that a more comfortable childbirth is possible. Also, such anesthetic modalities not only contribute to pain control but also to the levels of patient satisfaction rates and overall labor outcomes. Increasingly, some hospitals are currently exploring options like nitrous oxide to further expand the range of analgesia options, thus improving patient-centered care. Although the conventional methods are most common, the inclination towards the use of multiple modalities for pain management is evidence of the changing scenario in obstetric anesthesia, which necessitates ongoing education among practitioners to offer optimal care to pregnant women. A second clear indication for obstetric anesthesia arises when cesarean sections are conducted, either on the basis of choice or an emergency. Spinal and epidural anesthesia are most commonly employed to effectively manage pain during such surgical procedures. One of the key factors that was identified in later studies is the impact of the spinal needle type, as this determines the risk of postoperative complications such as headaches. Research indicates that some types of needles are linked to the development of mild headaches, pointing out the influence of technique in reducing side effects in the use of spinal anesthesia in cesarean section (Lakhe et al., 2024). Therefore, practitioners should consider these concerns in determining the appropriate anesthetic protocol for cesarean sections since it may significantly impact patient recovery and satisfaction. Secondly, educational campaigns have also shown to increase awareness toward alternative modes of anesthesia such as nitrous oxide for the relief of labor pain. Chronic documentation offers the following declining incidence within the United States, in contrast to other advanced nations. Recent studies have shown that provider training through specific modules can drastically change attitudes and practices in relation to the use of nitrous oxide in labor (Bhettay & Burger, 2024). Results in these trials are encouraging; following educational enhancements, high levels of practitioners indicated a willingness to make nitrous oxide part of their pain control armory. This shift is part of a broader movement toward diversifying obstetric anesthesia practice, ultimately to the benefit of laboring women with a more affluent choice of options and a superior overall birthing experience (Figure 3.7).

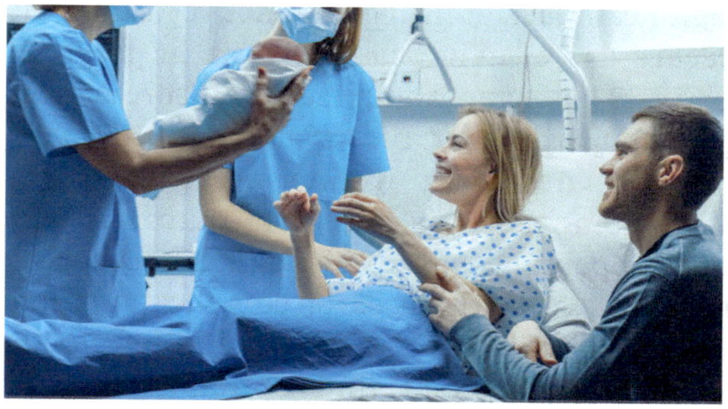

Figure 3.7. Indications for obstetric anesthesia.

Source: https://www.dailynurse.com/wp-content/uploads/2023/03/aana-updates-anesthesia-guidelines-web.jpg.

3.2.1. Pain Management During Labor

Effective pain relief during labor is essential for improved maternal and fetal outcomes and a generally improved childbirth experience for women. Of the many options, neuraxial analgesia, such as epidural and spinal anesthesia, has been the option of choice because of its efficacy and very few systemic side effects. The use of neuraxial analgesia allows women to experience strong pain relief yet remain awake and active during labor. Studies reveal that the method not only reduces labor pain but also provides greater patient satisfaction compared to other analgesic modalities. Strategic application of neuraxial analgesia should, however, consider patient-specific factors, including obstetric status and history, thus necessitating individualized approaches to maximize pain relief during this vulnerable period (Selvamani et al., 2024). Just as there are advantages of neuraxial analgesia, so is its application not without challenges and risks. One of the specific concerns is the danger of hematoma formation, especially in patients who have uncorrected bleeding disorders, thus making neuraxial techniques contraindicated in certain cases. The recent study demonstrates a significant lack of firm guidelines regarding the secure use of neuraxial analgesia in pregnant patients suffering from bleeding disorders due primarily to scant research data. Moreover, although numerous women are successfully undergoing neuraxial analgesia, outcomes may vary depending on specific clinical scenarios, for example, with cases of complications like obstetric emergencies. Ongoing research should fill those gaps and find optimal practices for the provision of neuraxial analgesia and charting out the potential interventions for minimizing the risks of its utilization in labor (Yi et al., 2023). Also, pain control in labor involves an interdisciplinary panel consisting of obstetricians, anesthesiologists, and hematologists, particularly in complicated cases. Expert communication is crucial in the improvement of patient outcomes, particularly when considering the numerous patient-specific variables involved. Such a multidisciplinary approach proves priceless where switching from epidural analgesia to general anesthesia is necessary, as in the case of unplanned cesarean sections. The use of local anesthetics and adjunct drugs together with the close monitoring of maternal and fetal well-being enhances the effectiveness and safety of pain relief processes. Lastly, ongoing research and innovation of pain relief strategies during labor will result in better, more individualized care, enabling women to be offered optimum analgesia without compromising their health or that of their infants (Selvamani et al., 2024) (Figure 3.8).

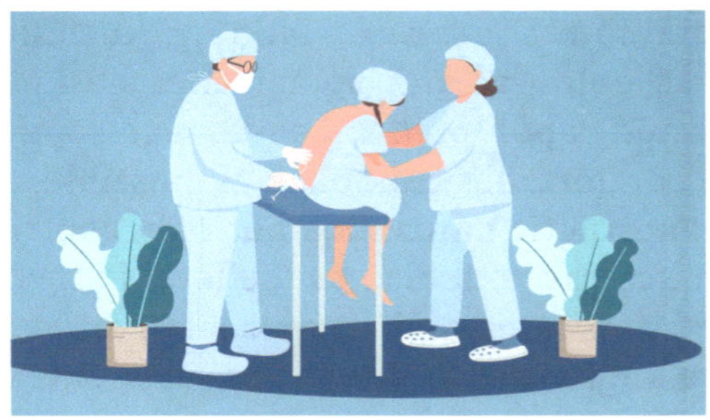

Figure 3.8. Illustration showing a patient receiving an epidural injection, assisted by medical professionals in a clinical setting.

Source: https://www.intimina.com/blog/wp-content/uploads/2021/04/pain.jpg.

3.2.2. Surgical Interventions Such as Cesarean Sections

Surgical interventions in obstetrics, including cesarean sections, are necessary for the mothers' and babies' safety during the childbirth process. As a surgical intervention, cesarean sections are employed to avoid danger from labor or complications of delivery. An indication for cesarean delivery may be necessitated by several factors, such as fetal distress, labor complications, or maternal issues. Understanding surgical risks, anesthesia practice, and postpartum recovery is the most critical, particularly in the development of protocols that enhance optimal patient outcomes. Obstetric anesthesia ensures vital care, enabling the management of pain and safety in cesarean section deliveries, to enable healthcare providers to establish a supportive environment for the surgeon and anesthetist, ultimately promoting the effectiveness of the procedure. While there are quite a number of benefits related to cesarean delivery, there are some complications that might arise during and after surgery. One of the significant ones is postpartum hemorrhage, which remains among the leading causes of maternal morbidity and mortality. This issue is exacerbated when the measurement of blood loss is estimated rather than by using precise measurement techniques. Adoption of quantitative blood loss (QBL) measurement in cesarean operations has potential benefits since research has demonstrated decreased rates of severe postpartum hemorrhage following the adoption of QBL. Intervention of such complications of surgery is essential since early diagnosis and management have a good probability of influencing maternal outcomes, adding to general recovery narratives, and resulting in safer obstetric practice that prioritizes patient well-being at the expense of nothing related to care quality. Furthermore, early skin-to-skin contact after cesarean section has been identified as a main practice to support bonding and breastfeeding. However, such integration is discouraged in operating rooms, particularly in the case of cesarean sections, due to a scarcity of early SSC opportunities. Findings identify that despite acknowledged benefits of SSC by obstetric nurses, various logistical and procedural challenges often prevent its use in the routine following cesarean deliveries. Overcoming these obstacles is essential in improving obstetric practice and allowing mothers and babies to benefit from the supporting care necessary to realize their best outcomes. Refining the surgery experience with maternal-infant-bonding facilitating practices is a key element of obstetric anesthesia, moving to balance surgical procedures like cesarean delivery with combined maternal and neonatal care strategies (Balatero, 2018; Barrier et al., 2022).

3.2.3. Special Considerations for High-Risk Pregnancies

In the obstetric anesthesia context, a few other factors must be taken into account in high-risk pregnancy because such cases are typically single and multiple issues. High-risk pregnancy involves an extensive array of issues like multiple pregnancies, maternal comorbidities (like hypertension or diabetes), and fetal anomaly, each requiring expert anesthetic management. Anesthesiologists must be most diligently observant of the maternal and fetal status throughout labor and delivery. The goal is to minimize risk to both mother and child and to allow effective pain relief. Maternal vital signs and fetal heart tones must be carefully monitored, as alterations may be indicative of distress and necessitate immediate intervention. Due to the potential for rapid alterations in clinical status, anesthesiologists must have a full understanding of the physiological changes that occur during pregnancy to provide safe and effective anesthetic care. With a pregnancy that is of high risk, multidisciplinary treatment is essential to procure maximum results. Involvement by obstetricians, anesthesiologists, and specialists assures the patient that there is a complete understanding of the treatment being pursued. For instance, a team might have to address orthopedic injuries that result in pregnancy, in which surgical intervention becomes the priority. Such situations, like in the described case of a patient requiring surgical fixation in a case of ankle fracture dislocation, require careful coordination and communication between obstetric and surgical teams. Heart tone monitors are important during the procedures to continuously monitor fetal well-being, as in this instance where emergency interventions had to be undertaken due to fetal distress (Sturges et al., 2013). Such intimate collaboration emphasizes the requirement of an interdisciplinary model of care to address the challenge of high-risk pregnancy successfully. Anesthetic practice must also be adapted to address the special requirements presented by high-risk pregnancy.

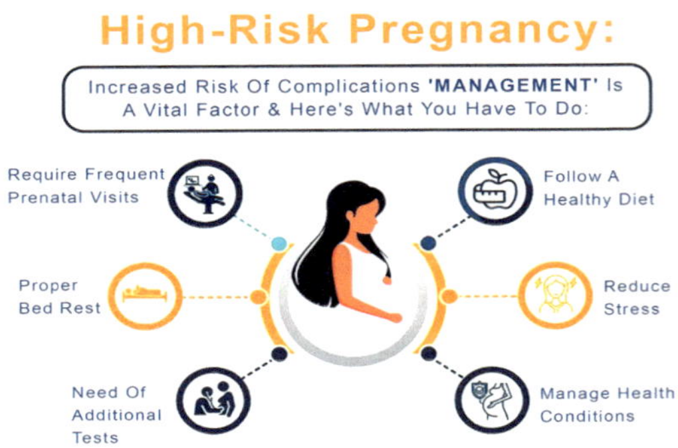
High-Risk Pregnancy:
Increased Risk Of Complications 'MANAGEMENT' Is A Vital Factor & Here's What You Have To Do:
Require Frequent Prenatal Visits
Follow A Healthy Diet
Proper Bed Rest
Reduce Stress
Need Of Additional Tests
Manage Health Conditions

Figure 3.9. Key management strategies for high-risk pregnancy, including prenatal visits, bed rest, healthy diet, stress reduction, and health condition monitoring.

Source: https://ik.imagekit.io/d7t01fhx21/Ovum_Hospitals/Blogs/Understanding%20High-Risk%20Pregnancies%20and%20How%20to%20Manage%20Them-01.jpg?updatedAt=1696332710809.

Regional anesthetic techniques such as epidurals and spinals, for example, can be used to effectively manage pain while maintaining minimal systemic effects on the mother and the fetus. Nonetheless, the clinician must weigh the risks closely, including hypotension and interference with uteroplacental perfusion. Proper patient positioning is also critical in preventing compromised blood supply since even slight variations can have severe maternal and fetal complications (Kuckowski & Van Zundert, 2007). Last, an anesthetic plan should first ensure the safety and comfort of both mother and fetus, and appropriate informed consent should be obtained after discussion of the risks and benefits associated with the modalities chosen. With evolving obstetric anesthesia, continued fine-tuning of technique and protocol remains essential to safeguard high-risk pregnancies (Figure 3.9).

Test Your Knowledge

1. What are the common indications for administering anesthesia during labor and delivery?
2. In which situations is general anesthesia indicated in obstetric patients?

3.3. Benefits of Obstetric Anesthesia

Learning Outcome

1. Enhanced maternal comfort
2. Improved fetal outcomes
3. Reduction of stress and anxiety during labor

The introduction of obstetric anesthesia has transformed the process of childbirth, with numerous good outcomes for both infants and mothers. Amongst the prominent advantages is the capability of pain control during labor and childbirth efficiently. Regional anesthetics, such as epidurals and spinal blocks, allow women to give birth with reduced pain, which provides a more pleasurable and manageable experience of labor. By alleviating pain, obstetric anesthesia enhances not just maternal satisfaction but also stands to improve maternal-infant bonding upon delivery. Moreover, anesthesia administration enables the administration of medical interventions that may be needed during complicated labor, thereby optimizing both maternal and fetal safety. Besides optimal relief of pain, obstetric anesthesia also enhances overall maternal and neonatal health. For instance, research has indicated a direct correlation between the use of epidural analgesia and decreased need for cesarean section since it allows mothers to conserve energy during prolonged labor. Moreover, obstetric anesthesia can reverse effects that would otherwise lead to unwanted outcomes. Although controversy exists as to the impact of directed pushing during the second stage of labor, it seems that proper utilization of obstetric anesthesia can encourage a less forceful and more natural manner of giving birth, which ultimately benefits both mother and child (Roberts & Hanson, 2007). Therefore, the role of anesthetics in obstetrics is not only limited to the modulation of pain but also to more general results related to the process of birth. Besides temporary benefits in labor, obstetric anesthesia has long-term influences on maternal mental health. Birth may be a significant stressor, and by diminishing pain, obstetric anesthesia may reduce the incidence of postpartum depression and anxiety. Evidence reveals that women who experience labor with no analgesia are at higher risk of having negative emotional outcomes (Balatero, 2018). By enhancing the labor experience through comfort and support, obstetric anesthesia may be responsible for improved psychological well-being. This correlation is noteworthy in its recognition of the importance of individualized care in labor; through tailoring anesthesia to suit each woman uniquely, caregivers can empower mothers, supporting a more positive perception of childbirth and leading to better mental health outcomes in the postpartum period (Figure 3.10).

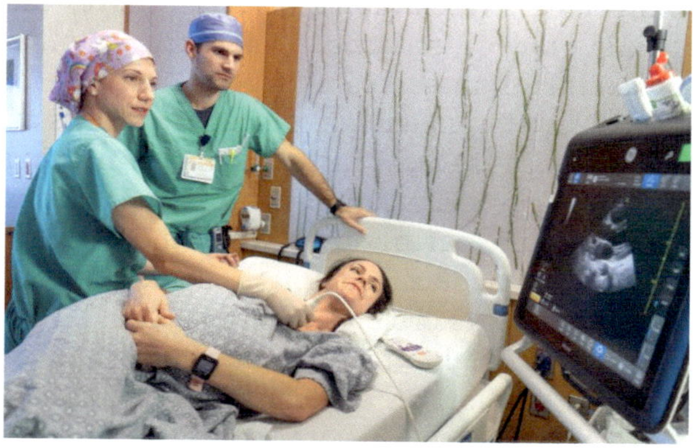

Figure 3.10. The introduction of obstetric anesthesia has significantly transformed the childbirth experience.

Source: https://cdn.atriumhealth.org/-/media/wakeforest/school/images/page-content/education-and-training/residencies-and-fellowships/obstetrics-anesthesiology/obstetric-anesthesiology-fellowship-wake-forest-school-of-medicine-ultrasound.jpg?w=100%25&rev=39c0260035e44da98278b544e392aaea&hash=9A8C688549BFA86CEE68F835223E905F.

3.3.1. Enhanced Maternal Comfort

The concept of enhancing comfort for the mother during delivery and labor has been a significant focus within the field of obstetric anesthesia. Comfort, albeit often regarded as an individualistic experience, still lies at the forefront of achieving a mother's whole process of giving birth. A recent study examined the effects of several alternatives to analgesics on mothers' comfort and satisfaction, showing the potential for intrapartum nitrous oxide as a real alternative to traditional epidural analgesics or to no analgesia at all. Findings on the comfort levels for female patients receiving nitrous oxide and those receiving other forms of analgesia indicated no significant difference, suggesting that how pain is relieved may not actually be a factor in maternal comfort during delivery (Such, 2020). These findings can inform clinical practice by showing the effectiveness and safety of different modalities for enhancing maternal comfort during childbirth. Furthermore, the shifting view of maternal preference for birth environments underscores the critical role of shared decision-making in obstetric care. As an illustration, research has shown that nursing students appreciate supporting labor positions and having the partner present during delivery, over a more medicalized option that a subset of medical students prefer (Tane et al., 2019). This disparity highlights the relevance of including maternal comfort in clinical practice because it is consonant with contemporary patient-centered care paradigms. It highlights the importance of healthcare workers encouraging patients to share pain management options and labor environments that facilitate comfort. By doing so, practitioners empower mothers to be actively involved in decision-making, thus improving their satisfaction and emotional state in the process of delivery. Lastly, the benefits of enhanced maternal comfort extend beyond mere short-term pain relief. A successful birth experience, characterized by sufficient comfort and support, has lasting implications for maternal mental health and infant bonding. Maternal satisfaction has been found to be related to optimal outcomes in maternal-infant relationships, which warrants a supportive labor environment. In addition, the realization that comfort and pain can coexist allows healthcare providers to reassess traditional childbirth practices. The integration of practices such as the administration of nitrous oxide, along with an understanding of individual comfort requirements, unlocks opportunities in a wider view of obstetric anesthesia, one where culture prioritizes the health of the mother and infant (Tane et al., 2019 Such, 2020) (Figure 3.11).

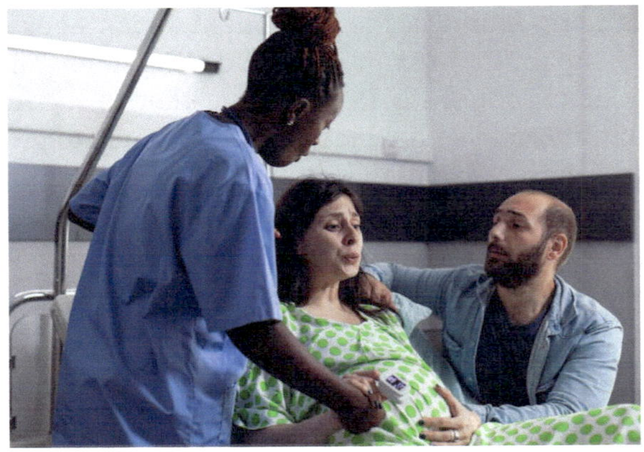

Figure 3.11. The concept of enhanced maternal comfort during labor.

Source: https://www.thevbpblog.com/wp-content/uploads/2023/12/pregnant-woman-pain-getting-medical-assistance.jpg.

3.3.2. Improved Fetal Outcomes

In obstetrical anesthesia, the success in achieving improved fetal results is of the highest priority to the health and well-being of both mother and child. Successful labor pain control can actually decrease maternal stress, which is significant since excessive levels of stress have been shown to negatively affect fetal health. As one example, the use of epidurals has been well-studied and has been shown to be exceedingly effective as a pain relief measure, improving the entire labor process. By facilitating a less painful delivery, mothers can engage more actively and remain alert during labor, reducing possible fetal distress. Evidence-based labor and delivery, like effective pain control methods, has a direct correlation with better fetal results, citing the importance of anesthetic interventions in obstetric care. Ultimately, research has indicated that certain practices of labor may be imperiling fetal well-being inadvertently. Notably, aggressive Valsalva bearing down attempts over the long term can have adverse fetal and maternal consequences, such as deoxygenation in the fetus and potential pelvic floor injury in the mother. Current practices still encourage aggressive pushing in supine positions, despite the evidence favoring an individualized approach that encompasses women's natural bearing down sensations. Shifting the emphasis to maneuvers like laboring down not only enhances maternal comfort but also allows the fetus to advance more naturally into the birth canal. With the integration of these evidence-based changes, clinicians can facilitate improved fetal outcomes and directly promote natural labor processes, which create a safer birthing environment. The availability of other analgesic options, such as nitrous oxide, is also essential to enhancing maternal comfort and fetal outcome. Nitrous oxide, whose use for the relief of labor pain has been longstanding, is no longer as universally available in the United States as it once was, reducing the choices for pain relief available to laboring women. Quality improvement initiatives have demonstrated the potential to change practice dramatically through increased education of anesthesia professionals on proper nitrous oxide use. After education, surveys indicated not only increased knowledge concerning nitrous oxide but also increased willingness among practitioners to offer this option to patients. By increasing the number of analgesic choices that can be offered to the patient during labor, clinicians can provide not only maternal comfort, but also protection of the fetus's safety and well-being, which ultimately leads to better fetal outcomes in obstetric management (Roberts & Hanson, 2007; Bhetta & Burger, 2024) (Figure 3.12).

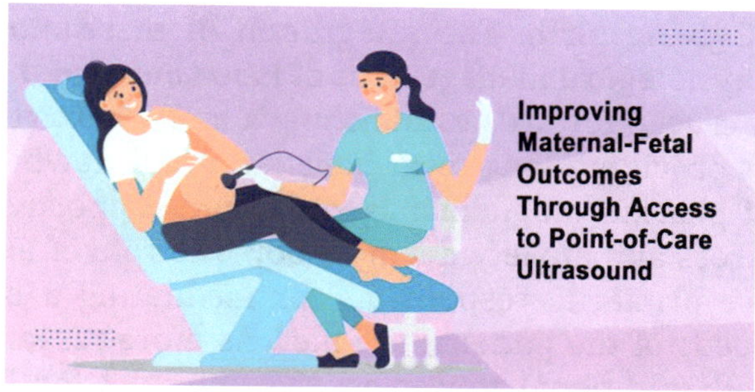

Figure 3.12. Improved fetal outcomes.

Source: https://www.pocus.org/wp-content/uploads/2024/06/2024_POCUS_Maternal_600x335_v2.jpg.

3.3.3. Reduction of Stress and Anxiety During Labor

Labor can be a very stressful experience for pregnant women; one filled with worry about pain relief and the health of their babies. Obstetric anesthesia is employed to relieve these anxieties through the elimination of pain as well as providing emotional consolation. The proof is that, by allowing the presence of a known person, such as a companion or support partner, during procedures like neuraxial labor analgesia, patients' anxiety levels can be significantly reduced. A survey of anesthesiologists in the United States indicated that majority of anesthesiologists support having a visitor during neuraxial technique placement, primarily due to reducing patient anxiety and addressing patient preference (Kumaraswami et al., 2018). This growing popularity speaks to the importance that is given to a holistic childbirth model in which emotional comfort is equally valued as pain management. Other than the emotional comfort delivered by loved ones, several nonpharmacological interventions have been shown to further alleviate stress and anxiety in labor. Complementary therapies in the form of massage therapy, acupressure, and reflexology have been found to be effective adjuncts to standard analgesia methods, providing an integrated intervention for managing pain (Yenter, 2024). These manual interventions have been observed to reduce labor pain in different stages effectively, ultimately leading to a more comfortable process of giving birth. The integration of these modalities in obstetric practice not only satisfies the physiological management of labor but also the psychological well-being of the mother. Integration is crucial towards establishing a more positive birth experience, which ultimately has the potential of providing long-term benefits to the newborn and mother. Last but not least, the combination of pharmacologic management and supportive care works to create a general plan for managing stress and anxiety during labor. The role of anesthesiologists is not just to administer drugs; they are primarily responsible for facilitating a calm environment and ensuring that the emotional needs of the patients are met. As more research comes out supporting the use of complementary and traditional therapies, the potential for better obstetric outcomes grows. Awareness of the multifaceted experience of pain during labor and its resultant fears not only leads to more satisfied patients but forms the basis for better maternal and newborn health outcomes (Kumaraswami et al., 2018; Yenter, 2024). With advancements in obstetric anesthesia, attention to these differing modalities will continue to hold a central role in sound labor management strategies (Figure 3.13).

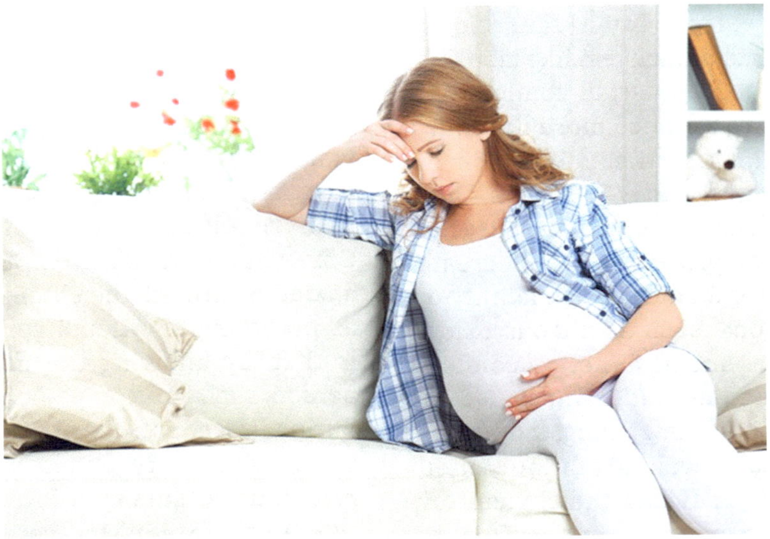

Figure 3.13. The process of labor can be a profoundly stressful experience for expectant mothers.

Source: https://news.sanfordhealth.org/wp-content/uploads/2016/11/Pregnant-woman-sitting-on-couch.jpg.

Test Your Knowledge

1. What are the common side effects associated with regional anesthesia in obstetric patients?
2. What complications can occur with general anesthesia during obstetric procedures?

3.4. Risks and Complications

Learning Outcome

1. Potential side effects for the mother
2. Risks to the fetus
3. Long-term implications of anesthesia use

In the field of obstetric anesthesia, awareness of the risks and complications is important for obtaining maximal maternal and fetal outcomes. Among the most distressing complications is amniotic fluid embolism (AFE), a rare and catastrophic condition that can occur during delivery or labor. Research indicates that AFE has a significant incidence rate of approximately 4.1 per 100,000 deliveries, predominantly in women who are having a vaginal delivery. The sudden onset of symptoms, such as loss of consciousness, fetal bradycardia, and respiratory distress, highlights the need for early identification and management of the emergency. Guidelines for AFE management emphasize the importance of specialized training among anesthesiologists in the management of maternal cardiovascular collapse, emphasizing the immediacy of preparedness within the obstetric setting, considering the cited 15% mortality danger of this complication (Skolnik et al., 2017). Complementing the risks associated with obstetric anesthesia are the concerns of anticoagulation therapy and its use close to operations. Recommendations suggest perioperative management of anticoagulated patients as an orderly process to prevent the risk of bleeding, yet provide sufficient protection against thromboembolic phenomena. Recent studies indicate that while oral anticoagulants can reduce thrombotic events substantially, they do so at the expense of an increased rise in postoperative or operative bleeding complications. The GRADE guidelines, when used in clinical guideline development, suggest the delicate balance between the continued anticoagulation of patients who have an established risk of thromboembolism and the urgency of hemostasis for invasive procedures (Keeling et al., 2016). Anticoagulation discontinuation is highly variable from patient to patient, observational studies show, and thus, having a well-informed and personalized approach to every case is essential. Moreover, the side effects of antiplatelet therapy also show the complexities in the management of obstetric patients subjected to anesthetic administration. Antiplatelet medication, especially dual antiplatelet therapy, has been linked with high incidences of postoperative bleeding, and therefore, much concern has been raised regarding the careful application of these drugs in the operating theater. Research has established that, while the continuation of low-dose aspirin may be possible for most surgical interventions, the concurrent use of more than one antiplatelet agent poses serious challenges. The strategic timing of discontinuation, optimally weighing perioperative thromboembolic complications against the risk of severe bleeding, is a component of preanesthetic assessment. Lastly, the balancing of these risks and complications in obstetric anesthesia requires perseverance, constant education, and mutually agreed decision-making among clinicians to ensure the safety and well-being of both mother and child.

3.4.1. Potential Side Effects for the Mother

The administration of obstetric anesthesia is associated with various potential side effects in the mother on both short-term and long-term health. Of these, spinal and general anesthesia are the most common anesthetic techniques applied during cesarean delivery, both of which carry their own set of risks. Spinal anesthesia, being less frequently utilized due to its safety profile, can lead to severe side effects such as hypotension, headache, and pain on injection site. These are caused by changes in fluid dynamics and neural responses elicited by local anesthetics. In addition, allergic reactions or heightened anxiety linked with the anesthetic procedures could happen in some women, and therefore, careful assessment and regulation by healthcare providers are necessary to avoid injury in the process of administration. Aside from side effects that appear immediately, obstetric anesthesia also has effects on the newborn. The choice of analgesia can determine neonatal outcomes, such as Apgar scores and initiation of breastfeeding. For instance, intrathecal or epidural drugs can transiently compromise maternal hemodynamics, which consequently impacts fetal circulation and oxygenation. Systemic use of opioids has been demonstrated to interfere with early skin-to-skin contact immediately after cesarean delivery—a key practice for maternal-infant bonding and breastfeeding achievement (Balatero, 2018). Therefore, obstetric anesthetists must weigh these potential side effects against the benefits carefully, delivering optimal anesthesia care and promoting maternal and fetal health. Moreover, the implications of anesthetic choices on maternal pain management and satisfaction remain an active area of consideration. Studies have shown that intrathecal medication, as well as buprenorphine use, can extend pain relief with minimal side effects and thus help improve the overall experience in postpartum care (Rabiee et al., 2014). However, if the anesthesia is not well controlled, mothers will likely experience chronic pain or delayed recovery, which will disrupt the ability to resume required postpartum activity and provide appropriate care for their newborns. Addressing such concerns underscores the necessity of personalized anesthetic plans tailored to the health condition and needs of each mother, ultimately ensuring improved quality of obstetric care and good outcomes for both mother and child (Figure 3.14).

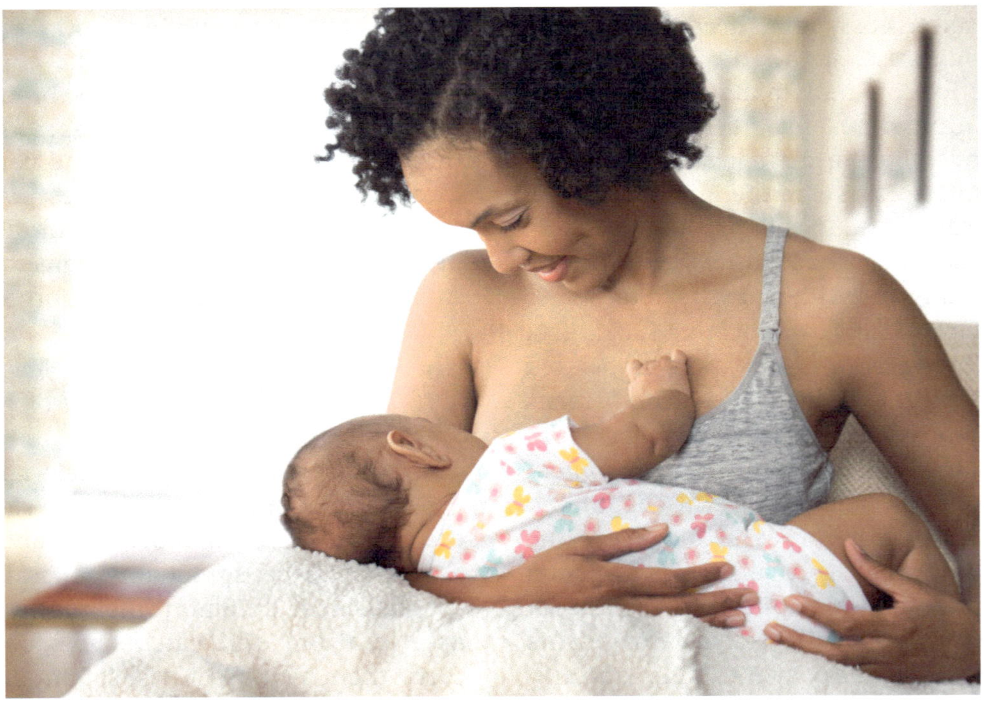

Figure 3.14. The administration of obstetric anesthesia.

Source: https://ucmscdn.healthgrades.com/eb/ba/e403574f485cb7a748a400a3a5cd/gettyimages-482136885.jpg.

3.4.2. Risks to the Fetus

In obstetric anesthesia, the first concern is to minimize the risk to the fetus, particularly under surgeries performed under surgery or anesthesia. Fetal distress may be due to many factors, including maternal position and the effect of anesthetic drugs. Surgical procedures, especially under traumatic injury, should take into account the physiological influence on the mother and fetus in a careful manner. For instance, when operating on a pregnant patient, it is essential to monitor fetal heart tones during surgery to pick up any distress at an early stage. An example scenario shows how important it is; a woman in the third trimester had fetal distress during surgery, prompting the emergency delivery by cesarean section, stressing the risks that are involved if surgical management is performed on pregnant patients (Sturges et al., 2013).

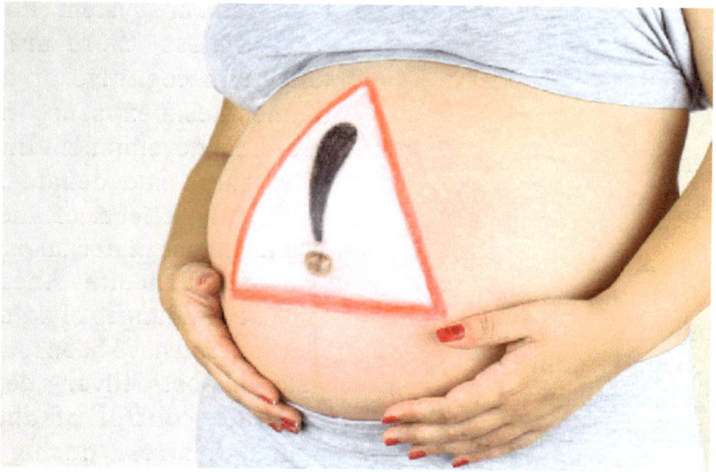

Figure 3.15. The risks to the fetus.

Source: https://shreeanshfetalcare.com/blog/wp-content/uploads/2018/07/Symptoms-of-High-Risk-Pregnancy.png.

Such occurrences compel anesthetic teams to adopt strategies to minimize risks and enhance outcomes for the fetus as well as the mother. Anesthesia delivery during delivery and labor also entails inherent risks to the fetus, particularly where the occurrence is complicated with preeclampsia. This hypertensive complication complicates analgesic and anesthetic management, calling for a precise understanding of how regional anesthesia techniques can affect fetal and maternal hemodynamic stability. Certified Registered Nurse Anesthetists (CRNAs) must be collaborative in ensuring that anesthetic methods do not hinder fetal health during labor. Investigations have shown that both spinal and epidural anesthesia are disadvantageous and advantageous in pain relief and hemodynamic stability, and excellent well-informed technique choice is the best way to prevent fetal injury (Potter et al., 2008). Pre-anesthetic assessment and continuous monitoring can reduce adverse effects on fetal well-being, emphasizing individualized regimens of anesthetics in obstetrics. Moreover, fetal risks extend beyond the immediate impact of surgery and anesthesia. Maternal disease processes, such as preeclampsia, can put the fetus at risk for fetal complications like intrauterine growth restriction and preterm labor. The attendant physiological stresses these maternal processes cause for the fetus must be considered when planning for anesthesia and analgesia during labor. Anesthetists must be careful about maternal health having an impact on fetal outcome, employing evidence-based practice guidelines in guaranteeing optimal care. Such a focus on holistic care reflects the interrelatedness between fetal and maternal well-being, necessitating concerted efforts by caregivers. As a core fact, minimizing risks to the fetus while administering obstetric anesthesia requires a collaborative effort that honors maternal safety while safeguarding fetal health (Figure 3.15).

3.4.3. Long-Term Implications of Anesthesia Use

The use of anesthesia in obstetric procedures, particularly cesarean sections, has significant long-term implications for mothers and babies. Anesthesia management affects not only the short-term surgical process but also long-term maternal outcomes. For example, studies have established that women undergoing cesarean sections through general anesthesia are likely to have a range of complications that accompany them even after they leave the facility long-term. These include complications like prolonged recovery, chronic pain, and psychosocial effects resulting from surgical trauma. As mentioned, even mild evidence for immediate skin-to-skin contact (SSC) following delivery is not always accessible to those who undergo cesarean deliveries, losing the critical moment of bonding, which can affect maternal-infant bonding and potentially give rise to longer-term emotional and psychological issues in both the mother and child (Balatero, 2018). In addition, improvement in obstetric anesthesia has greatly increased its safety and efficacy but not its long-term outcome. Efficacy of pain relief and anesthesia during delivery is critical to enhance maternal satisfaction and infant well-being. The anesthesia provider plays a critical role in the team of obstetricians, midwives, and neonatologists to maximize outcomes in mothers and neonates. Their skills, which are particularly applicable to resuscitation and critical care, are invaluable in tending to high-risk patients, as a symbiotic relationship with the healthcare system (Robert & Hanson, 2007). Nevertheless, there are concerns regarding long-term cognitive or developmental effects of anesthesia exposure in infants during times of critical development that remain a "hot topic" of research and debate within the discipline. Finally, the effects of anesthesia use continue to encompass maternal psychological well-being and mental health. Anesthesia complications and the challenges of adjusting to post-delivery motherhood have been found to lead to increased risks of post-delivery depression and anxiety. Accurate control of anesthesia can reduce pain and stress during delivery, potentially averting these adverse psychological outcomes. Furthermore, understanding the barriers to procedures like immediate SSC after cesarean delivery is crucial; these barriers may not only impede maternal physical recovery but also her emotional healing process. Taking these factors into account in obstetric anesthesia practice can enhance short- and long-term health outcomes of mothers and their infants, which reflects a need for continued innovation in anesthesia protocols and care methods (Balatero, 2018).

Test Your Knowledge

1. What are the key responsibilities of an anesthesiologist before, during, and after surgery?
2. How does an anesthesiologist ensure patient safety and pain management during surgical procedures?

3.5. Role of Anesthesiologists in Obstetric Care

Learning Outcome

1. Preoperative assessment and planning
2. Intraoperative monitoring and management
3. Postoperative care and pain management

Anesthesiologists' role in obstetric care is purely based on the unique requirements of childbearing and laboring patients. Anesthesiologists are responsible for administering relief from pain by various modalities, one of which includes the epidural and spinal anesthesia, which are now the standard in labor analgesia. These interventions not only decrease pain but also result in a more soothing birthing experience, thereby better maternal and neonatal outcomes. But their function is not to merely provide anesthesia; they also perform preoperative assessments, monitor hemodynamics during delivery, and monitor for complications. A comprehension of the physiological changes that occur in pregnancy allows anesthesiologists to predict issues and adjust their approaches to meet each patient's individual requirements, ensuring safety and efficiency in the labor process. Further, education and training of anesthesiologists are critical to their ability to manage obstetric patients effectively. While there is recognition by fellowship programs of the need for extensive training that addresses a variety of patient populations, recent studies indicate that gaps are present in integrating specific curricula of sexual and gender minority (SGM) health education into obstetric anesthesia. Program director surveys highlighted widespread recognition of SGM healthcare concerns, but few reported that they saw the value in incorporating this material into training curricula. The disconnect indicates possible avenues for growth in anesthesiology training because enhanced education of the trainees concerning SGM health issues would presumably extend to more competent, more diverse care protocols for obstetric care, eventually benefiting a wider range of patients during labor (MacCormick & George, 2020). In addition to clinical and educational roles, anesthesiologists contribute to obstetric care by collaborating with the broader healthcare team. Effective communication and interprofessional teamworking are required in the management of obstetric emergencies, such as uterine hemorrhage or fetal distress, where timely anesthesia management can be critical. Anesthesiologists typically collaborate with obstetricians, midwives, and pediatricians in formulating interdisciplinary care programs that are aimed at patient safety and comfort. Moreover, this team system aids in the assurance that the anesthetizing interventions harmonize with the general medical treatment of the patient during the process of labor. As care continues to emphasize personalized care, the role of the anesthesiologists in facilitating collaborative practices in obstetric care will be imperative to foresee and effectively respond to every individual childbirth experience (University of Iowa, 2011) (Figure 3.16).

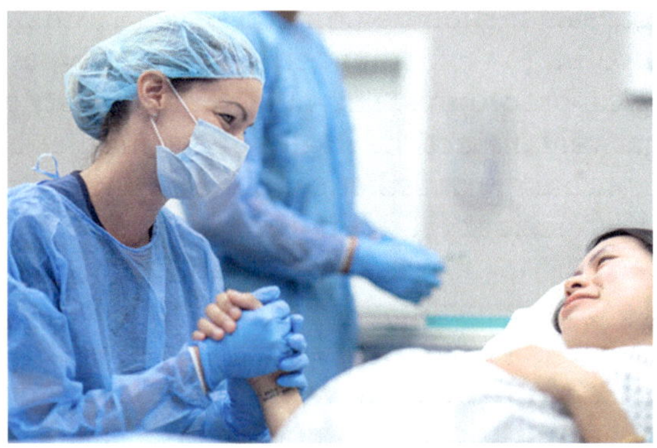

Figure 3.16. The role of anesthesiologists in obstetric care.

Source: https://health.ucdavis.edu/media-resources/contenthub/health-library/treatments/obstetric-anesthesia-marquee.jpg.

3.5.1. Preoperative Assessment and Planning

Ideal preoperative evaluation and planning are of utmost significance in obstetric anesthesia as they directly influence fetal and maternal outcomes in the operating room. Thorough assessment begins with an adequate medical history and physical examination because identification of any underlying conditions, such as hypertension or diabetes, may dictate anesthetic choice and reduce risk. In urgent surgery situations, such as those necessitated by trauma or complications, coordination between anesthesiologists, obstetricians, and surgeons becomes essential. Such multidisciplinary coordination ensures that all factors in the mother and the fetus are considered, with timely intervention to any intraoperative maternal or fetal status change. Further, positioning of the patient in the operating room should also receive special consideration to facilitate uteroplacental perfusion, an aspect that is significant in that it can play a significant role in fetal well-being and maternal safety (Sturges et al., 2013). Psychological problems, notably preoperative anxiety, form part of the preoperative assessment among obstetric patients. It has been found that women undergoing elective caesarean section demonstrate greater anxiety compared to women undergoing other types of surgical procedures. This heightened anxiety can negatively impact the health of the mother and complicate the anesthetic process. Identification of the patient at high levels of anxiety is important to inform appropriate coping skills and patient education, which assist in decreasing the fears associated with anesthesia and surgery. Also, understanding how past childbirth might influence a patient's attitude towards anesthesia can educate anesthesiologists in these interactions. By addressing these psychological factors, healthcare providers can create a more beneficial environment, which not only ensures the highest patient satisfaction but also results in improved surgical outcomes (Perumal et al., 2023). The presence of a robust preoperative assessment allows for creating customized anesthetic plans that consider both maternal and fetal well-being. The most critical factors to consider are the type of anesthesia employed—regional or general anesthesia—and the timing. For example, particular considerations must be made for timing administration of the anesthetic relative to fetal heart tones, well-known and gestational age, because any delay or accident could lead to serious risks. In addition, preoperative preparation should involve proper communication with the patient about the intended method, potential risks, and expected surgical experience to provide a concordant decision-making situation. Proper preoperative preparation allows the operating team to establish proper preparations against any obstetric complication, hence safeguarding both the mother and her child during the perioperative experience (Sturges et al., 2013).

3.5.2. Intraoperative Monitoring and Management

In obstetric anesthesia, intraoperative care and monitoring are essential aspects that ensure the safety and well-being of the mother and the fetus. During surgical interventions in pregnant patients, it is invaluable to maintain a continuous assessment of the patient's vital signs, such as blood pressure, heart rate, and oxygen saturation. These values provide significant information about the patient's hemodynamic status and general physiological stability. In addition, fetal heart rate monitoring has a two-fold purpose: not only does it evaluate fetal health, but it also warns the surgical staff about distress that is happening intraoperatively. The use of advanced monitoring methods not only optimizes maternal treatment but also allows timely interventions if there is unexpected complication, ultimately providing better results for both patients and babies, as has been stressed in clinical settings with specialized attention to critical surgical procedures in pregnant women

(Sturges et al., 2013). Obstetric anesthesia management of intraoperative complications requires an approach by collaborations involving anesthesiologists, obstetricians, and surgical teams. Good coordination and communication are essential in managing complex cases, such as when there is a pregnant patient with traumatic injury or operating emergencies. At this point, intraoperative monitoring is an important tool to identify signs of fetal and maternal distress. For example, when fetal heart tones signify distress, an emergency cesarean section may be required to expedite delivery and prevent injury to the fetus. The emphasis on teamwork among healthcare providers cannot be stressed too much, as it is majorly responsible for decision-making as well as the execution of timely surgical operations in emergency situations (Sturges et al., 2013). The multifaceted approach brings forth an environment where intraoperative decision-making is potent and quick, ensuring the safety of both mother and baby. Along with that, technological advancements in surgical techniques have also expanded the scope of intraoperative management options for obstetric patients. The concern must also be to face challenges posed by certain conditions, such as a morbidly adherent placenta (MAP), with the risk of inducing severe hemorrhage during surgery. Ground-breaking techniques like resuscitative endovascular balloon occlusion of the aorta (REBOA) have also become newer interventions in high-risk situations, equipping surgeons with tools to control hemorrhage appropriately. REBOA can maximize maternal safety and prevent transfusion risks in patients who may decline them due to personal principles, such as those of Jehovah's Witnesses. Application and familiarity with these advanced techniques in intraoperative care also reflect having the competence in managing complex obstetric patients while considering factors related to patients that can influence surgery results (Figure 3.17).

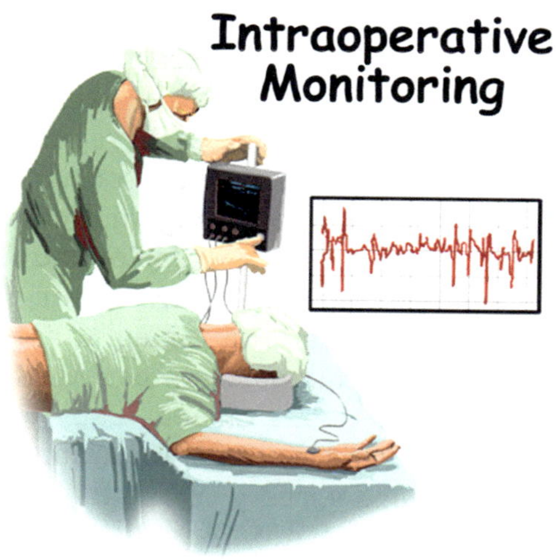

Figure 3.17. Intraoperative monitoring and management.

Source: https://eorthopod.com/sites/default/files/images/intraop_monitoring_intro01.jpg.

3.5.3. Postoperative Care and Pain Management

Effective postoperative care and pain control are integral components of good results from obstetric interventions, such as cesarean delivery. Pain control must be tailored to each patient based on her individual needs, taking into account factors such as type of anesthesia, patients' desire for pain relief, and anticipated side effects. Multimodal pain control, where several analgesic modalities are combined, has gained widespread popularity in recent years. Such methods may include intrathecal opioids, non-steroidal anti-inflammatory drugs (NSAIDs), and regional anesthesia techniques, ultimately providing improved pain control than the standard opioid-based regimen alone. Notably, studies have demonstrated that intrathecal buprenorphine combined with local anesthetics can significantly prolong the analgesic duration and reduce reliance on systemic opioids, thereby minimizing resulting side effects and enabling patient comfort (Rabiee et al., 2014). Moreover, postoperative pain assessment is important in evaluating the success of measures taken to relieve pain. Clinical practice uses an extremely helpful tool called the visual analog scale (VAS), whereby patients can effectively measure their pain level. Continual monitoring of patients' pain scores by health professionals is significant in that it allows timeliness in adjusting analgesia regimens and gauging overall satisfaction with relief from pain. In obstetric anesthesia, adequate postoperative control of pain has a direct impact on the patients' recovery, emotional well-being, and engagement with their baby. Practitioners, in turn, must be attentive to monitor pain intensity and factor in patients' preferred option and experience while designing integrated pain control strategies (Rabiee et al., 2014). Another significant characteristic of postoperative care is the integration of multidisciplinary teams to enhance patient outcomes. Multidisciplinary collaboration between obstetricians, anesthesiologists, and nursing staff ensures that the specific needs of both baby and mother are taken care of and prioritized, improving communication and team coordination. For example, in obstetric emergencies involving surgery, such as in trauma surgery, maintaining uteroplacental perfusion becomes a priority. This involves accurate patient positioning and continuous fetal monitoring, which will influence anesthesia planning as well as procedure timing. In general, having a protocol for postoperative care based on an awareness of general physical, emotional, and procedural concerns will result in better recovery experiences among obstetric anesthesia patients.

Test Your Knowledge

1. What are some recent innovations improving safety and pain relief in obstetric anesthesia?
2. How have modern techniques enhanced maternal and fetal outcomes during labor and delivery?

3.6. Current Trends and Innovations in Obstetric Anesthesia

Learning Outcome

1. Advances in technology and techniques
2. Research on safety and efficacy
3. Integration of multidisciplinary approaches

The field of obstetric anesthesia is evolving rapidly, spurred by advances in technology as well as increasing understanding of maternal and fetal physiology. Among the emerging trends is the increased use of ultrasound technology in the administration of regional anesthesia. Clinicians have historically relied on anatomic landmarks to place needles, which is challenging, especially in the obese patients. Current research highlights the effectiveness of ultrasound for enhancing the precision of epidural and spinal injections, particularly if anatomical landmarks are difficult to palpate. It was based on a survey of Student Registered Nurse Anesthetists (SRNAs) and Certified Registered Nurse Anesthetists (CRNAs) that the majority of practitioners came forward with confession to the use of ultrasound during such procedures and reported improved results when the technique was employed in obese patients who are prone to variation from normal visibility in anatomy (Loebig, 2020). Such a shift towards ultrasound-guided techniques is a seminal development in obstetric anesthesia practice. With advancing technology, the field has witnessed growing interest in patient-focused care and personalized anesthesia care. As parturients are increasingly keen on having an active participation in giving birth, those anesthetic choices that minimize side effects but maximize comfort are being brought to the forefront. This also reflects broader social trends towards medical practice personalization, where personal choice and preference become a priority. Enhanced recovery after surgery (ERAS) protocols are also becoming increasingly accepted as a foundation of this process, which includes customized anesthesia approaches eschewing excessive sedation and promoting early mobilization. ERAS protocols are also informed by ongoing research into the pharmacologic management of pain, which seeks to balance effective pain relief with reduced opioid use, thus addressing concerns about opioid addiction in the postpartum population. With facial trends running parallel to contemporary practice in healthcare, obstetric anesthesia development remains solidly based on improving patient outcomes.

Interdisciplinary collaboration and investigation are necessary to drive innovations in obstetric anesthesia. Facilities and institutions increasingly strongly recognize the necessity for multidisciplinary approaches to improving care delivery and management within the health sector. For example, the Indian Institute of Management, Ahmedabad (IIMA) has extended its research domains to the healthcare sector, exploring issues related to governance and management in urban and rural healthcare settings. By establishing interfaces between anesthesiologists, obstetricians, and healthcare management experts, there are opportunities to develop and translate models that enhance patient safety and procedural efficacy in anesthetic services during labor and delivery (Ramani et al., 2010). Moreover, ongoing education and training of the anesthesia practitioners are essential to a level that they remain proficient with new technologies and techniques. In this dynamic environment, it cannot be overemphasized that collaboration is important as it underpins the foundation of constant innovations in practices in obstetric anesthesia (Figure 3.18).

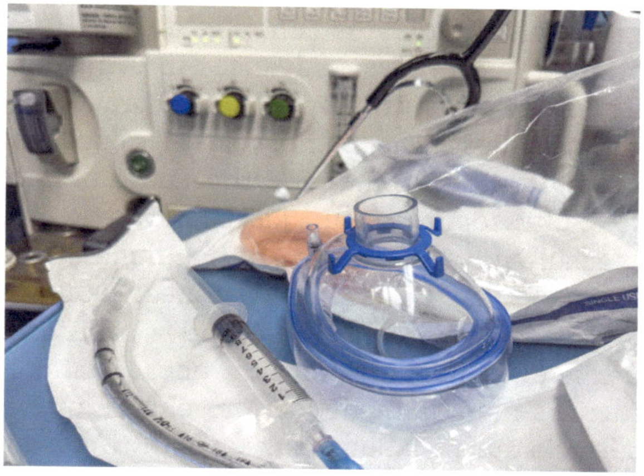

Figure 3.18. Current trends and innovations in obstetric anesthesia.

Source: https://world.skanray.com/wp-content/uploads/2023/09/anesthesia-mask-laryngoscope-represent-controlled-care-precise-intervention-hospital-airw-scaled.jpg.

3.6.1. Advances in Technology and Techniques

The landscape of obstetric anesthesia is constantly evolving, driven by advances in technology and innovative techniques that seek to enhance patient outcomes. A recent development is the application of resuscitative endovascular balloon occlusion of the aorta (REBOA) in managing profound obstetric hemorrhage secondary to conditions such as morbidly adherent placenta (MAP). Obstetric hemorrhage has been a significant problem in the past, with maternal morbidity and mortality being its most frequent cause globally. The REBOA technique allows for the control of non-compressible hemorrhage at once through a minimally invasive technique, which is particularly valuable in high-risk obstetric procedures. As the medical community accepts the potential for REBOA, it is increasingly necessary to establish a protocol for its implementation in obstetric care, especially where traditional therapies are not feasible because of resource or patient preference constraints, such as those in Jehovah's Witnesses (Chen et al., 2018). As an integrated process, advances in ultrasound technology are transforming the practice of obstetric anesthesia, namely, needle placement for epidural and spinal anesthesia. Adding the use of ultrasound imaging has been worthwhile, especially for the so-called difficult anatomical landmarks, i.e., the obese. With nearly 50% of the parturients being obese and a significant portion of them being morbidly obese, standard practices may be inadequate to ensure proper analgesia during labor. A survey of CRNAs found that most of them admitted to the advantages of using ultrasound for needle placement during epidural. Although there are continued impediments of limited access to devices and knowledge gaps, the majority indicated the merits of ultrasound in enhancing rates of procedural success and patient safety (Loebig, 2020). Secondly, the growing proficiency in multimodal analgesia and sedation techniques in obstetric anesthesia reiterates the emphasis on optimizing maternal care. These new practices are meant to minimize reliance on opioids, as well as optimize pain management methods, reducing possible side effects while enhancing recovery periods. Use of multimodal regimens can significantly reduce perception of pain along with the specific problems that occur in the obstetric population, and it is distinct from that of the general surgical population. With these practices picking up speed and evidence guideline recommendations being set, the profile of obstetric anesthesia will continue to evolve, providing practitioners with longer and more diverse options to ensure the health of mothers and their babies.

3.6.2. Research on Safety and Efficacy

Research into safety and efficacy in obstetric anesthesia has increasingly become critical, particularly with the management of complications related to widespread procedures like neuraxial anesthesia. One of the significant concerns is the occurrence of post-dural puncture headache (PDPH), an occurrence that will definitely impact patient comfort and recovery. Needle type and size have been shown by research to be among the factors that determine this complication. Furthermore, many demographic variables, including age, gender, and history of PDPH, raise risk in the obstetric population. It is important for practitioners to understand these nuances as they endeavor to balance the benefit of effective pain relief against avoiding excessive potential harm and thus aligning their practices with the best outcomes for patient safety in this vulnerable group. This information enables possible tailoring of anesthetic practices to avoid complications, thus enhancing the quality of care in obstetrics. Preventive treatment and novel modes of treatment are critical in the prevention of PDPH and its effects. Studies indicate that academic programs in anesthesia practitioners can efficiently increase their familiarity with novel treatment models, ascertaining the effectiveness of alternatives such as the sphenopalatine ganglion block (SPGB). The technique has been shown to be promising not only for pain relief but also for stemming reliance on more intrusive interventions such as the epidural blood patch. Through creating an environment where providers are trained on the uses and benefits of SPGB, the healthcare community is able to enhance patient outcomes through care. A well-trained strategy equips clinicians to make informed decisions for pain alternatives, leading to patient satisfaction as well as recovery rates after obstetric procedures. With increasing shifts in health systems, continuous examination of the safety and efficacy of anesthetic techniques still remains significant. Recent research stresses the importance of ongoing education of anesthesia providers, particularly in managing complications like PDPH. Increased training and awareness can lead to increased adoption of alternative methods, encouraging doctors to do less invasive procedures in the first place. It is a collective effort of the medical fraternity that not only contributes to improving the care of individual patients but also has advantages for broader health-related efforts towards patient safety and satisfaction. With the addition of evidence-based practice and focus on continuous learning, obstetric anesthesia has the capability to reduce complications by a significant amount and enhance overall levels of care for pregnant women undergoing various procedures. This commitment to continuous research and education is crucial in providing the best possible results for patients with regard to obstetric anesthesia (Figure 3.19).

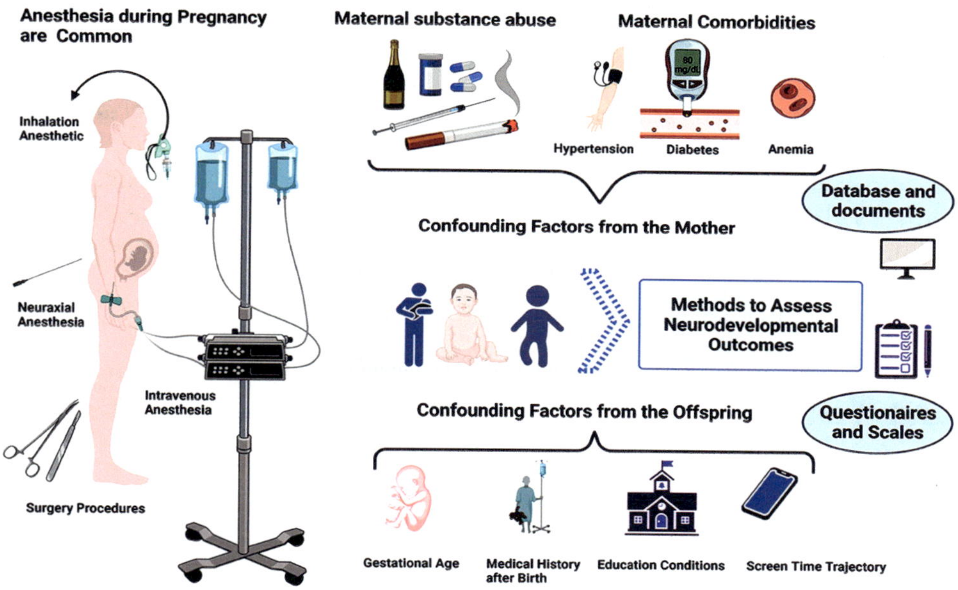

Figure 3.19. The research on safety and efficacy within obstetric anesthesia.

Source: https://images-provider.frontiersin.org/api/ipx/w=1200&f=png/https://www.frontiersin.org/files/Articles/1146569/fneur-14-1146569-HTML/image_m/fneur-14-1146569-g001.jpg.

3.6.3. Integration of Multidisciplinary Approaches

Multidisciplinary practice in obstetric anesthesia is essential for achieving maximum maternal and fetal outcomes during delivery. Multidisciplinary teamwork is necessary to address the complexity of obstetric care, with healthcare workers such as anesthesiologists, obstetricians, nurse-midwives, and neonatal specialists involved. This model guarantees that each member of the team utilizes his/her expertise in delivering the best care. For instance, on-site learning and educational interaction among medical students and certified nurse-midwives (CNMs) have determined that inter-professional learning enhances learning about each other's roles and thereby fosters a more cooperative healthcare setting. Greater knowledge concerning inter-professional practice significantly affects future healthcare professionals' preparedness to embrace teamwork in clinical practice, which, in turn, contributes to enhanced patient care outcomes (Hanson et al., 2005). Emergency cesarean sections present specific challenges that demand high-level interdisciplinary organization. They account for a substantial percentage of deliveries, so the necessity for highly organized team members able to respond rapidly to medical crises is especially critical. Good organization between obstetricians and anesthesiologists is essential, particularly where both maternal and fetal well-being are involved. Studies have indicated that multidisciplinary team functioning during emergency cesarean sections depends directly on the physical design and layout of the operating room (OR). Properly designed buildings can overcome workflow bottlenecks and facilitate better interspeciality interactions, thereby enhancing the operating team's overall efficiency (Sotto et al., 2021). This underscores the importance of integrating multidisciplinary approaches not only in treating patients but also in spatially organizing care centers. Furthermore, a culture of multidisciplinary practice in obstetric anesthesia can lead to remarkable clinical practice innovation. Through open minds and varied expertise from various disciplines, healthcare teams can innovate and improve anesthesia practices, pain control strategies, and emergency responses. Interdisciplinary training programs make healthcare workers interact and use teamwork skills, which result in improved communication and reduced errors in handling patients. Teamwork is particularly necessary in high-volume delivery centers where there is a requirement for rapid decision-making. With studies consistently finding the benefits of interdisciplinary practice, obstetric anesthesia can go further to support safer, more efficient care systems for pregnant women and neonates, ultimately shaping the future of obstetric anesthesia practice (Hanson et al., 2005).

Test Your Knowledge

1. What are the latest advancements in regional anesthesia techniques used in obstetrics?
2. How are new monitoring technologies improving safety for both mother and fetus during anesthesia?

SUMMARY

The obstetric anesthesia experience is a significant illustration of the subtle balance between optimal pain relief and maternal safety during parturition. Anesthesia using neuraxial, in the form of spinal anesthesia, is a foundation in anesthetic management of obstetrics, especially for patients undergoing cesarean delivery. Despite excellent evidence for the effectiveness of spinal anesthesias, their severe adverse effects, such as spinal-anesthesia induced hypotension (SAIH), are still concerns for both non-obstetric and obstetric patients. Prophylactic measures, such as the preoperative administration of ondansetron, have been investigated in a search for the prevention of such complications. However, current evidence remains contentious, and further study is necessary to find out the true effectiveness of such interventions in actually preventing the development of SAIH in a significant manner. Secondarily, resolution of the issue of hematologic screening in preeclampsia patients, as well as in other obstetric patients, becomes necessary for safe anesthetic provision. As indicated in recent literature, pre-neuraxial blockade (NB) platelet counts are not reliable or reproducible, which implies a consensus issue among anesthesiologists about acceptable hemostatic values. This variability has inherent risks to patients and underscores the necessity for standardized preoperative guidelines. Through promoting uniform testing and better-defined protocols, clinicians can enhance the safety of neuraxial blocks in high-risk patients and thereby advance obstetric patient outcomes. The ongoing evolution of the specialty of obstetric anesthesia demands attention to rigorous research and constant improvement of medical practice. Research regarding prophylactic measures and reconfirmation of hematologic tests' criteria directly affects maternal and neonatal safety under anesthesia. Upcoming activities must focus on coordinating research activity to produce more homogenized results that can safely be integrated into practice. With the encouragement of an environment of investigation and emphasis on collaboration among obstetric anesthesiologists, the underlying objective of optimizing patient care and protection in obstetric anesthesia can be achieved, positioning this specialty at the forefront of maternal healthcare advancements.

The specialty of obstetric anesthesia is characterized by a continued evolution in practice and awareness of maternal and neonatal well-being. Pain control in labor and delivery is one of the principal concerns for this specialty, and there exists a delicate balance to which a delicate ratio needs to be found to effect effective analgesia without compromising the safety of mother and offspring. The focus of recent research is the avoidance of maneuvers like prolonged Valsalva bearing-down attempts. These interventions, traditionally employed to enhance the second stage of labor, have been found to have negative effects, for example, potential fetal deoxygenation and maternal injury. The current consensus therefore, is for individualized care that promotes women's natural reflexes in labor, making bearing down more instinctual, diminishing risk, and enhancing maternal comfort and confidence (Roberts & Hanson, 2007). Apart from that, a crucial element of contemporary obstetric anesthesia is the broader health environment within which maternity care is delivered. The MacArthur Foundation project reflects an effort to enhance maternal and reproductive health by professional midwifery institutionalization in Mexico. The project reflects an awareness that professional midwifery can address gaps in traditional health models and end up enhancing mothers' health outcomes. By supporting the training and regulation of midwives, the program aims to offer high-quality care in congruence with the current practice in obstetric anesthesia. This is based on the integration of midwifery as a necessary supporting framework in the overall maternity care, with evidence to support the provision of an environment that prioritizes women's health and well-being (Atkin et al., 2017). Overall, the incorporation of modern practice in obstetric anesthesia testifies to a commitment towards enhancing the quality of care provided to women in labor. The transition from outmoded techniques to an individualized practice shows the evolving appreciation of physiological as well as psychological aspects of labor. Additionally, attempts to enhance midwifery practice constitute significant aspects in the development of maternal health. Such problems point to a growing recognition of evidence-based practice that will guarantee safe and respectful birth care in a way that addresses individual needs for each woman. Through consistent inquiry and implementation of these critical practices, the field of obstetric anesthesia can help shape effective and compassionate care for mother and baby.

KEY TERMS FROM THIS CHAPTER

Amniotic fluid embolism (AFE)
Emotional challenges
Fetal health
Maternal morbidity
Maternal-fetal monitoring
Neonatal health
Postpartum hemorrhage (PPH)
Certified Registered Nurse Anesthetists (CRNAs)
Epidural anesthesia
Global health
Maternal recovery
Medical efficacy
Obstetric anesthesia

Critical Thinking Questions

1. **Which of the following agents is contraindicated in obstetric general anesthesia due to its uterotonic effects?**
   a. Ketamine
   b. Propofol
   c. Nitrous oxide
   d. Methoxyflurane
2. **Which physiological change in pregnancy impacts anesthetic drug distribution?**
   a. Decreased plasma protein levels
   b. Increased renal clearance
   c. Increased cardiac output
   d. All of the above
3. **Which complication is unique to obstetric anesthesia?**
   a. Aspiration pneumonia
   b. Amniotic fluid embolism
   c. Post-dural puncture headache
   d. Nerve injury
4. **The most appropriate management for post-dural puncture headache (PDPH) is:**
   a. Intravenous fluids
   b. Caffeine administration
   c. Epidural blood patch
   d. Oral analgesics
5. **Why is spinal anesthesia preferred over general anesthesia for elective cesarean delivery?**
   a. Better pain control post-surgery
   b. Reduced risk of aspiration
   c. Maternal consciousness during delivery
   d. All of the above

Short Answer Questions

1. What are the risks of general anesthesia in obstetrics compared to regional techniques?
2. What is the most common complication of epidural anesthesia in obstetric patients?
3. What is the gold standard treatment for post-dural puncture headache (PDPH)?
4. How does pregnancy affect the minimum alveolar concentration (MAC) of inhalational anesthetics?
5. What is the role of nitrous oxide in obstetric analgesia?
6. What are the key steps to manage a patient with supine hypotensive syndrome?

Answer to Critical Thinking Questions

1. (c); 2. (a); 3. (d); 4. (a); 5. (a)

References

1. Bhettay, A., & Burger, R. (2024). Sphenopalatine ganglion blocks for post-dural puncture headache: A case report in a 3-year-old child. *Paediatric anaesthesia*, *34*(2), 182–184. https://doi.org/10.1111/pan.14785(accessed on 28th June 2025).
2. Rabiee SM, Alijanpour E, Jabbari A, Rostami S. Benefits of using intrathecal buprenorphine. *Caspian J Intern Med*. 2014;5(3):143-147.(accessed on 28th June 2025).
3. Allert, R., Brüggmann, D., Raimann, F., Zander, N., Louwen, F., & Jennewein, L. (2023). The influence of epidural anesthesia in pregnancies with scheduled vaginal breech delivery at term: A hospital-based retrospective analysis. *Archives of Gynecology and Obstetrics, 310*, 261–268. https://www.semanticscholar.org/paper/cddeb4a345b6469c50bb38b74a699e43ac9e37f8 (accessed on 28th June 2025).
4. Roberts, J., & Hanson, L. (2007). Best practices in second stage labor care: maternal bearing down and positioning. *Journal of midwifery & women's health*, *52*(3), 238–245. https://doi.org/10.1016/j.jmwh.2006.12.011(accessed on 28th June 2025).
5. Guenther S, Vrekoussis T, Heublein S, et al. Decidual macrophages are significantly increased in spontaneous miscarriages and over-express FasL: a potential role for macrophages in trophoblast apoptosis. *Int J Mol Sci*. 2012;13(7):9069-9080. doi:10.3390/ijms13079069(accessed on 28th June 2025).
6. Sotto, K. T., Hedli, L. C., Sie, L., Padua, K., Yamada, N., Lee, H., Halamek, L., Daniels, K., Nathan-Roberts, D., & Austin, N. S. (2021). Single-center task analysis and user-centered assessment of physical space impacts on emergency Cesarean delivery. *PloS one*, *16*(6), e0252888. https://doi.org/10.1371/journal.pone.0252888(accessed on 28th June 2025).
7. Eriko Tane, Yosie Umeno, Yoko Ishioka, Simon Peter Bahau, Roger Lord (2019). Comparison of perceived requirements for maternal delivery between medical versus nursing students. POJ Nurs Prac Res. 3(1):1-11. DOI: https://doi.org/10.32648/2577-9516/3/1/4(accessed on 28th June 2025).
8. Balatero, J. S. (2018). Obstetric nurses' perceived barriers to immediate skin to skin contact after cesarean birth. https://core.ac.uk/download/159401074.pdf (accessed on 28th June 2025).
9. Barrier, M. R. (2022). Improving maternal outcomes through quantifying blood loss in cesarean sections. https://core.ac.uk/download/534838705.pdf (accessed on 28th June 2025).
10. Breethaa Janani Selvamani, Kalagara, H., Volk, T., Narouze, S., Childs, C., Patel, A., Seering, M. S., et al. (2024). Infectious complications following regional anesthesia: A narrative review and contemporary estimates of risk. *Regional Anesthesia & Pain Medicine*. https://www.semanticscholar.org/paper/e5121a23791498b63705abac051b5baea1fdac7b (accessed on 28th June 2025).
11. Kumaraswami, S., Pothula, S., Inchiosa, M. A., Jr, Kubal, K. P., & Burns, M. A. (2018). Anesthesiologists' Preferences regarding Visitor Presence during Placement of Neuraxial Labor Analgesia. *Anesthesiology research and practice, 2018*, 3481975. https://doi.org/10.1155/2018/3481975(accessed on 28th June 2025).
12. Buttigieg, G., & Buttigieg, G. G. (2014). Medico-legal litigation: The clinical contractual nature

of the obstetric anesthetists–patient relationship. https://core.ac.uk/download/46602471.pdf (accessed on 28th June 2025).

13. Sultan, P., & Butwick, A. (2013). Platelet counts and coagulation tests prior to neuraxial anesthesia in patients with preeclampsia: a retrospective analysis. *Clinical and applied thrombosis/hemostasis : official journal of the International Academy of Clinical and Applied Thrombosis/Hemostasis, 19*(5), 529–534. https://doi.org/10.1177/1076029612441860(accessed on 28th June 2025).
14. Lakhe G, Shrestha P, Duwadi V. Postdural Puncture Headache after Spinal Anaesthesia in Parturients Undergoing Cesarean Section in the Department of Anesthesia in a Tertiary Care Center: A Descriptive Cross-sectional Study. *JNMA J Nepal Med Assoc*. 2023;61(261):417-420. Published 2023 May 1. doi:10.31729/jnma.8140(accessed on 28th June 2025).
15. Chen, H., Girda, E., Humphries, M. D., et al. (2018). Management of high-risk obstetrical patients with morbidly adherent placenta in the age of resuscitative endovascular balloon occlusion of the aorta. https://core.ac.uk/download/322437922.pdf (accessed on 28th June 2025).
16. Schwarzkopf, R., Gross, S. C., Coopersmith, A., & Gidumal, R. (2013). Ankle fracture surgery on a pregnant patient complicated by intraoperative emergency caesarian section. *Case reports in orthopedics, 2013*, 962794. https://doi.org/10.1155/2013/962794(accessed on 28th June 2025).
17. Vanhaesebrouck, E., Govaere, J., Smits, K., Durie, I., Vercauteren, G., Martens, A., Schauvliege, S., Ducatelle, R., Hoogewijs, M.K., Schauwer, C.D., & Kruif, A.D. (2010). Ovarian teratoma in the mare: a review and two cases. *Vlaams Diergeneeskundig Tijdschrift*.(accessed on 28th June 2025).
18. MacCormick, H., & George, R. B. (2020). Sexual and gender minorities educational content within obstetric anesthesia fellowship programs: a survey. Contenu éducatif traitant des minorités sexuelles et de genre au sein des programmes de fellowship en anesthésie obstétricale : un sondage. *Canadian journal of anaesthesia = Journal canadien d'anesthesie, 67*(5), 532–540. https://doi.org/10.1007/s12630-019-01562-x(accessed on 28th June 2025).
19. Habek, D., Medić, F., & Miletić, A. I. (2023). Što povezuje ginekologa/opstetričara s dišnim putom? https://core.ac.uk/download/587284782.pdf (accessed on 28th June 2025).
20. Hanson, L., Kirby, R. S., & Tillett, J. (2005). Medical students' knowledge of midwifery practice after didactic and clinical exposure. https://core.ac.uk/download/213085474.pdf (accessed on 28th June 2025).
21. Kearns, R. J., & Young, S. J. (2011). Transversus abdominis plane blocks; A national survey of techniques used by UK obstetric anesthetists. https://core.ac.uk/download/9387070.pdf (accessed on 28th June 2025).
22. Keeling, D., Tait, R. C., & Watson, H. G. (2016). Peri-operative management of anticoagulation and antiplatelet therapy. *British Journal of Hematology, 175*, 602–613. https://doi.org/10.1111/bjh.14344 (accessed on 28th June 2025).
23. Atkin, Lucille & Keith-Brown, Kimberly & Rees, Martha & Sesia, Paola. (2017). MACARTHUR FOUNDATION'S INITIATIVE TO PROMOTE MIDWIFERY IN MEXICO COMPLETE BASELINE REPORT. 10.13140/RG.2.2.10803.84002. (accessed on 28th June 2025).
24. Kuckowski, K., & Van Zundert, A. (2007). Anesthesia for pregnant women with valvular heart

disease: The state-of-the-art (Review). https://core.ac.uk/download/55881363.pdf (accessed on 28th June 2025).

25. Loebig, W. F. (2020). Nurse anesthetists' perceptions and use of ultrasound for epidural and spinal needle placement in obese parturient. https://deepblue.lib.umich.edu/bitstream/2027.42/156390/1/Loebig2020.pdf (accessed on 28th June 2025).
26. Ramani, K. V., Trivedi, P. & Malek, I. (2010). IIMA in healthcare management: Abstract of publications (2000–2010). https://core.ac.uk/download/pdf/6815495.pdf (accessed on 28th June 2025).
27. Mallawaarachchi, R., Pinto, V., & De Silva, P. H. D. P. (2020). Perfusion index as an early predictor of hypotension following spinal anesthesia for cesarean section. *Journal of Obstetric Anesthesia and Critical Care, 10*, 38–38. https://doi.org/10.4103/joacc.joacc_39_18 (accessed on 28th June 2025).
28. Marinelli, E., Montanari Vergallo, G., & Zaami, S. (2017). Assessing malpractice lawsuits for death or injuries due to amniotic fluid embolism. https://core.ac.uk/download/98348698.pdf (accessed on 28th June 2025).
29. McRae, J. (2018). Following epidural PCA use, do obstetric patients feel satisfied with their pain control. https://core.ac.uk/download/301292709.pdf (accessed on 28th June 2025).
30. Mills, L., O'Connor, J. C., & Valdes, J. (2022). An educational module for the utilization of sphenopalatine ganglion blocks as a treatment alternative for post-dural puncture headache: A quality improvement project. https://core.ac.uk/download/548486138.pdf (accessed on 28th June 2025).
31. Department of Anesthesia. University of Iowa. Spring 2011. https://core.ac.uk/download/18608347.pdf (accessed on 28th June 2025).
32. Nayan, A., Kumar, A. R., Prasad, A., Patil, C., Krishna Prasad, C. R., et al. (2024). Achieving surgical, obstetric, trauma, and anesthesia (SOTA) care for all in South Asia. https://core.ac.uk/download/604369984.pdf (accessed on 28th June 2025).
33. Perumal, M., Zainal Abidin, M. R. B., Gan, P. T., Krisnamurthy, N., Nagandran, E., Chua, S. K., Lim, P. S., et al. (2023). Prevalence of severe anxiety among elective caesarean section mothers and their perceived complications of anesthesia in Malaysia. https://core.ac.uk/download/599135835.pdf (accessed on 28th June 2025).
34. Potter, L. M. (2008). Spinal versus epidural anesthesia for the management of patients with preeclampsia undergoing elective or urgent cesarean section. https://core.ac.uk/download/567882393.pdf (accessed on 28th June 2025).
35. Rees, Q. (2018). Does prophylactic administration of ondansetron prior to spinal anesthesia decrease spinal-anesthesia induced hypotension in obstetric and non-obstetric patients? A literature review. https://core.ac.uk/download/346443661.pdf (accessed on 28th June 2025).
36. Skolnik, S., Ioscovich, A., Eidelman, L. A., Davis, A., Shmueli, A., Aviram, A., & Orbach-Zinger, S. (2017). Anesthetic management of amniotic fluid embolism–A multi-center, retrospective, cohort study. *The Journal of Maternal-Fetal & Neonatal Medicine, 32*, 1262–1266. https://doi.org/10.1080/14767058.2017.1404024 (accessed on 28th June 2025).
37. Such, T. (2020). Effects of intrapartum nitrous oxide use on comfort and satisfaction with the birth experience. https://core.ac.uk/download/352870167.pdf (accessed on 28th June 2025).

38. Xiao, F., Xu, W., Yao, H. Q., Fan, J., & Chen, X. (2021). A randomized double-blinded dose-dependent study of metaraminol for preventing spinal-induced hypotension in caesarean delivery. *Frontiers in Pharmacology, 12*. https://doi.org/10.3389/fphar.2021.608198 (accessed on 28th June 2025).

39. Yenter, E. (2024). Efficacy of complimentary manual therapies for labor pain management. https://core.ac.uk/download/617013176.pdf (accessed on 28th June 2025).

40. Yi, Y., Niu, B. T., Duffett, L., El-Chaâr, D., Tinmouth, A. T., Wang, T. F., & Khalife, R. (2023). Neuraxial analgesia in pregnant individuals with bleeding disorders: A comprehensive examination of obstetric anesthesia practices and outcomes. *Blood*. https://www.semanticscholar.org/paper/6a5583f47e5084f4721d0756869cc25ecc64f6bc (accessed on 28th June 2025).

PEDIATRIC ANESTHESIA

4

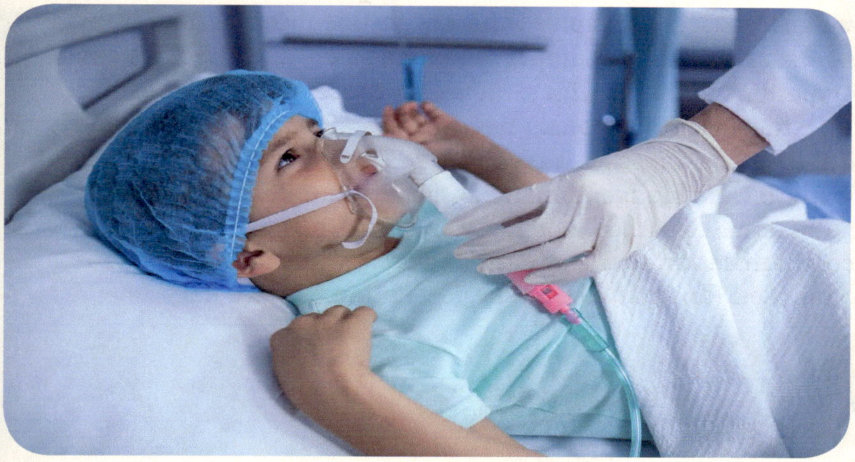

Introduction

Pediatric anesthesia is an important field of anesthesiology that is specifically crafted to address the unique physiological and psychological needs of children. With shifts in the environment of pediatric care, anesthesia practices must be adjusted accordingly to include the specific developmental considerations unique to pediatric populations. Anesthesia in children is not just scaled-down adult practice; it involves an intimate understanding of the development and pathways of rudimentary organ systems. These facts underscore the importance of training for this specialty and extensive experience in pharmacology and physiology, essential to safety and effectiveness in administering anesthesia to pediatric patients. Moreover, the growing body of literature, including studies presented in Smith and Aitkenhead's Textbook of Anesthesia, emphasizes the importance of individualized care that recognizes the wide range of medical conditions found in children, especially preoperative evaluation and treatment. Understanding the developmental biology of children is very

LEARNING OBJECTIVES

After studying this chapter, you will be able to:

1. Discuss the historical background
2. Explain the types of anesthesia used in pediatrics
3. Focus on physiological considerations
4. Know preoperative assessment
5. Understand intraoperative management
6. Explain the postoperative care

important to anesthesiologists because it has a direct influence on drug metabolism, physiological response, and potential side effects. For instance, as has been put into perspective by recent studies, including cerebral palsy (Facco & Zanette, 2017), the nature of various diseases brings to pediatric anesthesiologists an awareness of the need to grasp each child's individual health situation with a subtle approach. The interplay between the protocols of anesthesia and pediatric comorbidities, for instance, prematurity and genetic disorders, necessitates a multidisciplinary consideration so that intervention is holistic. Pediatric anesthetists must not only be technically skilled but also sensitive to the needs of children and their caregivers, so that anxiety is minimized and cooperation is maximized. This is a highly relevant factor in achieving trust and optimum patient experience for patients who are more apt to have higher fears about surgical interventions. The complexity of pediatric anesthesia highlights the importance of ongoing education and research, continuously refining techniques and results. The evidence-based principles inherent in this practice, driven by rigorous clinical studies and observations, ensure continuous improvement in safety and effectiveness. As indicated by the presence of new regulations and guidelines, including those found in texts like Smith and Aitkenhead's Textbook of Anesthesia, professionals need to remain updated with the newest developments in pharmacological care and anesthesia technology. These resources enhance the construction of a more profound body of knowledge, enhancing anesthesia delivery in many different surgical environments. Finally, effective anesthesia delivery in children is predicated on a synergy of experience, compassionate communication with patients, and commitment to continuous improvements in practices specifically tailored for this vulnerable population (Figure 4.1).

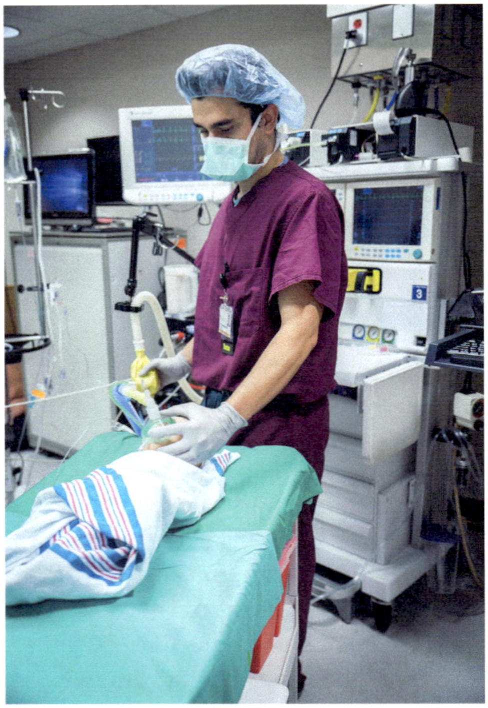

Figure 4.1. Pediatric anesthesia represents a crucial facet of anesthesiology.

Source: https://gme.medicine.uiowa.edu/sites/gme.medicine.uiowa.edu/files/wysiwyg_uploads/pediatric_anesthesia_residency_simulation.jpg.

Definition of Pediatric Anesthesia

Pediatric anesthesia is a sophisticated branch of anesthesia that addresses the unique physiological and psychological needs of infants, children, and adolescents undergoing surgical and exploratory procedures. It entails the intricacies of providing anesthesia to a population of patients that differs vastly from adults based on developmental stages, medication metabolism, and responses to anesthetic agents. The technique requires an intimate understanding of pediatric physiology, i.e., body weight factors and organ maturity, which are fundamental to determining appropriate dosages and forms of anesthesia administration. Beyond pharmacology, pediatric anesthesiologists must also confront the psychological and emotional issues, reassuring patients as well as their families throughout the perioperative process, thus making the experience less traumatic and safer for all concerned. A further level of pediatric anesthesia is the management of dental anxiety in pediatric patients, potentially with a dramatic impact on outcomes. Anxiety at the dental visit has origins in early psychological development and appears in a variety of forms, from mild apprehension to full-blown panic response, making care difficult. Pediatric anesthesiologists not only need to be well-skilled in pharmacologic choices for sedation but also skilled at applying non-pharmacologic techniques in lowering anxiety. Techniques such as iatrosedation and hypnosis are increasingly being viewed as a valuable tool, enabling practitioners to create a treatment setting with less reliance upon sedating drugs. This integrated approach is consistent with the model of holistic dentistry, focusing upon the importance of treating both emotional and physical facets of child patients who are being treated for procedures wherein anesthesia may be necessary (Facco & Zanette, 2017). Within the context of surgical operations, in pediatric cardiac surgery, the practice of enhanced recovery after surgery (ERAS) protocols becomes more relevant but is insufficient. ERAS aims to optimize recovery through the implementation of best practices in caring for the patient in preoperative, intraoperative, and postoperative phases. Though application of these principles in pediatric cardiac surgery is quite diverse, surveys conducted in recent times indicate an emerging appreciation of their relevance. Notably, a quantitative questionnaire revealed that few institutions have a formal approach to incorporating these protocols into the perioperative pathway, evidencing the potential for improvement in clinical practice (Meier et al., 2025). With the execution of ERAS protocols, pediatric anesthesiologists can maximize recovery results, minimize complications, and ultimately facilitate an easier readjustment for young patients to postoperative life, evidencing the evolving nature of pediatric anesthesia (Figure 4.2).

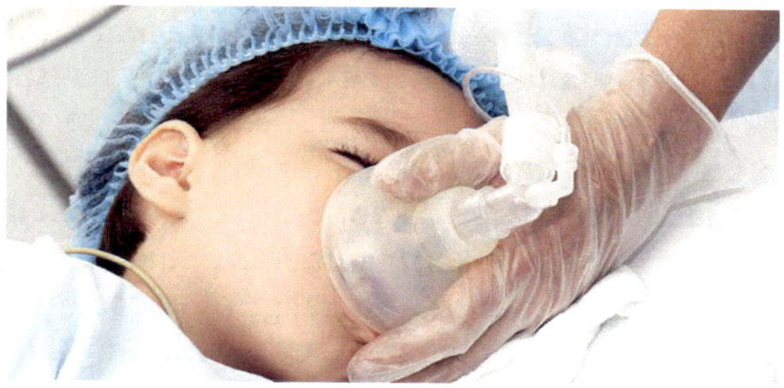

Figure 4.2. Pediatric anesthesia.

Source: https://external-content.duckduckgo.com/iu/?u=http%3A%2F%2Fanesthesiologyofmarin.com%2Fwp-content%2Fuploads%2F2016%2F07%2Fpediatricanesthesia.jpg&f=1&nofb=1&ipt=256eb5e9f93d4a74275a48a8413afd684d47b4860d982c44de69071dee650d98.

Importance in Pediatric Surgery

The role of pediatric surgery plays a critical role in the management of congenital defects and acquired medical illnesses in pediatric patients because the interventions can potentially significantly improve not only physical health but also the quality of life in pediatric patients.

Because the pediatric patient has unique anatomical and physiological characteristics, surgical procedures must be thoroughly planned and executed. Pediatric surgeons acquire the skills to adapt general surgical techniques to the unique needs of children in consideration of their smaller size, growth phase, and psychological status. This subtlety supports better clinical outcomes with fewer complications. The importance of this specialized surgical intervention is further heightened when one reviews the complex cases of medically impaired or developmentally disabled kids, as these sets of children would be more likely to require more specialized protocols for their safety and efficacy in surgery (Loyola-Rodriguez et al., 2009). Anesthesia is an important aspect of pediatric surgery, requiring a profound insight into the anesthetic process as modified to the specific physiological characteristics of children. Pediatric anesthesiologists not only ensure anesthesia administration but also ensure management of pain during and following surgery as per the special needs of pediatric patients. Due to the greater susceptibility of children to the effects of anesthetic drugs, preoperative assessment is essential. Pre-existing medical disease or undergoing intricate and lengthy procedures necessitates careful anesthetic planning and monitoring. This heightened vigilance is supported by ongoing studies into risks related to pediatric anesthesia, with the results showing that while deaths have decreased, the risk of preventable complications remains a challenge (Argo et al., 2019). Thus, an enhancement of anesthetic safety features becomes imperative in pediatric operating theaters to minimize risk. In addition, the interdependent nature of pediatric surgery and anesthesia operates to emphasize interdisciplinary collaboration. Surgeons, anesthesiologists, and nurses all must be work together so that every aspect of patient care is taken care of, from preoperative tests to postoperative care. This collaboration brings about a culture of safety where members are free to exchange ideas and concerns that facilitate tailoring care plans to each child's needs. The education from a multidisciplinary approach allows it to be possible to use of best practices that enhance surgical and anesthetic outcomes. Placing the emphasis on education and training in the identification and handling of potential surgical complications is essential. As pediatric surgery techniques and anesthesia continue to advance, ongoing evaluation of patient outcomes will remain a high priority in order to further optimize processes and protocols in pediatric surgery (Loyola-Rodriguez et al., 2009) (Figure 4.3).

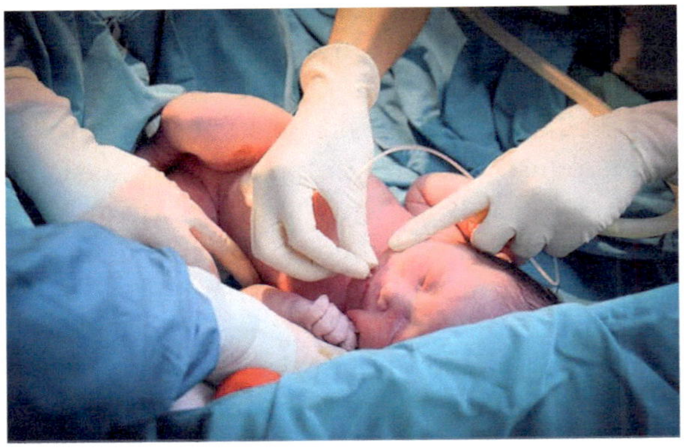

Figure 4.3. The role of pediatric surgery.

Source: https://mbpatelhospital.com/wp-content/uploads/2024/02/pediatric-surgery-card-img.jpg.

4.1. Historical Background

Learning Outcome

1. Evolution of anesthesia techniques
2. Milestones in pediatric anesthesia
3. Key figures in the development of pediatric anesthesia

The historical foundation for pediatric anesthesia is very well established in general advancements in medical practice and surgical methods in the 19th and 20th centuries. Surgery in the early times often was not afforded effective analgesia, particularly for susceptible groups such as children. It was not until the advent of general anesthesia in the mid-1800s that the trajectory of surgery truly began to shift, with the possibility of undertaking more complex interventions that were not only bearable but also safer for kids. Early anesthesia pioneers such as William Morton and James Simpson introduced ether and chloroform, respectively, to totally flip the practice on its head and extend the advantage of surgical intervention to all ages. The necessity for precision and close attention in the delivery of anesthesia to children specifically emphasized the necessity to develop distinct protocols according to their physiological and psychological needs, ensuring both efficacy and safety in what would be a growing subspecialty within anesthesiology practice. Pediatric anesthesia specialization became more evident in the mid-20th century, coinciding with increased comprehension of the distinct needs of children in a medical setting. This period saw the attitude change to recognize that children are not little adults but have their own anatomy and pharmacology that guide anesthetic management. As surgery evolved and became more complex, the need for specialized pediatric anesthetic methods was clear. Developments in drug formulations, delivery systems, and monitors followed as a consequence of this realization and resulted in pediatric anesthesia being a sub-specialty of anesthesiology. Important clinical advances involved guidelines for addressing specific challenges like airway management, calculation of doses, and recovery from anesthesia in children, which were critical to improving outcomes with this patient population and establishing a culture of safety in the operating room. Most important to the history of pediatric anesthesia is an acknowledgment of the lingering effect of unethical medical care observed during the Holocaust. The Nazi regime's notorious Tiergarten 4 project revealed the dark side of medical experimentation, as the suffering of marginalized communities was exploited in the interests of scientific research. This pernicious blot on history led to increased ethical awareness and numerous reforms in the practice of medicine post-war. As the science of anesthesiology kept evolving technologically, so too did it have to reconcile itself to the ethical lessons of history. As the practitioners honed their craft, ethical principles were used to ensure that patient interests were paramount, something that is still relevant to pediatric anesthesiology today. The creation of ethical codes and guidelines is a testament to the fact that the field has learned from the past while trying to ensure that the principles of beneficence and non-maleficence are paramount when treating pediatric patients (Argo et al., 2019).

4.1.1. Evolution of Anesthesia Techniques

The evolution of anesthetic techniques has significantly influenced the complexion of children's care, particularly in the area of surgical intervention. The early anesthesia agents, such as ether and chloroform, although groundbreaking in their era, were not highly specific and caused significant safety concerns. Over the decades, advances in pharmacology have made it possible to manufacture more tailored anesthetic drugs that take into consideration the patient's own biology and the developmental course of a child. This trend is significant, for the metabolic rate, respiratory distress, and anatomical differences of pediatric patients necessitate a more delicate level of anesthesia. Furthermore, the advances that have just occurred in monitoring technology provide for the direct observation in real time of pediatric patients' vital signs during procedures, improving safety and efficacy in pediatric anesthesia and paving the way toward an increasingly advanced practice prioritizing the outcome of the patient over the operative situation itself. The addition of new imaging technologies has also played a pivotal role in the evolution of anesthesia for pediatric populations, particularly in the management of complex cases that are usually associated with congenital heart disease (CHD). According to Ntsinjana et al. (2011), the application of cardiovascular magnetic resonance (CMR) has improved diagnostic and treatment alternatives for CHD patients among children. This technology not only provides accurate 3D anatomical images but also assesses physiological data, invaluable in the creation of multi-dimensional anesthesia plans. New anesthetic practices must adapt to these technological innovations, such that anesthesia is not simply a procedural adjunct, but a part of the preoperative and postoperative continuum of care. The combination of advanced imaging and anesthesia solidifies the trend towards a multidisciplinary approach, enhancing understanding and management of pediatric pathologies and enhancing anesthesia techniques to keep pace with contemporary clinical practice. Similarly, handling the complexities of difficult airways in children necessitates an ever-evolving approach to the techniques employed in the use of anesthesia. Pediatric patients are unique due to anatomical variations and conditions that make airway management complex. As discussed in Łepiket al. (2024), a keen understanding of such complexities lends itself to tailor-made approaches that combine traditional practices with emerging technologies. Current practices also utilize advanced airway devices and pharmacologic interventions tailored specifically for pediatric needs. All these developments are complemented by multidisciplinary team management such that appropriate management is addressed from initial assessment through the postoperative period. This progress not only enhances the quality of care during the instant moment but also reduces complications, demonstrating the necessity for ongoing research and refinement in pediatric anesthetic techniques to maximize safety and effectiveness in an ever-changing medical landscape (Figure 4.4).

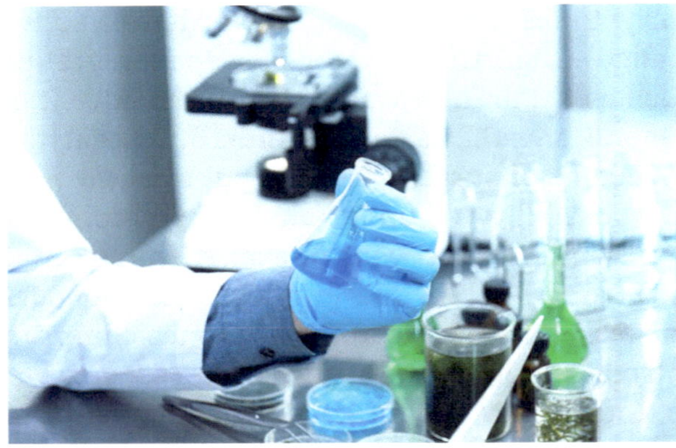

Figure 4.4. The evolution of anesthesia techniques.

Source: https://external-content.duckduckgo.com/iu/?u=https%3A%2F%2Fdrbrianblick.org%2Fwp-content%2Fuploads%2F2023%2F02%2Fpexels-photo-2280571.jpeg&f=1&nofb=1&ipt=ccdca61f0859c18152e85e262e02394b87f4c622e70577cf97677377d45a061e.

4.1.2. Milestones in Pediatric Anesthesia

Pioneers in the area of pediatric anesthesia have been marked with extraordinary breakthroughs that have greatly improved patient outcomes. The historical progress has been marred by problems, as children's physiological and psychological responses to anesthesia are very different from those of adults. Anesthesia in children at the beginning has often been accompanied by severe morbidity and mortality rates, primarily due to inadequate knowledge of pediatric anatomy and pharmacology. Over time, the recognition of these differences initiated the development of specialized anesthetic techniques and protocols to significantly enhance both safety and efficacy. As an illustration, the development of neuromuscular blockers and dosing techniques by age has facilitated more targeted management during surgery, ultimately resulting in increased recovery times and reduced complications. This kind of redirection in practice is typical of ongoing commitment to innovations focusing on the specialist needs of the pediatric patient. Yet another milestone area of interest in pediatric anesthesia is the use of multimodal analgesia (MA) as an essential foundation for perioperative pain management. MA, which targets numerous pain pathways at once, provides additive or synergistic pain relief and decreases opioid dependence with its association with adverse effects and addiction. Bibliometric analysis spanning 2013 to 2023 illustrates a crescendo of research on MA, confirming an epoch change in understanding pain management within pediatrics. The USA, China, and Canada have led among the most prominent nations, with contributions coming through key players, with their contribution further enforcing the acknowledgment of analgesic modality combinations. The growing body of evidence, including that which pertains to ERAS protocols, is in support of practice that includes individualized analgesic modalities more congruent with the holistic care of pediatric groups (Jiang et al., 2025). Furthermore, progress in the advancement of anesthetic devices and monitoring technologies is a critical milestone in the history of pediatric anesthesia. There have been remarkable developments across decades in child-tailored anesthesia delivery systems. Among the developments are reduced and precise dosing devices, advanced monitoring devices, and advancements in airway management equipment. Such developments not only render anesthetic administration more secure but also provide clinicians with the technology required to monitor patients' vital signs efficiently during procedures. The continuous advancement of apparatus, as well as enhanced understanding of pediatric pharmacology, has significantly contributed to reducing the risk of intraoperative complications. Through the focus on age-related medical technologies that cater to the unique physiological requirements of children, pediatric anesthesia practice continues to evolve, contributing to better surgical outcomes and enhancing the overall experience of children undergoing treatments (Kerby, 2022).

4.1.3. Key Figures in the Development of Pediatric Anesthesia

The development of pediatric anesthesia has been influenced directly by visionaries whose advancement and wisdom have informed practice today. Dr. Virginia Apgar was one such visionary whose work contributed to the assessment of newborn well-being in a meaningful way. Her Apgar Score, first created in 1952, revolutionized how clinicians monitor infants at and near birth, and influences pediatric anesthesia indirectly by assuring that anesthetic management sensitized to neonates is safe as well as effective. Apgar's focus on newborn physiological and behavioral responses has influenced anesthetic guidelines for pediatric patients, since familiarity with the unique considerations of this group became essential in creating anesthesia. Her presentation of her score system highlighted the importance of specialized care models that generate improved patient outcomes in pediatric anesthesiology and surgery. Dr. Alan C. H. Tan is another prominent figure in pediatric anesthesia. For his efforts in furthering research on pharmacological properties of anesthesia in pediatric patients, Dr. Tan has endeavored to learn about differences among adult and pediatric patients regarding drug dosing, safety, and efficacy. By employing rigorous studies on the unique metabolic profiles of children, he has fostered a sophisticated model for anesthetic techniques tailored for pediatric patients. His findings have been used in the development of guidelines that benefit anesthesiologists to provide safer, more personalized care during surgery. Through his campaign, Dr. Tan has brought into focus the crucial need for ongoing education and training in pediatric anesthesia, thereby ensuring that newer generations of practitioners in anesthesia are properly equipped with the right knowledge and skills. Moreover, Dr. Charles H. W. Wright's work supported pediatric anesthesia principles even further. By his work in implementing safe anesthesia practices on children at the earliest possible ages, he contributed considerably to minimizing surgical procedure-related risks. By pointing out the importance of monitoring and making precise alterations to anesthesia techniques based on the child's physiologic responses, Dr. Wright contributed to ensuring the practice was more precise and effective. The application of highly specialized equipment suited to pediatric applications under his guidance has enabled consistent provision by anesthesiologists of care sensitive to the unique anatomical and physiological dimensions of children. In conjunction with the achievements of Dr. Apgars and Dr. Tan, Dr. Wright's work itself demonstrates collaborative growth of pediatric anesthesia, once again emphasizing the multidisciplinary approach to improving pediatric surgical care outcomes (Figure 4.5).

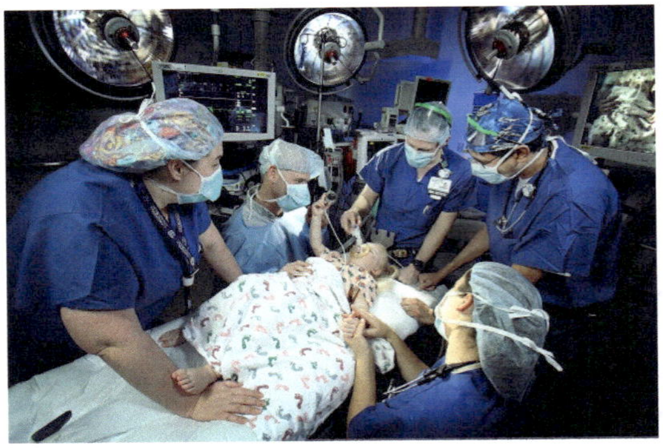

Figure 4.5. Key figures in the development of pediatric anesthesia.

Source: https://external-content.duckduckgo.com/iu/?u=http%3A%2F%2Fanesthesiology.hopkinsmedicine.org%2Fwp-content%2Fuploads%2F2016%2F07%2FPediatricFELLOWSHIPGirlDownMaskOnInOR.171820166.jpg&f=1&nofb=1&ipt=7731aa1972fb71d99c2040edd37c7757173a13d3407c347a28a43798959ad0ce.

Test Your Knowledge

1. What are the common types of anesthesia used in pediatric patients?
2. How does pediatric anesthesia differ from adult anesthesia in terms of technique and considerations?

4.2. Types of Anesthesia Used in Pediatrics

Learning Outcome

1. General anesthesia
2. Regional anesthesia
3. Sedation techniques

In pediatric anesthesia, various modes of anesthesia are employed in an attempt to make children comfortable and secure while undergoing surgical procedures. General anesthesia is also among the key modes that are applied with the patient being in a reversible state of unawareness. This mode is very effective for lengthy procedures or for surgical operations that induce a great deal of anxiety among children. Inhalational anesthetic administration, commonly in conjunction with intravenous anesthetics, allows for quick recovery and induction. The pediatric anesthesiologist must exercise utmost caution in analyzing the individual risk factors of each child, including age, history, and physical status, to tailor the anesthetic regimen suitably. The subtlety of cases in pediatrics often demands a team effort to realize optimum outcomes with a minimum of potential complications arising from anesthesia in children. Regional anesthesia is also a critical component of pediatric anesthesia, providing focal analgesia with low systemic exposure to anesthetic agents. Techniques such as nerve blocks and spinal anesthesia are commonly used in the ambulatory setting so that children can recover quickly and have less pain postoperatively. For instance, a postoperative regional block can significantly reduce the demand for opioid analgesics, thus reducing the risks of opioid exposure in children.

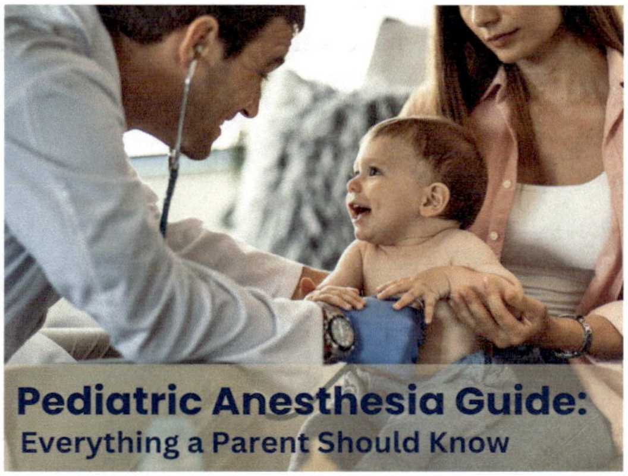

Figure 4.6. In pediatric anesthesia, several types of anesthesia.

Source: https://drapoorvakulkarni.com/wp-content/uploads/2023/12/Pediatric-Anesthesia-Guide-Everything-a-Parent-Should-Know-Dr.Apoorva-Kulkarni.jpg.

Regional application of anesthesia is crucial to interventions such as orthopedic and abdominal surgery, where pain control is essential during recovery. Further, regional success is widely marketed through various interventions, including the utilization of non-drug interventions such as Clown Doctors, which may help in minimizing anxiety among children and their parents undergoing surgery (Arriaga & Pacheco, 2016). In addition to general and regional anesthesia, sedation techniques are also valuable in pediatric anesthesia care, particularly in outpatient surgery. Sedation can range from superficial to deep, based on the type of procedure and the child's level of anxiety. Oral, intranasal, or intravenous sedatives employed allow practitioners to manage anxiety sufficiently while they administer patient cooperation and immobility for various diagnostic or therapeutic procedures. Research illustrates how the measurement of child behavior and cooperation is useful in establishing appropriate levels of sedation, for example, in caregiver and provider belief measurement (Staines, 2019). By observing the child's reaction to sedation cautiously and making proper adjustments to procedures, anesthesiologists are able to improve the overall process in the treatment of children, contributing heavily to improved surgery results and patient satisfaction (Figure 4.6).

4.2.1. General Anesthesia

In pediatric anesthesia, the application of general anesthesia involves utmost care owing to its special implications on younger patients. General anesthesia is particularly needed when working with children with a high degree of behavioral problems, making traditional procedures insufficient. For instance, non-cooperative patients, such as young children under four years old, may require a general anesthetic since they cannot be taught to cooperate during procedure time, hence posing a higher risk of complications if sedative techniques were employed alone. According to one study, general anesthesia is required for ASA III or higher children, again pointing to the importance of preoperative assessment to ensure safety and success in treatment for such vulnerable populations (da Silva et al., 2015). Pediatric dentists have to deal with these cases, and familiarity with the specifics of general anesthesia provides a foundation for achieving maximum patient outcomes while ensuring the highest standards of care. Choosing between general anesthesia and conscious sedation normally hinges on the individual character of pediatric patients, i.e., how developed they are and the nature of their specific illness. Conscious sedation can be effective in anxious or needle-phobic children since it offers a more managed form of pain and distress management. General anesthesia, nonetheless, can become a necessity in cases related to individuals with special needs or neurodevelopmental disorders that have poor communication skills, and those showing hyperemesis reflex (da Silva et al., 2015).

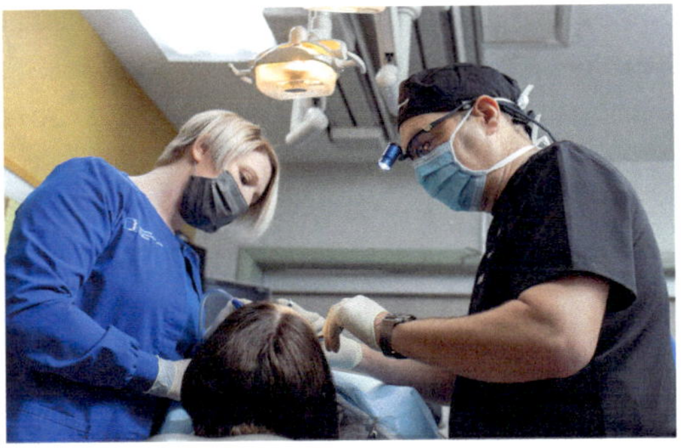

Figure 4.7. The application of general anesthesia.

Source: https://external-content.duckduckgo.com/iu/?u=https%3A%2F%2Fwww.aosillinois.com%2Fwp-content%2Fuploads%2F23-0308-Peoria-103-1024x683.jpg&f=1&nofb=1&ipt=db7c3ceb840174da5fe805a6937b24837f01cb1fe76b086fd55670ae584dc0c2.

This is a critical differentiation; it puts the onus on clinicians to be well aware of indications and contraindications for both modalities, which will ultimately guide choices regarding the safest and most efficient means of rendering dental care to children. As controversy surrounding pediatric anesthesia continues to evolve, concerns regarding the neurodevelopmental impact of general anesthetics have emerged as subjects of study and clinical concern. Recent literature has indicated that opioid-sparing interventions and regional anesthesia modalities can dampen some of the side effects traditionally associated with general anesthesia. This advancement demonstrates a decrease in the use of general anesthesia towards safer practice that aims at the long-term developmental outcome of pediatric patients. An awareness of the potential risk of general anesthesia coupled with an investigation into alternatives enables pediatric anesthetists to make informed decisions in the best interests of their patients. Continuing research into the effectiveness and safety of these approaches is essential, keeping the practice evolving with new information and enhancing the quality of care for children receiving surgery and dental treatment (Figure 4.7).

4.2.2. Regional Anesthesia

Regional anesthesia is now an important pediatric skill in the field of anesthesia, providing localized pain relief for most types of surgery. By anesthetizing part of the body instead of giving general anesthesia, the procedure eliminates systemic side effects and can lead to faster recovery times for kids. Regional anesthesia in pediatrics has been advocated through the expanding evidence base for its efficacy and safety relative to the conventional techniques. It also provides postoperative analgesia, which can dramatically enhance the quality of the experience for both parents and patients. This approach is particularly valuable in children's pain control during procedures such as hernia repair or limb procedures, where regional control is of great benefit to comfort and satisfaction post-procedure. Trending and evaluating regional anesthesia development is relevant in maximizing pediatric care and outcomes in clinical practice (DEPARTMENT OF ANESTHESIA, UNIVERSITY OF IOWA, 2011). Additionally, improvements in ultrasound technology have significantly revolutionized the administration of regional anesthesia, particularly in children. Ultrasound-guided techniques enhance the accuracy and efficacy of nerve blocks, which play a critical role in optimal pain management. Ultrasound allows anesthesiologists to visualize target nerves and surrounding structures, greatly reducing risks associated with blind techniques. Pediatrics, where anatomical variations can render routine anesthetic techniques challenging, benefits from ultrasound as a useful tool, enhancing safety and efficacy. Additionally, the real-time monitoring of local anesthetic distribution leads to clinicians receiving immediate feedback, thus improving the chances for successful anesthetic blockage. This breakthrough in regional anesthesia is vital to improving pediatric anesthetic care, reducing the trauma of procedures and increasing comfort for young patients (Angelo & Polyvios, 2018). The psychological impact of effective regional anesthesia on children should not be minimized since it quiets fear and worry traditionally associated with operations. Children are most afraid of needles and intrusive interventions that could undermine their willingness to undergo necessary treatments. Less intrusive techniques, such as regional anesthesia, address not only physiologic pain but also psychological distress. Its positive feedback of reduced pain and improved recovery results can instill confidence in the medical environment for children. Moreover, regional anesthesia's predominance over some of the more minimally invasive dental procedures emphasizes its suitability and effectiveness in most fields of medicine, such as dentistry. In conceptualizing child-centered practice in medicine, the successful application of regional anesthesia is a pivotal aspect of planning constructive healthcare outcomes for children (DEPARTMENT OF ANESTHESIA, UNIVERSITY OF IOWA, 2011) (Figure 4.8).

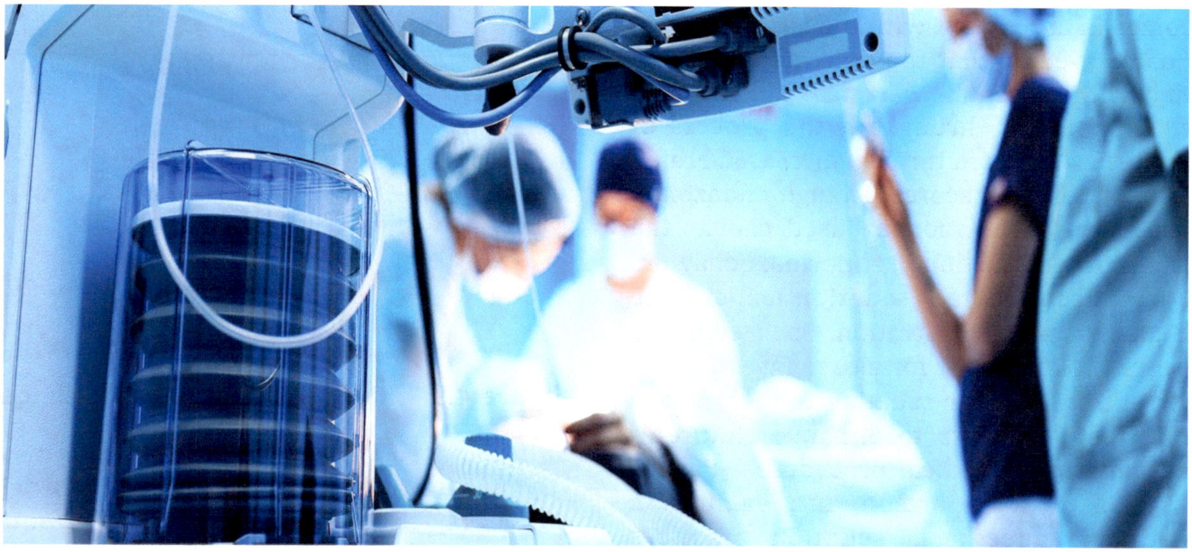

Figure 4.8. Regional anesthesia has emerged as a crucial technique in pediatric anesthesia.

Source: https://www.upstate.edu/anesthesiology/images/headers/header-pediatric-anesthesiology-home-1.jpg.

4.2.3. Sedation Techniques

The choice of sedation techniques under pediatric anesthesia plays a vital role in the treatment outcome as well as comfort of the child patients undergoing medical interventions. Among all the drugs utilized, benzodiazepines—diazepam and midazolam—are extensively studied to be very effective in reducing pain and anxiety during dental procedures. A randomized study assessing the combination of diazepam, meperidine, and hydroxyzine showed that the regimen with diazepam achieved a higher success rate than with midazolam. There was a significant difference found in Houpt sleep scores, which might suggest that diazepam does result in a less stressful postoperative experience for children who are treated in dental clinics. Thus, the application of diazepam as a component of sedation regimens can be central to enhancing patient satisfaction, even with continued scrutiny of its longer-term implications (Henderson, 2019). Further research into sedation practices confirms the importance of customization to individual patient requirements, particularly in children. A crossover pilot trial of oral sedation compared with hydroxyzine and meperidine, facilitated by either diazepam or midazolam, emphasized prominent behavioral outcomes in agreement with the sedative drug. The data revealed that the patients who were treated with diazepam were less anxious and more cooperative throughout the process of treatment, as reflected through increased Frankl and Houpt behavior scores. Though midazolam has been the conventionally used choice, the results show a reduction in abnormal behaviors and enhanced overall sedation experience with diazepam administration. Such evidence supports the argument for closer investigation of current practice for sedation to incorporate more effective agents to enhance children's preparedness for medical procedures (Parikh, 2017). Lastly, comparison and evaluation of pediatric anesthesia sedation practices emphasize further research to validate results and enhance patient care. While studies illustrate potential advantages in the utilization of diazepam, such as shorter recovery times and improved behavior with therapy, practice norms need to continue evolving based on empirical findings. Future research will have to employ larger sample sizes and diverse pediatric populations to identify determinative benefits of specific regimens of sedation. Furthermore, continued monitoring post-procedure remains important to control any adverse reactions and maintain the well-being of sedated children. Through the emphasis on evidence-based care and clinician feedback, the practice of pediatric anesthesia is able to enhance practices centered on both safety and comfort, with the trend moving towards improved outcomes for pediatric patients (Parikh, 2017; Henderson, 2019) (Figure 4.9).

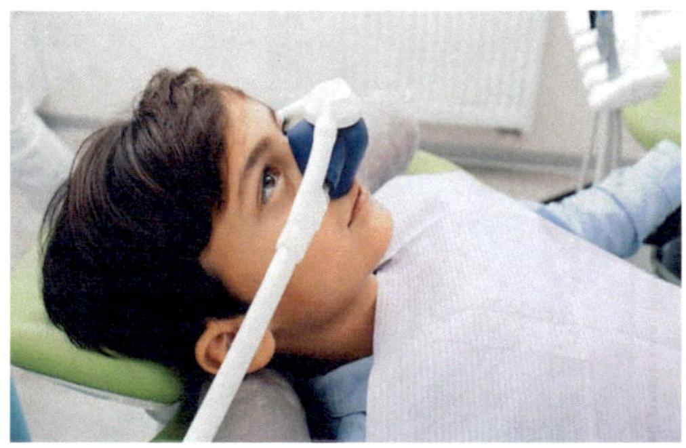

Figure 4.9. The choice of sedation techniques.

Source: https://www.joyfulsmilespediatricdentistry.com/3-commonly-used-dental-sedation-techniques-for-pediatric-dentistry/

Test Your Knowledge

1. Which types of anesthesia are commonly used in pediatric surgeries?
2. Why is general anesthesia more frequently used in children compared to regional anesthesia?

4.3. Physiological Considerations

Learning Outcome

1. Differences between pediatric and adult physiology
2. Drug metabolism in children
3. Impact of age on anesthetic choice

In pediatric anesthesia administration, a number of physiological factors are considered to maintain the efficacy and safety of the procedure. Children's anatomy and function differ from those of adults, affecting their pharmacokinetics and pharmacodynamics. For instance, the body surface area-to-volume ratio in children is much greater, which affects drug distribution and metabolism. Furthermore, drug clearance and organ system maturation, particularly of the liver and kidneys, are critical considerations in this context. Failure to understand them appropriately can lead to insufficient or overdosing, which causes side effects or inadequate anesthesia during operations. Clinicians must be experienced with age-related residual effects and clinical responses to anesthetics, which may differ substantially from those in adults, and hence require specialized pediatric anesthesia management techniques. Pain management is another important aspect of pediatric anesthesia, given the prevalence of pain caused by procedures in children. Lumbar punctures and bone marrow aspirations cause pain in children, and they impose significant physical and psychological distress (Liossi, 1999). Therefore, adequate assessment of pain and pain management strategies needs to be given due attention. Pharmacological interventions can include local anesthetics, conscious sedation, or general anesthesia, depending on the level of complexity of the procedure and the requirements of the individual child. Also essential are non-pharmacologic interventions—such as preparation, cognitive-behavioral therapy, and hypnosis—that can significantly alleviate anxiety and augment the child's perception of pain. A multi-modal strategy to pain management is essential, as it optimizes the child's experience and limits potential long-term psychological consequences associated with painful procedures. Dental anxiety (DA) control is another key concern in pediatric anesthesia. DA can have a profound impact on interfering with children's desire to receive necessary treatments, potentially leading to dental avoidance and overall risk for oral pathology (Facco & Zanette, 2017). Understanding the source of this fear, which can be linked to the fight-or-flight response, is crucial in the development of effective coping strategies. Interventions are most often a mixture of communication measures, such as preparation and information-provision, followed by pharmacological options, such as sedation when warranted. However, the role of non-pharmacological interventions such as hypnosis and iatrosedation cannot be ignored. These interventions can endow children with the ability to handle anxiety better and enable them to progress through dental treatment independently in the future. Comprehensive knowledge of physiological and psychological aspects of caring for pediatric anesthesia is essential for a satisfactory patient outcome and a good healthcare experience for the child patient.

4.3.1. Differences Between Pediatric and Adult Physiology

The physiological difference between children and adults is substantial, demanding special attention in pediatric anesthesia. The major difference is located in the cardiovascular system, with children and infants having an increased heart rate and reduced systemic vascular resistance as compared to adults. The result is reduced stroke volume with altered cardiac output dynamics, and hence, hemodynamic stability must be closely observed by anesthesiologists. Furthermore, the immaturity of the neonatal cardiovascular system can also further complicate anesthesia care with a high predilection toward hypotension and bradycardia. Understanding these cardiovascular differences is critical to the application of anesthetic drugs and techniques to pediatric care for successful and safe perioperative management. Apart from cardiovascular differences, respiratory physiology also shows significant differences between children and adults. Children have a higher metabolic rate, proportionally equivalent to greater oxygen demand and carbon dioxide production. They have smaller, more compliant airways that are more susceptible to obstruction and reactive airway disease. These facts necessitate modifications in airway management practice, including the utilization of appropriate endotracheal tube sizes and modes of ventilation. In addition, the use of noninvasive monitoring equipment has become inevitable in pediatric anesthesia, as indicated by advancements like near-infrared spectroscopy (NIRS), which offers real-time tissue oxygenation of regional tissues and can help in forecasting critical values like the anaerobic threshold in potential stress situations (Rao et al., 2012). Another significant factor in anesthesia is the management of thermoregulation among pediatric patients, particularly neonates and infants. With their larger surface area-to-volume ratio and less developed thermoregulatory mechanism, children are much more susceptible to hypothermia under the operation. Such susceptibility requires preventative approaches such as the use of warming devices and careful monitoring of core body temperature to prevent perioperative morbidity. In addition, the physiological response of anesthetic agents may be different between the adult and pediatric patient, with the latter eliminating some drugs faster, hence necessitating altered dosing regimens. An awareness of such differences not only optimizes anesthetic practice but also optimizes patient safety and outcomes in pediatric patients (Drucker et al., 2019) (Figure 4.10).

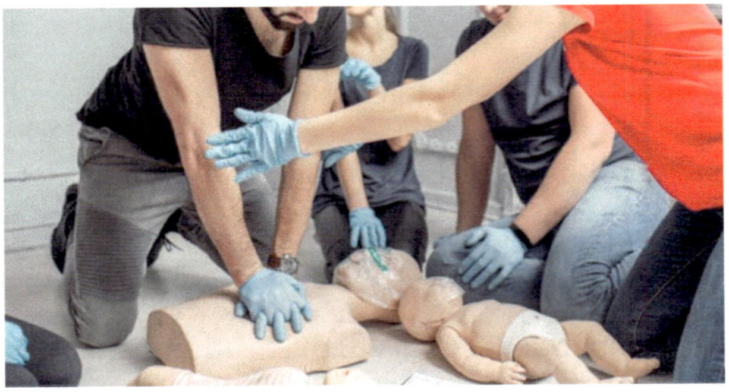

Figure 4.10. The physiological differences between pediatric and adult patients.

Source: https://cpraedcourse.com/wp-content/uploads/2023/08/Understanding-differences-between-adult-and-pediatric-cpr-post-img.webp.

4.3.2. Drug Metabolism in Children

The metabolism of drugs in children presents unique challenges that are distinctly different from adults and have a direct impact on pediatric anesthesia practice. Drug metabolism is the biotransformation process that changes pharmacologic substances into more water-soluble compounds for elimination. In children, particularly the neonate, these processes are still immature, and therefore, there is heterogeneity of drug clearance rates by age and developmental stage. This ontogeny influences the pharmacokinetics of anesthetic drugs and demands accurate dosing adjustments for the administration of effective anesthesia with minimal risks of toxicity. It must be noted that the metabolic pathways in children rise immensely during development, influencing the safety and efficacy of anesthetics with the course of time. Therefore, a proper understanding of ontogeny is critical for anesthesiologists to tailor anesthesia practice appropriately for children and provide the optimal perioperative outcome. Pharmacodynamics, or the effect of drugs on the body, also varies significantly in children compared to adults. As identified by recent studies, there is a considerable lack of information as to how children metabolize anesthetic drugs like propofol. Even though propofol pharmacokinetics in children have been well characterized, problems concerning their relative sensitivity and peak effect timing in this patient group remain mostly unsolved. The complexities involved in measuring drug effects during anesthesia, compounded by the practical limitations of existing monitoring equipment designed for adult subjects, introduce an additional layer of complexity into pediatric anesthesia care. It is thus crucial that medical professionals remain vigilant and well-informed about these differences to prevent potential adverse effects. The absence of standardized target-controlled infusion parameters for children complicates individualized anesthesia plans, highlighting the necessity for specialized pediatric pharmacological investigation. In addition to varying metabolic processes, children's physiologic differences are also likely to increase the risk of complications from anesthesia. Children have been found to have elevated perioperative cardiac arrest compared to adults, and this is most likely due to a wide range of different factors that include age, comorbid conditions, and the nature of the surgical procedure children are receiving. In particular, the majority of incidents occur during induction and maintenance of anesthesia and are usually followed by complications like bradycardia or hypotension. Recognition of such risk factors is essential to improve patient outcomes, as cardiac arrests tend to occur with no apparent prior signs. An understanding of the specific factors resulting in such critical events is essential to further design safety protocols in pediatric anesthesia and formulate adequate preventive measures. More training and alertness are essential in the fight against such challenges to decrease risks associated with children's anesthetic practice, mirroring the necessity of continued research in this crucial area of pediatrics.

4.3.3. Impact of Age on Anesthetic Choice

The influence of age on anesthetic choice in children is a subtle aspect of pediatric anesthesia care with a marked effect on patient outcome. Children are younger and have different physiological attributes than adults, such as increased metabolic rates and shifted pharmacokinetics, necessitating altered anesthetic regimens. These bodily differences may affect agent selection; for example, agents such as sevoflurane and desflurane, which are volatile anesthetics with a high onset and recovery profile, are often employed because of their rapid onset and recovery. The knowledge of age-related changes in drug metabolism and effect is of paramount importance, for poor selection may result in undesirable outcomes or complications, especially in susceptible groups like neonates and infants. The selection of appropriate anesthetic medications and techniques is most critical to ensure both efficacy and safety, requiring research that examines age as an important variable in pediatric anesthesia. With advancing age in pediatric patients, anesthetic selection has modifying effects. For instance, intraoperative management of older children has different problems and considerations. Age-related variations in the pharmacodynamics of anesthetic agents and in psychological factors in children undergoing surgery influence the variables in emergence agitation, a state of disorientation with alteration of behavior following anesthesia. Drugs like desflurane have been identified in the literature to produce quicker emergence but potentially higher rates of emergence agitation than sevoflurane (LaLande, 2008). This constitutes a vital consideration; the choice of anesthetics not only impinges on the clinical markers of recovery but also on the psychological well-being of patients who are children. The clinicians thus need to trade off pharmacological properties against behavioral outcomes while making decisions on anesthetics, affirming that age is a critical factor in anesthetic practice. In addition, understanding the impact of age on anesthetic choice extends to some anatomical and developmental features inherent in pediatric patients. For example, variations in the physiological and anatomical makeup of younger children necessitate careful consideration of airway management techniques and anesthetic delivery methods. Quoted in recent literature, the application of erythrocyte concentrates was linked with reduced recurrence-free survival in pediatric surgery for cancer, underlining the role of anesthetic and ancillary management in age-based interventions (Müller et al., 2024). Consequently, the meaning of anesthetic choice cannot be divorced; it involves an intricate interaction with the child's developmental stage and the entire surgical regimen. The developing evidence underscores the importance of child-focused anesthetic planning, with the understanding that age is more than a demographic feature but a pivotal determinant in modulating safe and efficacious anesthesia provision in children (Figure 4.11).

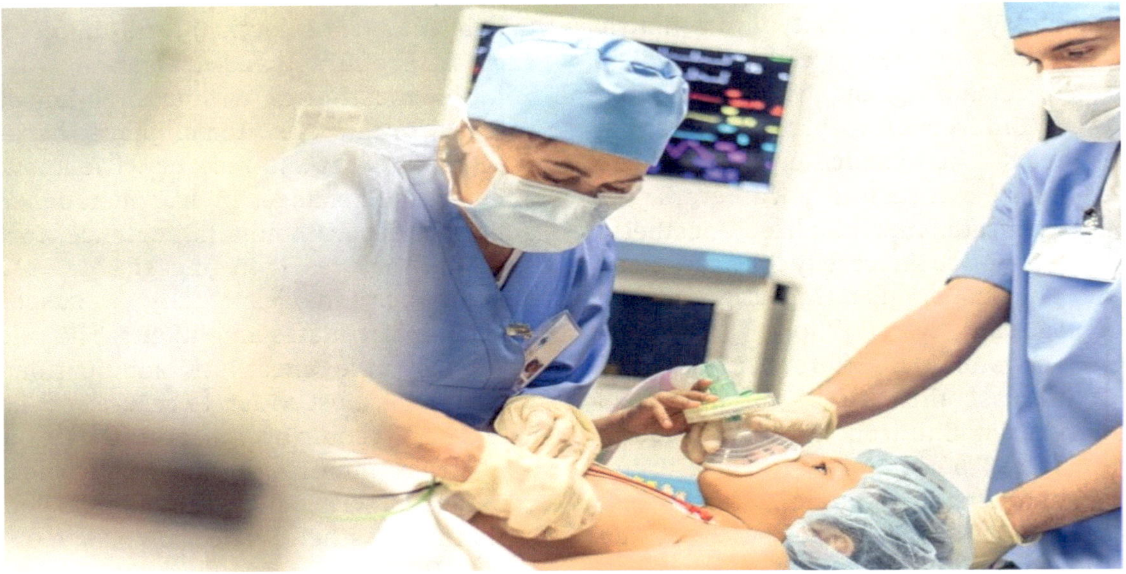

Figure 4.11. The relationship between age and anesthetic choice in pediatric patients.

Source: https://radiusanesthesia.com/wp-content/uploads/2024/11/pediatric-1024x684.jpg

Test Your Knowledge

1. How does respiratory function differ between pediatric and adult patients?
2. Why are drug dosages different for children compared to adults?

4.4. Preoperative Assessment

Learning Outcome

1. Importance of medical history
2. Evaluation of anesthetic risks
3. Parental involvement in preoperative planning

Preoperative assessment in pediatric anesthesia is a critical aspect that has a direct bearing on the safety and effectiveness of surgical procedures. Preoperative assessment consists of an overall examination of the child's past history, including associated conditions and those risks associated with anesthesia. Effective preoperative assessment is required to identify any abnormalities that might complicate anesthetic conduct. In addition, having a thorough concept of the child's development stage allows communication methods to be structured in a personalized way, thereby reducing anxiety and promoting cooperation. Consistent with current evidence, successful innovations in preoperative assessments have led to improved patient safety practices, as evident in many healthcare organizations (McCarthy & Blumenthal, 2006). These proactive measures not only make contributions to risk evaluation but also to the end surgical results by ensuring that both the medical and psychological needs of child patients are met prior to the procedures. An integral part of preoperative evaluation is preoperative anxiety, which is a typical condition among child patients. Literature reveals that preoperative anxiety has multiple deleterious effects, such as longer postoperative recovery and increased pain perceptions (Stant, 2025). To prevent these, it is crucial to integrate methods to decrease anxiety levels before surgery. It is possible to use tools like the modified Yale Preoperative Anxiety Scale to measure pediatric patients' levels of anxiety efficiently. In most cases, the pharmacologic interventions, such as administration of midazolam or dexmedetomidine, are employed to pre-emptively decrease anxiety and ease the surgery. How these concerns are addressed during the preoperative evaluation is paramount to ensuring that children not only tolerate a minimum of distress but also achieve maximal postoperative benefit. Moreover, the implementation of evidence-based guidelines in the preoperative assessment process is crucial in ensuring practice standardization among pediatric surgical centers. Most of the hospitals today lack sufficient protocols that reflect the multi-factorial aspect of anxiety among children, and hence variability in care (Stant, 2025). Using well-established frameworks, such as the Iowa Model, research can be incorporated into practice so that healthcare providers are provided with the most current knowledge and techniques. Clarity in such a procedural process is essential to enhance the quality of care provided to pediatric patients. Lastly, an orderly preoperative evaluation protocol not only reinforces the principles of patient safety but also underscores the intention of improving the overall experience in pediatric surgery in laying the course towards a more efficient conduct of anesthetic procedures.

4.4.1. Importance of Medical History

Appreciation of the importance of medical history in pediatric anesthesia is essential in ensuring safe and successful treatment. Accurate medical history includes knowledge of the child's past illnesses, surgery, and known drug or anesthetic allergy. This helps anesthesiologists assess potential risks and tailor anesthesia plans as appropriate. Additionally, various physiologies of children patients, particularly neonates and infants, call for a sensitive approach wherein pre-existing medical histories can play a significant role in their responses to anesthesia. This is an example of how detailed medical histories are not just paperwork; they are blocks that enhance decision-making phases with pediatric anesthesia protocols that ultimately minimize risks associated with anesthesia administration. Deeper still, the psychological and emotional aspects of a child's medical history must not be disregarded. History is more likely to reveal experiences that have the potential to shape a child's attitude toward medical procedures, including hospital visit-related trauma in the past. Medical personnel must be able to recognize these elements to maintain a trusting relationship with the patient and the patient family. For instance, if a child has had traumatic procedures or has been restrained during prior treatment, awareness of these prior experiences can assist anesthesiologists in making efforts to reduce anxiety and distress when administering anesthesia.

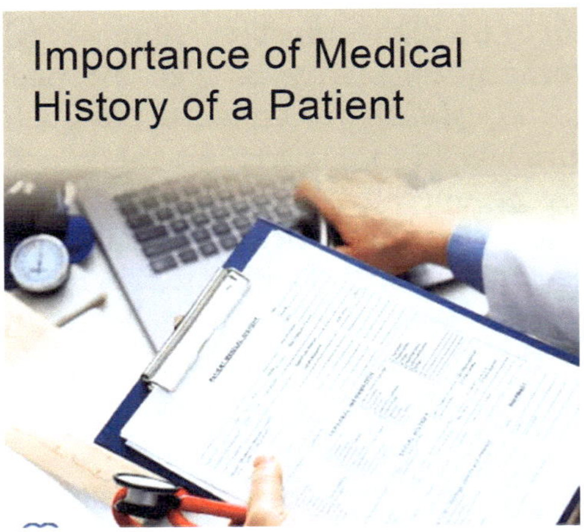

Figure 4.12. The importance of medical history in pediatric anesthesia.

Source: https://cdn-idoej.nitrocdn.com/krDFdMpwQAiOpICINhUhPAQgVbVPdUND/assets/images/optimized/rev-b15f48f/www.ambula.io/wp-content/uploads/2023/09/Screen-Shot-2023-09-28-at-21.58.13-400x399.png.

By valuing children's experiences and hearing their voices actively, as suggested by Bray et al. (2014), health professionals are able to increase compliance and satisfaction and thus have better outcomes for pediatric anesthesia. Furthermore, the ethical issues attendant to the handling of pediatric patients' histories are deep. It is not only the role of healthcare providers to acquire accurate information but also to ensure that information is conveyed in a child-sensitive manner. Literature reaffirms that the rights of children should be honored, such as hearing them and engaging them in decision-making around their care, and this is particularly relevant when it comes to prior medical history (Bray et al., 2014). A good medical history is not just a clinical tool; it is a basis for ethical decision-making. It gives strength to patients and families to be heard and influence treatment protocols. This combined response ultimately ensures pediatric anesthesia practice becomes aligned with ethical standards, raising overall quality of care for young patients (Figure 4.12).

4.4.2. Evaluation of Anesthetic Risks

Pediatric cases call for a nuanced understanding of patient health records, particularly when distinguishing between healthy and medically sick children. It has been proven that healthy children can require sophisticated procedures under general anesthesia with longer procedure time corresponding to greater anesthetic exposure. For instance, a study had revealed that normal children needed a median operating time of 161 minutes compared to 84 minutes for medically compromised or developmentally disabled children, a contrast in danger profiles and therapeutic needs as stark as it was (Loyola-Rodriguez et al., 2009). This differentiation necessitates an acute attention to baseline health status, as these variables will influence both the choice of anesthetic medications and the techniques employed to exclude risk in treatment. As more general anesthesia finds its way into pediatric dentistry, understanding these differences is critical in the development of effective safety protocols. When scheduling the administration of anesthetic medications, risks inherent in some medications must also receive careful consideration. Different anesthetic drugs have varying profiles regarding efficacy, safety, and side effects, commonly with disproportionate adverse effects on children. For example, ropivacaine and tetracaine local anesthetics have been established to be effective analgesic agents with minimal systemic effect when applied for short procedures like intravitreal injections (Pacella et al., 2015). This highlights the potential of individualized approaches to guarantee patient comfort and minimize side effects associated with deeper levels of anesthesia. Interestingly, the anesthetic technique to be used should also consider not only short-term effectiveness but also long-term implications, especially in at-risk categories like children with chronic illness. Secondly, the need for continuous monitoring under anesthesia cannot be overemphasized, given that children are at the highest risk of developing procedure-related complications. Due to their physiological variations from the adult patient, children require extra care of their vital signs and physiological reactions to anesthesia. The quality of anesthetic techniques must be weighed against the potential to manage intraoperative alterations promptly and effectively. Anesthesiologists must be prepared to reverse any unwanted effects that occur, demanding a comprehensive risk assessment process with preoperative assessment and ongoing real-time monitoring during the procedure. This alertness is important in ensuring that the benefits of surgery outweigh risks from anesthetics, thereby safeguarding pediatric patients' health in various clinical settings.

4.4.3. Parental Involvement in Preoperative Planning

Appropriate parental involvement in preoperative planning is critical in pediatric anesthesia since it can effectively minimize anxiety among children and parents before surgery. Preparing the family for the process of surgery involves thorough education on the upcoming operation, information about anesthesia, and postoperative care. Research shows that when parents are properly informed, they can support their children better, hence helping to decrease the level of preoperative anxiety (Yahya Al-Sagarat et al., 2017). Moreover, interventions using therapeutic play and interactive methods greatly enhance the readiness of the parents and children. These tactics pave the way for families to be open with healthcare professionals, enabling parents to bring up any concerns and be more educated about preparing their kids for surgery. Not only does this joint action boost family's comfort level, but also an atmosphere that makes kids feel safer and better educated when they undergo surgery. Besides psychological preparation, factors of operation, such as preoperative fasting instructions, are crucial during preoperative planning. Parents should be educated on the necessity for adherence to fasting regimes because prolonged NPO durations could evoke anxiety and have adverse health outcomes in children. A recent experiment revealed that preoperative education of parents on phone calls in advance significantly reduced average NPO times for infants undergoing outpatient surgery, indicating parental contribution to the best condition (Ward et al., 2023). Encouraging parents to encourage compliance with fasting orders can help healthcare workers advance best practices while ensuring consideration for safety. This initial awareness allows the parents to be active participants in their child's preoperative care so that both the child and the health team have an easier experience overall. Lastly, the healthcare professionals' ability to make effective parent involvement throughout the preoperative process possible is most critical. Nurse practitioners and other healthcare professionals are in a good position to establish a culture of parental involvement that enables them to access the resources and assistance to be actively involved in their child's care. Such collaboration is instrumental in ensuring optimal preoperative experience as it renders parents more active, not merely informed, with improved surgery outcomes (Yahya Al-Sagarat et al., 2017). Treating the individualized needs of parents with targeted educational programs enhances confidence and effective parent-advocacy abilities in parents, thereby decreasing preoperative anxiety. Through promoting a team-based approach, pediatric healthcare teams can enhance the psychosocial preparation of families to lead to an improved surgical experience and better recovery pathways in pediatric patients (Figure 4.13).

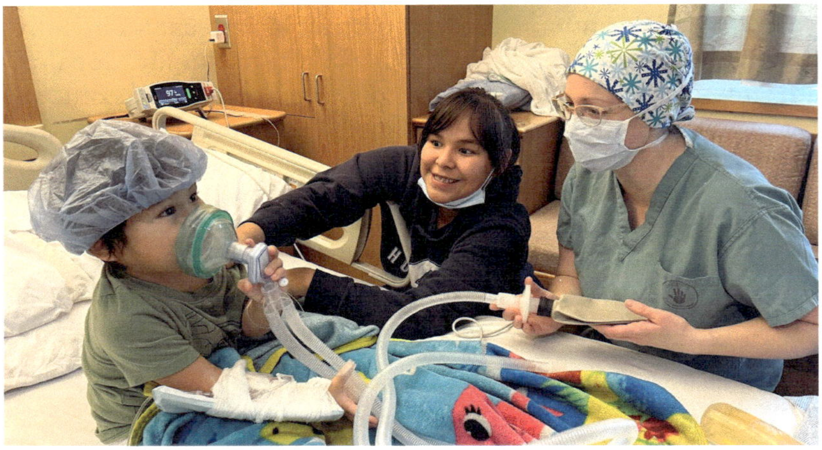

Figure 4.13. The parental involvement in preoperative planning is crucial in pediatric anesthesia.

Source: https://media.oralhealthgroup.com/uploads/2023/02/1a-1-e1675365018428.jpg.

Test Your Knowledge

1. How does drug metabolism differ in neonates, infants, and older children?
2. Why does age influence the selection and dosage of anesthetic agents in pediatric patients?

4.5. Intraoperative Management

Learning Outcome

1. Monitoring techniques for pediatric patients
2. Anesthetic administration protocols
3. Handling emergencies during surgery

Pediatric intraoperative care under anesthesia is a critical field that demands careful attention to the physiological as well as psychological needs of the child patient. Anesthesia providers must adapt their strategies depending on the age, weight, and general health status of the child, which necessitates careful preoperative assessment. Preoperative assessment enables planning for potential complications and selecting appropriate anesthetic agents. Besides, effective communication amongst the surgical team and between the caregiver and provider also increases a sense of safety for the parents and the child. Incorporating child-centered techniques, such as preoperative education and distraction, can efficiently minimize preoperative anxiety and thus enhance the overall experience and outcome of the operation. Intraoperative monitoring plays an important role in ensuring the optimal degree of patient safety and anesthesia effectiveness. Constant vigilance is required to detect any change in vital parameters, which may become a precursor to developing complications such as hypoxia or hemodynamic instability. Intraoperative monitoring technologies of today can provide real-time feedback, facilitating anesthesia personnel to make appropriate decisions on time. Secondly, knowledge of the idiosyncratic pharmacodynamics and pharmacokinetics of anesthetic agents in children is important, as children metabolize and respond to drugs differently than adults. These differences necessitate a dynamic anesthetic depth control and fluid management during surgery to offer individualized care suited to the child's needs. A crucial aspect of intraoperative care is the scientific assessment of factors that would compromise the safety of the patient, especially in complex surgical settings. Literature highlights the importance of the identification of human factors that could lead to complications in pediatric surgery. By integrating holistic safety interventions and frequent monitoring of such interventions, teams can significantly reduce the incidence of near misses and unintended complications during the procedure. The fluid working environment of the operating room necessitates ongoing training to enhance teamwork and communication between the medical teams. As emphasized by current evidence, ongoing and regular assessment of performance and safety practice plays a crucial role in improving intraoperative management skills in pediatric anesthesia, ultimately leading to enhanced patient outcomes and improved safety in this susceptible population (Schraagen et al., 2009; DEPARTMENT OF ANESTHESIA, UNIVERSITY OF IOWA, 2011).

4.5.1. Monitoring Techniques for Pediatric Patients

For pediatric anesthesia, appropriate monitoring techniques are the key to patient safety and achieving optimal outcomes from operations. Because of the unusual physiological characteristics of children, particularly anatomical and metabolic factors that distinguish them from adults, monitoring becomes mandatory. Children's vital signs, such as heart rate and breathing patterns, are variable, necessitating tailored methods with unique monitoring equipment. Advanced technologies such as pulse oximetry and capnography are applied consistently to follow oxygen saturation and exhaled carbon dioxide, respectively. These non-invasive monitoring techniques enable anesthesiologists to rapidly identify potential complications and adjust anesthesia plans accordingly. Continuous monitoring not only addresses immediate concerns but also results in reduced postoperative complications, thereby improving the overall experience and safety in children receiving anesthesia. The incorporation of transcutaneous carbon dioxide monitoring ($PtcCO_2$) is one example of an accurate method for enhancing the validity of respiratory screening in children. One investigation into the correlation between $PtcCO_2$ and arterial carbon dioxide pressure ($PaCO_2$) has shown promising results, indicating that $PtcCO_2$ can be a valuable ancillary tool. This modality offers real-time monitoring of carbon dioxide levels throughout procedures, particularly laparoscopic surgery, where physiologic alterations can quickly take place due to factors like pneumoperitoneum. In the study, the results offered a close relationship between $PtcCO_2$ and $PaCO_2$ values, validating the utilization of $PtcCO_2$ in standard monitoring protocols. These findings suggest that $PtcCO_2$ could increase the process of anesthesia management of pediatric patients, enhancing clinical decision-making and patient safety during operation (Wang & Argalious, 2023). Furthermore, the management of possible difficult airways in pediatric anesthesia is relevant when addressing monitoring practices. Anatomical differences in children pose peculiar challenges to them, which complicate airway management and predispose them to serious complications. In-depth comprehension of the etiology of difficult pediatric airways—both acquired and congenital—is enhanced through increased competency in the ability to predict emergencies among anesthesiologists. Interventions may involve the use of advanced airway devices, thorough evaluation, and multidisciplinary team care to optimize patient care. Monitoring needs to be continuous during and after airway intervention, as real-time observation of respiratory status is made available, hence timely intervention for complications such as hypoxia or airway trauma. Through emphasizing close watchfulness, in such cases, clinicians are able to minimize risk and provide better patient outcomes for pediatric patients under anesthesia (Lepik et al., 2024) (Figure 4.14).

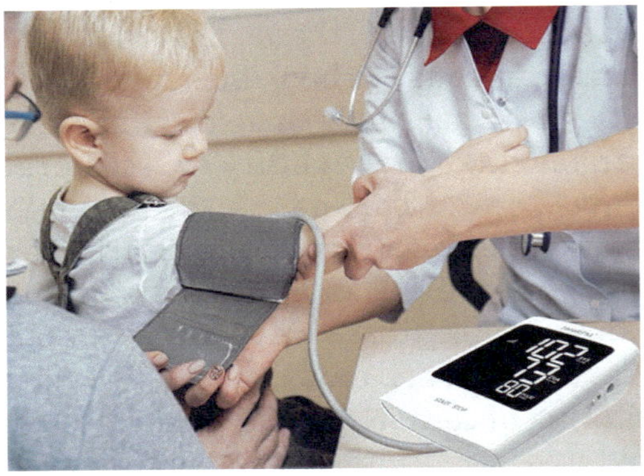

Figure 4.14. Monitoring Techniques for Pediatric Patients.

Source: https://www.transtekcorp.com/uploads/image/20240523/17/ensuring-accuracy-in-blood-pressure-monitoring-for-children-small-arm-circumference-solutions.webp.

4.5.2. Anesthetic Administration Protocols

Pediatric anesthesia administration demands strict protocols specific to the special physiological and psychological demands of children. In contrast to adults, children exhibit different degrees of anxiety and behavior, which can enormously influence the ease of cooperation during procedures. Therefore, uniform protocols need to be formulated to evaluate and treat these behavioral issues effectively. For instance, the use of behavior assessment tools, e.g., the Frankl Scale, may enable us to comprehend a child's temperament during dental treatment. One study evaluated the interrater agreement among dental providers, caregivers, and children in their ratings of cooperative behaviors and found 81% agreement among guardians and children but lower agreement with providers. This is an indicator of the all-encompassing role of behavior assessment in coming up with policies on anesthetic administration that prioritize the comfort and safety of the child during treatment (Staines, 2019). Additionally, such anesthetic administration policies ought to incorporate training health staff on emergency procedures for anesthesia-related complications. In child patients, in particular, risk from local anesthetic systemic toxicity (LAST) calls for cautious approaches that adopt precautionary protocols. The American Society of Regional Anesthesia and Pain Medicine is supportive of establishing a set of emergency guidelines documenting signs and therapies specific to LAST. A training session conducted within a rural hospital established that such training is possible, with substantial improvement in the knowledge and confidence of the providers to deal with LAST emergencies among the health professionals. By utilizing a grab-and-go LAST emergency response bag, medical professionals will be more likely to respond on time, with resultant improved patient outcomes. Utilization of these guidelines is essential not just for the prompt attention but also for developing a culture of safety in pediatric practice settings (Vaughn, 2024). The integration of optimal anesthetic practice into pediatric anesthesia is more than mere procedural compliance; it fosters a safe and trusting culture. Awareness of the psychological dimensions of anesthetic administration is paramount. By having an awareness of children's behavior patterns and proactively involving guardians during administration, anesthetic routes can be fine-tuned to achieve maximum experience This collaborative approach can prevent anxiety and assist in the development of a therapeutic relationship between the child, guardian, and medical staff. Routines that are established according to the child's stage of development and consistent communication assist in making sure each pediatric patient receives maximum care and attention. Overall, the combination of effective behavioral assessments with emergency readiness protocols can lead to a general anesthetic strategy that combines safety with comfort in pediatric anesthesia (Staines, 2019; Vaughn, 2024).

4.5.3. Handling Emergencies During Surgery

For pediatric anesthesia, emergency control within surgery is of critical value to ensure patient safety and success. The pediatric patient often presents special difficulties due to their dissimilar anatomy and physiology compared to adults. These differences require the acquisition of expertise and skill by surgical teams and anesthesiologists in responding to potential emergencies effectively. Emergency situations, such as respiratory compromise, cardiovascular instability, or anaphylactic shock, require immediate and decisive action. Adequate coordination among the anesthesia and surgical teams, adhering to standardized protocols, can minimize the risk of such emergencies. Moreover, monitoring of physiological parameters in real-time and the use of state-of-the-art technology can facilitate early detection of adverse occurrences so that timely intervention can be planned. Adequate planning and training in emergency response management are therefore central to pediatric anesthesia practice, ensuring that clinical teams are ready to deal with crises. Beyond this, open lines of communication between surgical teams can be a critical issue in managing emergencies during surgery. In the highly stressful environment of the operating room, clear and effective communication could easily prove the difference between a successful intervention and a disaster. All staff need to be sensitized to one another's roles and responsibilities, promoting a team ethos. During emergencies, the swift sharing of information regarding the patient's status, responses to treatment, and any alteration in vital signs is essential. In addition, simulation training exercises can play a pivotal role in preparing staff to handle emergencies, allowing them to practice reactions and build a mutual understanding of their roles. Ultimately, communication and teamwork culture in the operating room optimizes the capacity to handle emergencies, a natural part of pediatric anesthesia.

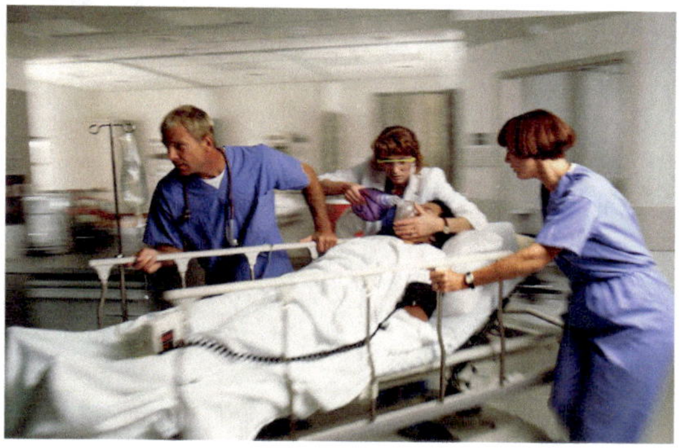

Figure 4.15. The ability to handle emergencies during surgery.

Source: https://www.verywellhealth.com/thmb/RbpigLVedvZy9mjtwUne4I-AoRY=/1500x0/filters:no_upscale():max_bytes(150000):strip_icc()/GettyImages-AB28669-1b5e340f5a0f4bc8b47f3e3b5902ccf8.jpg.

Utilization of non-physician anesthesia practitioners, such as nurse anesthetists, has become a strategy to enhance emergency handling for surgical patients, particularly in poor-resource settings. Research indicates that well-designed training schemes can produce capable nurse anesthetists who can deliver safe anesthesia care, as evidenced by Médecins Sans Frontières in Haiti, where such professionals played a crucial role in responses to surgical emergencies following disasters (Rosseel et al., 2009). Being able to train and integrate non-physicians into surgical teams not only increases capacity but also the diversity of skills for use in emergencies. Having trained nurse anesthetists present can help relieve some of the pressure on anesthesiologists, enabling them to concentrate on more complicated cases while assuring that emergency needs are addressed. This role of supportive assistance allows for enhanced overall efficiency in pediatric anesthesia, thus promoting patient safety and outcomes during operations (Figure 4.15).

Test Your Knowledge

1. What is the main goal of intraoperative management during surgery?
2. Why is continuous monitoring important during the intraoperative period?

4.6. Postoperative Care

Learning Outcome

1. Recovery room protocols
2. Pain management strategies
3. Long-term effects of anesthesia in children

Post-anesthetic care in pediatric anesthesia is crucial for ensuring the safety and well-being of pediatric patients following a surgical procedure. The recovery from the operating room to the recovery room after general anesthesia is most critical. The child's response to anesthesia may vary with age, weight, and current state of health. The monitoring will generally include assessment of vital signs, oxygen saturation, and response. Constant observation throughout this period is crucial since pediatric patients are at an increased risk of postoperative complications such as respiratory distress and hypoxia. A pediatric sedation review highlighted that the interaction of anesthetics can affect recovery times, with certain regimens of recovery within a shorter time while remaining safe, with the importance of having tailored postoperative care regimens to obtain the best possible outcomes and improve patient satisfaction (Ahmed et al., 2016). Management of pain is a key focus area of pediatric postoperative care. Given the heightened sensitivity to pain that occurs in children, health care providers must utilize age-appropriate pain assessment and medication management. Multimodal analgesia is the most guideline-recommended approach, wherein several classes of medications are combined to gain the greatest amount of pain control while limiting the possibility of side effects. For instance, the addition of drugs such as ketamine has been reported to reduce the total quantity of anesthetic drugs required, thus potentially resulting in reduced recovery times and better overall outcomes (Ahmed et al., 2016). Additionally, the existence of an extensive pain control regime post-surgery increases the likelihood of uneventful recovery experiences for children, fostering physical rehabilitation and emotional stability during their recovery process. Moreover, the influence of parental involvement in the postoperative care of children cannot be exaggerated. Parents and guardians must be entrusted with the task of identifying signs of distress and communicating them to health professionals effectively. The presence of a familiar person and reassurance can significantly reduce children's stress following surgery. Educational programs for parents regarding expectations of the postoperative period, pain control, and educating healthcare workers on potential complications can enhance the level of quality of care rendered. Hospital-parent collaborations also highlight best practices and disparities in access to postoperative care, particularly in low- and middle-income nations where surgery is less accessible. By prioritizing the key role of family in postoperative convalescence, health professionals are able to support children and their families during the recovery process with confidence and ease.

4.6.1. Recovery Room Protocols

Pediatric anesthesia recovery room protocols are significant in ensuring the safety and well-being of children following surgery. Protocols are designed to keep important signs such as vital signs, pain adequately controlled, and assessing the child's recovery from anesthesia closely. Throughout this period, clinicians follow a structured pattern that entails continuous assessment of oxygen saturation levels, heart rate, and respiratory function. Correct documentation of these parameters helps detect any complications in the early stages and enables timely interventions. The aim is to turn patients over from the anesthetic effect to full consciousness smoothly without posing a risk of harmful events like hypoxia. Age-specific assessment equipment used ensures that the health care providers can tailor recovery regimes according to the child patients' developmental needs to ascertain safety and effectiveness in this vulnerable treatment phase. Due to recent advances in sedation techniques, the recovery room guidelines may include adjunct medication to facilitate recovery. For instance, the inclusion of ketamine in a sedation protocol has been demonstrated to reduce recovery time without compromising safety (Ahmed et al., 2016). By allowing combinations of medications through protocols, clinicians can tailor the depth of sedation and enhance the postoperative experience for children. Comparative studies suggest that optimal control of the recovery room reduces complications and significantly improves patient satisfaction. Individualized recovery planning considering elements of age, the type of surgery, and prior health status can be useful. Understanding the drug interactions during recovery is critical to further enhance pediatric anesthesia recovery room practice. Further, healthcare provider participation in the recovery room cannot be overstated. Professionally qualified staff who can manage pediatric patients' unique issues create a comforting environment that maximizes the recovery process. For instance, coping strategies through timely and reassuring engagement ensure mental well-being, given that children develop anxiety after surgery (Balatero, 2018). Multidisciplinary intervention makes sure not just physical but also emotional needs are catered to in the recovery process. By establishing an atmosphere of reassurance and security, medical professionals can significantly influence the child's overall perception of their operative experience. Therefore, regular training and adherence to recovery room protocols are crucial to achieving improved outcomes in pediatric patients undergoing anesthesia (Figure 4.16).

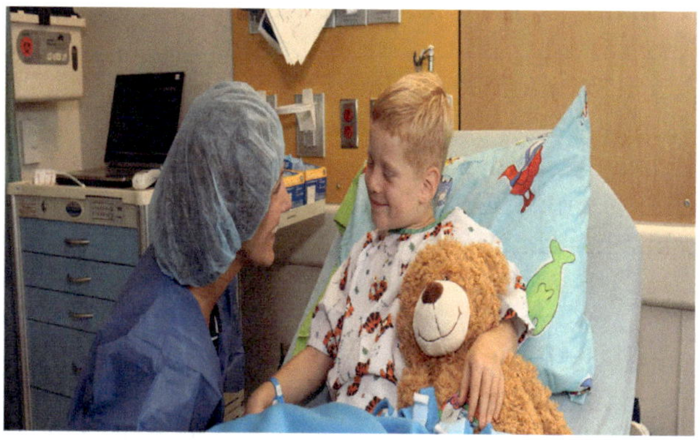

Figure 4.16. Recovery room protocols.

Source: https://www.pennstatehealth.org/childrens/services-treatments/anesthesia

4.6.2. Pain Management Strategies

Maximum pain control in children is necessary, particularly in cases of anesthesia, as inadequate pain control can cause immediate distress and long-term adverse psychological effects. Traditional methods of pain control, such as opioids, are often accompanied by a host of undesirable side effects like sedation and respiratory depression. Due to these complications, newer modalities such as regional anesthesia have gained popularity. For instance, thoracic epidural analgesia has been explored as a method of decreasing overall opioid requirements with substantive pain relief. Recent studies have demonstrated that in children with low-grade spina bifida who are undergoing lower urinary tract reconstruction, thoracic epidural placement significantly decreased opioid consumption (and had consistent pain levels), which implies the efficacy and safety of thoracic epidural as a pain control method in pediatric anesthesia (Roth et al., 2018). Along with regional methods, the psychological component of pain management must also be addressed, particularly in children who have pre-existing neurodevelopmental disorders like autism spectrum disorder (ASD). Children with ASD can present with difficult-to-manage behaviors when in pain, leading to less-than-optimal care experiences. Research has also indicated that integration of parent partnerships in developing individualized strategies can enhance such issues, with the child being offered timely and best pain control while minimizing distress (Johnson & Rodriguez, 2013). Strategies such as distraction, utilization of visuals, and creating a soothing environment can assist in optimizing the management of pain in pediatric patients with ASD. By bridging the difference between hospital care and the unique behavior of children with ASD, healthcare professionals can maximize overall effectiveness in pain management. Finally, the use of multimodal analgesia (MMA) has been a key tactic in pediatric pain management, wherein numerous analgesic drug classes have been used for the optimal control of pain and prevention of unwelcome opioid use. This technique may involve the addition of NSAIDs, acetaminophen, and regional anesthesia methods, effectively treating pain through different mechanisms. Through the use of MMA, health care providers can deliver effective analgesia without increasing risk for adverse opioid sequelae, an important consideration in pediatrics. The hope is that it will allow for the creation of individualized pain control regimens based on each patient's specific characteristics, e.g., age, history, and individual surgical outcomes. The present research into the effectiveness of such various methods sheds light on the worth of new methods to provide effective pain relief in pediatric anesthesia and then advance post-operative recovery and quality of life in pediatric patients.

4.6.3. Long-term Effects of Anesthesia in Children

The use of anesthesia in pediatric patients has also been well studied to establish whether it has long-term effects on children's cognitive and behavioral development. Research has established that exposure to general anesthesia during periods of brain development can increase the likelihood of neurocognitive disorders, influencing a child's ability to learn and behave in life. Research indicates that long-term changes in neuronal connectivity and synaptic plasticity, induced by anesthesia exposure, may underlie these cognitive deficits. Although the specific mechanisms are still very much under scrutiny, beginning to clarify such potentialities is critical to guiding clinical practice. As such, child anesthesiologists must weigh the immediacy of surgical intervention against the possible long-term consequences of anesthesia, showing both the immediacy of care needed and the long-term health of child patients. Compounding the challenge of this question is the growing body of literature exploring how age, anesthesia time, and type of procedure may all contribute to the long-term effects seen in children after anesthesia. Children three and under appear particularly vulnerable since their brains are undergoing significant development during this period. There have been studies demonstrating that repeated exposures to anesthesia have associations with higher risks of developmental disorders like ADHD and learning disabilities during later life. Conversely, there have been reports stating that less invasive techniques of anesthesia can potentially lower such risks. With progressive advances in anesthetic techniques, continuous research is required to assess the interaction of these variables intensively, thus presenting more distinct conclusions to respond to improvements in pediatric surgical procedures and anesthesia care. To make sure pediatric anesthetic practices are based on the most optimal results, it is vital to institute rigorous preoperative testing and monitoring following operations. The incorporation of formal pain management programs, as outlined by groups such as the European Society for Pediatric Anesthesiology (ESPA), dictates that a consideration be made for short-term pain as well as for the potential long-term effects of anesthesia on children's health. Interventions, including the employment of interventions to reduce levels of anxiety during surgery, can reduce children's and caregivers' levels of stress, which is essential in the context of anesthesia. Furthermore, evidence supporting preoperative clown interventions shows that enhancing the emotional environment of surgery has a positive influence on postoperative recovery experiences and, in turn, long-term health outcomes in children (Arriaga & Pacheco, 2016). With this as context, continued focus on more integrated practice in pediatric anesthesia can optimize care while remaining mindful of the long-term impact on cognitive as well as emotional development (Figure 4.17).

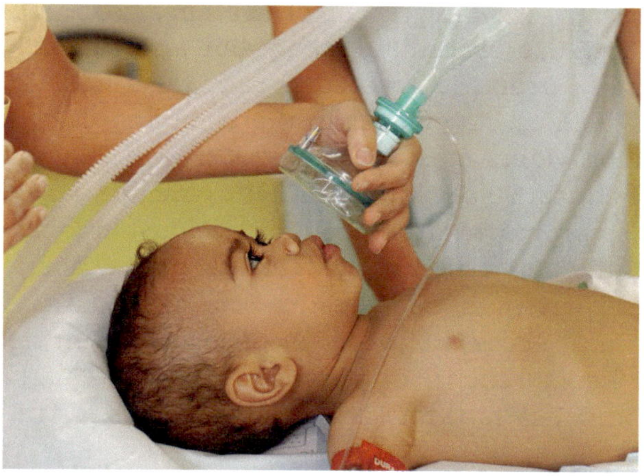

Figure 4.17. Long-term effects of anesthesia in children.

Source: https://theanesthesiaconsultant.com/wp-content/uploads/2018/07/am_150605_child_anesthesia_800x600.jpg.

Test Your Knowledge

1. What are the essential components of immediate postoperative care?
2. Why is monitoring vital signs important in the postoperative period?

Summary

Pediatric anesthesia is a highly evolved specialty that demands both clinical acumen and an ethical framework sensitive to the unique needs of children. Anesthesia delivery to pediatric patients necessitates thoughtful consideration of their physiological differences, psychological requirements, and the potential impact of procedures upon their developing bodies and minds. As the evidence indicates, children tend to become upset in therapeutic settings, often exacerbated by methods of restraint or holding them during therapy. This is an expression of an ethical predicament that arises from the effort of healthcare providers to reconcile the nature of emergent medical procedures with the imperative of maintaining children's rights. Yet, if things are not addressed in the right manner, then they might have long-term effects on trust within the health system and ultimately affect a child's overall well-being and inclination to use medical services in the future, as suggested by some reviews (Bray et al., 2014). Moreover, the need for continuous research and discussion on the subject cannot be overstated. The evolving attitudes of pediatric patients and anesthesia-induced reactions to them highlight the imperative necessity for evidence-based care encompassing medical efficacy and moral integrity. For instance, recent studies report a critical necessity to inform caregivers regarding the potential harms of extended breastfeeding and its association with oral health disorders in children, like early childhood caries (ECC) (Dean et al., 2018). These situational observations put more emphasis on interdisciplinary collaboration between pediatric healthcare areas to address both anesthesia procedures and the broader impact on children's health holistically. An integration of evidence from multiple studies can impact procedures that not only optimize procedural safety but also safeguard the psychological well-being of child patients. Finally, pediatric anesthesia calls for a holistic approach that prioritizes the voices of children and families. As evident in the emerging discourse of children's rights in clinical settings, healthcare providers must create a culture where children feel at ease and their voices heard. Integration of ethical values into anesthetic care not only decreases moral distress to healthcare providers but also promotes a therapeutic relationship founded on trust. By respecting children's autonomy within the interaction with medicine, practitioners can assist in constructing more favorable healthcare experiences, and thus ensure that results of treatment are no longer exclusively measured in clinical success but also in terms of acquiring improved quality of care and child experience. Such a comprehensive approach will set the platform for future advances in pediatric anesthesia and ultimately facilitate healthier outcomes for future generations.

The sophistication of pediatric anesthesia necessitates a detailed understanding of physiological variables and surgical intervention. One of the fundamental aspects of good anesthetic management involves knowing the unique individual physiological and developmental differences in children compared to adults. For instance, the pediatric patient's anesthetic plan needs to take into account factors such as reduced blood volume, altered pharmacokinetics, and changes in anatomy with age. These aspects highlight the importance of customized anesthetic strategies that ensure the best possible safety along with efficacy. Also, the role of preoperative investigations like hemoglobin estimation is crucial in minimizing intraoperative complications and optimizing postoperative outcomes. Incorporation of current blood-sparing modalities also emphasizes the shift towards more conservative handling strategies for pediatric surgical cases, especially in adolescent idiopathic scoliosis operations (Patel et al., 2014). Another extremely important element in pediatric anesthesia is the tendency and the process of blood loss and transfusion that occurs during and after operations. Research has shown that the use of sophisticated intraoperative blood-sparing methods can dramatically reduce the requirement for allogeneic blood transfusions and thereby improve patient safety. Through a retrospective case series of adolescents undergoing corrective spinal surgery, it was noted that a small percentage of patients needed transfusion after surgery, illustrating the effectiveness of such practices. The study pointed out a clinically significant fall in hemoglobin levels in the early postoperative period, which tends to stabilize later on. These findings validate the use of minimum preoperative hemoglobin values to ensure maximum safety in surgery. Finally, the ability to perceive and react to the trends in blood loss through physiological responses can lead to better clinical outcomes and more autonomous decision-making in pediatric anesthesia (Patel et al., 2014). The broader implications of the advances in pediatric anesthesia are also validated by ongoing collaboration among healthcare organizations. Effective safety innovations case histories are very important lessons in enhancing patient outcomes across various clinical settings. The deployment of multidisciplinary teams fosters a culture of safety that benefits both practitioners and patients. With the sharing of knowledge and experiences, organizations get to refine best practices and facilitate the adaptation of strategies that mitigate risks associated with anesthesia. These cooperative practices not only elevate the standard of care but also promote ongoing education for clinical teams, which is paramount in responding to the ever-evolving challenges in pediatric anesthesia. Through mutual ideas and recommendations, the medical community can build safer operating rooms, solidifying its dedication to excellence in pediatric care.

KEY TERMS FROM THIS CHAPTER

- Anesthesiology
- Anxiety
- Cardiovascular magnetic resonance (CMR)
- Congenital heart disease (CHD)
- Crucial milestone
- Enhanced Recovery After Surgery (ERAS)
- Hypnosis
- Iatrosedation
- Influencing anesthetic management
- Multimodal analgesia (MA)
- Orthopedic surgeries
- Pediatric anesthesiologists
- Pediatric population
- Pediatric surgery
- Pharmacological management
- Physiological

Critical Thinking Questions

1. **Which induction agent is most commonly used in pediatric anesthesia?**
   a. Thiopental
   b. Propofol
   c. Ketamine
   d. Sevoflurane
2. **What is the narrowest part of the airway in a pediatric patient under 8 years of age?**
   a. Epiglottis
   b. Glottis
   c. Cricoid cartilage
   d. Vocal cords
3. **Which of the following is a common side effect of inhalational induction in children?**
   a. Hyperthermia
   b. Laryngospasm
   c. Hypertension
   d. Bradycardia
4. **Which monitoring parameter is most sensitive for detecting apnea in a pediatric patient under anesthesia?**
   a. ECG
   b. Pulse oximetry
   c. Capnography
   d. Blood pressure
5. **Which premedication is commonly used to reduce anxiety in pediatric patients before anesthesia?**
   a. Midazolam
   b. Fentanyl
   c. Atropine
   d. Ketamine

Short Answer Questions

1. What are the main physiological differences between children and adults relevant to anesthesia?
2. What is the most commonly used induction agent in pediatric anesthesia?
3. How does a child's airway differ anatomically from an adult's airway?
4. What is the recommended dose of atropine for bradycardia in a pediatric patient?
5. What is the significance of using uncuffed endotracheal tubes in younger children?
6. How is fluid maintenance calculated for pediatric patients during surgery?

Answer to Critical Thinking Questions

1. (d); 2. (c); 3. (b); 4. (c); 5. (a)

References

1. Facco, E., & Zanette, G. (2017). The Odyssey of Dental Anxiety: From Prehistory to the Present. A Narrative Review. *Frontiers in psychology*, *8*, 1155. https://doi.org/10.3389/fpsyg.2017.01155(accessed on 28th June 2025).
2. Yahya Al-Sagarat, A., Al-Oran, H. M., Obeidat, H., Hamlan, A. M., & Moxham, L. (2017). Preparing the Family and Children for Surgery. *Critical care nursing quarterly*, *40*(2), 99–107. https://doi.org/10.1097/CNQ.0000000000000146(accessed on 28th June 2025).
3. Ahmed, N., Sheikh Sohail, R., Hedlund, M., Lauren, S., Hicks, T., Shawn, B., Nitu, C., et al. (2016). Propofol-based procedural sedation with or without low-dose ketamine in children. https://core.ac.uk/download/227054212.pdf (accessed on 28th June 2025).
4. Bray, L., Snodin, J., & Carter, B. (2015). Holding and restraining children for clinical procedures within an acute care setting: an ethical consideration of the evidence. *Nursing inquiry*, *22*(2), 157–167. https://doi.org/10.1111/nin.12074(accessed on 28th June 2025).
5. Argo, A., Buscemi, R., Karch, S. B., Lanzarone, A., Roccuzzo, R., & Zerbo, S. (2019). Perioperative and anesthetic deaths: Toxicological and medico legal aspects. https://core.ac.uk/download/224993621.pdf (accessed on 28th June 2025).
6. Arriaga, P., & Pacheco, C. (2016). Effects of clown doctors on child and caregiver anxiety at the entrance to the surgery care unit and separation from caregivers. https://core.ac.uk/download/46603912.pdf (accessed on 28th June 2025).
7. Balatero, J. S. (2018). Obstetric nurses' perceived barriers to immediate skin to skin contact after cesarean birth. https://core.ac.uk/download/159401074.pdf (accessed on 28th June 2025).
8. Jan Maarten Schraagen, Paul Barach and Josine van de Ven et al. Teams and Cardiac Surgery. 2009. DOI: 10.14236/ewic/NDM2009.14(accessed on 28th June 2025).
9. Meier, S., Borzel, J., Hellner, N., Catena, D., Beck, C. E., Schindler, E., & Kleine-Brueggeney, M. (2025). Enhanced Recovery after Surgery (ERAS) in Pediatric Cardiac Surgery: Status Quo of Implementation in Europe. *Journal of cardiothoracic and vascular anesthesia*, *39*(1), 177–186. https://doi.org/10.1053/j.jvca.2024.10.005(accessed on 28th June 2025).
10. McCarthy, D., & Blumenthal, D. (2006). *Committed to Safety: Ten Case Studies on Reducing Harm to Patients.* https://core.ac.uk/download/71350251.pdf (accessed on 28th June 2025).
11. Müller, S. D., Both, C. P., Sponholz, C., Voelker, M. T., Christiansen, H., Niggli, F., Schmitz, A., Weiss, M., Thomas, J., Stehr, S. N., & Piegeler, T. (2022). Association between Intraoperative Blood Transfusion, Regional Anesthesia and Outcome after Pediatric Tumor Surgery for Nephroblastoma. *Cancers*, *14*(22), 5585. https://doi.org/10.3390/cancers14225585(accessed on 28th June 2025).
12. Roth, J. D., Misseri, R., Whittaker, S. C., Monn, M. F., Horn, N. D., Cain, M. P., & Green, M. C. (2019). Epidural Analgesia Decreases Narcotic Requirements in Patients with Low Level Spina Bifida Undergoing Urological Laparotomy for Neurogenic Bladder and Bowel. *The Journal of urology*, *201*(1), 169–173. https://doi.org/10.1016/j.juro.2018.06.063(accessed on 28th June 2025).

13. Angelo, Z., & Polyvios, C. (2018). Alternative practices of achieving anaesthesia for dental procedures: a review. *Journal of dental anesthesia and pain medicine*, *18*(2), 79–88. https://doi.org/10.17245/jdapm.2018.18.2.79(accessed on 28th June 2025).

14. Jiang, W., Qin, Y., & Chen, L. (2025). Bibliometric analysis of multimodal analgesia research in the perioperative period: trends, contributions, and emerging areas (2013-2023). *Frontiers in medicine*, *12*, 1573112. https://doi.org/10.3389/fmed.2025.1573112(accessed on 28th June 2025).

15. Pacella F, Collini S, Turchetti P et al./ Senses Sci 2015; 2 (4):106-110 doi: 10.14616/sands-2015-4-10(accessed on 28th June 2025).

16. ŁEPIK, Michał, USZOK, Zofia, ROSIAK, Krzysztof, PŁESKA, Kacper, REGUŁA, Kacper, WALOCH, Kamil, WOJTANIA, Joanna, PIASZCZYŃSKI, Szymon, CZAJKA, Andrzej and SZYMAŃSKI , Bartłomiej. Difficult pediatric airway in anesthesia practice andfuture sport performance. Quality in Sport. 2024;18:50920. eISSN 2450-3118. https://dx.doi.org/10.12775/QS.2024.18.50920(accessed on 28th June 2025).

17. Rao, R. P., Danduran, M. J., Loomba, R. S., Dixon, J. E., & Hoffman, G. M. (2012). Near-infrared spectroscopic monitoring during cardiopulmonary exercise testing detects anaerobic threshold. *Pediatric cardiology*, *33*(5), 791–796. https://doi.org/10.1007/s00246-012-0217-8(accessed on 28th June 2025).

18. Dean, M. L., Fields, R., & Fritz, H. (2018). Got caries? Breast milk and early childhood caries? https://core.ac.uk/download/215483270.pdf (accessed on 28th June 2025).

19. Drucker NA, Jensen AR, Te Winkel JP, Markel TA. Hydrogen Sulfide Donor GYY4137 Acts Through Endothelial Nitric Oxide to Protect Intestine in Murine Models of Necrotizing Enterocolitis and Intestinal Ischemia. *J Surg Res*. 2019;234:294-302. doi:10.1016/j.jss.2018.08.048(accessed on 28th June 2025).

20. Fezeu F, Ramesh A, Melmer PD, Moosa S, Larson PS, Henderson F Jr. Challenges and Solutions for Functional Neurosurgery in Developing Countries. *Cureus*. 2018;10(9):e3314. Published 2018 Sep 17. doi:10.7759/cureus.3314(accessed on 28th June 2025).

21. Loyola-Rodriguez, J. P., Zavala-Alonso, V., Gonzalez-Alvarez, C. L., Juarez-Lopez, L. A., Patiño-Marin, N., & Gonzalez, C. D. (2009). Dental treatment under general anesthesia in healthy and medically compromised developmentally disabled children: a comparative study. *The Journal of clinical pediatric dentistry*, *34*(2), 177–182. https://doi.org/10.17796/jcpd.34.2.u665328k4g467pg2 (accessed on 28th June 2025).

22. Henderson, B. H. (2019). Comparison of triple combination oral sedation regimens for pediatric dental treatment. https://core.ac.uk/download/215487165.pdf (accessed on 28th June 2025).

23. Ntsinjana HN, Hughes ML, Taylor AM. The role of cardiovascular magnetic resonance in pediatric congenital heart disease. *J Cardiovasc Magn Reson*. 2011;13(1):51. Published 2011 Sep 21. doi:10.1186/1532-429X-13-51(accessed on 28th June 2025).

24. Johnson, N. L., & Rodriguez, D. (2013). Children with autism spectrum disorder at a pediatric hospital: a systematic review of the literature. *Pediatric nursing*, *39*(3), 131–141.(accessed on 28th June 2025).

25. Kerby, A. D. (2022). From madness to medicine: How Nazi medical experimentation morphed into today's medical field. https://core.ac.uk/download/534236610.pdf (accessed on 28th June 2025).

26. Kim, G. (2018). Impact of sensory adapted dental environment on children with developmental disabilities. https://core.ac.uk/download/215483212.pdf (accessed on 28th June 2025).
27. LaLande, C. (2008). Comparison of emergence behavior in pediatric dental patients undergoing general anesthesia with sevoflurane versus desflurane. https://core.ac.uk/download/51291258.pdf (accessed on 28th June 2025).
28. da Silva, C. C., Lavado, C., Areias, C., Andrade, D., & Mourão, J. (2015). Conscious sedation vs general anesthesia in pediatric dentistry–A review. https://core.ac.uk/download/143387708.pdf (accessed on 28th June 2025).
29. Łepik, M., Uszok, Z., Rosiak, K., Płeska, K., Reguła, K., Waloch, K., Wojtania, J., et al. (2024). Difficult pediatric airway in anesthesia practice and future sport performance. *Quality in Sport*. https://www.semanticscholar.org/paper/ca7a3743abe8dac45443ed1b3a15eb080e8a37b1 (accessed on 28th June 2025).
30. Liossi, C. (1999). Management of pediatric procedure-related cancer pain. https://core.ac.uk (accessed on 28th June 2025).
31. Rosseel, P., Trelles, M., Guilavogui, S., Ford, N., & Chu, K. (2010). Ten years of experience training non-physician anesthesia providers in Haiti. *World journal of surgery*, *34*(3), 453–458. https://doi.org/10.1007/s00268-009-0192-2(accessed on 28th June 2025).
32. Parikh, O. A. (2017). A comparison of moderate oral sedation drug regimens for pediatric dental treatment: A pilot study. https://core.ac.uk/download/84402545.pdf (accessed on 28th June 2025).
33. Patel, D. R., Neelakantan, M., Pandher, K., & Merrick, J. (2020). Cerebral palsy in children: A clinical overview. *Translational Pediatrics, 9*, S125–S135. https://doi.org/10.21037/tp.2020.01.01 (accessed on 28th June 2025).
34. Patel, D., Stephenson, J., Van Popta, D., Verma, S., et al. (2014). The pattern of blood loss in adolescent idiopathic scoliosis. https://core.ac.uk/download/30730023.pdf (accessed on 28th June 2025).
35. Staines, C. A. (2019). Perception of patient cooperation among dentist, guardian, and child. https://core.ac.uk/download/215487147.pdf (accessed on 28th June 2025).
36. Stant, W. R. (2025). Development of evidence-based clinical practice guidelines for pediatric preoperative anxiety. https://core.ac.uk/download/616421797.pdf (accessed on 28th June 2025).
37. Vaughn, R. (2024). Local anesthetic systemic toxicity: LAST protocol development, implementation, and evaluation for healthcare providers. https://core.ac.uk/download/621638204.docx (accessed on 28th June 2025).
38. Wang, M., & Argalious, M. (2020). *Smith and Aitkenhead's Textbook of Anesthesia* (7th ed., Vol. 130, e103–e104). *Anesthesia & Analgesia*. https://doi.org/10.1213/ane.0000000000004649 (accessed on 28th June 2025).
39. Wang, W., Zhao, Z., Tian, X., Ma, X., Xu, L., & Shang, G. (2023). Noninvasive carbon dioxide monitoring in pediatric patients undergoing laparoscopic surgery: Transcutaneous vs. end-tidal techniques. *BMC Pediatrics, 23*. https://www.semanticscholar.org/paper/53cf185114bd42f8150205e008c89b48a1296c65 (accessed on 28th June 2025).

40. Department of Anesthesia. University of Iowa. Spring 2011. https://core.ac.uk/download/18608347.pdf

41. Ward, J. C. (2023). Optimizing NPO times in infant outpatient surgical patients. https://core.ac.uk/download/568188831.pdf (accessed on 28th June 2025).

ANESTHESIA FOR ENT AND AIRWAY SURGERY

5

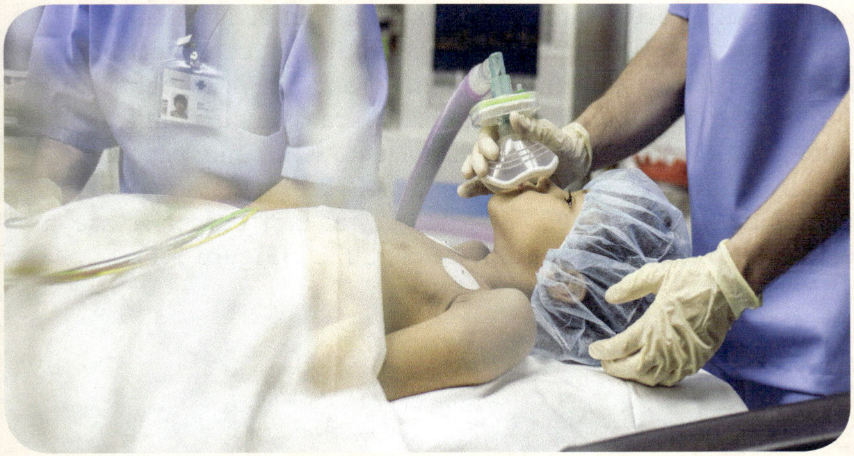

Introduction

Introduction of modern anesthetic techniques has dramatically changed the field of ear, nose, and throat (ENT) surgery. Traditionally, such surgeries were plagued with tremendous challenges considering the complexity of airway management and intraoperative complications. Against the background of recent advancements, surgeons and anesthesiologists are now operating in closer collaboration than ever before, optimizing patient advantages through better anesthesia management. Present studies indicate that as surgical knowledge advances through the shift towards less invasive surgeries, in the same way, there also appears to be a need for anesthetic practice that ensures the prevention of the dangers of bleeding and postoperative states like nausea and vomiting. The use of computer-aided navigation in such surgeries is another depiction of the impact of new technologies on anesthetic care, paving the way for precision-fine-tuned anesthetic practice in the field of patient safety and care (Salinding et al., 2022). The anesthetic management's decisive role in ENT and airway

LEARNING OBJECTIVES

After studying this chapter, you will be able to:

1. Discuss the types of anesthesia
2. Focus on preoperative assessment
3. Explain the anesthetic techniques for ENT procedures
4. Understand the anesthetic considerations for airway surgery
5. Know complications and risks
6. Learn about postoperative care

surgery cannot be overemphasized since the peculiar anatomical features of the upper airway call for specialized knowledge and skill. Anesthesia for the operations typically involves careful assessment of the patient's individual risk factors and co-morbid conditions, which can influence the anesthetic drug choice. Recent literature emphasizes the importance of an individualized approach in managing patients who are exposed to airway procedures, particularly in complex cases with difficult intubation conditions. For example, the administration of drugs like propofol and fentanyl can facilitate smoother induction, while inhaled agents like isoflurane provide adequate depth for surgery. Collectively, these issues place the role of anesthesiologists as integral members of the multidisciplinary team of ENT procedure treatment (Salinding et al., 2022). Understanding the long-term implications of anesthesia in ENT and airway surgery goes beyond the OR since it also includes patient satisfaction and postoperative recovery. Postoperative pain control is still an integral component of postoperative care, and this necessitates the utilization of effective analgesic practices to minimize pain and facilitate recovery. Furthermore, the potential for complications must be proactively controlled by careful monitoring and management. Trends in postoperative care also indicate that the selection of analgesic drugs, such as metamizole, can play a significant role in influencing recovery patterns among patients. Anesthesiologists are now not only expected to deliver effective anesthesia administration but also ensure that optimal recovery courses are obtained by patients, thereby further reinforcing the concept that successful ENT surgeries are contingent on proper anesthetic planning and execution (Salinding et al., 2022) (Figure 5.1).

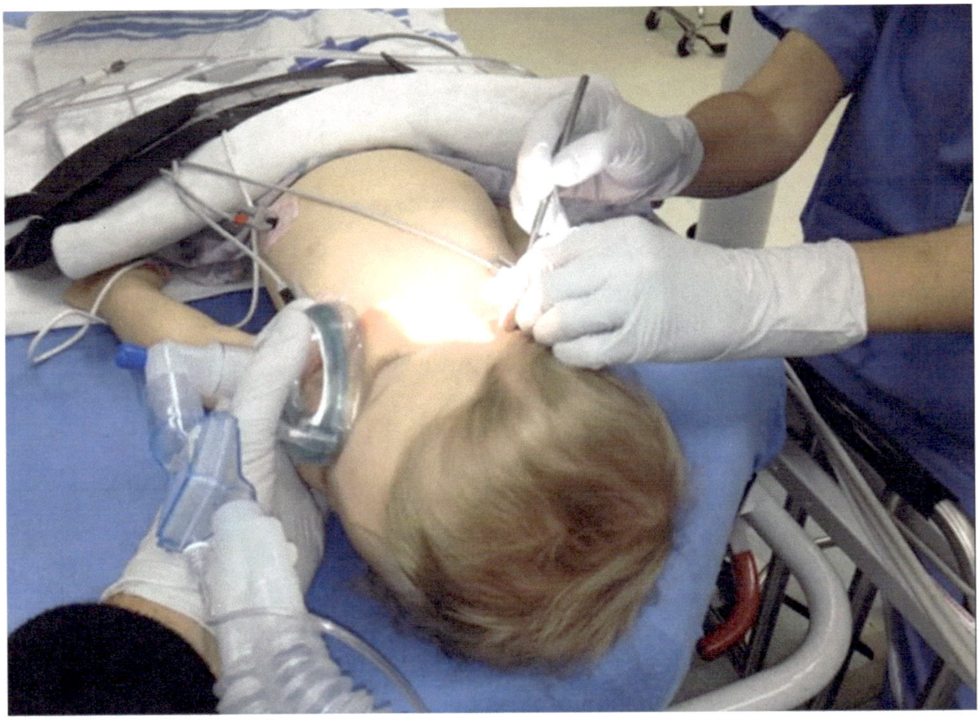

Figure 5.1. The advent of modern anesthetic techniques has significantly transformed the landscape of ear, nose, and throat (ENT) surgery.

Source: https://i0.wp.com/aneskey.com/wp-content/uploads/2022/11/f22-02-9780323829021.jpg?w=960.

Definition of Anesthesia

Anesthesia can be defined as a clinical technique that involves the administration of pharmacologic agents in order to create a state of insensibility and consciousness of pain during procedures or operations. The primary goal of anesthesia is the provision of comfort to patients by removing pain perception while simultaneously allowing surgeons to perform complex operations without interruptions caused by movement or discomfort of patients. This condition can be achieved by various means like general anesthesia, regional anesthesia, and local anesthesia, each being used according to the specific requirement of the surgery being performed. In ENT and airway surgery, where precision is of utmost concern, anesthesia plays a crucial role in achieving successful surgical outcomes with the least risk of airway management and patient discomfort. Besides, application of anesthesia within the field of ENT and airway procedures demands excellent knowledge of not only pharmacologic drugs but also guidelines for patient evaluation and airway management. Seasoned anesthesiologists apply advanced techniques to predict and manage expected problems with procedures, utilizing guidelines that render airway evaluations standardized. Current expert consensus has outlined the role of holistic evaluation methods using medical history, physical examination, and advanced technology to minimize risks in airway management, particularly in procedures where anatomy is expected to be obstructed or complex (Xia et al., 2023). Such a systematic approach is key to ensuring patient safety and optimizing the outcome of surgery in ENT, reinforcing the necessity for anesthesia to be an integral component in surgical planning and execution. Additionally, the evolving nature of anesthesia continues to encompass the acquisition of new technology and the incorporation of new management practices that can improve patient care even more. This entails a recognition of the need for interdisciplinary collaboration between anesthesia specialists, such as surgeons, anesthesiologists, and emergency physicians, to enhance the practice of anesthesia for patients undergoing ENT and airway operations. Best practice standards based on thorough reviews of the literature should be pivotal in formulating standards for directing clinical practice and safeguarding patient outcomes. These efforts delineate the need for continuous education and refining of techniques in the backdrop of changing complexities of patient health and operational requirements in order to achieve a whole platform for managing issues related to anesthesia in these subspecialties (Muschol et al., 2022). Consequently, a comprehensive understanding of anesthesia not only defines the practice but it also contributes to the overall efficacy and safety of ENT and airway surgical interventions (Figure 5.2).

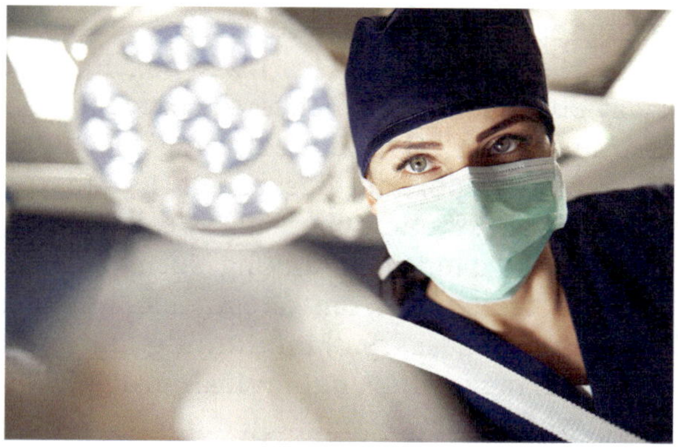

Figure 5.2. Anesthesia can be defined as a medical intervention.

Source: https://jasonsashfordmd.com/wp-content/uploads/2020/07/Anesthesia-Definition-and-Types.jpg.

Importance of Anesthesia in ENT and Airway Surgery

Anesthesia forms a vital part of ENT surgery, in addition to airway procedures. The delicate nature of these areas demands good precision and control from the anesthetic team. Quality anesthesia offers optimal conditions for surgery, minimizing patient movement and pain while also enabling surgeons to work efficiently. Especially in such procedures such as tonsillectomies or myringotomies, general anesthesia is applied to enable complete unconsciousness and pain relief. This ensures patient immobility and tranquility, giving rise to a more secure operative field. Proper use of anesthetic techniques directly influences the success and safety of the procedure, which stresses the significance of professional anesthesiologists in ENT clinics. Furthermore, the increasingly evident incidence of obstructive sleep apnea syndrome (OSAS) among surgical patients contributes to the importance of personalized anesthetic care in ENT surgery. OSAS, where diagnosed in up to 25% of those admitted for elective surgery, augments the risks of anesthesia, and indeed more so with respect to airway management and respiratory stability intra- and postoperatively. Undiagnosed OSAS patients are generally in greater danger of postoperative hypoxemia and airway obstruction, and hence, the prevention of these conditions after administering anesthesia is extremely important. Because of the sedative effect of an anesthetic, upper airway collapsibility is extremely dangerous among such patients, and thus vigilance from anesthesiologists is absolutely necessary. Maintaining patients' safety during otolaryngological procedures, under which airway management is always an issue of concern during the perioperative period (Vasu et al., 2012), is dependent upon the resolution of these problems. In conclusion, integration of anesthesia in ENT and airway procedures is more than merely sedation, but rather encompasses extensive considerations of preoperative assessment, intraoperative management, and postoperative care. Anesthesiologists play a vital role in assessing patient histories, identifying risk factors such as OSAS, and employing appropriate techniques that do not entail intrinsic risks of anesthesia in vulnerable patients. Besides, the advancements in anesthetic agents and techniques, such as regional anesthesia and multimodal analgesia, have played a crucial role in improving recovery profiles and minimizing opioid requirements, reducing side effects post-surgery. Improved understanding of these dynamics clearly highlights the multifaceted importance of anesthesia in delivering optimal outcomes in ENT and airway surgery, rendering it an indispensable part of surgical care (Prosser et al., 1998).

5.1. Types of Anesthesia

Learning Outcome

1. General anesthesia
2. Regional anesthesia
3. Local anesthesia

Anesthesia selection is paramount in ENT and airway surgery because it not only impacts patient safety but also the success of the procedure itself. One of the types of anesthesia that is used is local anesthesia, and it is particularly significant in minimally invasive surgery. Local anesthetics are usually used to anesthetize a localized area so patients do not have to be asleep or unconscious. This modality also reduces the risks of general anesthesia, such as airway obstruction or respiratory complications. Furthermore, local anesthesia is noted for excellent postoperative pain control and therefore reduces the consumption of opioids. Local anesthesia has also been paired with sedation by surgeons to enhance patient comfort and minimize anxiety with procedures like tympanostomy or nasal septoplasty. Lastly, the utilization of the correct form of local anesthesia for ENT operations ensures improved patient outcomes and experiences for less complicated surgical interventions. General anesthesia is also another essential form employed in ENT as well as airway surgery, especially for more invasive or complicated procedures. Under this technique, anesthetic agents induce a reversible unconscious state, enabling the surgeon to perform complicated surgeries without putting the patient at risk. For instance, some operations like tonsillectomy or laryngeal procedures might require general anesthesia due to the anatomical complexity as well as the requirement for patient immobility. The choice of general anesthesia not only ensures adequate analgesia but also allows control of the airway through intubation, which becomes crucial while dealing with procedures that have the potential to affect the airway in a direct way. However, general anesthesia is risky by nature with complications such as respiratory depression and allergic reactions, and therefore necessitates thorough preoperative evaluations and continuous monitoring during the surgery to ensure patient safety and minimize potential complications.

Monitored anesthesia care (MAC) has become increasingly popular in ENT practice as an intermediate between local and general anesthesia. This technique usually involves the administration of sedatives and analgesics by an anesthesiologist while providing a patient with responsiveness to verbal commands. MAC is most effective in operations such as flexible laryngoscopy or in the management of abscesses within the neck, where some patient responsiveness is required. Although patients are still somewhat aware of their surroundings, the administration of anxiolytics ensures that they will experience very minimal pain and stress. Furthermore, MAC can result in rapid recovery times, which in turn can promote decreased postoperative stays and more rapid hospital discharge. However, proper use of MAC will necessitate careful patient selection and skilled administration in order to benefit from its benefits without incurring associated risks, particularly in complex airway procedures (Mărginean et al., 2018) (Figure 5.3).

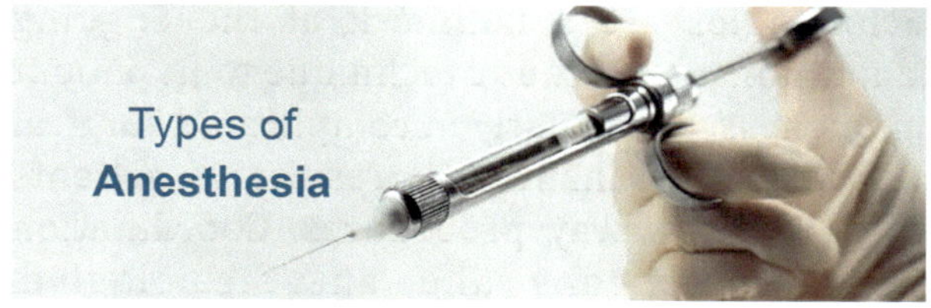

Figure 5.3. The selection of anesthesia is crucial in ENT and airway surgeries.

Source: https://www.medicoverhospitals.in/images/articles/types-of-anesthesia-begumpet.webp.

5.1.1. General Anesthesia

General anesthesia is a cornerstone in the field of otolaryngology, particularly in ENT and airway operations, where patient comfort and stability are paramount. Improvements in anesthetic techniques have significantly enhanced the safety and success of these procedures. During surgery, anesthesiologists must have careful consideration of airway management techniques, particularly for the high-risk patients. For instance, obstructive sleep apnea patients who are presenting with edema of the airway require careful planning not to cause laryngeal obstruction following intubation. The trade-off between deep extubation that inhibits airway reflexes and the need for continuous airway security is a testament to the complexity of general anesthesia in ENT surgery. Difficulty in mask ventilation scenarios complicates general anesthesia for laryngeal surgeries. For anesthesiologists, inability to provide adequate ventilation poses severe risks. In overcoming this problem, anesthesiologists often resort to awake extubation techniques, focusing on the convenience and safety of the patient. In a pediatric patient with tonsillar hypertrophy, the use of retrograde lidocaine spray permitted effective airway management with the prevention of laryngeal edema. These techniques not only minimized the risk of airway complications but also facilitated smoother transition from one stage of surgery to another. These new technologies are a hallmark of the ongoing adaptation of anesthetic technique to fit patient uniqueness, particularly in complicated surgical situations, to enhance the results of patients in ENT and airway procedures. Coordination between surgeons and anesthesiologists is necessary for the success of any airway management method employed in the conduct of ENT surgery. The shared goal of maintaining an unobstructed field for surgery with patient safety assurance calls for a concerted effort that leverages each discipline's strength. All considerations for the endotracheal tube, mode of ventilation, and oxygen enrichment are all active components that need coordinated efforts. As emphasized among anesthesiologists, general anesthesia is not just thought of as the provision of unconsciousness, but rather as a broad approach to physiological stability and the prevention of complications of surgery. This comprehensive approach is particularly important during surgery on delicate structures of the airway, where even a minor deviation may have disastrous adverse effects. The multifaceted requirements of anesthetic management in ENT and airway procedures emphasize the imperative nature of this interprofessional practice, ensuring enhanced safety and effectiveness for patients in these interventions (Radichkova & Mladenov, 2020; Alhaj et al., 2024).

5.1.2. Regional Anesthesia

In the setting of ENT and airway surgery, regional anesthesia has been an invaluable technique. Regional anesthesia involves the application of local anesthetics to specific nerves or regions, in effect, disrupting the sensory conduction. Through restriction of systemic drug administration, it curtails potential side effects of general anesthesia and hence is extremely useful to comorbid patients. Regional anesthesia also has a shorter recovery time, making patients able to resume normal activities sooner. Such a high rate of quick recovery is desirable in outpatient settings, where early discharge is targeted. As appropriately utilized, regional techniques not only provide effective analgesia but also a more comfortable overall patient-clinician interaction for ENT cases. The application of regional anesthesia is most self-evident in its application in most ENT procedures, such as tonsillectomy and sinus surgery. With the application of techniques like cervical plexus blocks or local infiltration, physicians can administer deep analgesia targeted at the area of surgery. Further, the use of ultrasound-guided techniques has been made available with a much improved nerve localization, thereby enhancing the efficacy of the blocks and reducing the chances of complications. Local anesthetic methods are employed for their analgesic effect in the postoperative period, resulting in decreased utilization of opioids. It is especially valid in today's time, with the urgent need to address the opioid epidemic in the healthcare sector. Regional anesthesia then not only provides maximal control of pain intraoperatively but also remains in concert with best practice, tending to optimize patient safety and comfort. One of the major advantages of regional anesthesia in airway surgery is its influence on airway management. The technique allows airway reflexes to be preserved without compromising proper analgesia, and it is therefore particularly beneficial in situations like fiberoptic intubation or laryngoscopy. Regional anesthesia provides a more cooperative pattern of breathing, and this is most critical in maintaining patients with complicated airway procedures adequately ventilated. As emphasized in recent coping strategies, local methods, supplemented by sedation, can offer a less stressful experience for patients, especially in the treatment that could result in anxiety or discomfort. Furthermore, with progress in endoscopic interventions, regional anesthesia continues to be the focal point for the attainment of successful results while maintaining patient safety and satisfaction in ENT surgery (Department of Anesthesia, University of Iowa, 2011) (Figure 5.4).

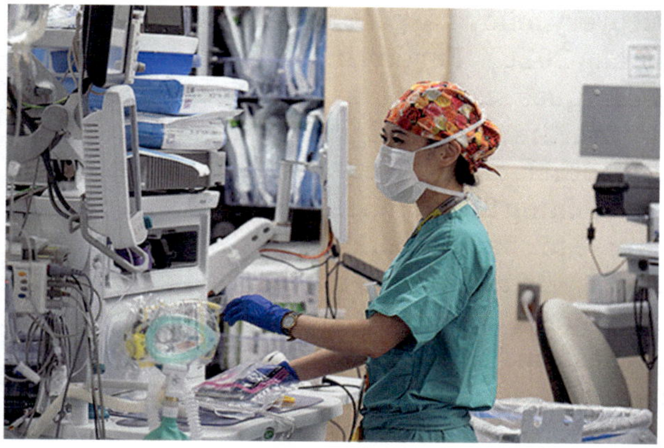

Figure 5.4. Regional anesthesia.

Source: https://health.ucdavis.edu/media-resources/contenthub/health-library/treatments/regional-anesthesia-marquee.jpg.

5.1.3. Local Anesthesia

Local anesthesia is an important component of ENT practice and airway surgery because it provides effective control of pain without causing significant systemic complications. Conscious sedation is possible using this modality, which proves beneficial in many procedures like nasal surgery, tonsillectomy, and several diagnostic procedures. Surgeons are able to do fine maneuvers in an awake and cooperative patient with the help of local anesthetics, which allow communication and immediate feedback regarding their comfort levels. Local anesthesia for outpatient surgery is also commonly employed because it allows for faster recovery and release to home from the hospital without a long period of postoperative observation. This technique not only enhances patient satisfaction but also makes sense of the surgery, making it an integral part of modern ENT practices. In deep neck infection procedures, local anesthesia can be particularly beneficial. Peritonsillar abscess or retropharyngeal infection often demands drainage procedures that, though invasive, can be performed under local anesthesia. This minimizes the risk of airway complications with room to allow good pain control. The local anesthetic, besides alleviating immediate pain, also provides some hemostasis by causing the blood vessels in the field to become smaller, reducing the risk of excessive bleeding during the procedure. Because such infections can lead to serious complications, including mediastinitis, and potentially life-threatening hemorrhage, precision afforded by local anesthesia raises efficacy and safety in the treatment of these conditions surgically, as attested by clinical procedures (Mărginean et al., 2018). In addition, psychological implications in surgery can play a significant role in patient outcomes in ENT and airway surgeries. Local anesthesia tends to minimize the procedure's invasiveness, and that can decrease anxiety and stress among patients, particularly those who are anxious about general anesthesia. Partial preservation of consciousness facilitates patient participation, with patients being more in control when they are being treated. It is particularly important in aesthetic cases; patients care about scarring after surgery and neck appearance in general after procedures. Patient education on the technique, outcome expectation, and complications is required to facilitate informed consent and reasonable expectations (Mărginean et al., 2018). Proper communication of the use of local anesthesia can also allay fears associated with the traumatizing nature of certain interventions, further increasing a satisfying surgical experience.

Test Your Knowledge

1. What are the main types of anesthesia used in medical practice?
2. What is the difference between general anesthesia and regional anesthesia?

5.2. Preoperative Assessment

Learning Outcome

1. Patient history and physical examination
2. Evaluation of airway anatomy
3. Assessment of comorbid conditions

There is a need for a complete preoperative assessment, including in the setting of ENT and airway anesthesia, because it directs the anesthetic plan and identifies possible risks. Following the initial assessment, clinicians must obtain a careful medical history, such as the patient's anesthetic past, comorbid conditions, and airway pathology that might make intubation challenging. It is particularly important to assess the airway anatomy since ENT procedures often involve complex anatomy. The use of fiber-optic or video laryngoscopy can also prove to be immensely helpful in locating a patient's airway during this assessment. Multidisciplinary collaboration of anesthetists, surgeons, and pediatric specialists is also essential in complex patients, as this permits a tailored approach to preoperative management and risk reduction, with the best outcomes at surgery and postoperatively, particularly in complex cases as in patients with Mucolipidosis (Scott-Warren & Walker, 2020). Preoperative assessment should also emphasize the evaluation of potential complications, particularly in at-risk patients. Patients with serious medical histories, such as cardiovascular or respiratory disease, require cautious scrutiny and often need further testing, including an echocardiogram or chest radiograph. Identifying these risks allows anesthetic practitioners to implement measures aimed at enhancing patient safety. Literature has highlighted the importance of preoperative optimization in minimizing perioperative complications like emergence agitation (EA), which might be observed during recovery following general anesthesia (Seok-Lee et al., 2020). Furthermore, the utilization of techniques such as total intravenous anesthesia or multimodal analgesia can minimize EA and other side effects to a significant level, highlighting the optimization of the perioperative course for patients undergoing ENT and airway surgery. In addition to clinical evaluation, strict communication with patients about the surgical process and anesthesia protocols is of greatest significance. Education can reduce anxiety levels and empower patients with the data required to better understand their involvement with the perioperative process. Such communication should incorporate potential risks, the nature of the anesthesia to be administered, and postoperative expectations so that patients can make well-informed decisions about their care. Moreover, parental presence during induction has been discovered to have a positive influence on patient cooperation and preoperative anxiety, particularly in the case of children undergoing ENT operations. Hence, preoperative assessment comprises clinical evaluation with patient-focused communication practices within a global plan aimed at ensuring safety as well as satisfaction for anesthesia in ENT and airway surgery (Figure 5.5).

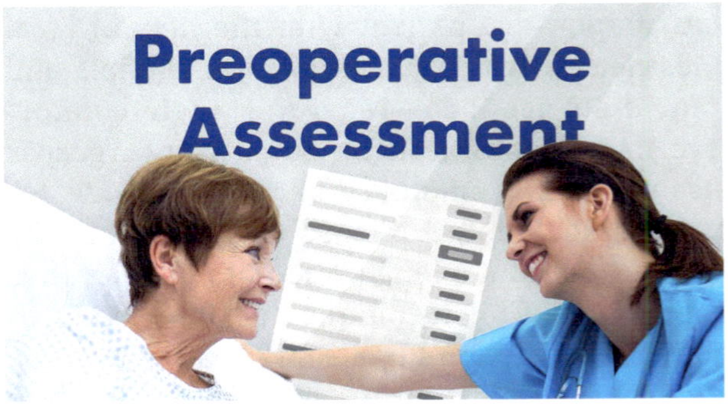

Figure 5.5. A comprehensive preoperative assessment.

Source: https://ausmed-images.s3-ap-southeast-2.amazonaws.com/ausmed.com/ausmed-course/COURSE122_01v2.0.jpg.

5.2.1. Patient History and Physical Examination

In ENT and airway surgery under anesthesia, patient history and physical examination are of utmost significance in order to attain the best results. Patient histories assist in detecting worthy information regarding existing medical conditions, medications, and past surgical experiences that could influence anesthesia care. Data on respiratory illnesses, such as asthma or chronic obstructive pulmonary disease, are particularly pertinent in the field of ENT, as these factors significantly impact airway management and choice of anesthesia. Moreover, an understanding of the past history of allergy and intolerance to anesthetic medications is critical in preventing risk during upper aerodigestive tract procedures, where mutual exposure to inhaled anesthetics occurs. This detailed patient history enables the anesthesiologist to tailor an anesthesia plan specifically to address known risks in each patient, safety and effectiveness are optimized. Physical examination complements patient history by enabling a direct measurement of relevant anatomical and physiological parameters. Special attention during ENT and airway surgery is given to inspecting the status of the upper airway because anatomical abnormalities can complicate intubation and ventilation. For instance, if the patient suffers from obstructive sleep apnea or anatomical problems, such as a reduced mandible, it can necessitate specific anesthetic techniques or the supply of alternative airway equipment. In addition, having a focused assessment allows clinicians to identify potential complications of the procedure, e.g., uncontrolled bleeding or airway obstruction. Through systematic evaluation of these factors, anesthesiologists are more likely to prepare for and prevent complications, ultimately enhancing the overall course of surgery and maintaining patient safety. Intense physical examination cannot therefore, be ignored in planning anesthesia. The conjunction of patient history and physical examination is even more critical in the backdrop of modern healthcare issues such as the COVID-19 pandemic, which intensified risks involved in aerosol-generating procedures common in ENT procedures. The requirement for incorporation of safety measures that are based on respiratory status and history of exposure captured the demand for adaptive examination protocols protecting both provider and patient safety. These concerns are underscored by guidelines developed during the pandemic that propose strict safety protocols and preoperative screening aimed at reducing infection risk to healthcare workers involved in direct patient contact (Givi et al., 2020). Furthermore, ongoing controversy as far as optimal anesthesia management practice is concerned echoes messages of multidisciplinary groups of specialists, echoing individualized care based on prior experience and physical examination findings for complex diseases like Mucopolysaccharidosis IVA, requiring accurate planning of anesthesia in surgical intervention (Akyol et al., 2019). Encapsulating these perspectives embodies a multi-faceted approach towards enhanced patient safety and surgical outcomes in ENT and airway surgery.

5.2.2. Evaluation of Airway Anatomy

A good understanding of the airway anatomy is of greatest significance to anesthesiologists and otolaryngologists involved in ENT and airway procedures. The intricate interactions between various components of the airway, including the nasal airway, pharynx, and larynx, must be extensively studied before any procedure. Effective evaluation of the airway ensures identifying potential complications that can impede intubation or ventilation during anesthesia. This anatomical evaluation not only enhances patient safety through the prevention of complications but also directs the anesthetic planning of anesthetic techniques tailored to each patient's unique airway characteristics.

Adapting the anesthetic technique to these variables significantly enhances the likelihood of successful surgical outcomes, especially in surgeries with delicate structures such as the trachea and larynx, where airway integrity must be maintained to ensure the patient's well-being (Parfianowicz et al., 2024). Use of imaging modalities like computed tomography (CT) and magnetic resonance imaging (MRI) has been of utmost importance in airway anatomy assessment. The imaging modalities give high-resolution cross-sectional images, which illustrate the spatial anatomy of airway structures in relation to surrounding tissues.

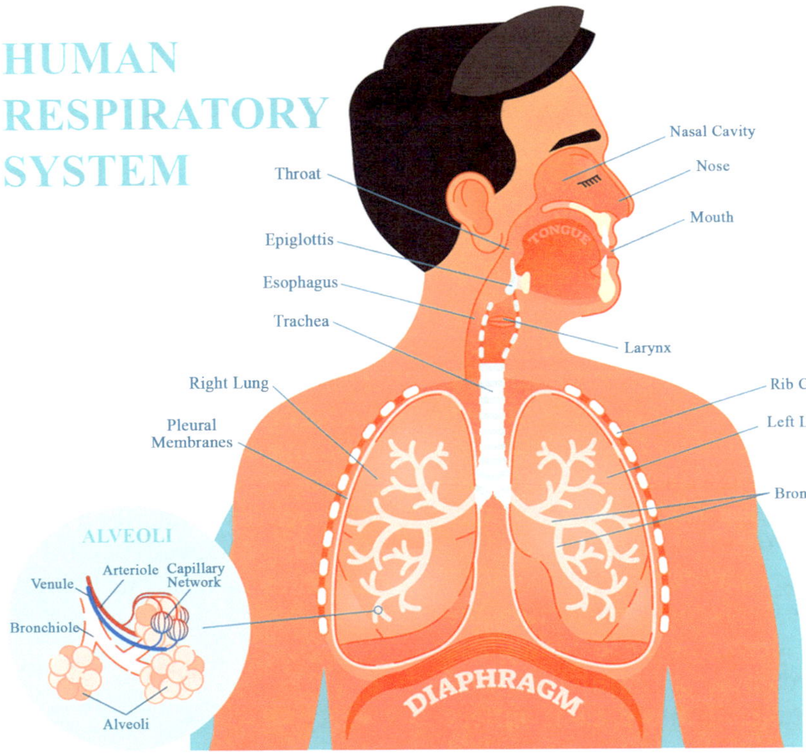

Figure 5.6. The anatomical structure of the airway is paramount for anesthesiologists.

Source: https://s3.us-east-2.amazonaws.com/medictests-production/ckeditor_assets/pictures/924/content_Human-Respiratory-System-anatomical-vector-illustration_-medical-education-cross-section-diagram-with-nasal-cavity_-throat_-lungs-and-alveoli.-923068560_1075x979.jpeg.

Such data have specific value in preoperative assessment as it is helpful in predicting potential complications such as airway obstruction or injury during surgery. Through the provision of a high-resolution picture of the airways anatomy, these imaging techniques make it possible for anesthesiologists to anticipate potential issues, thereby ensuring patient safety and surgical efficiency. Understanding these technologies facilitates improved cooperation between the surgical team and the anesthetic team and encourages a culture of interdependent care, reducing the risk of postoperative complications related to airway management (Singh et al., 2016). In addition to imaging, physical examination remains a vital component of airway assessment. It involves assessing the patients' history, clinical presentation, and anatomical findings that predict difficulty in managing the airway, e.g., Mallampati score or thyromental distance tests. Such assessments give anesthesiologists feedback about the patient's risk level in terms of potential airway obstructions so they can prepare strategies for effective intubation and ventilation. In addition, awareness of the patient's airway can guide anesthetic selection, either with a local anesthetic for outpatient procedures or with the expectation of general anesthesia in more complex ones. Lastly, thorough and proper investigation of airway anatomy enhances ENT interventions and provides the gateway to improved patient outcomes through informed anesthetic decisions (Parfianowicz et al., 2024) (Figure 5.6).

5.2.3. Assessment of Comorbid Conditions

Comorbid disease evaluation is an essential aspect of ENT and airway surgery planning and delivery of anesthesia. Meticulous consideration of a patient's overall health status is the foundation for anesthetic management since comorbidities have a significant bearing on both surgical outcomes and perioperative risk. For instance, patients with respiratory conditions such as asthma or COPD present special challenges during anesthesia, potentially making airway management more difficult and jeopardizing respiratory morbidity. Therefore, it is important that anesthesiologists possess an entire picture of all comorbidities by way of reviewing historical medical records, physical examination, and applicable diagnostic testing to inform their anesthesia plan and reduce risk associated with the procedure. In pediatric patients, the presence of comorbidities is observed to play a major role in the success of procedures such as supraglottoplasty, performed to correct pathologies such as laryngomalacia. Research estimates that up to 20% of patients with such conditions may develop severe comorbid medical conditions affecting postoperative results (Drummond et al., 2012). Such associated conditions, such as pharyngomalacia and gastroesophageal reflux disease, need careful observation during the procedure. The dynamic between laryngomalacia and its comorbidities illustrates the necessity of a tailored anesthetic plan that takes into account each patient's unique clinical environment. Thus, the evolved anesthetic plan in these patients needs to take into account how comorbidities might alter immediate and long-term success with surgery. The assessment of the comorbid conditions also extends beyond the immediate context of surgery into the plan for anesthetic management. For example, pulmonary hypertension (PH) is an important risk factor that might complicate airway surgery (Reinero et al., 2020). These patients pose the risk of greater postoperative morbidity due to hemodynamic instability, and hence careful preoperative screening and perioperative monitoring protocols are required. PH causes enable anesthesiologists to use customized therapeutic measures to decrease perioperative complications. Continuous re-evaluation of such comorbidities and their potential impact on the general physiology of patients is of utmost importance, underlining the pivotal position of efficient preoperative assessments in allowing safe and advantageous anesthesiology for ENT and airway procedures.

Test Your Knowledge

1. What key information is obtained from a patient's medical history?
2. Why is a physical examination important before treatment or surgery?

5.3. Anesthetic Techniques for ENT Procedures

Learning Outcome

1. Induction methods
2. Maintenance of anesthesia
3. Emergence and recovery

The practice area of anesthesiology for ENT operations encompasses a variety of techniques appropriate to the specific requirements of these operations. Due to the intricate physiology and anatomy of the speech and breathing systems, anesthesiologists must practice with each of the following specifics in mind. Local anesthesia, sedation, and general anesthetic techniques are the ones employed, each depending upon the complexity of the procedure and the personal health status of the patient. For instance, in minimal invasive procedures, local anesthetics may provide adequate analgesia without the need for general anesthesia, whereas more invasive procedures, such as tonsillectomy or sinus surgery, may demand general anesthesia to achieve patient immobility and unconsciousness during surgery. The choice of technique significantly influences the patient's comfort during the procedure and their postoperative course. Monitoring of physiological parameters during ENT surgery is crucial because of the close vicinity to the airway and the high risk of respiratory complications. The anesthetic method employed in the majority of cases would involve careful planning of airway management in patients with known difficult airways or anatomical pathology. Endotracheal intubation or the use of supraglottic airway devices may be employed to secure the airway safely and permit control of ventilation and oxygenation by the anesthesiologist. Techniques such as regional anesthesia have also gained popularity for some procedures, limiting the use of systemic drugs and allowing for quicker recovery times. For instance, in complex airway reconstruction, a combination of regional and general techniques is usually used to achieve maximum analgesia while keeping anesthetic exposure to a minimum and thus improving overall patient outcomes. Moreover, improvements in anesthetic techniques are being applied in clinical practice to enhance effectiveness and safety in ENT procedures. Improvements such as enhanced recovery after surgery (ERAS) protocols aim at multimodal analgesia through the combination of regional anesthesia with non-opioid adjuvants to reduce opioid dependence as well as minimize postoperative risk. These protocols have been shown to increase patient-reported outcomes and decrease recovery times, hence bridging the gap between the surgery procedure and the patient's overall experience.

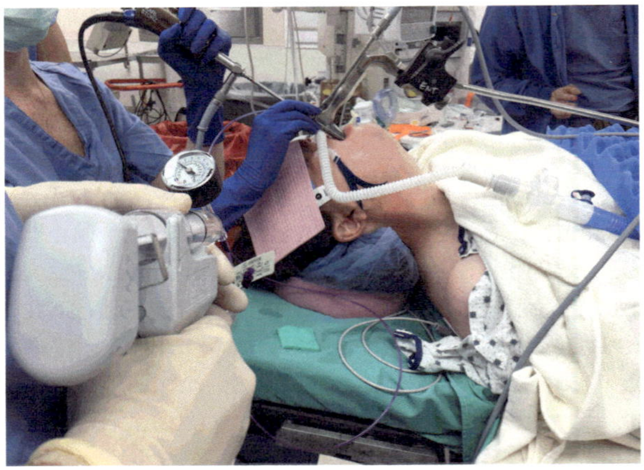

Figure 5.7. The realm of anesthetic techniques for ear, nose, and throat (ENT) procedures.

Source: https://static.cambridge.org/binary/version/id/urn:cambridge.org:id:binary:20201002023020199-0834:9781108303477:41953fig26_9.png?pub-status=live.

The value of incorporating a range of anesthetic strategies is emphasized by their influence on intraoperative management and postoperative recovery, most notably in procedures that affect swallowing and speech, as seen in research in cleft lip and palate repairs, where individualized anesthetic strategies played a role in successful surgical results (Luyten et al., 2013). These tips will help enhance your event-driven knowledge. The following evolution of techniques is imperative to ensure the highest possible standards of care in airway and ENT surgery (Figure 5.7).

5.3.1. Induction Methods

In airway surgery and ENT, selecting appropriate induction methods is the key to ensuring patient safety and optimal operating conditions. Induction is the period of time spent getting from an awake state to a controlled state of anesthesia, and selecting it can have a great impact on the challenges of managing the airway during the procedure. The most common techniques are intravenous (IV) induction, inhalation induction, and rapid sequence induction, each with its own advantage and consideration. IV induction allows for a rapid onset of anesthesia and is usually employed in controlled situations, while inhalational agents are frequently employed in pediatric patients due to their ease of administration and minimal cardiovascular effect. Lastly, the specific conditions of the operation, the patient's health status, and also any potential risk factors must guide the choice of the induction method. Of particular importance, when making a choice among the induction methods, are patients with comorbid illnesses, i.e., obstructive sleep apnea syndrome (OSAS). These patients possess greater collapsibility of their upper airway during sleep, thus elevating the risk of postoperative complications under anesthesia, particularly because sedation would additionally deteriorate their state. Research has indicated that sleep apnea is much higher in surgical candidates than in the general population, and thus careful preoperative assessment to identify high-risk patients is needed (Vasu et al., 2012). Its treatment may involve personalized anesthetic methods and adjunct therapy usage, emphasizing anesthesiologists' need to be sensitive to a patient's individual airway dynamics and attendant complications at induction. Also, the method of induction itself can have a direct effect on the overall airway handling during surgery. For instance, while rapid sequence induction is frequently used in urgent or in cases of high risk of aspiration cases, the successful achievement of that relies on acute sensitivity and skill in airway management. Application of neuromuscular blockers with this technique is used to aid intubation, but requires a sufficient understanding of the patients' respiratory dynamics and complications from their disease. With advancements in anesthesia continuing, investigation into induction methods will be critical to advancing technique and in offering ENT and airway patients the safest and most effective type of anesthesia care possible (Prosser et al., 1998).

5.3.2. Maintenance of Anesthesia

In ENT and airway surgery anesthesia, the maintenance of anesthesia is a critical stage that makes major contributions to the procedure outcome and patient safety. During this stage, the anesthesiologist seeks to maintain the patient in an optimal state of stable anesthesia during the procedure. This entails constant monitoring of such vital signs as heart rate, blood pressure, and oxygen saturation, in order to detect any alterations in physiology that may be a harbinger of developing complications. Dosage and mode of delivery of anesthetic agents must be constantly adjusted accordingly, while bearing in mind that factors such as patient age, health status, and some surgical requirements will determine these values. Understanding the pharmacodynamics of various anesthetic agents helps practitioners achieve a balance between sedation and wakefulness so that the patient remains comfortable without compromising safety protocols. Additionally, the sustainability of anesthesia demands utmost caution for the likelihood of complications, particularly in a high-tech specialty like ENT and airway surgery. These patients generally have unique anatomical considerations that will interfere with airflow and overall stability. For instance, the larynx and surrounding structures can be extremely sensitive to anesthetic agents and, as such, are susceptible to airway obstruction or hypoxic events if closely monitored. In a trial of neonatal and infant patients who underwent anesthesia, critical events such as hypotension or reduced oxygenation manifested in a high proportion of cases, emphasizing watchfulness during this time (Disma et al., 2021).

The anesthesiologist must be prepared to respond rapidly, employing methods such as ventilator setting manipulation or intravenous fluid administration, to preserve the patient's physiological stability while undergoing the procedure. Additionally, improved ERAS protocols are being increasingly utilized in ENT anesthesia care. ERAS protocols seek to optimize patient outcomes by minimizing anesthesia's effect and decreasing recovery times through a multifaceted approach. By incorporating multimodal analgesia methods, the incorporation of regional anesthetic techniques, and the utilization of sedation-sparing mechanisms, the severity of postoperative side effects can be reduced. This is particularly true in ENT surgery, in which postoperative nausea and vomiting (PONV) can significantly hamper recovery. Adding evidence-based practice is crucial, as there is evidence that supports increased complication risk for patients with existing comorbidities undergoing anesthetic procedures (Iorio-Morin et al., 2020). Thus, maintenance of anesthesia involves not just the technical achievement of anesthetic administration but also a broader view inclusive of patient-specific details and the general care continuum (Figure 5.8).

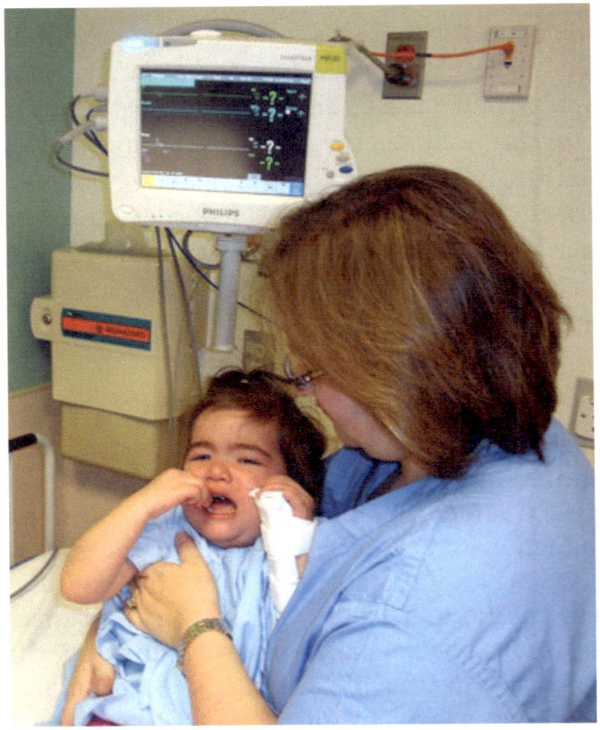

Figure 5.8. The maintenance of anesthesia.

Source: https://clinicalgate.com/wp-content/uploads/2015/02/B9780323066129000134_f13-06-9780323066129.jpg.

5.3.3. Emergence and Recovery

The process of emergence from anesthesia in ENT and airway surgery is a significant phase with a notable influence on the postoperative course of the patients. During this phase, anesthetists must monitor vital signs and neurological status very closely to make patients emerge safely and effectively from anesthesia. Multiple factors, like the type of anesthesia and the personal physiological responses of the patients, may affect the time and quality of emergence. Especially, middle ear surgery is prone to requiring special attention due to the particular anatomical and physiological intricacies. Local anesthesia is typically utilized by surgeons to enable recovery since it may have shorter emergence times without adding general anesthesia risks (Shyshchuk et al.,

2015). Understanding these dynamics allows anesthesiologists to modify their actions to allow for a smoother transition from surgical treatment to the postoperative condition. Recovery from anesthesia is not merely the rapid awakening but the gradual resumption of normal function over time. Patient recovery experience can have a real effect on patient satisfaction with the operation and their psychological well-being. This is especially so with ENT operations, where airway complications can arise in terms of anxiety or distress for the patient. Effective control of postoperative nausea and vomiting becomes important as such an occurrence may enhance discomfort as well as disrupt a patient's recovery process. Through the incorporation of practices such as the application of antiemetic medication, recovery results are enhanced. Moreover, through the provision of a complete understanding of principles in anesthesia and recovery, anesthesiologists can optimize their abilities and establish an environment that is supportive of patient recovery (Shyshchuk et al., 2015). Moreover, the emergence phase must be considered as part of the broad system of postoperative care measures based on ensuring patient safety and comfort. Greater vigilance over postoperative respiratory complications of ENT surgery should encourage anesthesiologists to adopt vigilant monitoring practices during recovery. Notably, recovery room staff are taught to observe airway patency and be prepared to intervene in potential emergency situations, thus ensuring a team approach to patient care. This collaborative effort is required to ensure that patients are adequately stabilized before discharge from the recovery room. Additionally, informing the patients about what they can expect during emergence and recovery can reduce anxiety as well as facilitate adherence to postoperative care. Lastly, catering to these areas can facilitate easier recovery, ultimately leading to improved surgical outcomes and patient satisfaction (Shyshchuk et al., 2015).

Test Your Knowledge

1. What anesthetic techniques are commonly used in ENT (ear, nose, and throat) surgeries?
2. What are the key airway management considerations during ENT procedures?

5.4. Anesthetic Considerations for Airway Surgery

Learning Outcome

1. Use of advanced airway devices
2. Challenges in airway management
3. Monitoring during airway procedures

A fundamental but essential aspect of anesthesia for airway surgery is an awareness of the unique challenge presented by upper respiratory tract anatomy and disease. Endotracheal intubation, which in these cases is normally necessary, presents added risk of airway difficulty, especially in such patients with preoperative syndromes like obstructive sleep apnea or extreme upper airway obstruction. Preparation of anesthesiologists for rapid sequence induction is necessary in order to decrease the time for apnea and aspiration risk. Moreover, patient position and head extension also matter since they can have tremendous influences on airway access and hemodynamic stability of patients during surgery. The use of advanced airway management techniques, including the use of fiberoptic intubation or supraglottic devices, may also enhance the safety of these procedures while minimizing mucosal trauma to the airway, thus lowering the risk of postoperative complications. Besides the problems of airway management, anesthetic agents must be selected with care in order to fulfill the individual needs of various patients and the needs of a particular surgery. Variables like the anticipated time of the procedure, intraoperative hemodynamic stability, and postoperative pain risk contribute importantly to the selection of anesthetic agents. For instance, propofol total intravenous anesthesia (TIVA) has been reported to decrease the occurrence of emergence agitation, a worthy consideration in younger patients receiving airway procedures. In addition, multimodal analgesia may optimize postoperative pain relief, accelerating recovery rates and decreasing hospital stays. The anesthesiologist also needs to consider the respiratory implications of some drugs, particularly for those whose airway integrity is compromised, weighing the anesthetic plan against the overall goals of surgery while maintaining patient safety during surgery. Besides, the occurrence of viral infections, such as SARS-CoV-2, has further emphasized infection control practices in airway surgery. The OR team must remain vigilant for perioperative routines, particularly in patients with known or suspected infections, in a way to prevent virus transmission in the operating room (OR). Following guidelines to mitigate against aerosol generation upon intubation and extubation is important, as both are high-risk times for transmission. Higher levels of personal protective equipment (PPE), including the use of N95 masks and face shields, must become an international norm for airway interventions. In addition, special ORs for COVID-19 confirmed cases with the corresponding ventilation systems serve to protect not only medical staff but also other patients from potential nosocomial infection. These practice modifications are in response to the evolving face of anesthetic issues that pertain to airway surgery, and there must be continual advancements in training and protocols to address emerging public health challenges (Figure 5.9).

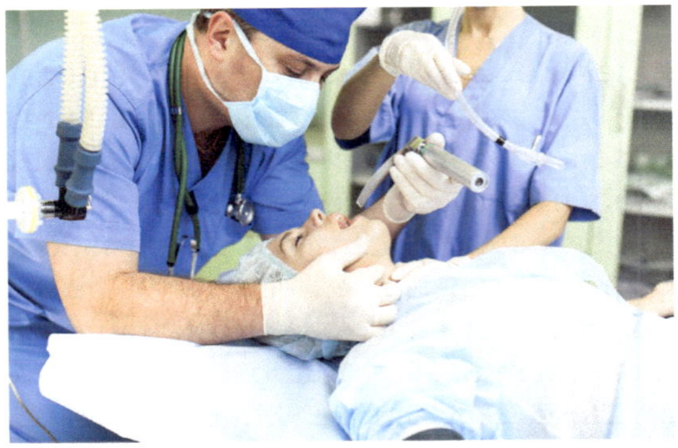

Figure 5.9. Anesthetic considerations for airway surgery.

Source: https://external-content.duckduckgo.com/iu/?u=http%3A%2F%2Fphotos.demandstudios.com%2Fgetty%2Farticle%2F99%2F128%2F489120943.jpg&f=1&nofb=1&ipt=be2e6f0404399fa66d044a88e41cee61262931fd9f417b9ebe8fa932f64abaec.

5.4.1. Challenges in Airway Management

Airway management is a complex issue, particularly in airway and ENT anesthesia procedures. The anatomical variability of the patient presents one of the main complications to the process of intubation. Other conditions such as juvenile-onset recurrent respiratory papillomatosis (JORRP) involve repeated operations to stabilize the airway and hence again increase the risk of complications. New data have implicated new techniques, such as transnasal humidified rapid-insufflation ventilatory exchange (THRIVE), for enhancing intraoperative oxygenation and reducing extubation rates. Through comparative analysis, application of THRIVE decreased the median number of extubations significantly, which equated to greater perioperative safety and efficiency. As physicians proceed with further development of airway management skills, it is important to critically evaluate these developments in order to maximize patient outcomes in ENT surgeries (Lei et al., 2025).

Another crucial challenge in airway management comes from anatomical abnormalities that complicate normal intubation techniques. An example of such a challenge is Mounier-Kuhn syndrome (MKS), characterized by pathological tracheal and major bronchial dilation. Such anatomic variations can be subtle and are not always evident in routine radiologic assessment, causing unforeseen difficulty during the administration of anesthesia. The patient, a 94-year-old woman, presenting with hemiarthroplasty, is one such case; despite an unremarkable respiratory examination, the dilation was apparent on preoperative chest X-rays. Keeping these complexities in mind, anesthesiologists must adopt a cautious preoperative evaluation strategy such that all potential anatomical challenges are addressed and tailored airway management protocols are formulated accordingly. Utilization of specialty airway devices, such as reinforced tracheal tubes, may also serve to preclude the hazards of airway administration in patients with conditions like MKS (Cheon et al., 2024).

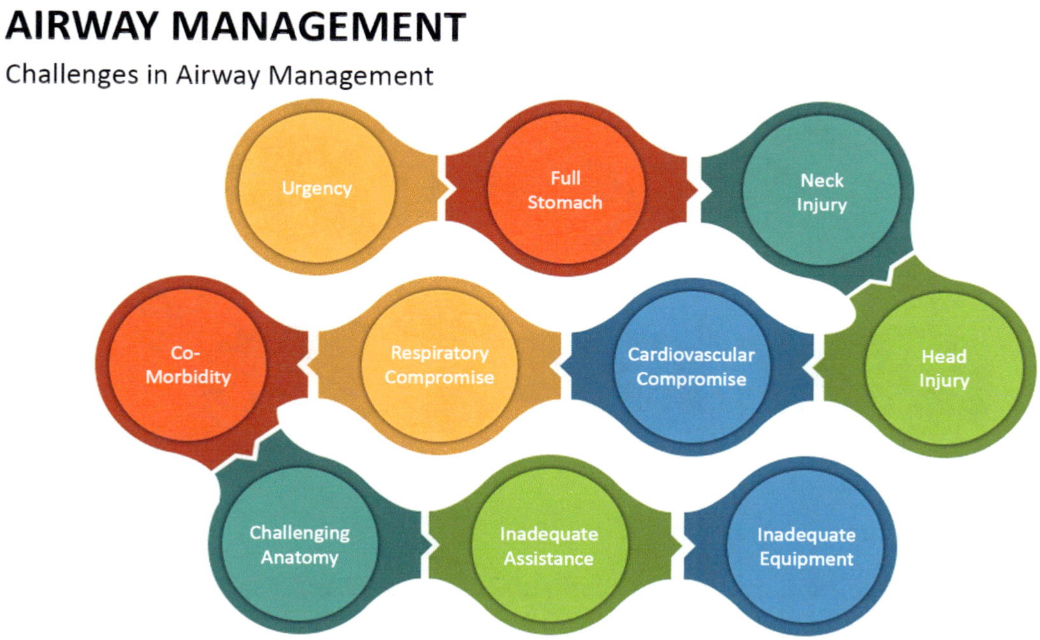
AIRWAY MANAGEMENT
Challenges in Airway Management
Urgency
Full Stomach
Neck Injury
Co-Morbidity
Respiratory Compromise
Cardiovascular Compromise
Head Injury
Challenging Anatomy
Inadequate Assistance
Inadequate Equipment

Figure 5.10. Airway management presents a complex set of challenges.

Source: https://www.collidu.com/media/catalog/product/img/d/5/d51a75ee35a5f01fe28a2624bbf48f0f0e8df9554b5a894ffb22442396e73102/airway-management-slide4.png.

Successful airway administration also requires continuous evaluation and adjustment during surgery. The dynamic nature of ENT surgeries can create sudden changes in patient status, and constant monitoring of ventilation and oxygenation is necessary. Even with newer methods like THRIVE, airway collapse or airway leakage can always be a risk in patients with specific anatomical characteristics. Hence, anesthesiologists are always expected to be adaptable and ready to convert plans based on intraoperative findings. Integration of new techniques, coupled with a precise understanding of patient's anatomical features, is essential to optimizing outcomes in airway management. As successive studies continue, novel approaches and methods are developed, and the practice of anesthesia for ENT and airway surgery can benefit from enhanced methods of ensuring patient safety and effective airway management in complex cases (Lei et al., 2025; Cheon et al., 2024) (Figure 5.10).

5.4.2. Use of Advanced Airway Devices

The application of advanced airway devices has revolutionized the practice of anesthesia, particularly in airway surgery and ENT. Application of advanced airway management techniques is important in the face of patients who may present with anatomical problems or a history of difficult intubation. Video laryngoscopy (VL) has greatly improved the success rate of tracheal intubation compared to direct laryngoscopy. Experience has proved that VL not only enhances first-pass success rates but also reduces complication rates of failed airway management (Law et al., 2021).

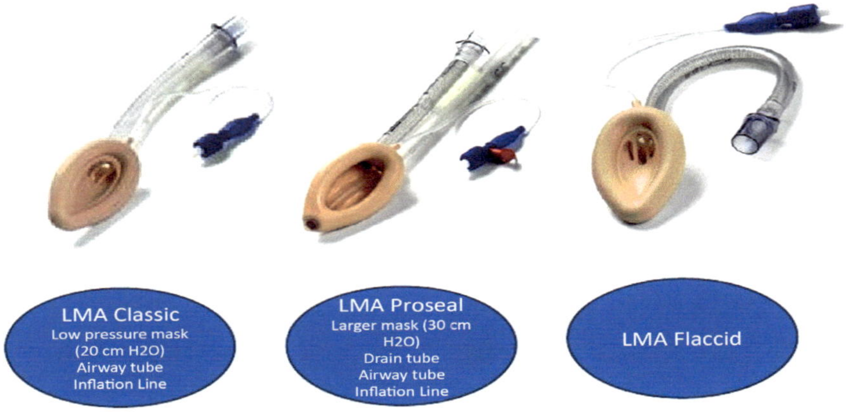

Figure 5.11. Use of advanced airway devices.

Source: https://external-content.duckduckgo.com/iu/?u=https%3A%2F%2Fimage.slidesharecdn.com%2Fdifficultairwaymanagement-090321143019-phpapp02%2F95%2Fadvanced-airway-management-in-the-intensive-care-unitfundamentals-of-intubation-and-difficult-airway-management-48-728.jpg%3Fcb%3D1237646834&f=1&nofb=1&ipt=95e61b1978bb4068f8e54731b1cd11ae7594639778b200682e62eebb02390d2a.

Therefore, VL application in routine practice is recommended as it provides anesthesiologists with a better view of the airway so that they can perform interventions more effectively. Additionally, higher technology airway devices, i.e., supraglottic airway devices (SGAs), are valuable adjuncts where tracheal intubation is not feasible. SGAs can help stabilize a patient's airway, particularly when rapid sequence induction is necessary or in emergency cases where stabilization of the airway has to be done immediately. Appropriate selection and use of these devices are of paramount significance, especially in populations at risk for airway complications, e.g., patients undergoing head and neck surgery. The Fourth National Audit Project highlights the frequency of airway complications in this population, stressing the availability of these sophisticated devices (Carin, 2019). By integrating SGAs with traditional methods, patient security can be improved and overall outcomes of airway management enhanced by anesthesiologists. In addition to optimizing primary airway management, the use of complex airway devices necessitates a clear insight into their limitations and complications. While devices like VL and SGAs enhance access and visualization, they are not flawless and can also fail in challenging conditions. Knowledge of other approaches is vital; for example, if repeated attempts at intubation fail, anesthesiologists must be able to implement a fallback strategy that might entail using maneuvers like front-of-neck access. In using systematic protocols of airway management, the risk of difficult intubations is minimized and good training among anesthesia practitioners is promoted (Law et al., 2021). This multi-modal strategy for the application of complex airway devices is essential in ensuring safety and effectiveness in the very complex practice field of anesthesia for ENT and airway surgery (Figure 5.11).

5.4.3. Monitoring During Airway Procedures

Successful monitoring during the conduct of airway procedures is crucial to maintaining patient safety as well as optimizing outcomes in ENT and airway surgery. Real-time monitoring of vital signs and respiratory function allows for the early recognition of potential complications, such as hypoxia or airway obstruction, that are particularly concerning in patients undergoing these advanced interventions. Application of complex monitoring techniques, including capnography and pulse oximetry, is now routine, which enables anesthesiologists and operating room staff to remain continuously vigilant during the process. In addition to enhancing situational awareness, these devices provide instantaneous feedback that can facilitate rapid intervention in the case of abnormal physiologic parameters. In addition, monitoring guidelines must be flexible so as to overcome the unique challenges present in airway procedures. The presence of anatomical abnormalities or a history of previous airway surgery may necessitate a more sophisticated approach, such as the utilization of extra monitoring modalities. A case in point is intraoperative neuromuscular monitoring, which can be instrumental in ensuring proper muscle relaxation, particularly in airway manipulation procedures. It is vital because residual neuromuscular blockade can lead to postoperative morbidity, such as respiratory failure, necessitating a very meticulous monitoring technique in the perioperative period. Individualized monitoring plans expansion is consonant with current evidence-based guidelines to improve surgical safety and patient outcomes. According to current literature and guidelines, for instance, in the management of multifactorial issues in airway management, it becomes necessary to firmly define and implement monitoring approaches that are evidence-based and consensus-driven. The importance of continuous monitoring is not only limited to respiratory and cardiovascular function, but also includes generalized considerations such as fluid management and drug interactions that may take place under anesthesia. These combined monitoring practices should find a place in clinical practice for facilitating team decision-making by multidisciplinary teams. The ongoing debate in the medical community regarding the evolution of monitoring techniques is a reflection of maintaining the quality of care in those undergoing ENT and airway surgery using anesthesia, with the final aim of enhancing clinical outcomes and patient safety (Prosser et al., 1998; Akyol et al., 2019).

Test Your Knowledge

1. Why is airway management critical during airway surgery?
2. What is a major anesthetic challenge in airway procedures?

5.5. Complications and Risks

Learning Outcome

1. Common complications associated with anesthesia
2. Specific risks in ENT and airway surgeries
3 Strategies for minimizing complications

Anesthesia for airway and ENT surgery has its very own unique set of risks and complications that call for careful consideration. One of them is the increased risk of postoperative complications in unsuspected OSAS patients. The prevalence of OSAS is much greater among surgical patients, and anesthesia has been shown to enhance collapsibility of the upper airway with attendant severe respiratory complications intraoperative and postoperative. Failure to recognize such patients preoperatively can result in inadequate management, and the probability of complications is higher. The association between anesthesia, sedation, and the REM sleep rebound process further underscores the need for screening for OSAS to minimize risk during the perioperative period. Special attention for this group is crucial in ensuring the successful management of airway surgery, with significance put on augmented preoperative evaluation and the implementation of tailored anesthesia protocols to guarantee patient safety (Vasu et al., 2012).

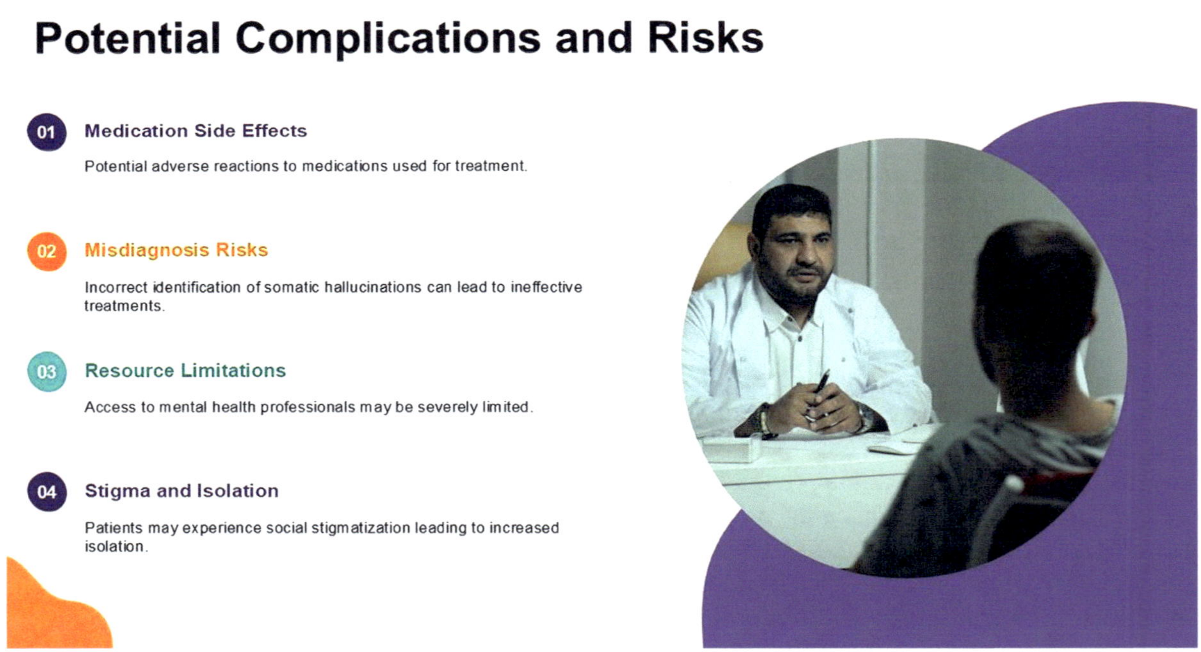
Potential Complications and Risks
01
Medication Side Effects
Potential adverse reactions to medications used for treatment.
02
Misdiagnosis Risks
Incorrect identification of somatic hallucinations can lead to ineffective treatments.
03
Resource Limitations
Access to mental health professionals may be severely limited.
04
Stigma and Isolation
Patients may experience social stigmatization leading to increased isolation.

Figure 5.12. Anesthesia for ENT and airway surgery presents a unique array of complications and risks.

Source: https://external-content.duckduckgo.com/iu/?u=https%3A%2F%2Fwww.slideteam.net%2Fmedia%2Fcatalog%2Fproduct%2Fcache%2F1280x720%2Fp%2Fo%2Fpotential_complications_and_risks_ppt_mockup_acp_slide01.jpg&f=1&nofb=1&ipt=c290d937570d925bfabc10264cf1be64f18456c01fc27f48603272caafd6ee0d.

Another significant factor in the complications presented in anesthesia is that of infection, particularly that of deep neck infections. Infections like these require a close understanding of the anatomical intricacy of the region involved and the potential complications they may pose intraoperatively. Extension of infection to the general region can lead to serious complications, such as mediastinitis and the risk of fatal hemorrhage. Demand for comprehensive surgical measures, at times multiple incisions for drainage, can have significant physical and psychological implications for patients. In addition, the fact that patients have tracheostomy and other treatments like nasogastric feeding can compound distress. Given these issues, surgeons and anesthesiologists must adopt a multidisciplinary approach to handling such cases by ensuring that there is patient information regarding the risks, benefits, and likely outcomes of the surgeries (Mărginean et al., 2018). Finally, the relationship between anesthetic and airway management in ENT surgery emphasizes the need for vigilance in observing and responding to potential problems. Anesthetics can cause unanticipated physiological effects, particularly in patients with preoperative respiratory illness. Therefore, intraoperative monitoring and preoperative planning must be established to allow prompt detection and correction of problems like airway obstruction or cardiovascular instability. Furthermore, the anesthetic technique greatly influences results. For instance, regional anesthesia may reduce the demand for general anesthetics and consequently reduce respiratory risks. With all these factors being so complex, there must be cooperation between the surgical team, anesthesia professionals, and nursing staff to maximize patient safety and minimize the occurrence of postoperative complications, thereby resulting in better surgical outcomes in patients with ENT and airway procedures (Vasu et al., 2012; Mărginean et al., 2018) (Figure 5.12).

5.5.1. Common Complications Associated with Anesthesia

Anesthesia plays a crucial role in ENT and airway surgery success, but it must be remembered that there are common complications in the process. Among the usual complications is an increased risk of respiratory issues, particularly in patients with OSAS, which is found in a high percentage of patients who are candidates for elective surgery. Sedative and anesthetic medications may exacerbate airway obstruction by increasing the collapsibility of the upper airway, leading to complications of the postoperative kind, such as respiratory distress and hypoxemia. The presence of undiagnosed OSAS among surgical candidates warrants full preoperative assessment and proper anesthetic management to avoid complications. Familiarity with the intricate relationship between anesthesia and respiratory function is vital in the pursuit of improving patient outcomes and ensuring safety in ENT and airway procedures (Vasu et al., 2012). Another important concern involving anesthesia is hemodynamic instability, which can have very serious effects on patients undergoing ENT and airway procedures. Anesthesia has effects on the cardiovascular system, particularly through the modulation of the autonomic response and vascular tone, potentially leading to alterations in blood pressure and heart rate. These hemodynamic changes may be particularly dangerous in patients with potential underlying cardiovascular disease or those undergoing long surgical procedures. Hemodynamic values need to be monitored and controlled with extreme care during anesthesia to prevent myocardial infarction or stroke under certain conditions. The effect of some drugs, particularly opioids, can also complicate hemodynamic stability and hence, tailored anesthesia management in high-risk patients is crucial (Mărginean et al., 2018). Deep neck space infections pose an additional challenge to both the surgical procedure and the administration of anesthesia. Peritonsillar and retropharyngeal abscesses have the potential to severely compromise the airway, necessitating urgent airway management intraoperatively. Infection of the deep neck has the potential to increase the risk of anesthetic complications, e.g., aspiration and airway obstruction. Anesthetic practitioners need to be able to foresee these complications and have strategies in place to deal with airway problems efficiently. Additionally, the risk of deep incisions and drainage necessary for these infectious complications carries a significant risk of postoperative pain and scarring, which can influence the overall recovery process for the patient. Thus, it is essential to address both the surgical and anesthetic aspects together for optimal outcomes for patients in the scenario of ENT and airway surgery (Mărginean et al., 2018).

5.5.2. Specific Risks in ENT and Airway Surgeries

ENT and airway surgeries carry unique risks and challenges that must be addressed adequately in an attempt to ensure patient safety. One of the risks involved is the danger of airway obstruction, a potentially severe complication that is exacerbated by the nature of procedures. Pre-existing conditions, such as OSAS, ensure that perioperative risks rise. ASOS prevalence in populations presenting for elective surgery works to emphasize the necessity of screening preoperatively because undiagnosed instances yield complications during the administration of sedation and anesthesia. The altered physiology of such patients, including the increased collapsibility of the upper airway with sedation, warrants cautious planning and management strategies for minimizing the risk of postoperative respiratory complications (Vasu et al., 2012). The second major risk in ENT and airway surgery is bleeding, particularly in those surgeries that involve the throat or nasal cavity, where there are numerous vessels and high risk of vessel injury. The challenge in hemostasis management is also enhanced by the likelihood of difficult intubation cases and the need for precise intraoperative airway management. Moreover, the use of medications such as anticoagulants or antiplatelet drugs can increase the risk of bleeding and make perioperative care more complicated. The effects of postoperative excessive bleeding are far-reaching, extending even beyond the direct surgical outcome, with longer recovery times and even lethal postoperative complications. Therefore, it is extremely important to have comprehensive knowledge about a patient's medication history and coagulation status in order to prevent side effects and maximize surgical outcomes (Akyol et al., 2019).

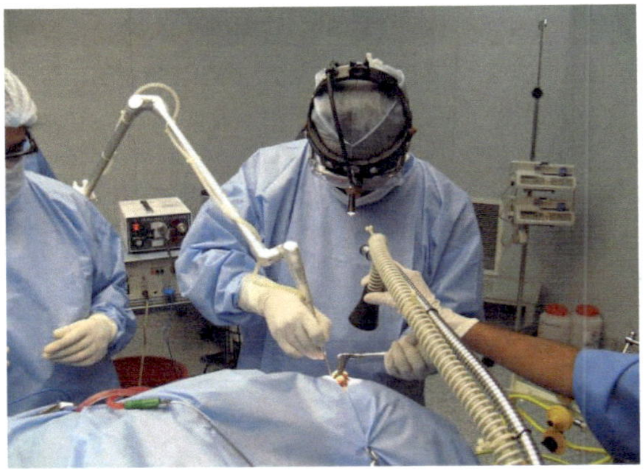

Figure 5.13. Specific risks in ENT and airway surgeries.

Source: https://external-content.duckduckgo.com/iu/?u=http%3A%2F%2Fwww.drpaulose.com%2Fwp-content%2Fuploads%2FLAPT.jpg&f=1&nofb=1&ipt=4ca799bd9b7608d0db9d84e73ddbb489696a57fe062bf20699ffa1cfa4c72720.

Lastly, aspiration risk is a primary consideration in the presence of anesthesia for airway and ENT procedures. The patient may present with a full stomach or gastric retention of emptying, increasing the chance of aspiration during induction or maintenance of anesthesia. Such a risk would be particularly significant in those presenting with airway structure manipulation procedures, where maintaining the patency of the airway would be difficult. Evidenced management procedures and techniques, including the use of rapid sequence induction and appropriate preoperative fasting, are essential in preventing this risk. Anesthesia providers must be attentive in assessing these risks for all patients and adjusting their anesthetic strategy to eliminate as much opportunity as possible for complications related to aspiration (Vasu et al., 2012) (Figure 5.13).

5.5.3. Strategies for Minimizing Complications

Effective methods for minimizing complications while patients are under anesthesia for ENT and airway surgery depend on appropriate preoperative assessment and the integration of innovative techniques. Accurate regard to the patient's history, including previous trouble with the airway, can warn the anesthesiologist of potential issues. Video laryngoscopy (VL) is an important advance in management of difficult airways. Studies have proven that VL significantly increases the success rate of first-attempt intubation and decreases complications when compared to direct laryngoscopy. Furthermore, the Canadian Airway Focus Group believes that VL must be the standard procedure for any anticipated tracheal intubations with the appropriate selection of blades to better visualize and minimize airway structural trauma (Law et al., 2021). Such anticipatory precautions improve airway management and also set up protocols through which intervention can be made promptly in the event of unexpected complications. Apart from preoperative assessment and the use of VL, standardized intervention during anesthesia is critical in minimizing complications among vulnerable populations like neonates and infants. The latest research showed that perioperative physiological instability under anesthesia in this patient group may evoke life-threatening events in need of urgent therapeutic intervention, mainly because of hypotension or inadequate oxygenation (Disma et al., 2021). The use of monitoring systems for the continuous observation of physiological parameters in real-time helps anesthesiologists react promptly to these derangements and thus, ensure that early corrective measures are adopted to stabilize hemodynamic and oxygenation variables. Furthermore, clinicians must establish unequivocal intervention thresholds from empirical evidence and collaborate closely with other medical specialists to formulate an integrated approach to the care of high-risk patients, especially those with underlying disease or congenital malformations. Finally, education and continuing education for anesthesia professionals are essential to enhance competency and minimize anesthetic risks in ENT and airway procedures. Repeated simulation-based training can prepare anesthesiologists for different airway management scenarios so that they might apply appropriate exit strategies in case of failed initial intubation. The CAFG emphasizes the need for designating an airway lead within institutions to organize training programs and assess the quality of airway management protocols. By creating a learning and adapting environment, anesthesiologists could enhance their ability and thus their performance to handle complex cases and deliver safer anesthesia outcomes and improved patient outcomes (Law et al., 2021). The preservation of continuous education and evidence-based guidelines would also go a long way in stemming the incidence of anesthetic procedure-related complications, reiterating the importance of preparedness to work in high-risk environments like ENT and airway surgery.

Test Your Knowledge

1. What is a common respiratory complication of anesthesia?
2. Why is monitoring important to prevent anesthesia-related complications?

5.6. Postoperative Care

Learning Outcome

1. Pain management strategies
2. Monitoring for complications
3. Discharge criteria and follow-up

Postoperative care is a significant component of the continuum of patient care following anesthesia for ENT surgeries. Understanding the nuances of anesthesia, especially in cases involving sedation or induction of general anesthetic, is crucial to prevent recovery complications. Postoperative monitoring is crucial to monitor the patient for respiratory distress or response to anesthetic agents, especially in view of the frequent airway problems encountered in the majority of ENT surgeries. This entails systematic assessment of oxygenation, ventilation, and overall hemodynamic stability. The development of anesthetic techniques, such as the use of short-acting agents, has been reported to improve recovery profiles and diminish complications like postoperative nausea and pain, once again highlighting the importance of customized postoperative protocols in achieving optimal patient outcomes in ENT surgery (Shetti, 2024). In airway management, no less significant is proper postoperative care. Because many ENT operations involve airway maneuvers, it is necessary to preserve airway patency and be aware of obstructions. The patient can have varying amounts of edema or swelling following surgery to complicate recovery. In this case, providers must be prepared to use specialized methods, such as fiberoptic intubation, to address unusual complications. By including specialized monitoring equipment, such as capnography, early respiratory compromise can also be detected. Additionally, postoperative care should include a multi-specialty plan incorporating intercommunication with surgical teams to transfer any intraoperative concerns, ultimately resulting in a seamless transition to recovery and improving the patient's overall experience (In et al., 2013). Moreover, patient and family education in the postoperative period cannot be overlooked. Providing clear instructions regarding complications, pain management, and follow-up visits is crucial to encourage patient confidence and understanding. Emphasizing the importance of adhering to postoperative regimens, including wound care and medication compliance, can profoundly influence recovery outcomes. In addition, assessing and addressing pre-discharge anxiety plays an important role in enhancing postoperative satisfaction. By fostering a culture of overall postoperative care, medical professionals not only facilitate patients' better recovery from surgery but also encourage them to appreciate follow-up as a way of preserving their well-being way beyond the operating room (Shetti, 2024) (Figure 5.14).

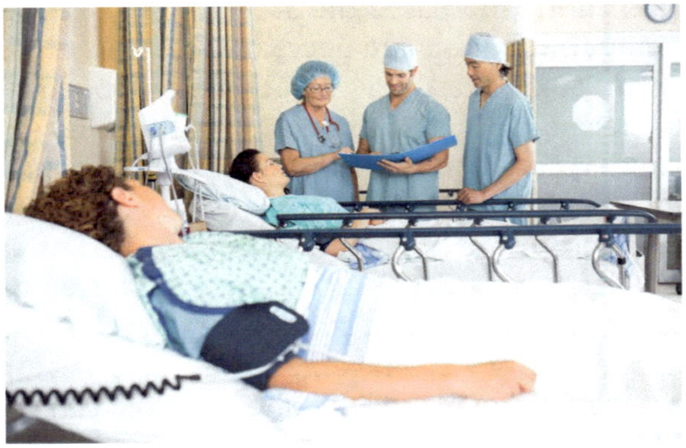

Figure 5.14. Postoperative care is a critical component in the continuum of patient management.

Source: https://external-content.duckduckgo.com/iu/?u=https%3A%2F%2Fassets.neurosurgicalatlas.com%2Fvolumes%2FATLAS%2F1-PRINCIPLES_OF_CRANIAL_SURGERY%2F25-Postoperative_Care%2FPCS_Postop_01.jpg&f=1&nofb=1&ipt=a1ae5a38508262179acde868c765b0748a0e49960a8e30e4a9fb716e847a7bb2.

5.6.1. Pain Management Strategies

Effective pain management in ENT and airway surgery is a multidirectional approach that demands a thorough understanding of patient-specific factors and surgical factors. The anesthesiologists' role includes developing a comprehensive pain management strategy that involves both pharmacologic and non-pharmacologic measures. For instance, the application of multimodal analgesia can significantly improve postoperative outcomes by including a variety of analgesics to treat multiple paths of pain. This approach not only reduces the demand for opioids but also lessens the danger of opioid-induced side effects. Augmenting interventions, such as nerve blocks, may be blended with systemic medication, yielding localized relief from pain targeted to the specific surgical procedure. In light of the multifaceted nature of ENT and airway procedures, involving typically tender anatomical structures, the implementation of these measures becomes a necessity for the best patient comfort and satisfaction (Disma et al., 2021). In addition to pharmacologic methods, non-pharmacologic methods also form a significant part of pain management measures in this surgical field. Interventions such as guided imagery, relaxation therapy, and educational therapy are perhaps useful in lowering anxiety as well as pain tolerance. These interventions allow the patients to actively participate in pain control, with resultant higher overall satisfaction in the delivered treatment. Integration of these interventions into the anesthesia care plan is also essential, particularly for pediatric patients, who perceive pain differently and psychologically process surgery. Patients and their families should also be taught by the anesthesia providers during the perioperative period about the pain management strategies, emphasizing mutual decision-making appropriate to the patient's preferences and expectations (Iorio-Morin et al., 2020). Monitoring of postoperative pain is necessary for maximizing pain management. Proper pain assessment using standardized scales, combined with open communication with the patient, enables medical personnel to actively adjust analgesic therapy based on differing pain experiences. Continual reassessment of pain severity offers an early chance for intervention, preventing undertreatment or overtreatment complications and ensuring relief. Special care may be needed for vulnerable populations, such as neonates and individuals with existing medical conditions, who develop altered responses to analgesics. Accordingly, a personalized adaptive pain management practice—integrating broad-spectrum assessments and evidence-based guidelines—can substantially enhance the quality of anesthesia care in ENT and airway surgery, ultimately benefiting improved patient outcomes (Disma et al., 2021) (Figure 5.15).

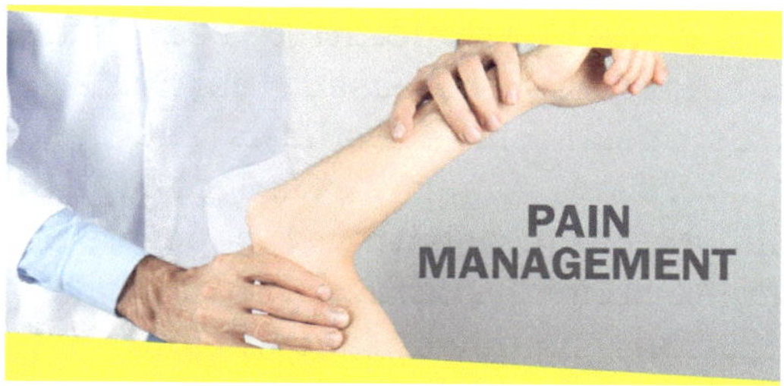

Figure 5.15. The pain management in ENT and airway surgery.

Source: https://external-content.duckduckgo.com/iu/?u=https%3A%2F%2Fwww.mostinside.com%2Fwp-content%2Fuploads%2F2022%2F04%2FPain-Management-Strategies.jpg&f=1&nofb=1&ipt=20d60eb4e27e4a59c2b660cc837ecc611f8cd7098b907016618e7ff71aa0d280.

5.6.2. Monitoring for Complications

Effective monitoring for anesthesia complications, particularly in ENT and airway surgery, is pivotal in maintaining patient safety. The nature of procedures required necessitates watchful monitoring since the case entails close contact of essential structures such as the airway, vocal cords, and vascular systems within close proximity. Continuous monitoring of vital signs such as heart rate, blood pressure, and oxygen saturation is important in identifying any physiologic aberrations that might be manifested during a surgical procedure. Furthermore, employing advanced monitoring techniques, such as capnography, allows anesthesiologists to monitor respiratory function in real-time, enabling them to detect likely airway-associated complications early. This proactive process is invaluable not only in preventing unwanted consequences but also in making the operating room environment ready to the best possible level for the operating team to facilitate an efficient teamwork environment that is critical in high-risk procedures. Patient-specific risk factors are also essential in the monitoring process. In OSAS patients, frequently not identified on preoperative assessment, the risk for perioperative complications is considerably increased, particularly as regards anesthesia. Anesthesia and sedation may increase upper airway collapsibility, raising the stakes within the perioperative arena. Awareness and understanding of such populations empower anesthesiologists to devise targeted intraoperative management strategies, minimizing risk. Efficient preoperative screening methods, like extensive medical history examination, facilitate adequate monitoring regimens and postoperative care depending on the unique needs of OSAS patients, as discussed in Vasu et al. (2012). This individualized approach addresses the importance of anesthetic management tailored to individual patients in order to prevent serious complications. Additional postoperative monitoring is especially important in eradicating potential risks that might be presented by anesthesia in ENT and airway procedures. After the surgical procedure, patients must be closely observed for signs of respiratory distress or airway obstruction because the latter occurs in a variety of forms, among which are stridor or desaturation. The use of continuous pulse oximetry in the recovery room allows for the earliest possible detection of hypoxemia, which can allow for immediate interventions in case of complications. Furthermore, opioid administration should be tightly controlled—useful as they are for postoperative pain control, they can also exacerbate airway complications, particularly in OSAS or other respiratory illnesses. Thus, a full system of monitoring not just encompasses intraoperative vigilance but also carries over to the postoperative period and makes sure that patients are provided with the safest and most effective care during their process of surgery, according to the information provided (Vasu et al., 2012) (Figure 5.16).

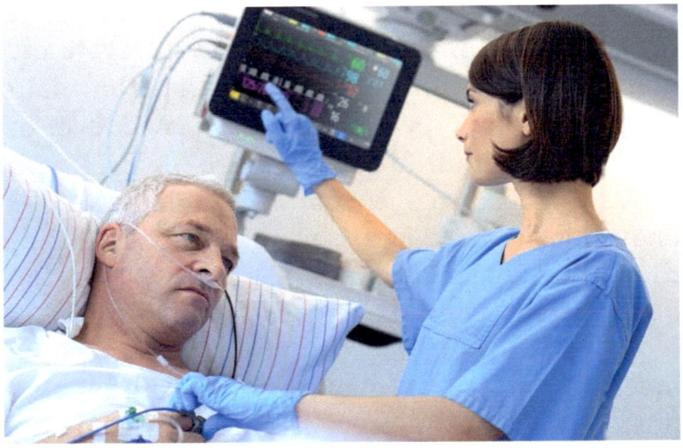

Figure 5.16. The monitoring for complications during anesthesia.

Source: https://external-content.duckduckgo.com/iu/?u=https%3A%2F%2Fwww.hhmglobal.com%2Fwp-content%2Fuploads%2Fnews%2F25165%2FPhilips_Patient_monitoring.jpg&f=1&nofb=1&ipt=de84544305802ea86b2cb3211402927db18ac028903ae7501afcb95927260ca0.

5.6.3. Discharge Criteria and Follow-Up

Effective discharge criteria and follow-up strategies are important parameters in ensuring patient safety and optimizing outcomes in ENT and airway anesthesia. Discharge from a surgical facility is typically directed by the recovery of the patient from anesthesia and overall physiological stability. Assessment is focused on vital signs such as blood pressure, pulse, oxygen saturation, and neurological examination. A structured protocol that establishes these criteria has the potential to significantly improve patient identification of risk for post-surgery complications. Complications such as hypotension and hypoxia, for example, which may present as low oxygen saturation, should be closely monitored after recovery. This holds especially true in pediatric and neonatal patients, where response to physiological changes could be vastly different, thus the imperative for an effective adaptation of discharge planning (Disma et al., 2021). Recovery from surgery is essential during follow-up care, especially in complicated airway management and procedures. A model discharge plan would not just offer home instructions on the taking of vital signs but also symptom protocols that mandate immediate attention. For patients undergoing procedures with inherent danger, such as mucopolysaccharidosis patients, an efficient follow-up timetable ensures that complications due to anesthesia are detected and treated in their early stages. The importance of multi-disciplinary involvement in the follow-up care process cannot be overstated, as it brings together the numerous expertise necessary for managing the unique needs of every patient. Such constant monitoring can help detect any late complications or issues related to anesthetic agents during surgery, ultimately ensuring patient safety and recovery outcomes (Moretto et al., 2018). Further, discharge and follow-up planning, patient education are also important. Teaching patients and their families the signs of potential complications can be empowering in that they will know how to access medical care in a timely fashion and avoid resultant adverse outcomes. What is learned needs to be clear, unambiguous, and at the level of understanding for the patients, considering the varied backgrounds of patients who are having ENT and airway surgery. It is also beneficial to assess the patient's level of access to support networks and health care, which could influence their ability to adhere to appointments and guidelines. By addressing these issues in an extensive way, medical practitioners can develop a more efficient discharge process and supportive aftercare scheme, ultimately ensuring a safer and more effective recovery for those patients who are undergoing anesthetic procedures (Disma et al., 2021).

Test Your Knowledge

1. What is the role of analgesics in anesthesia?
2. Name one non-pharmacological method used for pain management.

Summary

Administration of anesthesia for airway and ENT surgery is a complicated practice that demands a similarly complicated understanding of both the operation and the specific anesthesia technique involved. The intricacy involved in trying to manage airway access, particularly in infections like deep neck infections, reflects the need for multidisciplinary practice. ENT surgeons must also be adequately trained to deal with potential complications, such as mediastinitis and septic shock, that are likely to arise due to the dissemination of infections from primary sites in the neck. These conditions are not just demanding of expert technical skill but also meticulous preoperative assessment and postoperative observation to minimize anesthesia risks, eventually leading to better prognosis in this sensitive branch of medicine (Mărginean et al., 2018). Moreover, the psychological and aesthetic impact of ENT procedures cannot be underestimated. With surgery tending to introduce significant alteration in the morphology of the neck, patients can tolerate heightened distress and anxiety regarding scarring and need for postoperative interventions such as tracheostomy or nasogastric tubes. Thus, informed consent becomes important. Ensuring that patients are adequately educated on what to expect with their surgical intervention helps to build trust and provides for a better patient-provider relationship. By providing patients with an honest and comprehensive view of both the risks involved with surgery and the benefits of anesthesia, healthcare providers can maximize patient satisfaction and cooperation during the perioperative period (Mărginean et al., 2018). Finally, as we move forward to acknowledging anesthesia's role in these complex procedures, there should be an introduction of evidence-based standards for the care of anesthesia, similar to how this has been achieved in the formulation of integrated care protocols in diseases like mucopolysaccharidosis. The integration of experts' consensus in clinical use can optimize outcomes and make anesthesia practices safe as well as efficient. This interactive process, in which not only surgeons but also anesthesiologists and other experts are involved, is central to understanding the intricacies involved in ENT procedures. There is more research to be done in the future to address new methodologies and refine current guidelines, keeping intact the commitment to delivering quality care but assuring patient safety and comfort during these critical procedures.

In evaluating the complexities of ENT and airway surgery anesthesia, it is evident that an adequate understanding of potential complications as well as measures for risk reduction is necessary. One of the major risk elements is airway fire, a still-preventable complication of surgical procedures. Depending on the guidelines in place, minimization of the volume of oxidizing agents, especially oxygen, goes a long way in preventing it. It is critical that anesthesia practitioners are informed about such mitigation practices, as evidenced by a quality improvement project whose aim was to enhance provider knowledge and therefore reduce the volumes of supplemental oxygen administered in high-risk surgeries, underscoring the significance of continuous education and adherence to safety protocols in clinical practice (Patel et al., 2020). Difficult tracheal intubation (DI) is yet another risk particular to ENT surgery, especially in patients undergoing thyroid surgery. The incidence of DI is markedly greater on the basis of anatomical variations, such as thyromegaly. A strict preoperative airway evaluation is warranted, as highlighted by a study involving 2,379 patients, in which parameters such as neck circumference and history of DI have emerged as significant predictors. The research indicates that "although tracheal dislocation was a high predictor," it does not work independently of other predictors, so a more multi-factorial strategy for risk assessment is needed. This observation captures the importance of individualized assessment in planning anesthesia for thyroid surgery patients, thereby enhancing patient safety and surgical outcomes overall (Tošković et al., 2016). Lastly, effective anesthesia management of ENT and airway surgery needs to have an interdisciplinary practice of patient care from preparation, during performance, to post-operative monitoring. Emphasis should be placed on understanding the unique physiological concerns posed by airway-altering illnesses and thus require specially adapted anesthesia techniques. Among the major lessons of recent studies is the necessity for anesthesiology professionals to become more adept at conducting airway exams and in contemplating complications. This dedication to total preoperative evaluation and adherence to evidence-based practice ensures not only the minimization of adverse events but also the optimal postoperative recovery for patients of advanced ENT procedures. Overall, adherence to current guidelines and commitment to education are at the heart of effective anesthesia management for this specialized area of surgery.

KEY TERMS FROM THIS CHAPTER

- Anxiolytics
- Hypoxemia
- Landscape
- Meticulous anesthetic planning
- Monitored anesthesia care (MAC)
- Obstructive sleep apnea syndrome (OSAS)
- Surgical planning
- High-quality anesthesia
- Intubation scenarios
- Medical intervention
- Minimally invasive techniques
- Obstruction
- Safeguard patient outcomes

Critical Thinking Questions

1. **What is the primary concern during anesthesia for tonsillectomy?**
   a. Hypotension
   b. Airway obstruction
   c. Bleeding
   d. Bronchospasm
2. **Which of the following techniques is commonly used for airway management in microlaryngeal surgery?**
   a. Endotracheal intubation
   b. Jet ventilation
   c. Laryngeal mask airway (LMA)
   d. Nasopharyngeal airway
3. **During tracheostomy under general anesthesia, when is the most critical period for airway management?**
   a. During skin incision
   b. After the trachea is opened but before the tracheostomy tube is placed
   c. During suturing of the tracheostomy tube
   d. After the procedure is complete
4. **What is the most effective way to prevent airway fire during laser airway surgery?**
   a. Using high oxygen concentrations
   b. Employing a closed circuit ventilation system
   c. Avoiding nitrous oxide and reducing oxygen concentration
   d. Applying petroleum-based lubricants
5. **Which local anesthetic technique is commonly used for awake fiberoptic intubation in ENT surgery?**
   a. Glossopharyngeal nerve block
   b. Superior laryngeal nerve block
   c. Recurrent laryngeal nerve block
   d. All of the above

Short Answer Questions

1. What are the key considerations for airway management in microlaryngeal surgery?
2. Describe the role of jet ventilation in airway surgeries.
3. What are the challenges of anesthesia in patients with obstructive sleep apnea (OSA)?
4. Why is controlled hypotension used during endoscopic sinus surgery?
5. Which nerve blocks are commonly used for awake fiberoptic intubation in ENT surgery?
6. How is aspiration of blood prevented during nasal surgery?

Answer to Critical Thinking Questions

1. (d); 2. (c); 3. (b); 4. (c); 5. (a)

References

1. Reinero, C., Visser, L. C., Kellihan, H. B., Masseau, I., Rozanski, E., Clercx, C., Williams, K., Abbott, J., Borgarelli, M., & Scansen, B. A. (2020). ACVIM consensus statement guidelines for the diagnosis, classification, treatment, and monitoring of pulmonary hypertension in dogs. *Journal of veterinary internal medicine*, *34*(2), 549–573. https://doi.org/10.1111/jvim.15725 (accessed on 28th June 2025).

2. Akyol, M. U., Alden, T. D., Amartino, H., Ashworth, J., Belani, K., Berger, K. I., Borgo, A., Braunlin, E., Eto, Y., Gold, J. I., Jester, A., Jones, S. A., Karsli, C., Mackenzie, W., Marinho, D. R., McFadyen, A., McGill, J., Mitchell, J. J., Muenzer, J., Okuyama, T., ... MPS Consensus Programme Co-Chairs (2019). Recommendations for the management of MPS IVA: systematic evidence- and consensus-based guidance. *Orphanet journal of rare diseases*, *14*(1), 137. https://doi.org/10.1186/s13023-019-1074-9(accessed on 28th June 2025).

3. Alhaj, Z., Almubaid, Z., Irshad, O., Choucair, G., & Mohamed, S. (2024). Retrograde lidocaine spray for awake extubating in pediatric ENT surgery: Optimizing tonsillectomy and adenoidectomy outcomes. *Cureus, 16.* https://www.semanticscholar.org/paper/c7452989b693dbae605cc1d6edf785d41b673d6b (accessed on 28th June 2025).

4. Mărginean, E., Egor, S., Venter, C., Pantiș, A., Vălenaș, O., Sorban, I., Domuța, M., Bălălău, C., Scaunasu, R., & Popescu, B. (2018). Management of Deep Space Infections of the Neck. *Journal of Mind and Medical Sciences*, *5*(1), 53-58. https://doi.org/10.22543/7674.51.P5358(accessed on 28th June 2025).

5. Luyten, A., Bettens, K., D'haeseleer, E., De Ley, S., Hodges, A., Galiwango, G., Vermeersch, H., & Van Lierde, K. (2013). Impact of early synchronous lip and palatal repair on speech. *Folia phoniatrica et logopaedica : official organ of the International Association of Logopedics and Phoniatrics (IALP)*, *65*(6), 303–311. https://doi.org/10.1159/000362501(accessed on 28th June 2025).

6. Boukari, B. M., Maikassoua, M., Rabiu, M. B., Abdoulaye, M. B., Niandou, A. O., et al. (2021). Review of anesthesia for ENT, oral and maxillofacial surgery at the National Hospital of Niamey: Situational analysis in limited resource setting. *Anesthesia and Critical Care.* https://www.semanticscholar.org/paper/3da9f4aa72efccd7bfeda38a9d4e39ba2a438b6d (accessed on 28th June 2025).

7. Parfianowicz, A., Surma, A., Jaworski, A., Grajnert, F., Plizga, J., Głuszczyk, A., ... Holdun, N. (2024). Local anesthesia as an alternative to general anesthesia in ENT surgery – a review of selected procedures. *Quality in Sport*, *17*, 53354. https://doi.org/10.12775/QS.2024.17.53354(accessed on 28th June 2025).

8. Cheon, B., Lee, J. H., Kim, J. H., & Hwang, S. (2024). Airway management of a patient with Mounier-Kuhn syndrome during general anesthesia–A case report. *Anesthesia and Pain Medicine, 19*, 156–160. https://www.semanticscholar.org/paper/3e67e155ae6d336ef0e6e1de4bf79f9f4fcd5630 (accessed on 28th June 2025).

9. Givi, B., Schiff, B. A., Chinn, S. B., Clayburgh, D., Iyer, N. G., Jalisi, S., Moore, M. G., Nathan, C. A., Orloff, L. A., O'Neill, J. P., Parker, N., Zender, C., Morris, L. G. T., & Davies, L. (2020). Safety Recommendations for Evaluation and Surgery of the Head and Neck During the

COVID-19 Pandemic. *JAMA otolaryngology-- head & neck surgery, 146*(6), 579–584. https://doi.org/10.1001/jamaoto.2020.0780(accessed on 28th June 2025).

10. Disma, N., Veyckemans, F., Virág, K., Hansen, T. G., Becke, K., Harlet, P., Vutskits, L., et al. (2021). Morbidity and mortality after anesthesia in early life: Results of the European prospective multicenter observational study, neonate and children audit of anesthesia practice in Europe (NECTARINE). *British Journal of Anesthesia, 126*, 1157–1172. https://doi.org/10.1016/j.bja.2021.02.016 (accessed on 28th June 2025).
11. Singh, H., Vogel, R. W., Lober, R. M., Doan, A. T., Matsumoto, C. I., Kenning, T. J., & Evans, J. J. (2016). Intraoperative Neurophysiological Monitoring for Endoscopic Endonasal Approaches to the Skull Base: A Technical Guide. *Scientifica, 2016*, 1751245. https://doi.org/10.1155/2016/1751245(accessed on 28th June 2025).
12. Vasu, T. S., Grewal, R., & Doghramji, K. (2012). Obstructive sleep apnea syndrome and perioperative complications: a systematic review of the literature. *Journal of clinical sleep medicine : JCSM : official publication of the American Academy of Sleep Medicine, 8*(2), 199–207. https://doi.org/10.5664/jcsm.1784(accessed on 28th June 2025).
13. Drummond, R. L., Hermes, F. S., Krumenauer, R. C. P., Netto, A. P., et al. (2012). Laryngomalacia surgery: A series from a tertiary pediatric hospital. https://core.ac.uk/download/pdf/81110246.pdf (accessed on 28th June 2025).
14. Hagberg, C. A. (2019). Combined fellowship training in head and neck anesthesia and advanced airway management. *Journal of Head & Neck Anesthesia, 3*, e9–e9. https://doi.org/10.1097/hn9.0000000000000009 (accessed on 28th June 2025).
15. In, J., Park, M., & Han, J. (2013). Temporary solution for one lung ventilation with isolated bronchial blocker of Univent® tube. *Korean Journal of Anesthesiology, 64*, 187–188. https://www.semanticscholar.org/paper/8a6a1abe495c4c52a3ebe7ae4bc35f0691aa0c4a (accessed on 28th June 2025).
16. Iorio-Morin, C., Hodaie, M., Sarica, C., Dea, N., Westwick, H. J., Christie, S., McDonald, P. J., et al. (2020). Letter: The risk of COVID-19 infection during neurosurgical procedures: A review of severe acute respiratory distress syndrome coronavirus 2 (SARS-CoV-2) modes of transmission and proposed neurosurgery-specific measures for mitigation. *Neurosurgery, 87*, E178–E185. https://doi.org/10.1093/neuros/nyaa157 (accessed on 28th June 2025).
17. Kelly, J. W. (1977). *Administrative Manual for Schools of Nurse Anesthesia: A Research and Development Study.* https://core.ac.uk/download/618329673.pdf (accessed on 28th June 2025).
18. Law, J. A., Duggan, L. V., Asselin, M., Baker, P., Crosby, E. T., Downey, A., Hung, O., et al. (2021). Canadian Airway Focus Group updated consensus-based recommendations for management of the difficult airway: Part 1. Difficult airway management encountered in an unconscious patient. *Canadian Journal of Anesthesia/Journal Canadian Anesthesia, 68*, 1373–1404. https://doi.org/10.1007/s12630-021-02007-0 (accessed on 28th June 2025).
19. Lee, S. J., & Sung, T. Y. (2020). Emergence agitation: Current knowledge and unresolved questions. *Korean Journal of Anesthesiology, 73*, 471–485. https://doi.org/10.4097/kja.20097 (accessed on 28th June 2025).
20. Lei, G., Yang, S., Wu, L., Yin, Y., Xi, C., Xiao, Y., & Wang, G. (2025). Improved tubeless airway management in JORRP surgery: Comparative analysis of pre- and post-THRIVE implementation.

Therapeutics and Clinical Risk Management, 21, 647–654. https://www.semanticscholar.org/paper/8b0feffe671e0844ae5024bd746bff56aff9100c (accessed on 28th June 2025).

21. Moretto, A., Bosatra, M. G., Marchesini, L., & Tesoro, S. (2018). Anesthesiologic risks in mucopolysaccharidoses. *The Italian Journal of Pediatrics, 44.* https://doi.org/10.1186/s13052-018-0554-1 (accessed on 28th June 2025).
22. Muschol, N., Giugliani, R., Jones, S., Muenzer, J., Smith, N., Whitley, C. B., Donnell, M., et al. (2022). Sanfilippo syndrome: Consensus guidelines for clinical care. *Orphanet Journal of Rare Diseases, 17.* https://doi.org/10.1186/s13023-022-02484-6 (accessed on 28th June 2025).
23. Shyshchuk, V. D., Ohiienko, M. M., Redko, S. I., & Огиенко, et al. (2015). *General Questions of Anesthesiology.* https://core.ac.uk/download/141448194.pdf (accessed on 28th June 2025).
24. Patel, D., Smith, K., & Woodmansee, S. (2020). Airway fire prevention in the operating room. https://core.ac.uk/download/491320079.pdf (accessed on 28th June 2025).
25. Prosser, D., Friesen, M., Allman, P., Grassby, P., & Streisand, J. (1998). Oral transmucosal fentanyl. https://core.ac.uk/download/17353596.pdf (accessed on 28th June 2025).
26. Radichkova, V., & Mladenov, B. (2020). Difficult airways in ENT surgery. *16*, 24–28. https://www.semanticscholar.org/paper/a5b59653c6ef0ac1aadeb7caf2ad543ea40a3148 (accessed on 28th June 2025).
27. Salinding, A., Wahyudi, W., & Pradipta, A. (2022). Anesthesia and analgesia management profile for airway surgeries at Dr. Soetomo General Academic Hospital Surabaya. *Indonesian Journal of Anesthesiology and Reanimation.* https://www.semanticscholar.org/paper/6f40ff5d07b86cd667ad67ea49b6cd2ad173a43e (accessed on 28th June 2025).
28. Scott-Warren, V., & Walker, R. A. (2020). Perioperative management of patients with Mucolipidosis II and III: Lessons from a case series. *Pediatric Anesthesia, 31*, 260–267. https://doi.org/10.1111/pan.14090 (accessed on 28th June 2025).
29. Shetti. (2024). Sedation and anesthesia in ambulatory ENT procedures–A review. *IP Journal of Otorhinolaryngology and Allied Science.* https://www.semanticscholar.org/paper/a0cca46ee17823575a80cec96ece5aaaf3ecedde (accessed on 28th June 2025).
30. Tošković, A., Miličić, B., Marković, D., Stevanović, K., Stojanović, M., Kalezić, N., Sabljak, V., et al. (2016). Prediktori zbrinjavanja otežanog dišnog puta u kirurgiji štitnjače: Petogodišnja opservacijska prospektivna studija u jednom centru. https://core.ac.uk/download/33293370.pdf (accessed on 28th June 2025).
31. Department of Anesthesia. University of Iowa. Spring 2011. https://core.ac.uk/download/18608347.pdf
32. Xia, M., Ma, W., Zuo, M., Deng, X., Xue, F. S., Battaglini, D., Aggarwal, V., et al. (2023). Expert consensus on difficult airway assessment. *Hepatobiliary Surgery and Nutrition, 12*, 545–566. https://doi.org/10.21037/hbsn-23-46 (accessed on 28th June 2025).

ANESTHESIA FOR UROLOGIC AND RENAL SURGERY

6

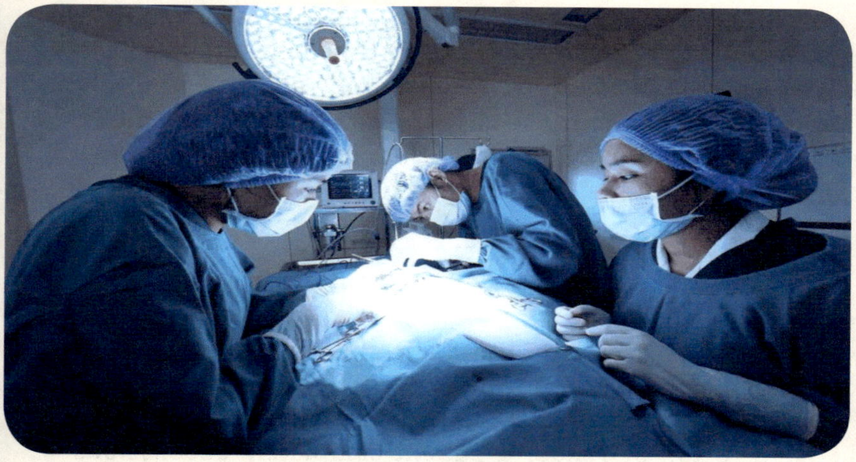

LEARNING OBJECTIVES

After studying this chapter, you will be able to:

1. Discuss the types of anesthesia
2. Focus on preoperative assessment
3. Understand anesthetic techniques in urologic surgery
4. Explain the anesthetic techniques in renal surgery
5. Know intraoperative management
6. Learn about postoperative care

Introduction

In urologic and renal surgery, anesthesia plays an important part in patient protection and comfort during the procedure. Technical necessities of these procedures involve a thorough comprehension of various anesthetic techniques, indications and contraindications, and correlation with surgical outcomes. It is essential to acknowledge the specific requirements of urologic operations, ranging from transurethral resections to nephrectomies, which dictate diverse anesthetic approaches tailored to optimize intraoperative conditions. Adequate anesthesia not only alleviates pain but also minimizes physiological stress response, thereby improving recovery and lessening perioperative complications. The importance of meticulously planning anesthesia protocols cannot, therefore, be overestimated since it directly affects surgical outcome and patient satisfaction. Besides, the perioperative environment is unique in the sense that it presents certain challenges, particularly regarding the prevention of potential complications like venous thromboembolism (VTE). VTE has been found to be a huge source of morbidity and mortality among surgical patients, necessitating prophylactic measures. According to the guidelines prescribed by the American Society of Hematology (ASH), individualized urologic procedural VTE prevention plans are essential in preventing postoperative care-related risks (Nelson et al., 2019). Utilizing evidence-based methods, anesthesiologists and the surgical team can cooperate to enhance patient outcomes by effectively dealing with complications well ahead of time. This approach not only highlights the imperatives of individualized care but also the growing intersection of anesthetic practice and broader-based considerations in surgery. In addition, ongoing innovation in anesthetic technique and technology continues to enrich their use in urologic and renal surgery. New agents, such as long-acting local anesthetics and adjuvants, have transformed multimodal analgesia approaches, enabling decreased use of opioids and improved postoperative recovery pathways. In addition, more recent evidence shows that direct oral anticoagulants (DOACs) are also useful in surgical patients, ushering in a paradigm shift for perioperative anticoagulation management (Nelson et al., 2019). Implementation of the innovation in practice underscores the need for ongoing education and training among anesthesia providers to assure safe and effective practice. As the science continues to advance, collaboration between anesthesiologists, surgeons, and other physicians will remain vital for continuing to fine-tune anesthesia for urologic and renal surgery in order to ultimately enhance patient safety and surgical efficacy.

Definition of Anesthesia

Understanding of anesthesia is at the heart of its application in urologic and renal surgery since it entails a set of techniques employed to block pain, induce unconsciousness, and ensure patient safety during medical procedures. In essence, anesthesia is a specialty in medicine that employs pharmacologic drugs to locally anesthetize a region or render a patient completely unconscious during surgery. The decision between general anesthesia, regional blocks, and local anesthetics relies on a variety of considerations, including the character of the surgical intervention, patient history, and postoperative recovery expectation. Each of these anesthetics bears intrinsic benefits as well as risks that have direct implications for surgical success. or failure, thereby identifying the importance of careful anesthetic planning and management unique to each patient. For urologic and kidney surgeries, anesthesia is critical to deliver optimal patient comfort and avoid postoperative issues. General anesthesia entails techniques such as making the patient completely unconscious for surgeries such as nephrectomy, while regional anesthesia is applied in less complex procedures to manage pain while not keeping the patient awake. Anesthetist' role goes beyond simple sedation; it involves a basic role in the control of physiological functions during surgery, like cardiovascular stability and respiratory status. Notably, the choice of anesthetic agents may influence courses of recovery since research has shown that selection between neuromuscular blockade reversals significantly influences the incidence of complications, for instance, significant pulmonary complications among patients undergoing noncardiac surgery (Kheterpal et al., 2020). Further, modern practice within anesthesia utilizes evidence-based guidelines to ensure safety and efficacy, notably with regard to the prevention of venous thromboembolism during surgery. Anesthetics do affect the hemodynamics, and prevention of venous thromboembolism (VTE) is especially relevant in urologic surgery, where there is exposure to immobilization and vascular stasis. Recommendations from expert bodies, such as those established by the American Society of Hematology, provide guidelines regarding prophylactic care unique to urologic surgery, encouraging mechanical preventive action and pharmacologic prophylaxis as appropriate (Nelson et al., 2019). By acknowledging the overall role of anesthesia in surgical care, clinicians are not only able to enhance patient outcomes but also reduce postoperative complications, placing a priority on customized anesthetic methods in urologic and renal procedures (Figure 6.1).

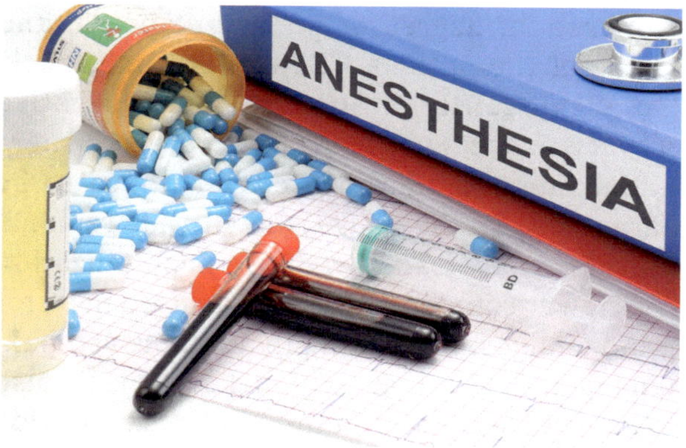

Figure 6.1. The anesthesia.

Source: https://external-content.duckduckgo.com/iu/?u=https%3A%2F%2Fpix4free.org%2Fassets%2Flibrary%2F2021-03-25%2Foriginals%2Fanesthesia.jpg&f=1&nofb=1&ipt=055f92ce13eb2b307ce74553cea60b58e8787ec28371b46bc381e517cdc01ade.

Importance of Anesthesia in Urologic and Renal Surgery

Anesthetic administration in urologic and renal surgery is of the utmost importance due to the complex nature of interventions being performed and the peculiar physiological factors of the urinary apparatus. In interventions such as radical cystectomy or nephrectomy, the patient is often subjected to comorbidities such as hypertension, renal insufficiency, or diabetes that can complicate anesthesia management. Good anesthesia not only gives the patients comfort but also minimizes the risk of complications during surgery. Specifically, individually tailored anesthetic regimens can optimize cardiovascular stability and renal perfusion, which is paramount in preserving kidney function during the course of surgery. The ability to customize anesthetic procedures according to the individual requirements of patients reflects a holistic approach that is important for maximum outcomes in these risk-prone settings (Gohad et al., 2025). Also, the choice of anesthetic technique has a significant influence on post-operative recovery and overall surgical success in urological and renal interventions. Multimodal analgesia, the combination of general anesthesia with regional techniques such as epidural analgesia, has been proven to improve pain control and reduce opioid use. It is especially important in patients with established renal disease, where the use of opioids may result in postoperative dysfunction, including renal impairment.

In addition, regional techniques can provide improved analgesia and hemodynamic stability during and after the procedure, enabling an expedited recovery process. The selective selection and implementation of these anesthetic approaches reinforce the significant role anesthesia plays in optimizing patient outcomes for urologic procedures (Assimos, 2019). Lastly, post-anesthesia care remains pivotal to achieving the best outcomes among patients experiencing urologic and renal procedures. Renal function and vital signs must be monitored continuously, especially in patients with pre-existing kidney disease or those who are having major surgery such as radical cystectomies. Effective anesthesia care avoids postoperative morbidity and allows early mobilization, greatly affecting pathways of recovery. For instance, early identification of any underlying issues in relation to renal function or pain control is achievable using stringent postoperative monitoring, which is one of the key considerations regarding maintaining patient safety. Overall, the multi-directionality of anesthesia, from preoperative to postoperative, highlights its irreplaceable contributions to the success of urological and renal surgical interventions (Gohad et al., 2025) (Figure 6.2).

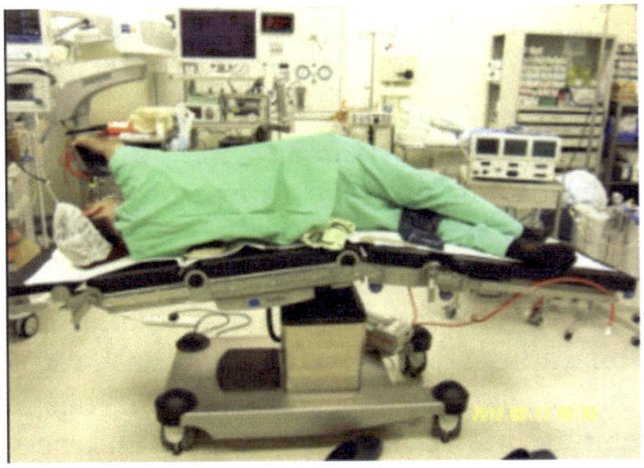

Figure 6.2. The administration of anesthesia in urologic and renal surgery.

Source: https://ars.els-cdn.com/content/image/1-s2.0-S1472029921001168-gr1.jpg.

6.1. Types of Anesthesia

Learning Outcome

1. General anesthesia
2. Regional anesthesia
3. Local anesthesia

Anesthesia plays a significant role in patient comfort and successful surgery during urologic and kidney surgery. The three most important types of anesthesia utilized are general anesthesia, regional anesthesia, and local anesthesia, each depending on the character of the surgical procedure and the needs of the patient. General anesthesia renders a patient unconscious, leading to generalized pain relief and muscle relaxation, which is particularly beneficial for complex procedures like nephrectomies or prostatectomies. Yet it has built-in dangers, such as respiratory distress and cardiovascular instability. Regional anesthesia, however, like spinal or epidural methods, blocks sensation in a particular area of the body, resulting in effective analgesia with patients conscious. This type is useful for brief procedures, avoiding systemic effects and maximizing recovery rate. Local anesthesia is only used for minor ambulatory procedures, targeting only the operative area to relieve pain. The selection between these two forms is based on a variety of factors, including time of operation, degree of pain anticipated, and history of the patient. The form of anesthesia also significantly influences post-operative recovery, particularly in urologic surgery, where patient mobilization and recovery have to be guaranteed. Studies have shown that regional anesthesia may lead to reduced hospitalization stays, fewer complications, and reduced need for opioid analgesia, resulting in an improved pain management regimen. Regional anesthesia also has advantages such as better patient satisfaction and a faster return to normal activities. Of special note, findings confirm that maximum reduction of opioid use through effective regional approaches can help provide fewer risks of side effects and complications associated with prolonged recovery periods. The necessity for adaptation of anesthetic schemes to the operative requirements of the patient and unique physiological characteristics is validated through guidelines provided by urological specialists. As there are continuous advancements in anesthetic techniques and medication, clinicians find themselves increasingly compelled to adopt an individualized approach in their practice of anesthesia for urologic and renal surgery with a view to providing improved patient outcomes and protection. Another significant aspect on the utilization of various types of anesthetics relates to patient comorbidities and the possibility of venous thromboembolism (VTE), which is a very risky risk factor in surgical settings. Surgery patients, especially cancer surgery patients, may be at higher risk of VTE and may need careful consideration and prophylaxis in anesthetic management. Anesthesia-related risk of VTE in high-risk patients, i.e., cancer or other comorbid conditions, requires meticulous monitoring, including drug thromboprophylaxis with the use of low-molecular-weight heparin.

Of note, revised guidelines have been published regarding the use of direct oral anticoagulants in VTE treatment of cancer patients, focusing on the importance of individualized management in anesthetic patients (Nelson et al., 2019). Thus, anesthetic selection and management plans must include consideration of special patient factors, perioperative risks, and potential thromboembolic complications to achieve maximum safety and efficacy in urological and renal surgery cases (Figure 6.3).

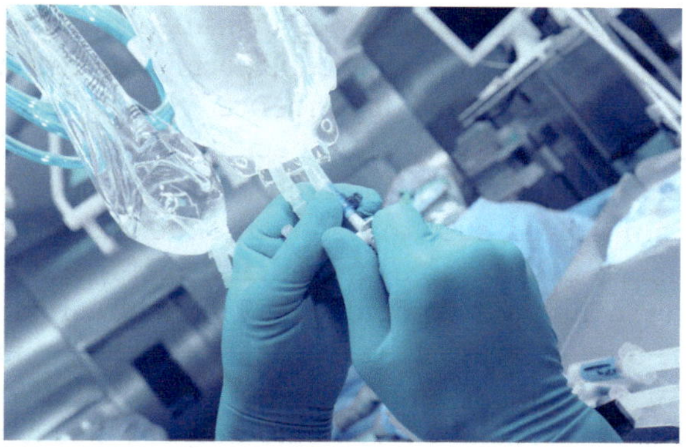

Figure 6.3. Anesthesia plays a pivotal role in ensuring patient comfort and surgical success.

Source: https://external-content.duckduckgo.com/iu/?u=https%3A%2F%2Fmyoms.org%2Fwp-content%2Fuploads%2F2019%2F10%2Ftypes_of_anesthesia.jpg&f=1&nofb=1&ipt=f8125347ad2f850717fd1f4014b002b045b855f4a45c5d5a5f7eff13452776e2.

6.1.1. General Anesthesia

General anesthesia is a key component in urological and renal surgery, ensuring a pain-free and controlled surgical condition. General anesthesia induces reversible loss of consciousness by administering intravenous anesthetics and inhalational anesthetics, thus ensuring patient safety and comfort throughout invasive and intricate procedures. The anesthetic drugs to be utilized must be chosen after a thorough consideration of specific surgical needs, depending on the duration of the operation, the patient's history, and potential drug interactions. Anesthesiologists should be in charge of keeping the patient hemodynamically stable and managing potential adverse effects of general anesthesia, particularly in procedures conducted with delicate organs like the kidneys and urinary tract. In addition, the position of patients during urologic procedures presents certain challenges to anesthetic management. The patient usually needs to be placed in variable positions, such as lithotomy or lateral decubitus, which interfere with respiratory mechanics and hemodynamics. Therefore, the anesthesiologists need to undertake adequate preoperative evaluation to identify any anatomical or clinical abnormalities that may complicate positioning and anesthesia administration. Moreover, they need to be vigilant throughout the procedure in order to regulate anesthetic depth and monitor vital signs accordingly. Such dynamic management of anesthesia for urologic procedures highlights the critical role played by the anesthesiologist in applying a paradigm that encompasses both preoperative and intraoperative factors with the advent of robotic-assisted surgical procedures that pose additional challenges in the management of the patient (Kaye et al., 2013). Furthermore, postoperative management plays a significant role in achieving optimal results following general anesthesia for urological procedures. The patients are susceptible to a range of complications like pain, nausea, and neurological dysfunction, which necessitate individualized postoperative management protocols. Anesthesiologists should work together with surgery teams to implement comprehensive pain management regimes that may involve the administration of opioids, nerve blocks, or non-steroidal anti-inflammatory drugs (NSAIDs) based on the extent of surgery. The inclusion of robust postoperative monitoring protocols is also crucial, especially in the case of robotic-assisted surgery, which could complicate hospital stay and recovery duration. Knowing the implications of general anesthesia in such cases ensures that anesthesiologists prepare well for all facets of care, thereby increasing patient safety and satisfaction in the increasingly large, intricate arena of urologic and renal surgery (Nova Southeastern University, 2024) (Figure 6.4).

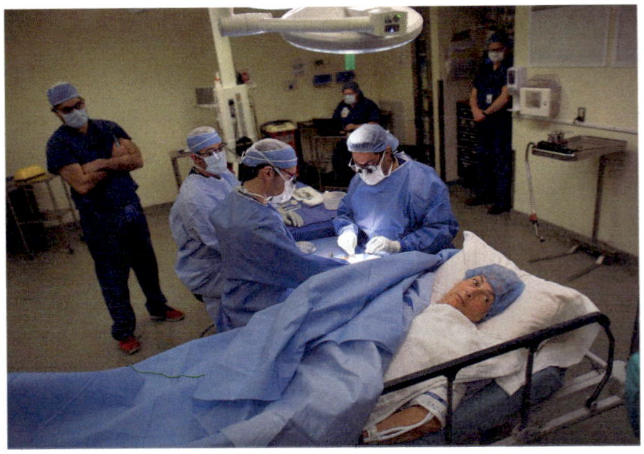

Figure 6.4. General anesthesia plays a pivotal role in urologic and renal surgeries.

Source: https://external-content.duckduckgo.com/iu/?u=https%3A%2F%2Fstatic01.nyt.com%2Fimages%2F2017%2F03%2F25%2Fscience%2F26AWAKE4%2F26AWAKE4-superJumbo.jpg&f=1&nofb=1&ipt=e7609fd8f1d21581818699c350f83dc75329d83f912fbcd3d714d363cfbe28f2.

6.1.2. Regional Anesthesia

Regional anesthesia applied in urologic and renal surgery is one of the major innovations to secure the patient's comfort and safety during procedures. General anesthesia keeps patients completely under, whereas regional anesthesia offers the local anesthetizing of a particular body area through the use of techniques such as spinal or epidural blocks. This technique is particularly helpful with urologic procedures, where the pelvic and lower abdominal regions are generally engaged. By minimizing systemic drugs, regional anesthesia can significantly lower the risk of complications, such as respiratory disorders and nausea, enhancing recovery and shortening hospital stay, in line with modern surgical philosophy for improved patient outcomes and satisfaction (Lerner et al., 2021). Therefore, the inclusion of regional anesthesia in urologic surgery is no longer a matter of choice but a changing standard of care that responds to an overarching paradigm shift toward minimizing patient invasiveness while maximizing recovery efficiency. Assessing the efficacy and safety of regional anesthesia across urologic and renal surgery uncovers multiple inherent advantages that make surgical practice better. Studies have indicated that patients in whom regional anesthesia is used for procedures have decreased pain scores and reduced needs for opioids during the postoperative period, a factor of significant value considering the current war against opioid dependence (Nelson et al., 2019). Additionally, the specificity of regional anesthesia allows for extended analgesia to be administered, such that the patient experiences a more comfortable immediate postoperative course. Enhanced postoperative control of pain not only improves the quality of recovery but also promotes more efficient mobilization, which is crucial in urologic surgery because timely ambulation can reduce the risk of complications, such as deep vein thrombosis or pulmonary embolism. The tailored aspect of regional anesthesia, as well as the decreased systemic drug exposure, further optimizes its use as an optimal anesthetic modality for such sensitive procedures. Moreover, regional anesthesia in urologic and renal surgery has support from evolving guidelines favoring its application among specific patient populations. For instance, patients with severe comorbidities or at higher risk for complications of general anesthesia could particularly benefit from regional approaches (Lerner et al., 2021). Furthermore, guidelines by prestigious urological societies suggest that regional anesthesia should be employed, especially in elective procedures, to ensure adequate pain control with minimal systemic sedatives. The individually tailored approach can then balance the hazards of anesthesia with acceptable localized pain relief. Therefore, with improved surgical techniques and patient preference increasing its significance, the employment of regional anesthesia is again on the rise. Its application in urologic and renal procedures not only adheres to clinical best practice, but it is also an investment in continuing patient-centered care in the operating room.

6.1.3. Local Anesthesia

In renal and urologic surgery, local anesthesia plays a key role both in successful pain control and in the facilitation of a wide range of procedures. Unlike general anesthesia, which makes the patient unconscious, local anesthesia is focused on specific parts of the body and keeps patients alert and awake. By successfully minimizing systemic effects and recovery time, this modality maximizes surgical efficiency and improves patient comfort. Procedures such as transurethral resection of the prostate and renal biopsies have used local anesthetic techniques with success, which have been shown to reduce postoperative discomfort significantly as well as improve patient satisfaction overall. The success of local anesthesia, particularly when combined with sedation, has been guaranteed by evidence demonstrating that it can make outpatient procedures feasible without significantly reducing general anesthetic complications. The application of local anesthesia for urologic surgeries is also supported by evolving clinical guidelines that adopt a patient safety and optimization of recovery strategy. According to evidence-based guidelines, certain types of surgical procedures are facilitated by the use of local anesthetic medication, which helps avoid the complications of venous thromboembolism (VTE) in the perioperative period. As highlighted by the American Society of Hematology, local anesthetic protocols complement VTE prevention guidelines since urological patients may have typical risk factors associated with lower extremity mobility (Nelson et al., 2019). Through the use of local anesthesia, operating surgeons are able to provide sufficient pain control and follow mechanical prophylaxis recommendations, all with the goal of improving patient outcomes and facilitating rapid return to normal activity. With these benefits, however, also come consideration of the limitations and possible complications of local anesthesia in urologic surgery.

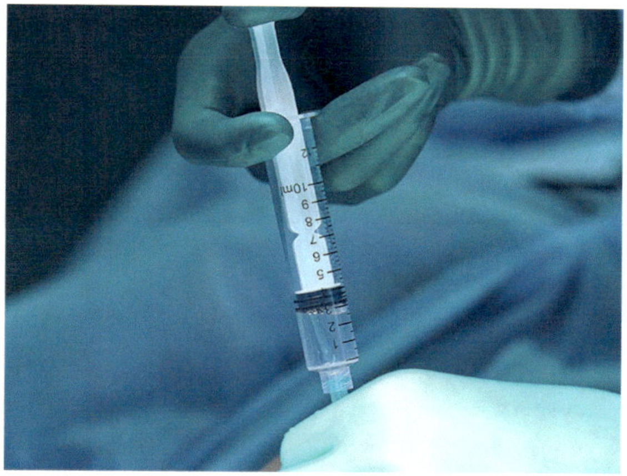

Figure 6.5. Local anesthesia plays a pivotal role in providing effective pain management while facilitating a wide range of procedures.

Source: https://external-content.duckduckgo.com/iu/?u=https%3A%2F%2Fwww.apsf.org%2Fwp-content%2Fuploads%2Fnewsletters%2F2020%2F3501%2Flocal-anesthetic-featured.jpg%3Ft%3D5fd60f1b3c048&f=1&nofb=1&ipt=818318953b2d242afc89fe2560ebd62428098c0bd83164de2a538051bcd33df7.

While uncommon, complications can include inadequate analgesia, allergy, and, infrequently, systemic toxicity of the anesthetic agent. Further, the choice of anesthetic technique must also be carefully individualized depending on the patient's requirements, with consideration given to concomitant comorbid conditions, as well as procedure complexity. For instance, the enhanced recovery after surgery (ERAS) guidelines emphasize the importance of the individualized pathways of care in the perioperative management of patients undergoing urologic procedures (Nelson et al., 2019). The guidelines demand awareness of the importance of integrating local anesthesia with multimodal analgesia in order to achieve optimal pain control suited to the specifics of the surgical procedure and the overall health of the patient (Figure 6.5).

Test Your Knowledge

1. Which type of anesthesia is commonly used for urologic and renal surgeries?
2. When is regional anesthesia preferred in these procedures?

6.2. Preoperative Assessment

Learning Outcome

1. Patient medical history
2. Risk factors specific to urologic and renal surgery
3. Anesthetic plan formulation

Comprehensive preoperative assessment is critical to optimizing patient outcomes in renal and urologic surgery, particularly in anesthetic management. The evaluation often includes a comprehensive review of the patient's medical history, including comorbidities that may impact the operative and anesthetic plans. Key considerations are cardiovascular stability, respiratory function, and history of venous thromboembolism, which have been linked with intraoperative risk. There is evidence to indicate that good preoperative assessment is significant in the detection of patients who will likely develop complications and hence assists clinicians in individualizing anesthesia plans according to the individual medical and surgical circumstances. For instance, conditions such as COPD and hypertension demand equipoised anesthetic practices that take into consideration both the benefits and risks associated with various anesthetics within the context of the perioperative care continuum, with immense priority being placed on comprehensive preoperative assessment. Preoperative diagnostic tests can effectively direct the selection of an anesthetic approach and surgical procedure. Routine practices include the laboratory values, such as complete blood count and electrolyte levels, and imaging studies when needed to assess renal function and anatomy. These studies play a significant role in interpreting the patient's physiological status, enabling the anesthesia personnel to anticipate complications and select suitable anesthetic drugs. Research has also shown that certain tests, such as post-void residual (PVR) measurements and imaging of prostate size, have a direct effect on anesthetic considerations and surgical planning for benign prostatic hyperplasia (BPH) treatments (Lerner et al., 2021). Through preoperative testing expected to inform possible complications, anesthesiologists can work in harmony with surgeons to ensure patient safety and surgical success. Patient education is an essential aspect of the preoperative assessment because it empowers the patient and prepares him or her for the future surgical process. More informed patients are more likely to be actively involved in their care, understanding the necessity of preoperative procedures such as fasting protocols and what anesthesia options mean. It is essential to discuss risks associated with anesthesia, especially for renal surgery, where existing comorbidities might complicate the recovery process. Evidence-based counseling of the patient has been promoted by recent guideline recommendations, emphasizing the requirement of thorough assessments and informed discussion to enhance clinical results (Nelson et al., 2019). Lastly, successful preoperative testing, both in medical evaluation and patient teaching, serves as a foundation for optimal anesthesia care of urological and renal surgeries, paving the way to improved recovery and decreased complication rates.

6.2.1. Patient Medical History

Within the context of urologic and renal anesthesia, there must be an understanding of the patient's extensive medical history of the patient. Preoperative assessment must consist of an extensive history of the patient's past health, operative history, and current medication. Diabetes, hypertension, and respiratory disease are long-standing conditions that have implications both for the anesthetic technique and postoperative recovery. Furthermore, knowledge of previous responses to anesthesia can guide anesthesiologists to adjust their technique accordingly and avoid complications. As the trend towards individualized medicine continues, incorporating patient-specific data into the anesthetic plan will make a huge difference in outcome, as anesthesiologists are better suited to deal with anticipated difficulties. The second important aspect to consider is the impact of a patient's medical history on the postoperative risk of complications. For example, patients who have a prior history of venous thromboembolism (VTE) require a strict assessment, as they have a higher tendency to develop complications from the surgical procedure and the anesthetic maneuvers used. The American Society of Hematology emphasizes the importance of risk stratification in its guidelines by advocating careful prophylaxis regimens according to the specific requirements of individual patients. Understanding the patient's medical history enables surgical teams to make educated decisions regarding the application of mechanical or pharmacological prophylaxis, which can significantly help avert risks and facilitate recovery. The integration of medical history, thus, in surgical and anesthetic decision-making helps in making the environment safer for urologic and renal patients. Multimodal pain management also relies significantly on patients' medical history. The anesthesiologists need to consider factors such as prior pain control history and chronic pain illnesses when designing an analgesic plan. Evidence has proven that regional anesthesia techniques, if well applied, can improve postoperative outcomes by achieving effective pain control and shortening recovery periods. However, their success also partly lies in proper knowledge of the patient's individual medical history, which governs the most appropriate nerve blocks or analgesic management to apply. Therefore, the availability of pain control customization not only enhances recovery but also is a current measure of anesthesia standards of practice in favor of more integrated patient care models for renal and urologic surgery (Chitnis et al., 2020). In addition, adhering to guidelines, for example, that of the American Society of Hematology for VTE prophylaxis, is important in patient's safety as well as in optimizing surgical outcomes (Nelson et al., 2019) (Figure 6.6).

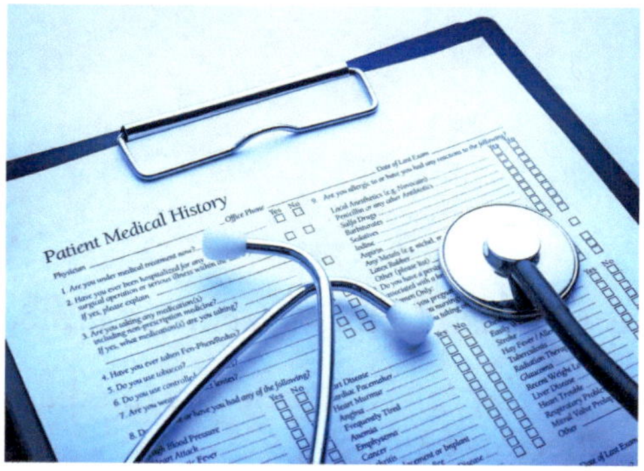

Figure 6.6. Patient medical history.

Source: https://external-content.duckduckgo.com/iu/?u=https%3A%2F%2Fwww.taproot.com%2Fwp-content%2Fuploads%2F2019%2F11%2Fpatient-history-medical-concept_125607485-1024x759.jpg&f=1&nofb=1&ipt=90c3ef2b7aa86add5bfa6e6491e9fe2acba2e0cee0fb836d9018add95370acab.

6.2.2. Risk Factors Specific to Urologic and Renal Surgery

The urologic and renal surgery background natively presents unique anesthetic management issues under a broad spectrum of risk factors. Obstructive sleep apnea syndrome (OSAS) is a significant one, with it being extremely common among the surgical population. The undiagnosed form has been shown to be particularly common in patients receiving elective urologic surgery, where it becomes vital to diagnose this syndrome prior to surgery. In patients with OSAS, anesthesia and sedation will exacerbate airway collapsibility, significantly enhancing postoperative risk. As surgery is often followed by the use of opioids, further depressing respiratory status, careful preoperative assessment is necessary. OSAS patients give anesthesiologists the chance to individualize their perioperative strategy in a patient-specific manner, having the proper interventions available to reduce the incidence of both intra- and postoperative complications (Vasu et al., 2012).

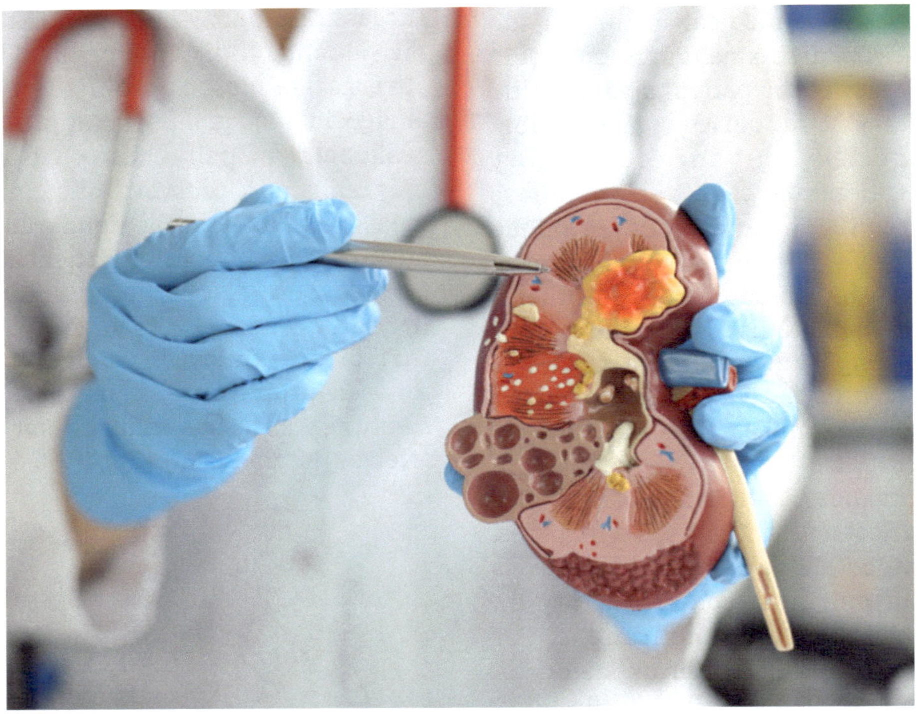

Figure 6.7. Risk factors specific to urologic and renal surgery.

Source: https://onewelbeck.com/media/4vsozeac/ureteric-stent-insertion.png?rmode=max&width=751&height=536.

Metabolic control problems of urolithiasis are yet another significant consideration during urologic surgery. The history of stone production in patients may be a reflection of underlying disturbances in metabolism that need to be thoroughly evaluated before anesthesia. The clinical management needs to identify not only the immediate danger of anesthesia, but also the long-term influence of renal function on surgical outcome. Stones in the ureters, for example, may have anesthesia-related complications in relation to fluid resuscitation and renal perfusion. Thus, steps essential to achieve maximal hydration and metabolic derangement correction should be utilized.

Advances such as medical expulsive therapy and advanced surgical techniques provide maximal patient safety and comfort options that facilitate the delicate balance between optimal care and anesthetic risk management (Rosa et al., 2013). Lastly, the physiological response of the patient with urologic and renal surgery cannot be overlooked. Intraoperative time may be defined by acute hemodynamic alterations that come with surgical manipulation of renal structures, again complicating anesthesia management. Intraoperative maneuvers and anesthetic drugs must be titrated correspondingly to correct these effects, particularly in preoperatively compromised patients, i.e., hypertension or diabetes mellitus. Renal protective maneuvers and careful monitoring of renal function during surgery must be done, especially in preoperatively compromised patients. In this context, anesthesiologists need to adopt a multi-disciplinary perspective with close collaboration between urologists and other specialists to ensure the highest outcomes and least perioperative risks (Vasu et al., 2012; Rosa et al., 2013) (Figure 6.7).

6.2.3. Anesthetic Plan Formulation

Planning an anesthetic for renal and urologic surgery necessitates a thorough understanding of the patient's clinical status and the procedure-specific individual needs. Anesthetic care depends on numerous factors, including the patient's history, underlying conditions, and the anticipated complexity of the procedure. For instance, a patient with significant comorbid conditions such as coronary disease or diabetes should be taken into account while developing an anesthetic plan. In one such reported case at Ben Taub Hospital, a patient with Fitch right renal cell carcinoma and underlying coronary artery disease was the subject of joint planning by a multidisciplinary team. This emphasizes the importance of anesthesiologists performing thorough preoperative assessments to avoid hazards associated with anesthesia in potentially high-risk procedures, effectively pursuing a best result that guarantees patient safety and postoperative recovery (Gashler et al., 2023). Furthermore, choosing the modality of anesthesia—general anesthesia, regional anesthesia, or a combination of the two—should be based on the surgical procedure and patient needs. Regional anesthesia possesses the possibility of conveying significant analgesic benefits, reducing systemic opioid requirements and accelerating recovery, but is especially significant for those patients experiencing very long renal procedures. Clinical factors should take into account variables such as expected blood loss, procedure length, and patient tolerance for specific anesthetic methods. Significance of this multi-aspect decision-making is best brought to light in anesthetic management of patients with complex disorders when the anesthesiologist has to weigh safety and effectiveness in order to enhance postoperative outcomes as well as minimize complications (Shyshchuk et al., 2015). Finally, continued intraoperative monitoring and application of advanced technologies, such as transesophageal echocardiography (TEE), are significant factors in successful anesthesia management of kidney surgeries. These interventions facilitate timely intervention, particularly in high cardiac risk patients, as seen in the above case study where TEE guided anesthetic management during tumor resection. Such individualized management not only improves the anesthetic experience but also underscores the importance of proactive and flexible anesthetic planning. In general, planning an anesthetic for renal and urologic surgery requires an assembly of clinical information, patient-specific considerations, and the implementation of state-of-the-art monitoring methods, all with the shared objective of attaining peak surgical results (Gashler et al., 2023) (Figure 6.8).

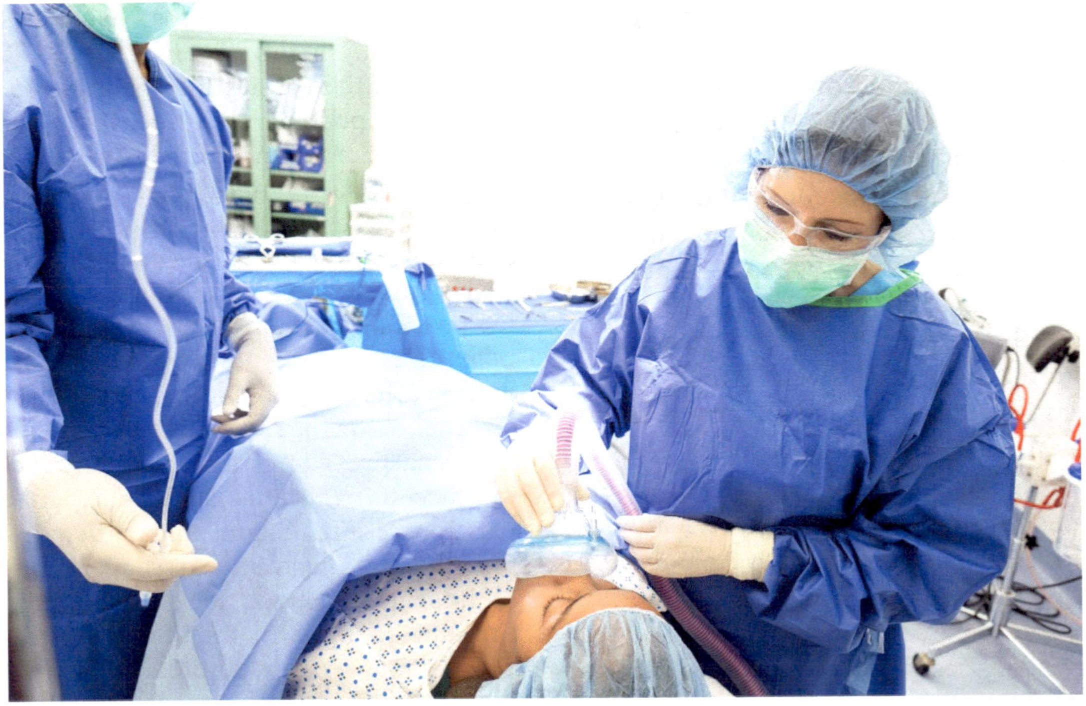

Figure 6.8. The formulation of an anesthetic plan for urologic.

Source: https://external-content.duckduckgo.com/iu/?u=https%3A%2F%2Fwww.verywellhealth.com%2Fthmb%2FZKvmXiUv0Lafxx8NDUJuAUZRiE8%3D%2F2121x1414%2Ffilters%3Afill(87E3EF%2C1)%2FiStock-489040642-5944169b3df78c537bc7c045.jpg&f=1&nofb=1&ipt=1b0cbb8f26b360018c6b42a7cc42eb30690671355de64fadb66bf2135b8fc084.

Test Your Knowledge

1. How does impaired kidney function increase surgical risk?
2. Why is fluid and electrolyte balance important in urologic and renal surgery?

6.3. Anesthetic Techniques in Urologic Surgery

Learning Outcome

1. Indications for general anesthesia
2. Use of spinal anesthesia
3. Considerations for laparoscopic procedures

The anesthetic technical challenge of urologic surgery demands a multi-disciplinary understanding of varied anesthetic techniques, which have a significant impact on outcomes in such patients. For robotic-assisted procedures, the anesthesiologist will have to take into account the distinct needs of the robotic system, the specialty positioning of the patient's anatomy, as well as pre-existing co-morbidities. The growing application of robotic surgical techniques emphasizes the necessity of tailoring anesthetic care to accommodate such factors. Accurate preoperative assessment is required to identify potential complications that may arise as a consequence of patient positioning or the employment of equipment during surgery. As portrayed in contemporary literature, careful positioning and specialty monitor use are essential to ensure maximum patient safety and optimal surgical outcome (Kaye et al., 2013). This increased complexity also brings with it a greater demand for anesthesiologists who are experienced in the newer technologies of urologic procedures. Additionally, anesthetic agent selection for use during urologic surgery may be strongly interdependent on procedure type and duration. General anesthesia is one of the more frequently used methods, which facilitates extensive surgical exposure and patient immobilization, and regional anesthesia, which can provide excellent pain relief with minimal systemic impact. The decision between these modalities typically depends on factors like anticipated operating complexity and the general health of the patient. Recent studies have shown the effectiveness of multimodal analgesia that involves the use of multiple analgesic approaches to decrease opioid use and improve postoperative recovery (Tekgül et al., 2017). This approach not only enhances pain relief but also minimizes the formation of postoperative complications caused by traditional analgesics. All anesthetic choices must be carefully considered, keeping in mind the unique needs of the patient and the procedure to yield optimal outcomes. As anesthesiology continues to evolve, the anesthetist's role in urologic surgery is becoming increasingly complicated. Continued advances in robotic and minimally invasive procedures necessitate continued learning and adaptation for anesthesiologists.

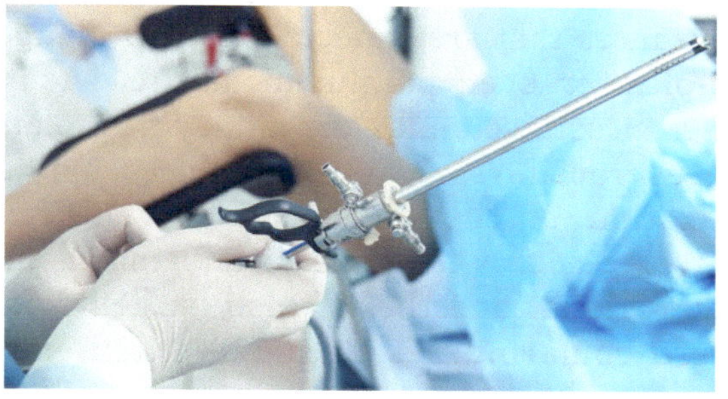

Figure 6.9. The complexity of urologic surgery necessitates a comprehensive understanding of various anesthetic techniques.

Source: https://transform.octanecdn.com/crop/1600x900/https://octanecdn.com/advancedhealthenginesites/advancedhealthenginesites_289847675.jpeg.

Practical exposure to the new technology and a clear grasp of widespread best practices keep anesthesiologists from being bogged down by the complexity that attends these procedures. A concentration on enhanced communication between surgical and anesthetist teams places both surgical results and patient safety on the rise. Also, the majority of institutions now put a high priority on interdisciplinary collaboration, understanding that everyone's acquaintance with surgical procedures increases the anesthesiologists' capability to prepare for potential issues during surgeries. As is evident from the literature, comprehensive training in both the technical specifics of the surgery as well as the perioperative role of anesthesia is essential in the enhancement of the quality of care for urologic and renal surgery (Kaye et al., 2013; Tekgül et al., 2017) (Figure 6.9).

6.3.1. Indications for General Anesthesia

In renal and urologic surgery, the selection of general anesthesia is based on a multitude of clinical indications with the purpose of ensuring patient safety and enhancing surgical results. General anesthesia is frequently utilized in procedures that are expected to be prolonged, complex, or even painful in nature, such as radical prostatectomies and kidney transplants. These procedures typically require complete relaxation of the muscles and ventilation control, easier with general anesthesia than with regional anesthesia. Also, patients with severe comorbidities or major intervention requirements typically have illnesses such that it is necessary to utilize general anesthesia to achieve an environment of controlled and stable physiology during the process. In-depth reflection on these patient-specific variables underscores the need for a strategy of anesthesia in accord with surgical goals alongside the unique traits of every patient (Lerner et al., 2021). A second significant justification for general anesthesia in urologic procedures relates to anatomical issues that could potentially make surgery difficult using localized anesthesia. For example, surgery on the bladder or ureters is technically challenging, and the need for sensitive instrumentation generally necessitates a state of general anesthesia. The technique allows surgeons to perform intricate movements without interference from patient motion or pain, otherwise compromise surgical precision. In procedures such as laparoscopic nephrectomies, where a great deal of manipulation of intra-abdominal organs is required, general anesthesia ensures ready access to the site of surgery and reduces the risk of inadvertent trauma to nearby structures. Thus, the complexity of the operative technique and the requirement for maximum visualization are the deciding factors in choosing general anesthesia in such cases (Ficarra et al., 2020). Moreover, patient comfort and procedure efficacy are the most important factors in determining general anesthesia suitability. The patients can report anxiety towards surgical procedures, particularly those that involve invasive procedures. General anesthesia not only helps reduce patient anxiety but also produces an amnestic effect that allows patients to tolerate surgical procedures without recalling uncomfortable experiences. Such psychological factors play a significant role in enhancing patient compliance preoperatively and postoperatively, facilitating easy passage through the surgical journey. Additionally, general anesthesia allows for speedy emergence, which enables patients to recover quickly as well as minimizing disturbances to the surgical process. Overall, all these facts vindicate the argument of general anesthesia being a crucial element in achieving favorable outcomes within the practice of urologic and renal surgery (Lerner et al., 2021).

6.3.2. Use of Spinal Anesthesia

Spinal anesthesia for urological and renal surgery has been of special interest as it may have more benefits over general anesthesia. One of the major benefits may be reduced postoperative complications, particularly respiratory complications, which might be the most important concern for patients with underlying disease. As explained in recent publications, spinal anesthesia, that is, segmental thoracic spinal anesthesia, has been demonstrated to be faster in onset compared to other techniques and has given rise to a less complicated anesthetic management protocol.

The specificity of spinal anesthesia provides uniform operative conditions with fewer opportunities for hemodynamic instability. This technique, therefore, not only meets the immediate needs of the operation but also prioritizes patient recovery and safety, and hence it is a suitable choice in the branch of urological surgery, particularly in high-risk patients (Hassan et al., 2025). The quality of analgesia produced by spinal anesthesia is also a key aspect to be discussed. Compared to conventional epidural techniques, spinal anesthesia is more likely to be linked with successful relief of pain with fewer injections of local anesthetic agents. This is specifically relevant in and following procedures like percutaneous nephrolithotomy, which are infamous for postoperative issues of pain. Success of analgesia achieved with spinal anesthesia can considerably influence patient comfort and satisfaction throughout the recovery process. Moreover, studies contrasting spinal anesthesia with other types, i.e., epidural blocks, have proven to be similar in their results for pain alleviation but with less ease of administration and fewer complications. Therefore, the application of spinal anesthesia would greatly enhance postoperative care for patients undergoing urological procedures (Prabeena et al., 2023). The addition of spinal anesthesia to the perioperative guidelines in renal surgery is an expansion of more patient-specific and tailor-made practice within the operating theater. It not only minimizes risks posed by general anesthesia, such as respiratory complications and prolonged recovery, but also aligns with enhanced recovery after surgery (ERAS) guidelines. By highlighting multimodal analgesia that includes spinal anesthesia, health care providers are able to optimize patient outcomes for patients needing procedures as significant as nephrectomy up to stone removal procedures. The mounting evidence indicates that the addition of this kind of anesthesia can lead to improved patient satisfaction and accelerated return to baseline function. Thus, spinal anesthesia does not only come as a technical possibility, but as a strategic therapy that reinforces the general goals of modern surgical treatment (Prabeena et al., 2023; Hassan et al., 2025) (Figure 6.10).

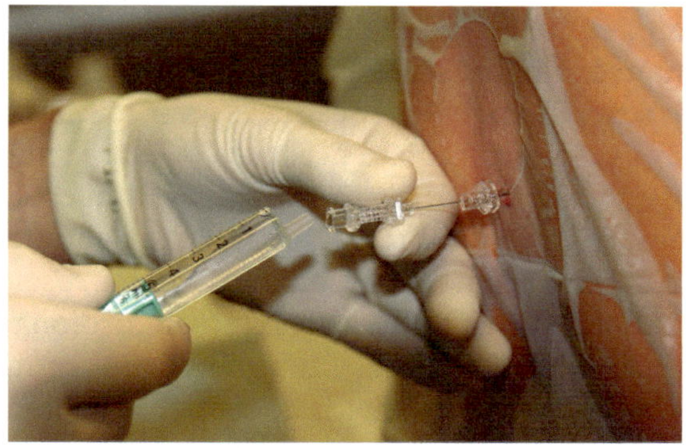

Figure 6.10. The use of spinal anesthesia in urologic and renal surgeries.

Source: https://upload.wikimedia.org/wikipedia/commons/e/e5/Liquor_bei_Spinalanaesthesie.JPG.

6.3.3. Considerations for Laparoscopic Procedures

The advent of laparoscopic surgery has revolutionized urologic and renal surgery with diverse benefits such as less postoperative pain, decreased recovery times, and minimal wounds. These advantages have special anesthetic considerations that demand serious consideration by the anesthesiologist. First, carbon dioxide insufflation in laparoscopy causes high intra-abdominal pressure, and this can impact hemodynamics by reducing venous return and cardiac output. An effective anesthetic management plan should thus incorporate cardiovascular complication monitoring, as well as fluid resuscitation strategy modifications. Furthermore, awareness of physiological alterations due to pneumoperitoneum is essential in ensuring patient safety and maximizing outcomes of surgery. Anesthesiologists can effectively guarantee the success of urologic and renal laparoscopic surgery by foretelling these issues. Patient positioning is also a critical component of anesthetic care for laparoscopic procedures. Given the complex nature of urologic procedures, several position maneuvers are used, each with its unique set of risks and complications. Trendelenburg positioning, for instance, which is commonly employed during laparoscopic pelvic procedures, can lead to an increase in intracranial pressure or impairment of respiration. Anesthesiologists must take precautions in monitoring patients for potential positional trauma, such as nerve compression or skin erosion, that may result from prolonged exposure to an unusual situation. Also essential is close interaction with the operating team to provide optimal positioning, alignment of the surgical field, and unobstructed access to all necessary monitoring devices throughout the case. This multidisciplinary approach enhances patient safety and facilitates early detection of complications, which, in the context of laparoscopic urologic and renal surgery, is important. Lastly, the evolution of robotic-assisted laparoscopic surgery demands a full comprehension of the uniqueness of anesthetic considerations involved. With evolving robotic technology, anesthesiologists must remain current regarding new techniques and devices that can influence intraoperative management. The dynamic relation between robotic surgical instruments and anesthetic agents is able to modulate medication dosing and delivery, highlighting the necessity of personalized anesthetic plans for every patient and case. Furthermore, as robotic surgery in the urological realm gains popularity, practitioners must overcome the obstacles of dynamic patient positioning and prolonged-duration surgeries that are both effects and causes of varied physiological responses. Proper preparation to handle such technologies must be done through continued education and perusal of the literature. Most importantly, rigorous study of anesthetic factors in robotics is essential for improving outcomes in patients (Kaye et al., 2013; Tekgül et al., 2017).

Test Your Knowledge

1. What types of anesthesia are commonly used in urologic surgery?
2. Why is spinal or regional anesthesia often preferred for some urologic procedures?

6.4. Anesthetic Techniques in Renal Surgery

Learning Outcome

1. Role of epidural anesthesia
2. Advantages of general anesthesia in nephrectomy
3. Monitoring and management during renal surgery

In renal surgical practice, anesthetic technique is essential to ensuring safety in the patient and optimizing surgical outcome. Planning for premedication, e.g., with anxiolytics, can be initiated to alleviate preoperative anxiety and facilitate induction of anesthesia. Careful choice of anesthetic drugs is necessary to consider the unique physiological demands that patients with renal disease present, as their renal function affects drug clearance and metabolism. Also, techniques such as regional anesthesia, such as lumbar plexus blocks, decrease the requirement for systemic opioids, thereby shortening postoperative pain and recovery duration. These considerations are indicative of the importance of personalized anesthetic technique according to both the type of surgery and patient variables. Through this, anesthesiologists can optimize renal surgery perioperative care and eliminate complications resulting from standard practice. Along with the progression in surgical techniques are the modifications in anesthetic approaches to renal surgery. Advances in technology, such as the use of laparoscopic and minimally invasive techniques, necessitate a re-evaluation of traditional anesthetic approaches. Transitions to single-incision laparoscopic nephrectomy, for instance, have been a viable alternative as a substitute to conventional techniques and come with decreased postoperative discomfort and better recovery outcomes (Repassy et al., 1996). This method requires anesthetic planning that is designed to provide the particular operating environment, typically needing general anesthesia with a focus on accelerated recovery protocols. Also, enhanced recovery after surgery (ERAS) protocols increasingly find their way into renal surgical care, with a focus on multimodal analgesia and minimizing opioid use. By synchronizing anesthetic techniques with these advances in surgical technique, patients would benefit from improved clinical outcomes, including reduced hospital stay and speedier return to function. In addition, advances in medical technology and techniques have revolutionized the management of urolithiasis and other renal diseases, which in turn influence anesthetic planning.

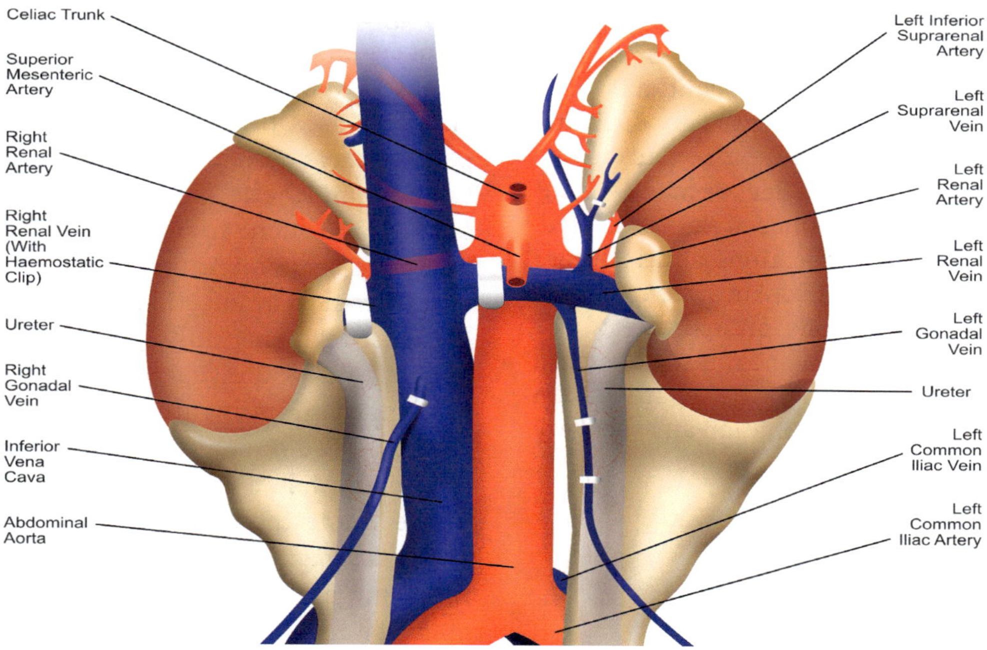

Figure 6.11. The anesthetic techniques play a pivotal role in ensuring patient safety and optimizing surgical outcomes.

Source: https://pub.mdpi-res.com/jcm/jcm-13-04188/article_deploy/html/images/jcm-13-04188-g001.png?1721223600.

Present research highlights the need to understand the complexity of nephrolithiasis treatment, including developments such as robotic-assisted ureterorenoscopy (Rosa et al., 2013). Such new techniques are demanding a thorough analysis of anesthesia strategies to follow the enhanced surgical skills, as well as patient safety. On the other hand, the incorporation of new technologies facilitates more accurate pain control methods and tailored anesthetic approaches in view of the specific requirements of renal patients. With continuous advancements in the urology field, it is teamwork between great surgeons and anesthesiologists that comes into the forefront while refining patient care in renal operations, eventually reaching for the best in both the operation and recovery process (Figure 6.11).

6.4.1. Role of Epidural Anesthesia

Epidural anesthesia is an important instrument in managing postoperative pain in urologic and renal surgeries, with significant advantage for pain control and patients' global recovery. It is a technique by which local anesthetic is administered into the epidural space for prevention of sensory nerve conduction to specific regions of the body. The outcome is reduced intraoperative pain and lower postoperative pain scores. Effective management of acute pain is essential since, if not controlled, pain can result in complications and interfere with recovery efforts. Also, initiation of pain management interventions preoperatively, for example, through epidural anesthesia, creates a better postoperative climate where patients can participate earlier in rehabilitation and recovery programs (Wenzel et al., 2016).

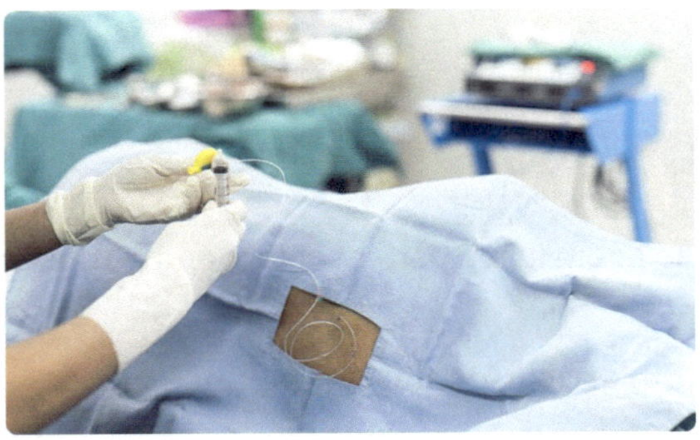

Figure 6.12. Role of epidural anesthesia.

Source: https://www.news-medical.net/image-handler/picture/2017/8/shutterstock_358075328.jpg.

The benefits of epidural anesthesia extend beyond mere pain alleviation; they include better respiratory function and less opioid consumption. In urologic and renal surgery, where patients are usually presenting with pre-existing complications of kidney damage, minimizing opioid consumption serves to prevent the risk of complications associated with opioids. Epidural anesthesia not only decreases the need for excess opioid dosing but also negates risks of opioid drug-related side effects, such as respiratory depression and prolonged recovery times. This philosophy aligns with the current practices trending towards improved ERAS protocols with emphasis on multimodal strategies to analgesia that enhance optimal recovery and patient satisfaction (O'Dwyer et al., 2015). Additionally, epidural anesthesia also enhances the immune modulation in the perioperative period. New findings indicate that various anesthetic modes, including regional anesthesia such as epidurals, are able to modulate the immune responses with effects on outcomes such as infection rates and recurrence of cancer following surgery. Epidural anesthesia use has the potential to counteract stress response and mitigate immunosuppression resulting from surgical procedures. Hence, it is essential to understand the interaction between anesthetic methods and the immune system to maximize outcomes in urological and renal surgery, pointing to the central place of epidural anesthesia. Such an interdisciplinary pain management strategy emphasizes the importance of anesthesiologists embracing integrated analgesic plans within perioperative practice (O'Dwyer et al., 2015; Wenzel et al., 2016) (Figure 6.12).

6.4.2. Advantages of General Anesthesia in Nephrectomy

General anesthesia for nephrectomy has a number of advantages that enhance surgical outcomes and safety. To begin with, general anesthesia induces profound muscle relaxation and complete unconsciousness, allowing surgeons to perform intricate urologic operations without anxiety about the possibility of patient movement, which would compromise surgical precision. This is particularly important in nephrectomy, where fine dissection and removal of renal structures are essential. Apart from this, general anesthesia enables better control of the airway to ensure that the patient is stable hemodynamically during the operation. Hence, the removal of physiological response to stress and facilitation of ventilation can lead to a more favorable postoperative recovery course, minimizing the associated risks of respiratory complications because of regional anesthesia techniques. General anesthesia also facilitates easier management and administration of analgesics in intraoperative monitoring. The ability to use inhalational agents and intravenous anesthetics allows for easy adjustments of the depth of anesthesia to be made within a short period, customized to the needs of the operation as it evolves. This facility is particularly valuable in nephrectomy, where variable blood loss and fluid shifts are anticipated. Further, general anesthesia also has the effect of reducing the need for postoperative analgesia, since the controlled environment of surgery restricts the stress response that is responsible for pain following surgery. Through effectively controlling pain early on, general anesthesia can lead to improved patient satisfaction as well as the expedited postoperative recovery, and this has broad ramifications for healthcare resources and patient throughput in the surgical environment. With regard to safety and efficacy, general anesthetic techniques have been found more successful in the procedure of nephrectomy compared to regional techniques. Studies have revealed that patients undergoing nephrectomy with general anesthesia have fewer intraoperative complications and overall lower morbidity. This is particularly important where renal tumors are being dealt with since precision in the removal of damaged tissues is crucial. In addition, general anesthesia offers space for thorough preoperative assessments and observation of comorbidities, which are critical for patients with comorbid conditions to assist in determining the appropriate types of surgery. As quoted in literature, these operating rooms are better served by utilizing highly evolved imaging modalities to better visualize tumors and thus supplement the overall success of general anesthesia in achieving the best possible surgical results (Nagaya et al., 2017). The complementarity of these factors emphasizes the advantages of using general anesthesia as a standard procedure in nephrectomies, optimizing patient management and clinical results in renal and urologic surgery (Finelli et al., 2017).

6.4.3. Monitoring and Management During Renal Surgery

Good monitoring and management intraoperatively during renal surgery are critical factors in the anesthesia care of urologic patients. This phase begins before the surgical operation, in which careful preoperative assessment is conducted to evaluate patient comorbidities and other risk factors associated with renal surgery. Anesthetic technique may be different depending on the operation type—whether nephrectomy, nephron-sparing surgery, or endourologic procedure. With the high likelihood of blood loss during renal surgery, fluid management becomes essential. The anesthesiology staff must continually observe hemodynamic status, thereby allowing the anticipation and correction of hypovolemia or hypotension on time. Thus, patient-tailored anesthetic regimens are crafted to optimize oxygen delivery such that surgery can be safely done with minimal complications. Renal function and drug nephrotoxicity must be handled with special care in renal surgery. Monitoring of renal perfusion is essential, especially when hypotension is a risk factor for surgery, because renal ischemia may lead to postoperative renal failure or acute kidney injury. Preoperative risk assessment using laboratory tests and medical imaging enables anesthesiologists to make informed decisions about anesthetic agents as well as dose. Those medications that are potentially risky to renal function, such as some anti-inflammatory drugs or some antibiotics, must be selected carefully, particularly among patient groups with pre-existing renal impairment. Equally important is the continued monitoring of urine output following surgery to ensure the preservation of renal function as well as immediately respond to any indication of dysfunction, thus safeguarding patient outcomes during the perioperative period (Nelson et al., 2019). Intraoperative management guidelines, particularly for patients to undergo surgery for kidney surgery, should have strategies for minimizing venous thromboembolism (VTE) risks. These are high-risk surgeries due to illnesses like cancer and immobilization and hence need prophylaxis like the administration of low molecular weight heparin (LMWH). The trend now is towards personalizing the VTE prophylaxis and emphasizing continuous monitoring of the requirement for anticoagulation in these high-risk procedures (Dean et al., 2016). Effective monitoring of coagulation factors, as well as vigilant observation for postoperative complications, is essential for ensuring patient safety. This total approach to monitoring and management in renal surgery ultimately enhances the efficacy of anesthetic care with fewer risks involved, providing a sound basis for successful surgical outcomes (Figure 6.12).

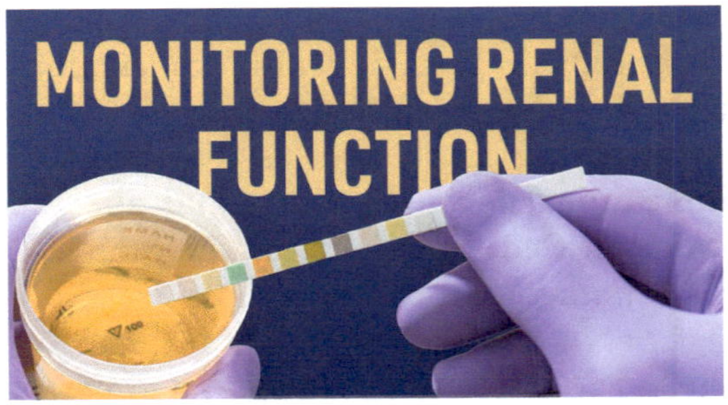

Figure 6.13. The monitoring and management during renal surgery.

Source: https://cdn-images.ausmed.com/ausmed-articles/20181008_cover_V2.jpg.

Test Your Knowledge

1. Which type of anesthesia is commonly used in renal surgery?
2. Why is careful fluid management important during renal anesthesia?

6.5. Intraoperative Management

Learning Outcome

1. Monitoring vital signs
2. Fluid management strategies
3. Pain control methods

Intraoperative management of urologic and renal surgery involves strict monitoring of various physiological parameters to achieve optimal results in the patient. Blood pressure, heart rate, and fluid balance should be monitored by anesthesia staff as a matter of extreme importance, given the liability of renal function to hemodynamic stress. The levels of mean arterial pressure (MAP) must be kept within optimal parameters because reductions below 60 mmHg have been linked with acute kidney injury (AKI). Investigation underscores that persistent hypotension, as reflected in episodes extending for more than ten minutes with critically low MAP values, potentially increases AKI risk substantially. Hence, anesthetic care and fluid management must be individualized based on patients' preoperative renal function and the complexity of planned surgery. This proactive intraoperative management step directly addresses reducing postoperative complications and ensuring postoperative recovery. The selection of anesthetic medications also has implications for urologic and renal surgery. For instance, volatile anesthetics may pose renal effects that must be appropriately evaluated. Intraoperative hemodynamic stability, particularly with renal manipulation, is important to maintain perfusion. Regional anesthesia techniques, such as paravertebral or spinal blocks, can produce excellent analgesia with the promise to decrease opioid-related side effects that may compromise renal perfusion. Moreover, intraoperative urine output monitoring constitutes an integral part of intraoperative management since it is a dynamic index of renal perfusion. Parameters of urine output offer the potential for real-time measurement of renal function and thus also play a significant role in the avoidance of complications with such sophisticated operations. Optimal practice in anesthetic management thereby functions to provide favorable outcomes in urologic and renal surgery. The inclusion of augmented reality protocols within intraoperative management has the potential to reshape postoperative outcomes for patients undergoing urologic and renal surgery. The ERAS guidelines emphasize multimodal analgesia and restricted use of opioids as part of a holistic perioperative care plan.

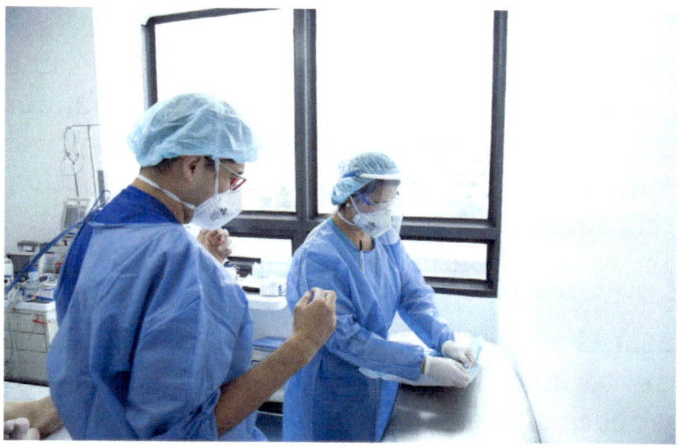

Figure 6.14. Intraoperative management during urologic and renal surgery.

Source: https://www.pdacademy.asia/sites/g/files/ebysai3471/files/2022-05/Image%201_0.jpg.

There is evidence that the strict adherence to such protocols leads to improved pain control, shorter hospital stay, and lower rates of complications. The impact of intraoperative variables, such as fluid resuscitation and hemodynamic optimization, is a critical determinant of ERAS success. In particular, the avoidance of euvolemia by individually tailored fluid administration and close monitoring can prevent hazards related to intraoperative hypotension. With proof from the latest consensus guidelines, including intraoperative care pathway suggestions geared towards best practice optimization, operating teams well-equipped to start these interventions are better placed to enhance patient outcomes while curtailing the risk of postoperative renal complications (Nelson et al., 2019) (Figure 6.14).

6.5.1. Monitoring Vital Signs

Careful monitoring of vital signs during anesthesia for renal and urologic surgery is the most important factor in patient safety and optimal surgical outcome. The critical vital signs that contain important data regarding the patient's physiological state during surgery are heart rate, blood pressure, and oxygen saturation. During the procedure on the table, fluctuations in these parameters are common and may signify imminent complications such as hypovolemia or inadequate blood oxygenation. Continuous monitoring allows anesthesiologists to respond promptly when abnormalities from baseline are detected, hence avoiding the hazards of adverse cardiovascular instability due to anesthesia. Furthermore, real-time feedback allows individualized anesthetic care, in which fluid replacement and drug dosing can be titrated according to the patient's changing status, thus optimizing the overall effectiveness of the anesthesia plan. In the field of urologic and renal surgery, some factors specifically underscore the importance of monitoring vital signs. Because the procedures are prone to involve instrumentation of the urinary tract and renal anatomy, the risk of intraoperative complications, e.g., bleeding or hypotension, is present. Intraoperative hypotension (IOH) is predisposed to cause severe morbidity, e.g., renal hypoperfusion and subsequent postoperative AKI. It has been proven in research that extended hypotension is followed by a greater incidence of AKI, and thus the tracking of vital signs is more than an official requirement—it is a critical aspect of patient care in this surgical arena. Forewarned detection of hypotensive episodes allows the operating team to implement ways of maintaining proper MAP necessary in guaranteeing renal function in and after surgery, corroborating the need for vigilant monitoring in such delicate procedures. Along with that, the integration of advanced monitoring technology enhances the accuracy of vital sign monitoring, allowing for better patient outcomes in renal and urologic surgery anesthesia. The addition of continuous arterial blood pressure monitoring, for instance, can permit immediate feedback about hemodynamic stability, reducing the reliance on sporadic measurement.

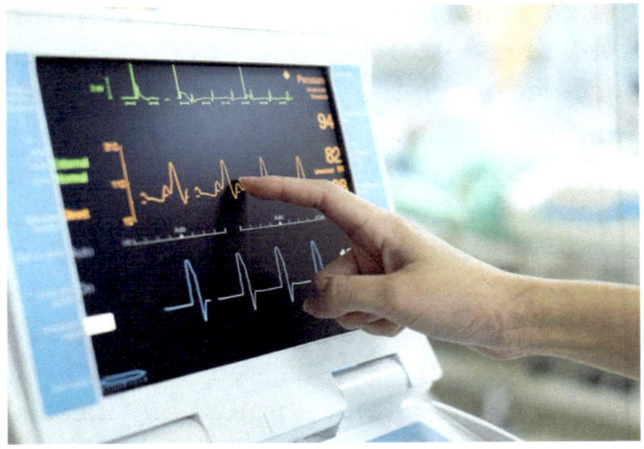

Figure 6.15. Monitoring vital signs on a digital display, highlighting heart rate and other critical parameters.

Source: https://activeplushomehealth.com/wp-content/uploads/2022/05/Hand-pointing-to-vital-signs-monitor.jpg.

Beyond these, capnography and advanced non-invasive monitoring systems can offer information about the patient's respiratory function and global metabolic status. When clinicians have a comprehensive view of important signs, they are in a better position to tailor anesthetic care to individual patient needs, ultimately yielding reduced morbidity and improved recovery profiles. Such advances in monitoring not only represent best practice guidance but also represent a patient-centered approach within the challenging field of urologic and renal surgical anesthetics (Nelson et al., 2019) (Figure 6.15).

6.5.2. Fluid Management Strategies

Anesthesia fluid management strategies in urologic and renal surgery are crucial in optimizing patient outcomes as well as minimizing complications. The nature of these surgeries, from patient position changes to potential fluid shifts during the process, calls for a thorough understanding of patients baseline fluid status and surgical requirements. Anesthesiologists must carefully assess preoperative hydration and modulate intraoperative fluid administration to account for hemodynamic stability and perfusion of organs. Furthermore, vigilant monitoring and modulation during the procedure is similarly essential in order to prevent, detect early, and treat blood loss properly, particularly because blood loss is widely variable in terms of amount based on the case and the method used. Such thoughtful care not only minimizes dangers of intraoperative hypotension but also accelerates recovery in the postoperative period. Within the context of robotic-assisted urologic surgery, there are certain fluid management issues. Robotic surgery has revolutionized the practice of urologic surgery but has also brought certain unique issues to the attention of anesthesiologists. Due to the intrinsic technical restraint of the robotic apparatus and a potential for creating a steep Trendelenburg position, careful fluid balancing takes the highest priority. The venous access and fluid replacement protocols must be revised to account for posture-related hemodynamic effects. Kaye et al. (2013) indicate that information regarding risks associated with robotic equipment and patient positioning directly influences the anesthetic plan and identify that this information is a critical component of ensuring successful surgical outcomes. In addition, postoperative fluid therapy continues to be a key component of the recovery process following urologic and renal surgery. Effective postoperative hydration has the potential to significantly enhance renal function and facilitate anesthetic drug elimination. Anesthesiologists should closely collaborate with surgery teams to design protocols to maximize fluid intake based on each patient's personalized requirements. Weaning from intravenous to oral fluid should be carefully monitored to prevent fluid overload or electrolyte imbalances. Balancing proper fluid delivery with prevention of postoperative complications becomes more critical as advances in surgical technique, such as minimally invasive and robot-assisted surgery, continue to mold the practice of urologic surgery, underscoring the critical importance of effective fluid management strategies.

6.5.3. Pain Control Methods

The effective treatment of pain following and during urologic and renal surgery is paramount to patient recovery and satisfaction. Various mechanisms of pain management have been developed and utilized to mitigate pain, particularly for open and laparoscopic techniques. For instance, regional anesthetic procedures such as spinal or epidural anesthesia have gained more attention due to their greater analgesia with the advantage of decreased reliance on systemic opioids. These methods not only avoid pain but also restrict the extent to which opioid-related side effects, such as nausea and constipation, can occur, thus retarding recovery. Besides, multi-modal analgesia strategies utilizing different classes of analgesics like non-steroidal anti-inflammatory drugs and acetaminophen have been seen to enhance pain relief with reduced opioid consumption. This multi-modal approach is crucial to the attainment of post-operative comfort and aiding in the process of healing. Recent improvements in surgical techniques have also played a significant role in better pain relief. For example, one has a new method to supplant the traditional laparoscopic procedure, allowing minimal access via a tiny skin cut. Not only does the method allow direct visualization of the surgical area, but it also lowers tissue trauma, with resultant minimized postoperative pain and morbidity to levels comparable to laparoscopic procedures. Using the JakoscopeTM probe and high-intensity fiberoptic light, surgeons can now perform complex operations more quickly and with more focus on patient comfort. The emphasis on less invasive techniques aligns with the current endeavors of maximizing patient outcomes and points to the importance of tailored pain control strategies in anesthesia for renal and urological surgery (Frang et al., 2011). Other patient groups, such as OSAS, are also of particular interest in pain control strategies. The prevalence of OSAS in surgical patients, particularly the elective population, is estimated to warrant meticulous preoperative assessment to offer these patients effective care. As the collapsibility of the airway is exacerbated by sedation and anesthesia, culminating in increased postoperative morbidity, early identification of such patients and applying certain anesthetic practices is imperative. They could involve avoiding the use of particular sedatives or opioids, using regional anesthesia if it is possible, and close monitoring of the postoperative course. Overall, one should appreciate the intricate balance of pain management and comorbidities in patients like OSAS to optimize anesthetic care in urologic and renal surgeries, ensuring safety and satisfaction in all patients (Vasu et al., 2012) (Figure 6.16).

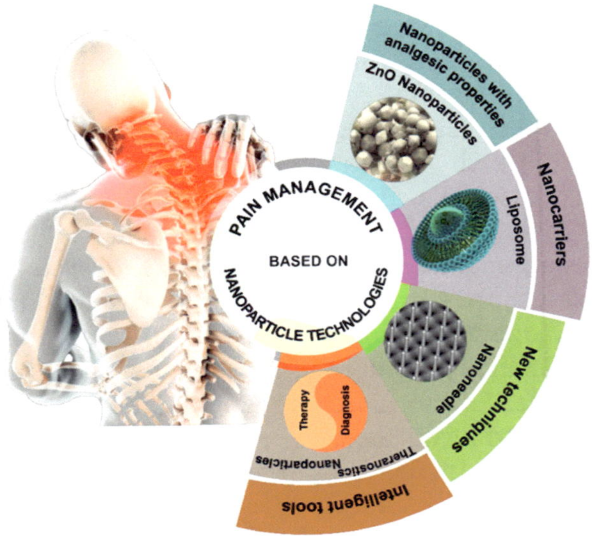

Figure 6.16. Pain control methods.

Source: https://media.springernature.com/lw685/springer-static/image/art%3A10.1186%2Fs12951-022-01473-y/MediaObjects/12951_2022_1473_Figa_HTML.png.

Test Your Knowledge

1. Why is fluid balance important during anesthesia?
2. What types of fluids are commonly used during surgery?

6.6. Postoperative Care

Learning Outcome

1. Recovery from anesthesia
2. Pain management protocols
3. Complications and their management

Postoperative care is a vital component of renal and urologic surgery, contributing significantly to patient recovery and ultimate outcomes. Appropriate management begins as soon as the surgical procedure concludes, with a strong emphasis on monitoring vital signs and physiological status for the detection of any incipient complications or abnormalities. This is when checking for evidence of bleeding, infection, or reaction to anesthesia is usually part of the assessment, necessitating monitoring by both nursing staff and anesthesia personnel. Pain management strategies must also be implemented early in order to make the patient comfortable, utilizing pharmacologic as well as non-pharmacologic methods. National guidelines, such as those from authoritative bodies, recommend a multimodal approach to pain relief that limits the use of opioids while keeping effectiveness at its peak, thereby paving the way for a smoother recovery process. Another fundamental element in postoperative care is the encouragement of ambulation and mobility as early as possible. Early mobilization has been shown to reduce the incidence of postoperative complications such as VTE and improve the recovery of gastrointestinal function. The patients must be encouraged for light physical activity, which not only contributes to reducing the risk of VTE but also enhances the satisfaction of overall recovery. Education is integrated into postoperative care; patients have to learn the importance of mobility and the dangers of bed rest. As is well documented in many studies, postoperative education translates directly into patient compliance and satisfaction, ultimately resulting in improved surgical outcomes. Furthermore, observation and evaluation of possible complications in the postoperative period should involve close screening for VTE signs in patients who have had significant urologic surgery. Pharmacologic prophylaxis with drugs like low-molecular-weight heparin (LMWH) or direct oral anticoagulants (DOACs) in high-risk patients can help prevent these risks. There is evidence to support individual patient risk factor and surgical profile-guided thromboprophylaxis strategies with reliance on clinician judgment to decide the best prophylactic intervention. Guidelines state that a comprehensive approach to evaluating VTE risk, along with patient-specific education regarding signs and symptoms, can significantly decrease complications of urologic and renal procedures, resulting in improved postoperative results (Nelson et al., 2019; Lerner et al., 2021).

6.6.1. Recovery From Anesthesia

Recovery from anesthesia, and particularly so in the context of urologic and renal surgery, is significant to the outcome in the patient. Anesthesia induces a status that necessitates ongoing monitoring during recovery so that complications can be appropriately managed. Side effects from patient recovery from anesthesia may present as nausea, confusion, and gradations of mental defect. The duration and mode of anesthesia employed may impact such effects. Because older patients are often exposed to urologic surgery, there is a need to be aware of their specific recovery needs, particularly because post-anesthesia complications can be amplified by age-related factors. Appropriate monitoring and management of patients during recovery can avoid complications, enhancing patient satisfaction and outcomes. Cognitive recovery is also a critical parameter in post-anesthesia care. Literature confirms that anesthetic agents can cause differential effects on cognition, particularly among elderly patients. For instance, the choice between agents such as desflurane or sevoflurane can yield differential levels of postoperative cognitive dysfunction, and this emphasizes the need for individualized anesthesia strategies in urologic and renal surgery (Department of Anesthesia, University of Iowa, 2011). Potential for transient cognitive impairment is especially important; while most patients return to normal function within hours, the ability to appreciate these dynamics allows for enhanced preoperative counseling and postoperative care planning.

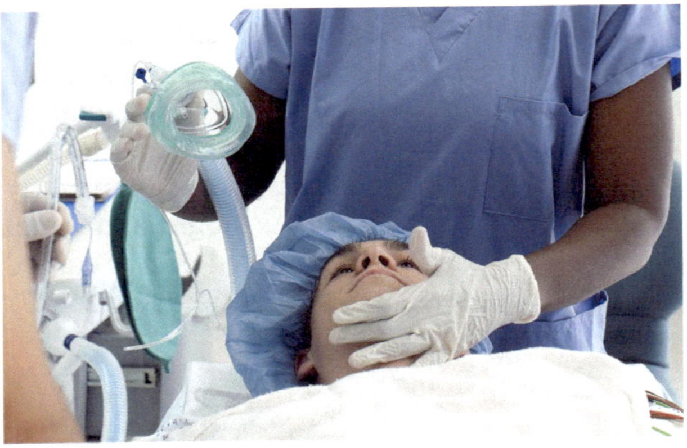

Figure 6.17. The recovery process following anesthesia.

Source: https://www.verywellhealth.com/thmb/CHgmB9UEHBgdRq34qSwCVlAw3cI=/1500x0/filters:no_upscale():max_bytes(150000):strip_icc()/86510584-56a9126e5f9b58b7d0f7db1d.JPG.

Operative room personnel and anesthesiologists must be proactive in promoting cognitive recovery, adapting style to the patient's individual profile to achieve an optimal recovery experience. Communication during the recovery phase, not only for managing clinical outcome but also for managing expectation and anxiety of the patient, is important. Postoperative patients may become disoriented or anxious, influencing their perception of pain and satisfaction from the operation. This emphasizes the importance of offering clear information regarding what is occurring during recovery, timeframes, and potential side effects (Department of Anesthesia, University of Iowa, 2011). Preoperative consultation with patients and relatives can generate an environment that is helpful to a smooth recovery process. Besides, utilizing recovery pathways with standardized assessment tools can enable the recovery from anesthesia to postoperative care to be more streamlined so that patients may receive timely intervention and care according to their individual requirements in urologic and renal surgery (Figure 6.17).

6.6.2. Pain Management Protocols

For renal and urologic surgery, the development of pain management plans is important to drive patient outcomes and postoperative recovery. Multimodal analgesia remains the cornerstone in modern practice, where various analgesic medications are utilized in a synergistic approach to maximize pain relief with fewer side effects. For example, the utilization of regional anesthesia techniques, such as nerve blocks, has been shown to significantly reduce the need for systemic opioids, thereby reducing the risk of opioid-related complications. This movement towards a more comprehensive pain control strategy is a reflection of an evolving understanding of pain pathways and the need for individualized protocols, eventually leading to improved patient satisfaction and reduced hospital stays. Recent studies have shown the effectiveness of non-pharmacologic interventions as valuable supplements to standard analgesics in the course of pain management regimens. Clinical data have shown that measures such as cognitive-behavioral therapy and acupuncture can achieve decreases in pain intensity scores and analgesic consumption in postoperative patients. These techniques must be implemented in urologic and renal surgery because they not only reduce drug dependence but also reduce the incidence of adverse effects on pharmacologic therapy. Also, with the use of patient-controlled analgesia (PCA) systems, patients are able to control their pain more effectively and have a sense of control, improving overall patient satisfaction. This holistic approach to pain management deals with physical as well as psychological aspects of pain, ultimately culminating in more robust recovery trajectories. Constant evaluation and update of pain management strategies become necessary in order to endorse their worthiness and safety in the postoperative setting. Research aiming for knowledge about patient responses to various modes of pain management becomes foremost. For instance, studies like that presented in Mongia et al. (2024) have shown the extensive range of results for pain with varying intervention methods, which all serve to strengthen the need for individualized treatment regimens. By implementing the practice of systematic assessment of pain protocols, including pain intensity scores and patient satisfaction, medical professionals can adapt their approaches to better suit the requirements of heterogeneous patient populations. The early and proactive implementation of such high-tech pain management practices within urologic and renal surgery has the twofold advantage of maximizing patient comfort as well as targeting the ultimate desideratum of improved clinical results in surgical care (Figure 6.18).

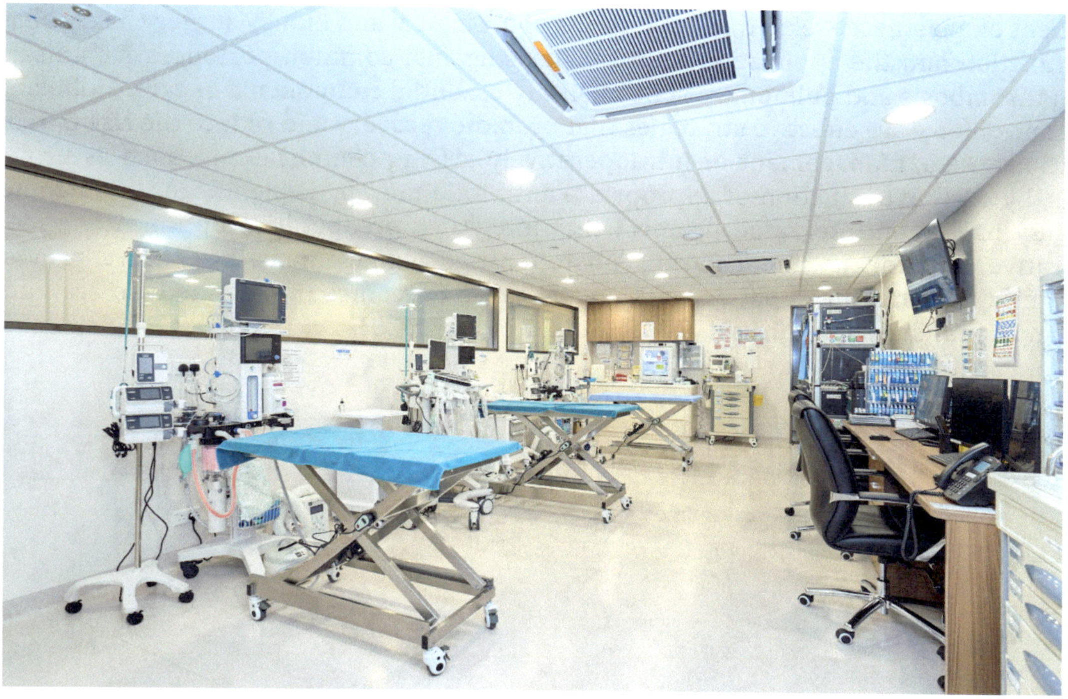

Figure 6.18. Pain management protocols.

Source: https://hvseh.com.hk/wp-content/uploads/2025/02/LCS04434-1-1.jpg.

6.6.3. Complications and Their Management

Anesthesia delivery in renal and urologic surgery carries risks per se, and awareness of potential complications is crucial for proper management. Preoperative assessment is crucial, particularly renal function, as impaired renal status can enhance postoperative risk for complications. For instance, patients with chronic renal disease are more likely to be susceptible to nephrotoxicity from surgery with agents, necessitating individualized anesthetic planning. Accurate patient positioning during surgery is also one such area where things can go wrong, from nerve damage and shift of respiration due to improper alignment or prolonged pressure on specific segments of the body. Therefore, an individual approach in anesthesia—having both procedure nature and patients' overall state of health in mind—is critical in avoiding risks and enhancing results in urologic and renal surgeries (Türksal, 2025). In more complex procedures, such as radical cystectomy with diversion, the interaction between chronic illnesses such as hypertension and chronic kidney disease demands a complex anesthetic plan. Management of such high-risk patients is a multi-factorial process that is not only concerned with anesthesia provision but also includes prevention of potential complications. For instance, application of invasive monitoring techniques, such as arterial blood pressure and monitoring of urinary output, is essential to guide hemodynamic control and ensure proper renal perfusion during the perioperative period. A multimodal opioid-sparing analgesic regimen can effectively manage postoperative pain without impairing the kidneys. This practice technique emphasizes the importance of careful management of complications, indicating the relevance of observation and modification of anesthesia technique based on the patient's response throughout the procedure (Gohad et al., 2025). Post-operative care is another essential phase in the management of anesthesia-related complications of urological and kidney surgery. Wary observation of renal function and the application of prophylaxis against common postoperative nuisances like deep vein thrombosis and pulmonary atelectasis are essential components of care. Mobilization and incentive spirometry are effective strategies that promote recovery and reduce the risk of respiratory complications. Also, management of intraoperatively arising complications, such as urinary tract infections, by early introduction of appropriate antibiotic therapy is significant in outcome during recovery. By having an integrated protocol that integrates preoperative optimization, meticulous intraoperative monitoring, and rigorous postoperative management, healthcare providers are able to significantly minimize patient risk and enhance outcomes in patients who are undergoing urologic and renal surgery (Türksal, 2025; Gohad et al., 2025).

Test Your Knowledge

1. Why is fluid balance important during anesthesia?
2. What types of fluids are commonly used during surgery?

Summary

The overview of an analysis of anesthesia in renal and urologic surgery brings together the most innovative of surgical techniques and the necessity of tailored anesthetic approaches. As surgeries become increasingly intricate, the anesthetic treatment must keep pace with the added complexity and multiple surgical procedures. In-depth analysis of more recent publications highlights a focus on integrating newer methodologies and technologies to optimize patient therapy and outcomes. These advancements not only impact surgical efficacy but also demand more understanding of the patient's physiological response to these intricate procedures. Anesthesia methods must adapt to these advancements to ensure safety as well as efficacy, thereby resulting in improved surgical outcomes and patient satisfaction. The successful use of combined surgical methods, such as total coronary artery bypass grafting and nephrectomy, also highlights the significance of anesthetic planning during the surgery with complex anatomies and pathologies. When more than one surgical procedure is performed at the same time, the anesthetic plan must encompass total cardiovascular support and careful monitoring of renal function. This dual focus allows greater security in high-risk procedures that otherwise would demand phase separation of treatment. These efforts are particularly relevant now as they represent a transition to integrated views for the handling of compounded medical cases, and they promote the necessity of anesthetic expertise and coordination within the surgical team (Budrikis et al., 2012). Lastly, the development of anesthetic techniques and perioperative strategies maximizes renal and urologic operation management. As reported in the literature, the continued study into the efficacy of medical expulsive treatments and advancing technology will continue to inform anesthetic guidelines specific to individual patient populations. This innovation is notably imperative in managing the variable presentations of urolithiasis as well as other urologic conditions, which require fluid responses from anesthetic care providers. The incorporation of new knowledge will facilitate greater understanding of patient needs, better pain management strategies, and better surgical outcomes. As the science develops, commitment to ongoing education and development in anesthetic practice will be required in the merging of these advancements with traditional techniques to ultimately enhance the quality of care in urologic and renal surgery (Rosa et al., 2013).

Anesthesia in urologic and renal surgery is crucial in ensuring patient safety and optimal outcomes of surgery. Selection of the most critical anesthetic points, of which selection of anesthetic technique is a significant one, will rely on the nature of the surgery to be done, patient factors, and the time expected in surgery. General anesthesia is usually reserved for complicated cases that might involve extensive tissue manipulation or prolonged surgical duration, while regional anesthesia might be of value in some cases, limiting systemic exposure to anesthetic drugs and postoperative pain. Proficiency in the selection of the appropriate anesthetic technique requires discerning knowledge of pharmacologic agents in addition to how they interact with varying patient factors, including age, comorbidities, and individual responses to anesthesia. This individualized approach to anesthetic care brings about improved patient satisfaction and decreased complications in favor of its establishment in urologic surgical practice. Management of potential complications, most significantly local anesthetic systemic toxicity (LAST), is another significant factor in the arena of anesthesia for urology procedures. Since the increasing application of ultrasound-guided regional anesthetic methods, LAST patterns have evolved, leading to delayed symptom onset and a higher incidence of complications related to fascial plane block. The shift entails wide-ranging education for all anesthesiologist staff so that they can identify and manage emerging dangers involved with anesthetic medications. More awareness needs to be created in a bid to create effective risk management tactics with an emphasis on vulnerable populations, such as those with existing hepatic or cardiovascular diseases. Such prevention can help decrease the incidence of LAST, and henceforth the need for ongoing professional development in anesthetic practice (Macfarlane et al., 2021). Incorporation of advanced technologies in pre-procedure planning also forms a key component of modern urologic anesthesia. Advances in technology like 3D printing have transformed the way complex cases are handled by anesthetic practitioners, with the ability to offer detailed, patient-specific anatomy that will allow accurate preoperative planning. The technology will allow one to simulate procedures and enhance training and education in surgery, ultimately increasing overall proficiency in handling difficult cases. These technologies find application in the development of custom surgical guides, patient-specific implants, and comprehensive counseling procedures for patients and ultimately enhance the results of operations. By applying such advanced procedures, anesthetists can enhance the standard of care in renal and urologic surgery by optimizing operative efficiency and patient satisfaction. The adoption of these methods into clinical practice is a key milestone towards even more individualized and effective anesthetic care (Macfarlane et al., 2021).

KEY TERMS FROM THIS CHAPTER

- Cardiovascular stability
- Evidence-based protocols
- Hemodynamics
- Nephrectomy
- Respiratory function
- Venous thromboembolism (VTE)
- Complexity
- Hematology
- Nephrectomies
- Renal surgery
- Urologic

Critical Thinking Questions

1. **Which anesthetic technique is commonly used for transurethral resection of the prostate (TURP)?**
   a. General anesthesia
   b. Regional anesthesia (spinal or epidural)
   c. Local anesthesia with sedation
   d. None of the above
2. **What is the primary complication associated with excessive absorption of irrigation fluid during TURP?**
   a. Hypertension
   b. TURP syndrome
   c. Bradycardia
   d. Pulmonary edema
3. **Which irrigation fluid is most commonly used for TURP to minimize the risk of TURP syndrome?**
   a. Normal saline
   b. Distilled water
   c. Glycine solution
   d. Lactated Ringer's
4. **What is the preferred anesthetic approach for extracorporeal shock wave lithotripsy (ESWL)?**
   a. Local anesthesia
   b. General anesthesia
   c. Regional anesthesia or sedation
   d. No anesthesia required
5. **What is the most significant anesthetic consideration for renal transplant surgery?**
   a. Maintaining hemodynamic stability
   b. Using nephrotoxic drugs
   c. Avoiding hyperglycemia
   d. Delayed emergence

Short Answer Questions

1. What are the anesthetic considerations for patients undergoing renal transplant surgery?
2. How does renal dysfunction affect the pharmacokinetics of anesthetic drugs?
3. What is the preferred regional anesthetic technique for transurethral resection of the prostate (TURP)?
4. Why is continuous irrigation used during TURP, and what complications can arise from it?
5. What are the risks associated with pneumoperitoneum during laparoscopic urologic surgery?
6. How is fluid balance managed during major urologic surgery?

Answer to Critical Thinking Questions

1. (b); 2. (b); 3. (c); 4. (c); 5. (a)

References

1. O'Dwyer, MJ; Owen, HC; Torrance, HDT (2015). The perioperative immune response. https://core.ac.uk/download/42490691.pdf (accessed on 28th June 2025).
2. Allard, M., Anderson, D., Applegate, R. L., Azer, T. E., et al. (2014). Cognitive dysfunction following desflurane versus sevoflurane general anesthesia in elderly patients: A randomized controlled trial. https://core.ac.uk/download/323070409.pdf (accessed on 28th June 2025).
3. Kaye AD, Vadivelu N, Ahuja N, Mitra S, Silasi D, Urman RD. Anesthetic considerations in robotic-assisted gynecologic surgery. *Ochsner J.* 2013;13(4):517-524.(accessed on 28th June 2025).
4. Anderson, D. R., Morgano, G. P., Bennett, C., Dentali, F., Francis, C. W., García, D., Kahn, S. R., et al. (2019). American Society of Hematology 2019 guidelines for management of venous thromboembolism: Prevention of venous thromboembolism in surgical hospitalized patients. *Blood Advances, 3*, 3898–3944. https://doi.org/10.1182/bloodadvances.2019000975 (accessed on 28th June 2025).
5. Assimos, D. (2019). Re: Comparison of ketamine with midazolam versus ketamine with fentanyl for pediatric extracorporeal shock wave lithotripsy procedure: A randomized controlled study. *The Journal of Urology, 201(1)*, 26. https://www.semanticscholar.org/paper/68140ee82173c5bc142294555222207d0f2abc93 (accessed on 28th June 2025).
6. Assimos, D. G., Krambeck, A. E., Miller, N. L., Monga, M., Murad, M. H., Nelson, C. P., Pace, K. T., et al. (2016). Surgical management of stones: American Urological Association/Endourological Society guideline, PART I. *The Journal of Urology, 196*, 1153–1160. https://doi.org/10.1016/j.juro.2016.05.090 (accessed on 28th June 2025).
7. Wenzel, J. T., Schwenk, E. S., Baratta, J. L., & Viscusi, E. R. (2016). Managing Opioid-Tolerant Patients in the Perioperative Surgical Home. *Anesthesiology clinics, 34*(2), 287–301. https://doi.org/10.1016/j.anclin.2016.01.005(accessed on 28th June 2025).
8. Bhardwaj, A., Deep, A., Chadha, A., & Kumar, Y. (2025). Advances in pain management in oral surgery. *Journal of Academy of Dental Education.* https://www.semanticscholar.org/paper/71c2a4b841ea69e235c3da0d26da94a929829d53 (accessed on 28th June 2025).
9. Rosa M, Usai P, Miano R, et al. Recent finding and new technologies in nephrolitiasis: a review of the recent literature. *BMC Urol.* 2013;13:10. Published 2013 Feb 16. doi:10.1186/1471-2490-13-10(accessed on 28th June 2025).
10. Budrikis, A., Jievaltas, M., Al Assaad, S., & Kinduris, S. (2012). Simultaneous nephrectomy and coronary artery bypass grafting through extended sternotomy. https://core.ac.uk/download/pdf/81076561.pdf (accessed on 28th June 2025).
11. Chitnis, S., Tang, R., & Mariano, E. R. (2020). The role of regional analgesia in personalized postoperative pain management. *Korean Journal of Anesthesiology, 73*, 363–371. https://doi.org/10.4097/kja.20323 (accessed on 28th June 2025).
12. Vasu, T. S., Grewal, R., & Doghramji, K. (2012). Obstructive sleep apnea syndrome and perioperative complications: a systematic review of the literature. *Journal of clinical sleep medicine : JCSM : official publication of the American Academy of Sleep Medicine, 8*(2), 199–207. https://doi.org/10.5664/jcsm.1784(accessed on 28th June 2025).

13. Ficarra, V., Novara, G., Abrate, A., Bartoletti, R., Crestani, A., De Nunzio, C., Giannarini, G., et al. (2020). Urology practice during the COVID-19 pandemic. *Minerva Urological e Nephrological, 72.* https://doi.org/10.23736/s0393-2249.20.03846-1 (accessed on 28th June 2025).

14. Finelli, A., Ismaila, N., Bro, B., Durack, J. C., Eggener, S., Evans, A., Gill, I. S., et al. (2017). Management of small renal masses: American Society of Clinical Oncology clinical practice guideline. *Journal of Clinical Oncology, 35*, 668–680. https://doi.org/10.1200/jco.2016.69.9645 (accessed on 28th June 2025).

15. Repassy, D. L., Frang, D., & Jako, G. J. (1996). Minimal and direct access surgery in urology. *Diagnostic and therapeutic endoscopy, 3*(2), 99–105. https://doi.org/10.1155/DTE.3.99 (accessed on 28th June 2025).

16. Gashler, K. R., Ritchie, A. K., Hood, R., & Ibekwe, S. O. (2023). Anesthetic Management of Renal Cell Carcinoma With Level 3 Inferior Vena Cava Extension in a Patient With Severe Coronary Artery Disease. *Cureus, 15*(8), e44180. https://doi.org/10.7759/cureus.44180(accessed on 28th June 2025).

17. Gohad, R., Jain, S., & Paul, A. (2025). Anesthetic management and perioperative care in a high-risk patient with bladder cancer, hypertension, and chronic kidney disease undergoing radical cystectomy with ileal conduit urinary diversion: A case report. *Multidisciplinary Science Journal.* https://www.semanticscholar.org/paper/2190998a0e7eeeb0d4d61b58aa1124625e3d6c80 (accessed on 28th June 2025).

18. Hassan, A. H., Mahmoud, M. A., Ahmed, I. M., & Soliman, F. I. (2025). Spinal versus epidural anesthesia for patients with chronic obstructive pulmonary disease undergoing supine percutaneous nephrolithotomy for management of renal stones: A prospective double-blind randomized clinical trial. *The Egyptian Journal of Hospital Medicine, 98*, 1029–1038. https://ejhm.journals.ekb.eg (accessed on 28th June 2025).

19. Tekgül ZT, Horsanali BÖ, Horsanali MO. Anesthesia for Urological Surgery [Internet]. Current Topics in Anesthesiology. InTech; 2017. Available from: http://dx.doi.org/10.5772/66197(accessed on 28th June 2025).

20. Key, N. S., Khorana, A. A., Kuderer, N. M., Bohlke, K., Lee, A. Y. Y., Arcelus, J. I., Wong, S. L., et al. (2019). Venous thromboembolism prophylaxis and treatment in patients with cancer: ASCO clinical practice guideline update. *Journal of Clinical Oncology, 38*, 496–520. https://doi.org/10.1200/jco.19.01461 (accessed on 28th June 2025).

21. Kheterpal, S., Vaughn, M. T., Dubovoy, T., Shah, N., Bash, L. D., Colquhoun, D. A., Shanks, A., et al. (2020). Sugammadex *versus* neostigmine for reversal of neuromuscular blockade and postoperative pulmonary complications (STRONGER). *Anesthesiology, 132*, 1371–1381. https://doi.org/10.1097/aln.0000000000003256 (accessed on 28th June 2025).

22. Lerner, L. B., McVary, K. T., Barry, M. J., Bixler, B. R., Dahm, P., Das, A. K., Gandhi, M. C., et al. (2021). Management of lower urinary tract symptoms attributed to benign prostatic hyperplasia: AUA guideline part II—Surgical evaluation and treatment. *The Journal of Urology, 206*, 818–826. https://doi.org/10.1097/ju.0000000000002184 (accessed on 28th June 2025).

23. Macfarlane, A., Gitman, M., Bornstein, K., El-Boghdadly, K., & Weinberg, G. A. (2021). Updates in our understanding of local anesthetic systemic toxicity: A narrative review. *Anesthesia, 76*, 27–39. https://doi.org/10.1111/anae.15282 (accessed on 28th June 2025).

24. Meyer-Szary, J., Luis, M. S., Mikulski, S., Patel, A., Schulz, F., Tretiakow, D., Fercho, J., et al.

(2022). The role of 3D printing in planning complex medical procedures and training of medical professionals—Cross-sectional multispecialty review. *International Journal of Environmental Research and Public Health, 19*, 3331–3331. https://doi.org/10.3390/ijerph19063331 (accessed on 28th June 2025).

25. Mongia, J. S., Tejaswee, A. S. S., Marella, V. G., Srilakshmi, D., Almasri, M. A., Tenglikar P., & Dayanithi, B. (2024). Evaluation of post-operative pain management techniques in oral surgery. *Journal of Pharmacy & Bioallied Sciences, 16*, S2360–S2362. https://www.semanticscholar.org/paper/37413d856a6b665f3b29474ba4d9df63793b767b (accessed on 28th June 2025).

26. Nagaya, T., Nakamura, Y., Choyke, P. L., & Kobayashi, H. (2017). Fluorescence-guided surgery. *Frontiers in Oncology, 7.* https://doi.org/10.3389/fonc.2017.00314 (accessed on 28th June 2025).

27. Nelson, G., Bakkum-Gamez, J. N., Kalogera, E., Glaser, G., Altman, A. D., Meyer, L. A., Taylor, J., et al. (2019). Guidelines for perioperative care in gynecologic/oncology: Enhanced Recovery After Surgery (ERAS) Society recommendations—2019 update. *International Journal of Gynecological Cancer, 29*, 651–668. https://doi.org/10.1136/ijgc-2019-000356 (accessed on 28th June 2025).

28. Nova Southeastern University. (2024). *NSU Health Professions Division 2023–2024 course catalog.* https://core.ac.uk/download/639220891.pdf (accessed on 28th June 2025).

29. Prabeena, B., Ananthi, J., Meeran, M. M., & Vasu, K. (2023). Comparison of ultrasound-guided dual transverse abdominis plane block (subcostal and posterior) vs epidural block by using 0.25% ropivacaine with fentanyl for patients undergoing open nephrectomy under general anesthesia: Randomised clinical study. *International Journal of Academic Medicine and Pharmacy, 5(6)*, 1364–1368. https://academicmed.org/Uploads/Volume5Issue6/281.%20[2066.%20JAMP_Mohamed%20Ali]%201364-1368.pdf (accessed on 28th June 2025).

30. Sun, L. Y., Wijeysundera, D. N., Tait, G. A., & Beattie, W. S. (2015). Association of intraoperative hypotension with acute kidney injury after elective noncardiac surgery. *Anesthesiology, 123*, 515–523. https://doi.org/10.1097/aln.0000000000000765 (accessed on 28th June 2025).

31. Türksal, E. (2025). Anesthesia for urological procedures. *Eurasian Journal of Anesthesiology and Intensive Care.* https://www.semanticscholar.org/paper/a5c22922b78e14939dbb18c33e2792a10047243d (accessed on 28th June 2025).

32. Department of Anesthesia. University of Iowa. Spring 2011. https://core.ac.uk/download/18608347.pdf

ANESTHESIA FOR ORTHOPEDIC AND TRAUMA SURGERY

7

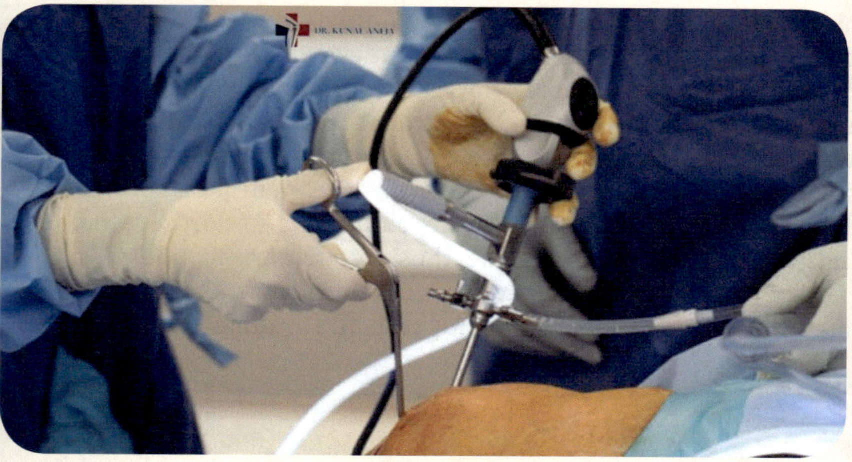

Introduction

Aesthetic anesthesia in trauma and orthopedic surgery calls for a foundational understanding of both the complexity of the surgery itself and the variations in patient physiology. Anesthesia is crucial to patient comfort, safety, and the best surgical outcomes during orthopedic procedures, which typically involve intricate maneuvers of the musculoskeletal system. Because of the character of trauma cases, with need potentially dictating initial decision-making, anesthetic care must be formulated to accommodate not only the nature of the surgery but also the severity of the injury and the patient's underlying medical status. For example, the use of effective regional anesthesia techniques can contribute heavily to pain management with a general reduction in opioid analgesics, in accordance with contemporary goals of minimizing opioid use during surgery. Understanding these dynamics is critical for anesthetists to be able to successfully operate in the intricate landscape of orthopedic and trauma surgery. Furthermore, advances in anesthesia technology hold paramount importance

LEARNING OBJECTIVES

After studying this chapter, you will be able to:

1. Discuss the types of anesthesia
2. Focus on preoperative assessment
3. Explain the anesthetic techniques in orthopedic surgery
4. Understand anesthetic techniques in trauma surgery
5. Know monitoring during surgery
6. Learn about postoperative care

for the post-recovery of the patient and surgical success. Anesthetic agents and regional anesthesia techniques have transformed traditional practices, providing practitioners with new avenues for improving postoperative results. Regional anesthetic methods, such as nerve blocks and peripheral anesthesia, are increasingly valued for their benefits, including a decrease in systemic complications and enhanced postoperative pain relief. These technologies hold particular significance in orthopedic surgery, where analgesia directly affects rehabilitation and patient satisfaction. The use of multimodal analgesia methods also reflects a broader trend toward comprehensive anesthetic care, controlling intraoperative as well as postoperative pain. The practitioners must understand these developments since they are central in determining anesthesia modalities in orthopedic settings, hence elevating the quality of care provided to patients. Also, education and competency base of anesthesia providers are imperative to the larger picture of orthopedic and trauma surgery. Successful administration of anesthesia relies not simply upon the technical proficiency of the anesthesiologists but also upon institutional structures underlying these positions. In low-resource settings, where anesthesiologists may be scarce, innovative training programs have been implemented to empower nurse anesthetists and non-physician anesthetists. For instance, Médecins Sans Frontières has demonstrated how granting nurse anesthetists the authority of safe anesthesia administration can have a substantial impact on the delivery of surgical service, particularly during emergency conditions following disasters. Such developments underscore the importance of ensuring adequate training and equipment for anesthesia providers in line with best practice in the practice of orthopedic surgery. Thus, education and supervision as priorities are at the core of propelling the volume of anesthesia care for orthopedic and trauma surgery in varied healthcare settings (Figure 7.1).

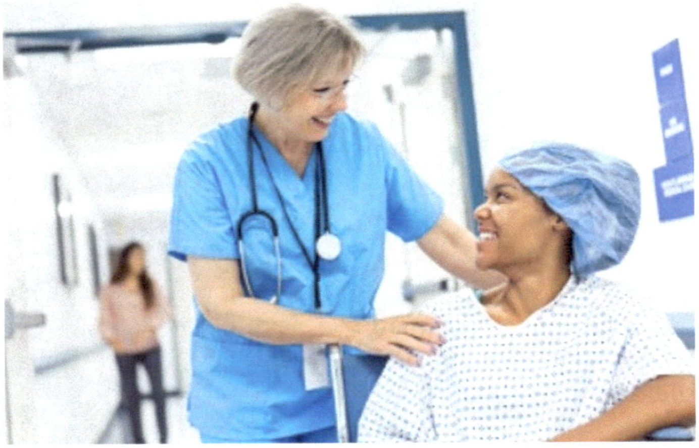

Figure 7.1. The practice of anesthesia for orthopedic and trauma surgery.

Source: https://www.bidmc.org/-/media/rich-text-images/beth-israel-org/centers-and-departments/orthopaedic-surgery/ortho-trauma-surgery/orthopaedic-trauma-surgery.jpg?h=233&w=350.

Definition of Anesthesia

Anesthesia is a key component of modern surgical practice, employed to facilitate procedures by inducing a controlled state of unconsciousness or insensitivity to painful stimuli. Anesthesia can be defined as a wide range of techniques employed by clinicians that allow invasive procedures to be performed while ensuring patient comfort and safety. For orthopedic and trauma surgery, anesthesia is often tailored to suit the patient and surgical requirements. This customization can include local, regional, or general anesthesia; each has specific advantages and handling methods. Regional anesthesia, for instance, can provide targeted analgesia without decreasing systemic exposure to medication, which can counteract continued concerns of opioid administration in postoperative care. To this extent, it is essential to know the definition of anesthesia because it not only identifies the multiplicity of techniques available but also emphasizes their strategic use in enhancing patient welfare during and subsequent to surgical procedures. The efficacy of anesthesia transcends the immediate requirements of surgery, having a significant impact upon perioperative management of the patient. As anesthetists collaborate with operating room teams to most effectively optimize intraoperative circumstances, likewise, they have a crucial role to play in planning and directing postoperative analgesia regimens. The shift towards multimodal analgesia is a recent instance of this collaborative process wherein several strategies for pain relief are employed concurrently to enhance the effectiveness of analgesics and reduce opioid dependence. This practice is particularly relevant in trauma surgery and orthopedics, where postoperative pain may be severe and complex. According to evidence documented in recent research, these techniques can significantly decrease opioid consumption and minimize harms from prolonged opioid use, which indicates the importance of an interdisciplinary approach to patient management in surgical practice (Schwenk et al., 2018). Furthermore, anesthesia is assisted by clinical practice and theoretical advancements that guide the decision-making in surgery. Theoretical surgery, as a concept, shows the contribution of scholarly research in guiding the knowledge and application of anesthesia techniques. Inter-professional research collaborations—among surgeons, scientists, and technical experts—deploy evidence-based practices to enhance surgery outcomes, exemplifying the need for inter-disciplinary discourse in optimizing the application of anesthesia (Lorenz & Rothmund, 1989). Such a working environment facilitates technological innovation and methodological progress in anesthesiology, keeping anesthesia both a science and an art, responsive to the diversity of patient requirements for orthopedic and trauma procedures. When stakeholders engage actively with each other, the definition and parameters of anesthesia continue to broaden and evolve, encompassing growing knowledge of its implications for patient health and recovery (Figure 7.2).

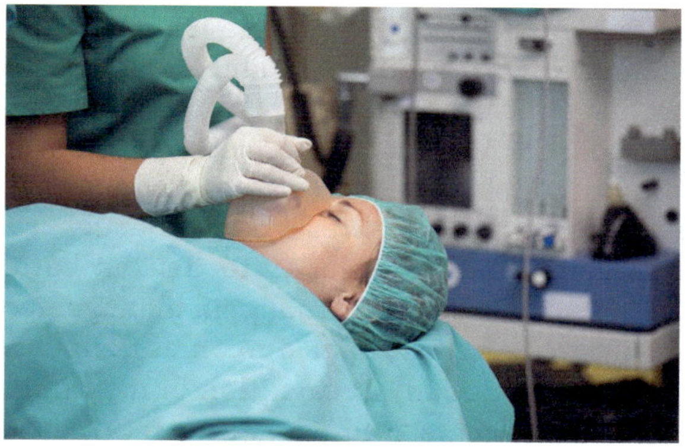

Figure 7.2. Anesthesia is a critical component of modern surgical practice.

Source: https://external-content.duckduckgo.com/iu/?u=https%3A%2F%2Fwww.online-sciences.com%2Fwp-content%2Fuploads%2F2016%2F01%2FAnesthetic-5.jpg&f=1&nofb=1&ipt=23babb41c3b63ac2a7aa3e800ed8c6538ff602b5305bc87cc4d7cb2265c80729.

Importance of Anesthesia in Orthopedic and Trauma Surgery

The role of anesthesia in trauma and orthopedic surgery extends far beyond sedation; it is critical to optimal operative results and patient safety. Intraoperative pain control and effective anesthesia protocols diminish physiological reaction to surgery, particularly relevant to patients who need advanced procedures. For instance, concerning total hip arthroplasties and spinal fusions, the anesthesia utilized has far-reaching effects on postoperative recovery and the risk for complications such as postoperative delirium (POD). Studies show that some anesthetic choices will reduce the risk for POD, particularly among older adults, demonstrating the necessity of effective planning with anesthetics to reduce unwanted effects and promote recovery (Urban et al., 2020). Also, please note that anesthesia choice has a major impact on postoperative pain relief quality, analgesic requirement, and patterns of recovery in general. For patients undergoing procedures such as total knee arthroplasties, regional anesthetic technique can optimize pain relief with reduced reliance on systemic opioids, which may be a contributing cause in delayed recovery as well as side effects. Use of multimodal analgesia, which combines the use of regional as well as systemic drugs, can potentially enable surgeons to deliver better patient care through optimal pain management and improved functional outcomes following surgery. Additionally, recognition of modifiable risk factors such as old age and comorbidities can guide anesthetic regimens based on the specific needs of the individual patient, thereby minimizing potential complications and improving surgical success rates (Urban et al., 2020). Lastly, the critical role of anesthetic procedures in orthopedic and trauma surgery should not be underestimated in view of the particular difficulties associated with such procedures, particularly in emergency cases. Orthopedic emergency procedures, such as in the case of patients with broken limbs, require speed-anesthetic interventions that are sure to alleviate pain and achieve patient stabilization. In such risky cases, the agility and expertise of the anesthesiology staff are most important to ensure that the procedure is as safe and effective as possible. The nuances of anesthesia not only add to the successful achievement of surgical objectives but also ensure a smoother post-procedure for patients, as evidenced by enhanced stability and pain management in complex cases. This interconnectedness of anesthesia and surgical outcome underscores the extremely important role that anesthesia plays in orthopedic and trauma surgery.

7.1. Types of Anesthesia

Learning Outcome

1. UGeneral anesthesia
2. Regional anesthesia
3. Local anesthesia

The selection of the mode of anesthesia is paramount to the efficacy and safety of orthopedic and trauma surgery. Among the most commonly practiced methods are general anesthesia, regional anesthesia, and local anesthesia. General anesthesia that renders the patient completely unconscious and insensitive to sensations is usually utilized in major surgeries such as total hip or knee arthroplasty. This technique allows the surgeon to perform extensive, movement-free procedures without patient awareness, thus enhancing surgical accuracy. Despite this, general anesthesia must be chosen with utmost discretion, particularly in the elderly, as studies have shown that there are several risk factors for postoperative complications, such as POD, which are influenced by both surgery type and the anesthetic used (Urban et al., 2020). Regional anesthesia consists of techniques like spinal and epidural block, which provide localized anesthesia to a specific body area. Regional anesthesia is particularly useful for orthopedic surgery of the lower extremities since it provides suitable analgesia with low systemic effects. In addition to pain relief, regional anesthesia can also lead to reduced blood loss and faster recovery. Significantly, its use has been correlated with a lower rate of POD compared to that of general anesthesia, and therefore, it represents an option that can be utilized in groups of patients at high risk for such a complication. Regional methods not only decrease postoperative pain better but can also shorten the length of hospital stay, which points to their role in enhancing surgical results in orthopedic settings (Urban et al., 2020). Local anesthesia, while less often used in major orthopedic procedures, remains a mainstay for minor procedures or in conjunction with other types of anesthesia. It describes the use of anesthetic agents in a local area, facilitating procedures that do not involve systemic anesthesia. Its applications include some fracture stabilizations and outpatient orthopedic interventions, where rapid recovery is achieved. In addition, as health systems continue to expand access to surgery globally, understanding the worth of different anesthetic approaches becomes increasingly critical in low-resource settings. Effective training and implementation of viable surgical programs within these settings can bring significant improvements in surgical care and outcomes and demonstrate the adaptability of anesthesia in the modern practice (Figure 7.3).

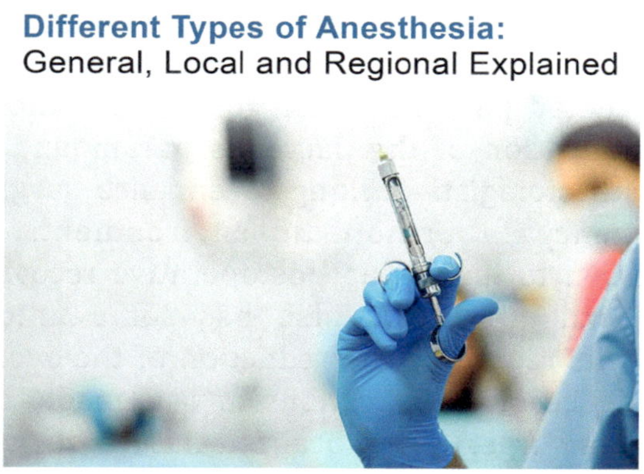

Figure 7.3. The selection of anesthesia type.

Source: https://www.parkhospital.in/storage/app/public/upload/i0eMpPcLdTQv9tzU7lIryus7J7KG9uPY0W02cZ8o.jpg.

7.1.1. General Anesthesia

General anesthesia plays a central role in offering the patient comfort and ensuring surgical precision in orthopedic and trauma surgery. When applied, it guarantees deep unconsciousness, hence preventing perception of pain during invasive treatments. General anesthesia also enables muscle relaxation, which is particularly beneficial in high-risk orthopedic procedures, where precision and controlled movement by the patient are crucial for successful surgical outcomes. Through the provision of a controlled environment, anesthesiologists can monitor vital signs closely and titrate anesthetic depth accordingly, which is important in operations involving critical anatomical structures and needing a long operational duration. Postoperative complications, like postoperative delirium (POD), may impact patient recovery and outcome to a great extent. It is revealed that general anesthesia as such is not a primary risk factor for POD, but is an entwined factor with other intrinsic patient factors that determine recovery patterns. For instance, in high-volume specialized orthopedic facilities, findings have indicated that emergency surgery, such as femoral and pelvic fractures, has higher rates of POD, which demonstrates both the overlap of surgical urgency and the intricacy of anesthesia care. It is the recognition of these relationships that becomes of most significance, as it allows for the formulation of ways to minimize risks and further enhance recovery routes within the environment of trauma and orthopedic surgery (Urban et al., 2020). Furthermore, the choice of anesthetic approach is very much patient profile and specifically procedure-dependent. Modern trends in anesthesia emphasize the multimodal regimen, where regional and general anesthesia are combined to oppose pain and reduce complications. Use of adjuncts such as intravenous patient-controlled analgesia in addition to general anesthesia has been discovered to influence postoperative results positively. As indicated in various studies, certain groups, particularly older persons, are more vulnerable to complications following procedures under general anesthesia. This points towards the necessity of adequate preoperative assessment to identify modifiable risk factors that may influence recovery (Gjeltema et al., 2017). With technological advances, ongoing research is essential to enhance safety and efficacy in anesthesia for orthopedic and trauma surgery (Figure 7.4).

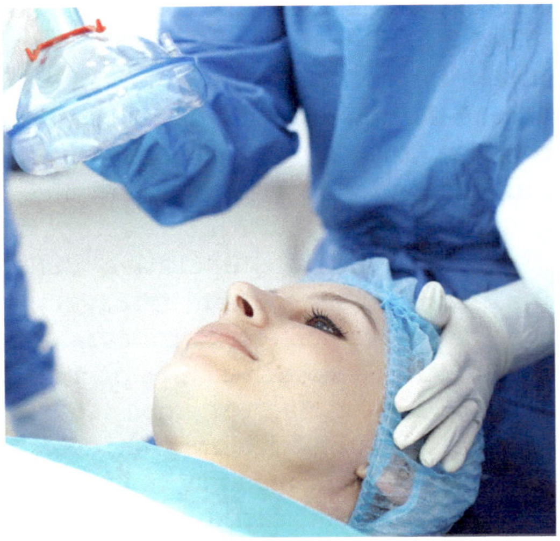

Figure 7.4. The general anesthesia serves as a pivotal component in ensuring patient comfort.

Source: https://ysm-res.cloudinary.com/image/upload/ar_1:1,c_fill,dpr_3.0,f_auto,g_faces:auto,q_auto:eco,w_500/v1/yms/prod/555930d3-576c-4328-8d3c-8667b6c7eb3f.

7.1.2. Regional Anesthesia

Regional anesthesia has emerged as an orthopedic and trauma surgery bedrock technique, and it has a number of advantages over general anesthesia. By targeting specific neural structures, regional anesthesia allows for effective control of pain at the time of and after surgery, reducing the quantity of systemic opioids consumed and thus the resulting opioid-related morbidity. Studies have shown significant decreased rates of POD in patients who have received orthopedic surgery when regional techniques are employed, particularly among elderly individuals. POD in patients receiving regional anesthesia was significantly lower at 1.2%, and studies revealed that early ambulation and multi-modal regional anesthesia are highly significant in minimizing this complication rate (Urban et al., 2020). This enhancement of patient results underscores the importance of selecting appropriate anesthesia techniques suited for the operating environment as well as the patient populations. The decision to use regional anesthesia for orthopedic procedures is based on various issues, including surgery type and the general health status of patients. Spinal and epidural anesthesia, for instance, are employed extensively in lower limb surgeries due to their ability to bring about profound analgesia as well as muscle relaxation. A retrospective study in Dr. Hasan Sadikin General Hospital revealed that 55% of orthopedic patients who were operated on were operated on under regional anesthesia, and the most common epidural procedures given were (Mudia et al., 2016). Such evidence shows that regional anesthesia not only enhances the level of patient comfort during surgery but also allows for a faster recovery process, where patients are able to engage in mobility exercises sooner compared to sedated patients under general anesthesia. Identification of this factor is paramount for anesthesiologists seeking to enhance surgical efficiency in orthopedic environments. In addition to improving postoperative recovery, regional anesthesia also has some unique benefits regarding the reduction of the overall incidence of complications in orthopedic and trauma surgery. The localized nature obviates the need for very potent systemic analgesics, which can produce unwanted side effects like respiratory depression or over-sedation. Moreover, the reduction of the stress response involved with less invasive anesthesia can enable quicker operating times and minimize the risks entailed. Importantly, the application of regional anesthetic techniques has not been discovered to harbor a higher risk for POD in cohort studies looking at the number of cases undergoing surgery, thereby confirming their place as a safe and effective alternative to managing surgical anesthesia (Urban et al., 2020). Through the incorporation of these techniques, health workers can enhance surgery for patients while further influencing critical outcomes pertaining to pain management and recovery time (Figure 7.5).

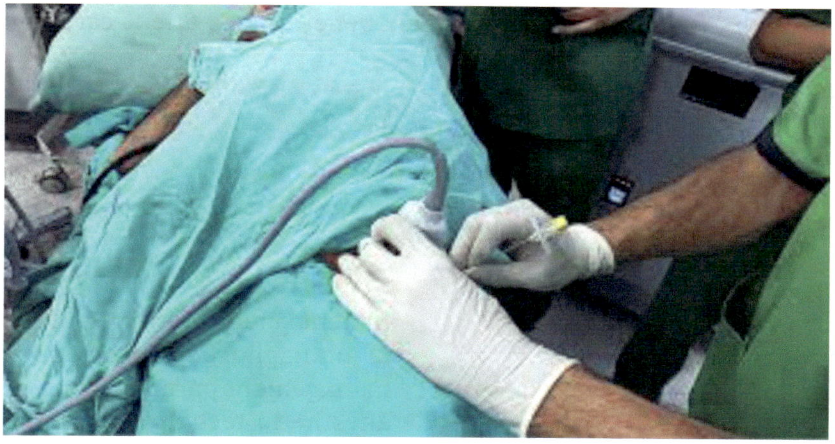

Figure 7.5. Regional anesthesia has emerged as a cornerstone technique.

Source: https://encrypted-tbn0.gstatic.com/images?q=tbn:ANd9GcSr6yA0MuNXEetjZ2QlGVU7KA-loEwGczV1kw&s.

7.1.3. Local Anesthesia

Local anesthesia is a major contributor to orthopedic and trauma surgery pain control, with some benefits over general anesthesia. Local anesthesia inhibits nerve impulse transmission at the location of the surgery, ensuring regional analgesia with minimal systemic effects, thereby accelerating patient recovery and minimizing the possibility of postoperative complications. Used appropriately, local anesthetics can significantly reduce the requirements of opioids, which under normal circumstances go along with side effects and addictions. During fracture fixation or arthroscopic surgery, the success of local anesthesia allows recovery at increased speeds and shorter hospital stays, resulting in orthopedic patient care efficiency. The effect of local anesthesia extends to short-term surgical outcomes; postoperative outcomes are also influenced, particularly in vulnerable populations. For instance, elderly patients who present with hip fracture surgery can be assisted using regional methods of anesthesia, which can promote postoperative management of pain and postoperative mobilization. Systemic reductions in exposure to anesthetic agents have proven to promote safety in patients, particularly those with comorbidities that complicate anesthesia management. Also, successful local anesthetic may lead to expedited mobilization—essential for preventing complications such as deep vein thrombosis and expediting rehabilitation in operated patients, as emphasized in more current literature that underscores the importance of anesthetic approaches designed for the individual patient risk for complications (Waller, 2012). With orthopedic trauma, the method of delivery of anesthetic may also exert some impact on shaping the intraoperative environment and patient course. Methods such as awake hand surgery, founded on local anesthesia, have become well-liked for allowing the surgeon to perform procedures on an awake and alert patient. Not only does it allow for the prevention of risks associated with general anesthesia, but it also facilitates increased precision in surgery through instantaneous feedback and collaboration between patient and surgeon. As pain management continues to evolve, the application of local anesthesia in orthopedic medicine reflects a refinement in patient-centered care, enhancing outcomes without sacrificing patient needs and desires (Department of Anesthesia, University of Iowa, 2011). With continued studies and applications, local anesthesia's impact on orthopedic surgery will only rise, providing further benefits for patient care.

Test Your Knowledge

1. Which types of anesthesia are commonly used in orthopedic and trauma surgeries?
2. When is regional anesthesia preferred in orthopedic procedures?

7.2. Preoperative Assessment

Learning Outcome

1. Patient medical history
2. Physical examination
3. Risk factors specific to orthopedic and trauma patients

A thorough preoperative assessment is essential in assessing the safety and appropriateness of anesthesia among patients undergoing orthopedic and trauma surgery. Not only does the assessment help understand the patient's medical history, but it also uncovers likely risk factors that can complicate surgical as well as anesthetic outcomes. For instance, certain patient populations, such as age and comorbidities, have been associated with varied risks of postoperative complications. Notably, greater than a single medical comorbidity and older age have been described as significant risk indicators for the development of POD among patients undergoing total hip arthroplasty (THA) and total knee arthroplasty (TKA) (Urban et al., 2020). In this way, attention to preoperative evaluation enables anesthesiologists to risk-stratify and create customized anesthetic plans—ultimately ensuring surgical efficacy and patient safety. Moreover, preoperative diagnosis of undiagnosed conditions may alter patient management parameters, especially concerning anesthetic techniques and perioperative care. Obstructive sleep apnea syndrome (OSAS), for instance, is prevalent in surgical patients and carries increased risk during anesthesia. The anesthetic agents' collapsibility tendency of the lower airway underscores the need for early diagnosis of such conditions (Vasu et al., 2012). Preoperative assessment tools need to actively screen for OSAS and other sleep-related disorders so that anesthesiologists can anticipate issues and revise perioperative plans in response. By incorporating comprehensive preoperative assessments that take both medical and psychosocial factors into account, anesthetic care providers can better minimize risk and optimize outcomes, leading to a healthier surgical environment. Finally, the data obtained through preoperative testing can significantly influence the choice of anesthesia technique, ultimately impacting postoperative recovery. Anesthesiologists can employ multimodal analgesia and regional anesthesia techniques to reduce opioid dependency, especially in at-risk patients identified through screenings. The impact of opioid administration on postoperative complications, such as POD, has been emphasized, prompting the formulation of a patient-specific anesthetic regimen that reduces opioid utilization (Urban et al., 2020). This is not only in line with contemporary practice to limit opioid-induced adverse events but also underlines the need for rigorous preoperative assessment. By identifying not just potential complications, but also modifiable risk factors, anesthetic specialists can facilitate more uneventful recoveries and improve overall patient outcomes in orthopedic and trauma surgical cases (Figure 7.6).

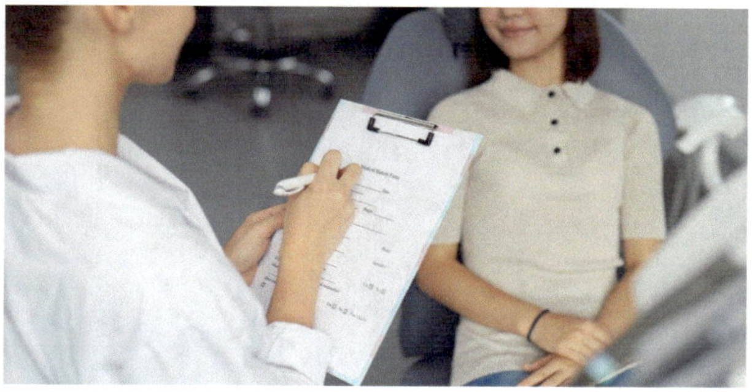

Figure 7.6. A comprehensive preoperative assessment.

Source: https://external-content.duckduckgo.com/iu/?u=https%3A%2F%2Fuksedation.com%2Fwp-content%2Fuploads%2F2021%2F05%2Fpreoperative-assessment-tool.jpg&f=1&nofb=1&ipt=3379f12170290bbff63b45c683f74134c6df48ecfdb59195c658903816d24025.

7.2.1. Patient Medical History

The significance of a patient's history cannot be overstated in planning anesthesia for orthopedic and trauma surgery. Anesthesiologists are alerted to risks and complications in the perioperative period through preexisting conditions known to them. Patients with a history of chronic pain, drug dependency, or anxiety, for instance, may be at greater risk for postoperative pain and opioid use. As described in recent literature, preoperative opioid use, along with psychological factors, is a strong predictor of chronic opioid dependence post-surgery. Through thorough assessment of these factors, anesthesiologists can better plan for reducing analgesic regimens via opioid exposure, which is consistent with newer multimodal practice guidelines for analgesia intended to maximize recovery and minimize dependence (Schwenk et al., 2018). This enhanced appreciation allows medical professionals to adapt plans of anesthesia, thus ensuring optimal results while efficiently controlling patient-specific risk. Moreover, the need for early intervention, particularly among elderly patients with orthopedic interventions such as fixation of hip fractures, further underscores the role of medical history in anesthesia management. Geriatric patients, who come more frequently with comorbidities and are usually on anticoagulant therapy like clopidogrel, require careful assessment in consideration of their increased risk for postoperative complications. It has been observed that while early surgery is critical in maximizing the success of surgery, patients on clopidogrel risk being at increased bleeding if surgery is performed too soon. Current research advocates for the use of personalized approaches that balance the need for surgery with risks presented by these medications, whereby patient history serves as the intermediary of decision-making in surgical urgency and anesthesia planning (Waller, 2012). These personalized approaches guarantee less mortality and better general patient safety. Lastly, understanding a patient's medical history allows the implementation of more vigorous recovery routes that will allow for faster recovery and release from hospital stay following surgery. Such routes can be through advanced techniques of anesthesia, including regional blocks, that have been found to effectively reduce opioid use and pain control effectively. Surgeon-anesthesiologist communication in developing an all-encompassing, tailored perioperative plan has a significant impact on patients' outcomes following recovery. Through the integration of patient histories, including elements from previous results in surgery to psychosocial elements, medical professionals can employ an anticipatory approach in managing anesthesia. Lastly, integration of comprehensive medical histories into anesthetic practice results in optimal patient outcomes and improves adherence to modern guidelines that emphasize opioid minimization while optimizing recovery (Schwenk et al., 2018) (Figure 7.7).

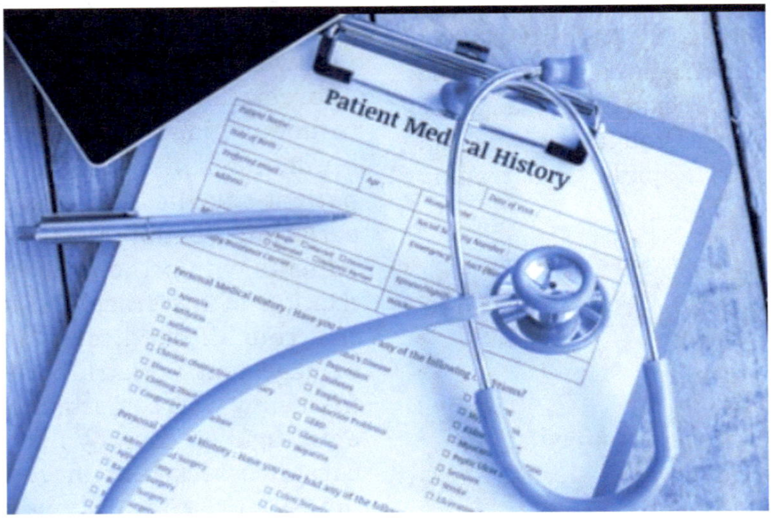

Figure 7.7. The significance of a patient's medical history.

Source: https://www.shutterstock.com/image-photo/patient-medical-history-on-clipboard-260nw-414285820.jpg.

7.2.2. Physical Examination

Extensive physical examination is the basis for correct anesthesia management in trauma and orthopedic surgery. This critical process begins with a comprehensive assessment of the patient's surgical history, responses to anesthesia, and other existing conditions that would influence surgical results. In physical examination, clinicians not only inspect the affected areas but also the other systems to give a comprehensive view of the person. For orthopedic surgery, assessment of the range of motion and mobility of the limb is most critical, as any underlying musculoskeletal abnormality can interfere with anesthesia techniques and recovery after surgery. Close consideration of potential complications of the surgical site is important, thereby allowing anesthesiologists to formulate tailored strategies that minimize risks, optimize pain control, and enhance patient safety. Furthermore, the need for obtaining important vital signs cannot be overstressed with respect to orthopedic and trauma anesthesia. Its monitoring for heart rate, blood pressure, and oxygen saturation establishes a clear baseline for control of anesthetics. Each of these abnormally occurring vital signs is indicative of underlying physiological issues, such as hypovolemia or cardiovascular instability, which need to be addressed before induction. For these purposes, the physical examination is taken beyond the surgical site to cover evaluation of the patients' general stability and fitness for anesthetic induction. Furthermore, screening for possible drug interactions among premedicant or anesthetic drugs is facilitated by this examination to ensure optimal pharmacologic management according to the patient's personalized requirements and health status. An essential component of the physical examination is also the evaluation of patient's airway and respiration, particularly in orthopedic surgery, where position may be harmful to ventilation. A thorough examination of the airway is able to show anatomical differences or obstructions unfavorable to intubation and ventilation. Thus, anesthesiologists can pre-emptively map out their methods based on these parameters. Moreover, in cases of traumatic injury, special care must be exercised in the observation of spinal and neurological examination to ensure that no complications arise during the surgical procedures. The pairing of these tests, Leicht brought about by surgical specificity in animal operations, i.e., avian patients (Gjeltema et al., 2017) and perioperative procedures used in veterinary practice (McKune et al., 2014), speaks about the necessity of acquiring knowledge regarding individual anatomical traits and overall impact on anesthesia efficiency in orthopedic clinics (Figure 7.8).

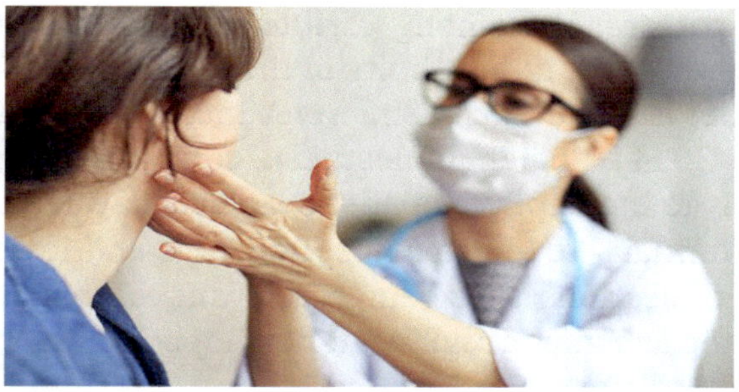

Figure 7.8. A comprehensive physical examination.

Source: https://external-content.duckduckgo.com/iu/?u=https%3A%2F%2Fhealthtips.ph%2Fwp-content%2Fuploads%2F2022%2F12%2FPhysical-Examination.jpg&f=1&nofb=1&ipt=a78f5a1a97e5c6b25844de5e07487ba29d7bfd03fe9a808c9bab7a88bb053400.

7.2.3. Risk Factors Specific to Orthopedic and Trauma Patients

Trauma and orthopedic patients demand anesthesia management that has an in-depth understanding of the specific risk factors that may influence perioperative outcomes. Surgical intervention being undertaken is one such significant risk factor. For example, research indicates that the incidence of POD in many of the orthopedic procedures is significantly variable. Patients undergoing spinal fusions carry a much higher rate of POD (3.3%) than patients with total hip arthroplasties (THA) (0.8%) or total knee arthroplasties (TKA) (1.2%)—a difference that reflects the severity of spine-involving procedures (Urban et al., 2020). In addition, emergent orthopedic procedures, such as the treatment of femoral and pelvic fractures, also reflect a much higher rate of POD at 7.2%. These findings illustrate how operative severity not only affects anesthetic care but also necessitates postoperative individualized care strategies to avert the occurrence of complications. Patient-related factors such as age, comorbidities, and preoperative health status, apart from the nature of the surgical procedure, significantly influence perioperative risks among orthopedic patients. Advanced age is consistently linked to increased occurrence of POD, with odds ratios suggesting about fivefold increased risk among older patients receiving THA compared to those younger (Urban et al., 2020). Other relevant risk factors include an American Society of Anesthesiologists (ASA) classification score of three or more, greater than one medical comorbidity, and pre-existing conditions like alcohol and chronic opioid dependence. These comorbid conditions not only complicate the anesthetic management but also may necessitate multidisciplinary preoperative evaluation. Thus, proper preoperative evaluation with a focus on these points is necessary in order to ensure safety and obtain improved anesthetic outcomes. Special analgesic techniques applied also introduce a risk factor for orthopedic and trauma patients. Research points to intravenous patient-controlled analgesia as being highly correlated with increased risk of susceptibility to POD in patients undergoing THA (Urban et al., 2020). In addition, certain medications given during the perioperative phase, such as parenteral diazepam, have been linked with increased incidences of delirium and complications, particularly in older patients (Urban et al., 2020). Pain management is a fundamental component of care postoperatively, especially with orthopedic surgery, where the quality of analgesia directly impacts recovery time. Thus, it is the responsibility of anesthesiologists to balance the merits and demerits of various modalities for analgesia so that they can individualize their approach according to the patient's profile as well as the procedure being performed.

Test Your Knowledge

1. How does blood loss increase risk in orthopedic and trauma patients?
2. Why is patient mobility a concern in these cases?

7.3. Anesthetic Techniques in Orthopedic Surgery

Learning Outcome

1. Indications for general anesthesia
2. Use of regional blocks in lower limb surgeries
3. Considerations for upper limb procedures

Orthopedic surgical anesthetic techniques are crucial in ensuring safety for the patient, minimizing pain, and ensuring maximum surgical success. Various modalities are employed, ranging from general to regional anesthetic techniques, such as spinal and epidural anesthesia. General anesthesia, although effective in major surgeries such as total hip arthroplasties, comes with some risks, among which is POD, particularly in older patients. Studies have shown that spinal fusion patients exhibit a greater incidence of POD than those with total hip arthroplasties, and the risk is significantly lower (Urban et al., 2020). To address these issues, the selection of the anesthetic method needs to consider the age of the patient, comorbidities, as well as the nature of the operation to reduce postoperative complications. Regional anesthetic techniques such as nerve blocks have gained prominence in orthopedics due to their ability to provide localized pain relief with reduced systemic use of narcotics. These regional anesthetic techniques, for example, interscalene or femoral nerve blocks, are beneficial in outpatient surgery with quicker recovery and decreased postoperative pain scores. A local anesthetic line block study detected no statistically significant difference in pain results among various control groups; however, the applicability of the method to pain relief is still of increasing relevance (McKune et al., 2014). Regional anesthesia contributed not only to the improved patient experience but also potentially to shorter hospital stays and fewer complications, thus being a relevant component of the anesthetic regimen for orthopedic surgery. In addition, the application of multimodal analgesia, or the use of multiple anesthetic modalities together, is now a standard technique in orthopedic procedures. The technique aims to optimize analgesia by using various mechanisms of action of various classes of analgesics to improve pain management and minimize opioid dependency. For instance, the combination of local anesthetics and nonsteroidal anti-inflammatory drugs or acetaminophen has been shown to significantly enhance analgesic effect with diminished opioid-related side effects (Urban et al., 2020). Moreover, the early ambulation protocols that are combined with an effective anesthetic technique have been shown to decrease POD's incidence to 1.2%, underscoring the importance of patient-tailored anesthesia regimens incorporating both pain management and postoperative recovery. Generally, the evolution of anesthetic techniques continues to improve outcomes in orthopedic surgery, reflecting an ongoing interaction between surgical innovation and anesthetic technology (Figure 7.9).

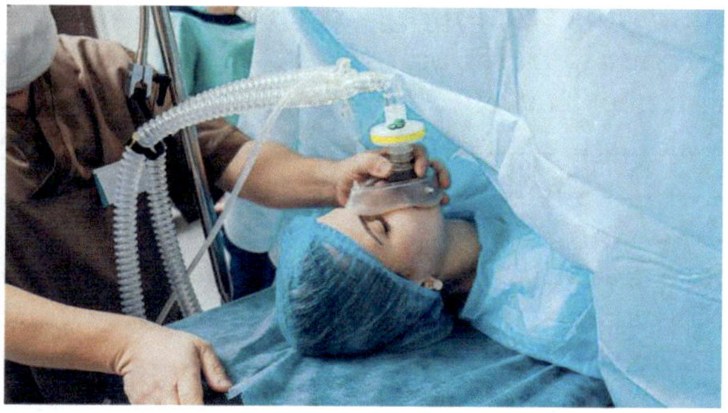

Figure 7.9. Anesthetic techniques in orthopedic surgery play a critical role in ensuring patient safety.

Source: https://docteurphilipperoure.com/static/8582c3951766ee91ff7e8d141a090ddf/7d509/anesthesie-chirurgie-orthopedique.jpg.

7.3.1. Indications for General Anesthesia

The role of general anesthesia in trauma and orthopedic surgery is not replaceable, especially when surgery involves massive manipulation of bones and soft tissues. General anesthesia provides an uninterrupted state of unconsciousness, analgesia, and muscle relaxation that is critical for patient comfort and protection during invasive orthopedic procedures. When repairing fractured bones or fixing joint injuries, surgeons must have a clear line of sight and complete control over the surgical field, which is facilitated by the muscle-relaxant action of general anesthesia. It also minimizes patient movement, which is critical in delicate procedures. Problems involving a large range of motion or of greater danger of pain, such as femur fractures or complex joint reconstructions, typically also make the use of general anesthesia appropriate to ensure optimal operation outcomes. In trauma surgery, whether or not to use general anesthesia can be based on the level of injury of the patient. Traumas in multiples can create polytrauma and require extensive surgeries. General anesthesia is indicated when quick action is necessary, such as in sėvere hemorrhage or compromised respiratory function, where quick cycles of intubation and stabilization are needed. Conditions that cause increased intracranial pressure, such as traumatic brain injury, can also be managed with general anesthesia for controlled ventilation and neurologic monitoring. Such a multi-modal approach is critical because it preserves the patient's physiological processes while allowing the surgeon to perform complex and life-saving surgeries with optimal efficiency and accuracy. In addition, multimodal methods of analgesia have transformed perioperative pain management, supporting the function of general anesthetics in trauma and orthopedic surgery. By merging many pharmacological classes that work through different pathways of pain, physicians can design more analgesics with fewer unwanted side effects of opioid administration. These regimens can combine opioids, non-opioid analgesics, and local anesthetics administered through regional block techniques, creating more integrated pain control regimens specifically tailored for patient needs. Apart from allowing faster recovery, this process may reduce hospital stays. However, problems such as drug shortages necessitate persistent lobbying by anesthesiologists to secure required medication for adequate pain management throughout the surgical continuum (Schwenk & Mariano, 2018). This points towards the essential link between the choice of anesthesia and postoperative outcomes, enhancing the overall quality of care in trauma and orthopedic surgery.

7.3.2. Use of Regional Blocks in Lower Limb Surgeries

In lower limb procedures, regional blocks are becoming a widely sought-after effective method of anesthesia, enhancing patients' outcomes and reducing complications. Regional methods of anesthesia, such as fascia iliaca blocks and popliteal nerve blocks, provide site-specific analgesia and reduce systemic opioids. The site-specific application not only guarantees a smoother recovery but also helps facilitate earlier rehabilitation and recovery. Literature advocates for the use of these methods because they result in fewer opioid-related side effects, which are imperative in the management of pain postoperatively. By using regional blocks, anesthesiologists can create tailored pain management protocols that suit particular patient needs, which ultimately results in greater satisfaction and fewer complications of lower limb surgeries. This change in anesthetic practice is one aspect of a broader movement towards multimodal analgesia strategies focused on patient-centered care and optimal pain relief. Regional anesthesia has a function that extends beyond the operating theatre and is a valuable tool in both preoperative and postoperative settings. Regional blocks, best practice now recommends, should be implemented as part of enhanced recovery pathways in optimizing lower limb surgical outcomes for patients. Regional anesthesia not only permits pain management in invasive interventions but also ensures maximum postoperative analgesia. This combined approach avoids the risks of opioid use, which may lead to chronic dependency and side effects. As emphasized in military experience, regional blocks are not just used in ordinary operating rooms but can be used for the management of acute pain in trauma situations. By using these practices in prehospital and early care settings, anesthesiologists are in a better position to offer enriched overall therapeutic environments for their patients, afford rapid relief, and establish the foundation for subsequent recovery phases (Wu et al., 2011). Furthermore, interactive dynamics between anesthesiologists and surgeons also greatly contribute to the optimization of regional blocks in the application of orthopedic surgical procedures. Effective pain management modes involve coordination and collaboration between the perioperative team when they design multimodal analgesia regimens combining regional anesthesia and non-opioid adjuvants. There is some evidence that multidisciplinary cooperation in managing analgesic plans can significantly minimize the use of opioids while concurrently addressing patients' pain management needs more holistically. Thus, individualized use of analgesia not only ensures patient safety but is also consistent with modern-day paradigms of anesthesia to reduce opioid consumption after surgery in general. Enhanced recovery pathways with a planned approach to pain management, including the expertise of anesthesiologists in regional anesthesia, result in enhanced patient outcomes for those undergoing lower limb operations, thus fostering a more effective and efficient healthcare environment (Schwenk et al., 2018) (Figure 7.10).

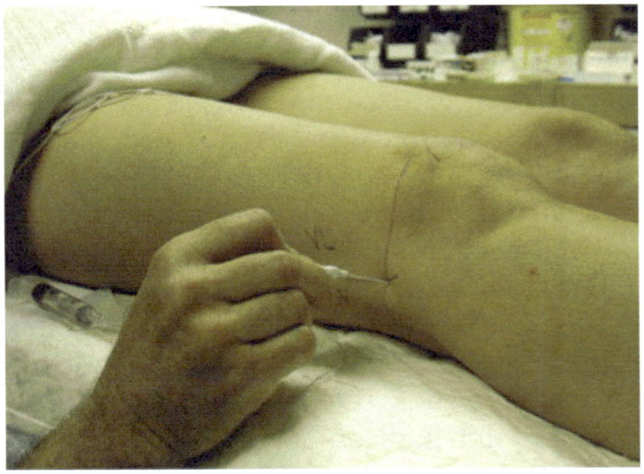

Figure 7.10. Use of regional blocks in lower limb surgeries.

Source: https://ars.els-cdn.com/content/image/1-s2.0-S1472029907000288-gr4.jpg.

7.3.3. Considerations for Upper Limb Procedures

For the management of upper limb surgery, the choice of anesthesia is of paramount importance to achieve the greatest benefit for the patient and to prevent complications. Among a spectrum of techniques, regional anesthesia is increasingly preferred for its ability to provide a selective block with reduced systemic opioid use. In addition to its enhanced pain control, it obviates the side effects of opioids, an important concern during the postoperative period. The implementation of multimodal analgesia protocols that involve agents like local anesthetics and non-opioid analgesics is beneficial. The protocols have vast potential to decrease total opioid consumption and, as a result, reduce the risk of chronic postoperative pain, which ultimately leads to faster recovery rates and improved patient satisfaction (Schwenk et al., 2018). Anesthesiologists, in collaboration with surgeons, are best suited to tailor these anesthetic strategies to meet the specific needs of individual patients and the special case requirements. One must also consider the special anatomical and functional considerations of the upper limb when planning orthopedic surgery anesthesia. For example, shoulder, elbow, or hand surgery can require specific anesthetic techniques that are appropriate for the character of the procedure and the specific physiological makeup of the patient. It is facilitated by familiarity with brachial plexus neuroanatomy to safely and effectively deliver regional blocks with greater analgesia and preservation of motor function as required. In addition, proper attention needs to be given to comorbidities, such as vascular or neurological disease, so that intraoperative and postoperative complications can be averted. The anesthetic plan should be integrated, addressing intraoperative positioning and postoperative care so that complications are not precipitated, creating a seamless transition of care throughout the perioperative interval (White et al., 2014). Finally, with the onset of evolving surgical techniques and advancement in anesthetic techniques, an active preoperative planning and patient education process is paramount. Involvement of the patient in an anesthetic choice discussion facilitates informed consent and enhances overall satisfaction with the surgical procedure. This is particularly true when undertaking upper limb surgery, when the patient is specifically anxious about pain relief and restitution of function. Furthermore, post-surgical patient observation and assessment of pain persistence or complications permit anesthesiologists to act early when something is wrong. With early intervention, as asserted by current research, medical practitioners can clearly prevent long-term opioid dependence while improving the outcome of patients who undergo upper limb surgery (Schwenk et al., 2018). Finally, a multidisciplinary effort is paramount to get the best outcome in anesthesia for trauma and orthopedic surgery, especially in the case of upper limb procedures.

Test Your Knowledge

1. What types of anesthesia are commonly used in orthopedic surgery?
2. Why is regional anesthesia often preferred for limb surgeries?

7.4. Anesthetic Techniques in Trauma Surgery

Learning Outcome

1. Challenges in emergency settings
2. Rapid sequence induction
3. Use of sedation in trauma patients

Proper selection of anesthetic techniques in the case of trauma surgery plays an instrumental role in optimizing patient outcomes. Not only does proper anesthesia address the issues related to pain relief, but it also has a critical role to play in assisting surgical operations. Having a proper knowledge of patients condition, including the extent and type of injury, is important in formulating anesthetic plans. For instance, intraoperative stability and postoperative analgesia can be influenced significantly by the choice between general anesthesia or regional blocks. In traumatic cases where rapid intervention is crucial, general anesthesia may be preferable because of its rapid onset of action as well as better control of physiological responses. However, the evolution of multimodal analgesia, which can be combined with regional anesthesia, has the possibility of providing benefits in the form of reduced opioid usage, minimizing side effects, and better recovery, particularly in elderly patients, because they are more likely to develop anesthesia-related complications (Urban et al., 2020). In recent years, the application of regional anesthesia in trauma surgeries has also gained prominence, with the focus being laid on its safety and efficacy. Techniques such as nerve blocks enable pain to be administered in a controlled manner, with patients being able to remain more alert and functional post-surgery. Regional anesthetic techniques such as nerve blocks or epidural anesthesia have been associated with lower postoperative pain scores and reduced hospital stays. Secondly, evidence shows that incorporating regional anesthesia can lead to a decrease in postoperative complications such as delirium among geriatric patients who are admitted for orthopedic surgery (Urban et al., 2020). Through managing pain at the point of injury and minimizing systemic opioid use, regional techniques yield improved patient satisfaction and results, making them a desirable option for trauma surgeons. Despite the advantages offered by regional techniques, their use will rely on a judicious assessment of risk factors and the suitability of the patient.

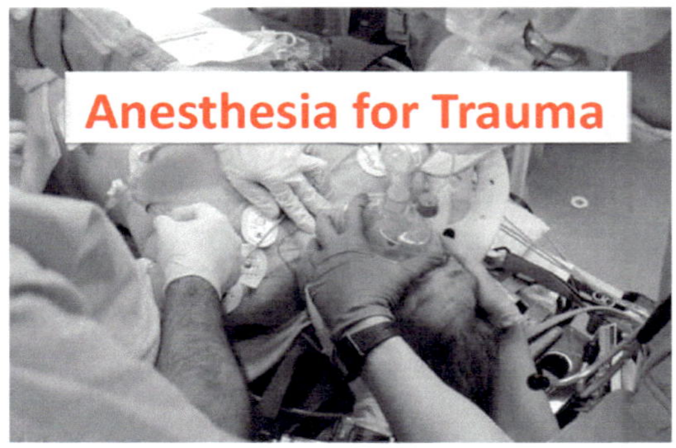

Figure 7.11. Anesthetic techniques in trauma surgery.

Source: https://cdn.slidesharecdn.com/ss_thumbnails/anesthesiafortraumamillerchapter72-131225153242-phpapp02-thumbnail.jpg?width=640&height=640&fit=bounds.

For example, not all patients will be candidates for nerve blocks, particularly those with certain comorbidities or anatomical issues. Furthermore, urgency for operation will typically necessitate a speeded-up process of decision-making, where general anesthesia may take precedence. A general understanding of the risks and advantages of various anesthetic techniques is required for anesthesiologists and trauma surgeons. Both must make the best out of the balance between addressing acute pain and minimizing risks associated with postoperative complications, such as respiratory depression or delay in recovery, mainly in the case of patients with advanced age or severe medical histories. Therefore, a delicate balance, specific to the individual patient's needs, is essential to enhance outcomes in trauma surgery anesthesia (Figure 7.11).

7.4.1. Challenges in Emergency Settings

In emergency conditions, particularly in poor-resource settings, anesthesia delivery for trauma and orthopedic surgery is especially daunting. Perhaps one of the major challenges in this regard is access to trained anesthesia staff. In most circumstances, anesthesia care is provided by non-physician personnel such as nurses who are usually inadequately trained or irregularly supervised. As emphasized by efforts such as those of Médecins Sans Frontières, training nurse anesthetists has proven critical to bridging this deficit, especially in Haiti, where 79% of the graduates remain engaged in their field following intensive training. These education programs emphasize the need to establish strong training structures that produce strong training systems that build a competent human resource base that is able to administer anesthesia safely under high-stress situations (Rosseel et al., 2009). In addition, the infrastructural and logistical constraints inherent within the emergency setting only add to the challenges of delivering anesthesia for surgical procedures. The availability of equipment and consumables needed is typically suboptimal, with older or less advanced technology being relied upon in such settings. Within settings like Somalia, where Médecins Sans Frontières operates, the necessity of speed in surgical procedures inevitably conflicts with the absence of up-to-date operating facilities, resulting in difficulty in the delivery of care resulting. Higher-level procedural techniques become unmanageable, necessitating changes in practice that increase the risk for adverse consequences. Provision of adequate resources to administer anesthesia is thus a matter of urgency, as illustrated in the surgical model established by organizations committed to providing care in such conditions of deprivation (Ford et al., 2011). Moreover, psychological and physical workload for both patients and caregivers cannot be exaggerated in emergency settings. Multiple traumas and varying degrees of shock in trauma patients increase the complexity of managing anesthesia. The psychological stress that doctors and other healthcare professionals operate under in such high-stress situations can also lead to burnout and decreased performance. Effective communication and collaboration help overcome the challenges. Organization of an effective operative team that can react with swiftness and competency to emergencies is crucial in ensuring timely patient safety and optimal outcomes. Planning and provision of anesthesia care in these circumstances, therefore, not only require technical proficiency but also sensitivity to the wider systemic problems at stake, thereby affirming the multi-faceted nature of emergencies (Rosseel et al., 2009).

7.4.2. Rapid Sequence Induction

Rapid sequence induction (RSI) is a critical technique employed in the management of orthopedic as well as trauma anesthesia, particularly in cases where the challenge of airway security is crucial. RSI is a technique whereby a combination of paralytic and sedative drugs is employed to reduce the risk of aspiration during intubation. The necessity of the majority of orthopedic and trauma surgery—typically prompted by acute trauma—cements the importance of RSI, as it not only allows for rapid intubation but also enhances patient safety. Intraoperative issues can be significantly reduced with the rapid administration of anesthetic agents, allowing for rapid airway control.

Anesthesiologists' proficiency in performing RSI is thus paramount for those who practice in high-acuity settings such as trauma centers, where patient status can rapidly change. An effective RSI protocol would generally involve agents that permit a rapid onset and quick recovery, such as etomidate or etomidate and succinylcholine. Selection of the analgesia and induction agent are key consideration, with certain agents impacting hemodynamic stability, particularly in traumatized patients. For instance, the use of ketamine has been controversial due to its effect on intracranial pressure (ICP), but recent studies show that it is effective in traumatic brain injury patients without having to increase ICP (DiLoreto, 2023). Conversely, propofol administration is, in most cases, acceptable for induction because it is hemodynamically stable and reduces inappropriate intracranial peaks. These aspects are crucial in optimizing the anesthetic approach to trauma patients for maintaining them stable physiologically during surgery. Rapid sequence induction has its risks and challenges, especially in trauma. The anesthesiologist should always consider the patient's individual characteristics, including the type of injury and his or her pre-existing health status. Adherence to standard protocols—such as those framed for the management of anesthetic care in trauma—empowers the practitioner to deal with the complex issues pertaining to anesthesia administration and airway management (Vaglio et al., 2016). Ongoing education and simulation training also play an important role in refining the competency and performance of practitioners at administering RSI, thus ensuring enhanced outcomes for the patient in orthopedic and trauma surgeries. The integration of contemporary evidence-based practice and greater understanding of pharmacological drugs is of paramount significance in the refinement of the process of rapid sequence induction within the specialty of trauma anesthesia (Figure 7.12).

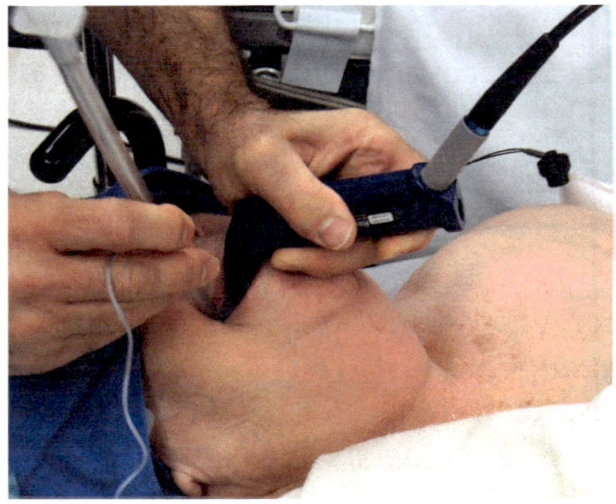

Figure 7.12. Rapid sequence induction (RSI).

Source: https://www.jonathandownham.com/wp-content/uploads/2016/09/Glidescope_02.jpg.

7.4.3. Use of Sedation in Trauma Patients

In orthopedic and trauma anesthesia, the position of sedation in trauma patients is key to obtaining maximum outcomes. Sedation is particularly significant in emergent cases where patients typically present with extreme pain and agitation due to their injuries. Through pain relief and sedation, patients' cooperation during diagnostic imaging and intervention improves. In addition, the depth and form of sedation can differ depending on the condition of the patients; for example, light sedation is most commonly used in situations where the patient needs to be evaluated quickly, whereas deeper sedation can be necessary during surgical interventions. This tactical application not only increases patient comfort but also ensures easier workflow for the surgical team, thus maximizing operational efficiency in trauma centers. A retrospective review of postoperative complications, including POD, underscores the importance of careful sedation management in the elderly trauma population. Research has clearly confirmed that POD prevalence is particularly marked in such a group, especially following non-ambulatory orthopedic surgery, with marked incidence rates being significantly elevated. Some procedures, such as spinal fusion, illustrate an even greater vulnerability to POD and mandate appropriately modified sedation practices. Interestingly, general anesthesia was not listed as a high-risk factor for POD, but other factors like age, medical comorbidities, and certain analgesic protocols were found to significantly influence outcomes. This information guides the need for vigorous monitoring and adjustment of sedation protocols to prevent the risk of postoperative complications like POD in trauma patients (Urban et al., 2020). The application of intra-articular anesthesia, as in the case of veterinary medicine diagnostic lameness, demonstrates the potential benefits of local sedation techniques that can be applied to human orthopedic procedures. Intra-articular anesthesia, when coupled with sedation, has shown strong success in locating the cause of joint pain with accuracy, similar to the case of trauma surgery, where directed intervention is crucial. The same approach in human medicine would improve patient outcomes, especially with the management of pain-containing joint trauma. Through maximization of sedation methods and multimodal anesthesia protocols, surgeons are in a better position to deliver improved pain control, reduce the incidence of undesirable events, and allow for faster recovery times among traumatic patients. The changing model of sedation and anesthesia in trauma therapy thus holds immense advantage in terms of improving patient safety and surgery efficiency (Van Vynckt et al., 2012).

Test Your Knowledge

1. What anesthetic technique is commonly used in trauma surgery?
2. Why is sedation used in trauma patients?

7.5. Monitoring During Surgery

Learning Outcome

1. Vital signs and hemodynamic monitoring
2. Neuromuscular function assessment
3. Depth of anesthesia monitoring

Intraoperative monitoring is an important component of anesthetic care in trauma and orthopedic surgery, where outcomes and patient safety hinge heavily on close observation. Anesthesia monitoring is an integrated process that includes the assessment of vital signs, oxygenation, ventilation, and hemodynamic stability intraoperatively. Continuous monitoring allows anesthesiologists to detect early alterations in physiological parameters, which makes it possible for them to intervene early to avoid unnecessary complications. Utilization of new monitoring equipment, such as capnography, pulse oximetry, and electrocardiography, enhances the anesthesiologist's vigilance in response to anesthetic depth changes and intraoperative risk control. Therefore, adherence to existing guidelines of monitoring is essential in delivering safer patients and optimizing surgical outcomes. As the expanding orthopedic and trauma surgery complexity keeps rising, careful monitoring cannot be overestimated because it is a vital safety mechanism against the development of anesthesia-related complications. Besides usual vital sign monitoring, multimodal analgesia approaches are also now equally acknowledged as an orthopedic best practice. By combining analgesic and regional anesthesia techniques, anesthesiologists can decrease the use of opioids and enhance postoperative pain relief. This method not only minimizes the risk of opioid-related complications but can also reduce the risk of developing chronic postoperative pain, which is one of the problems pointed out by recent studies. The anesthesiologists' contribution, in this case, is vital outside the operating room, as they collaborate with surgical teams to personalize intraoperative medication regimens based on patient requirements. This comprehensive management post-and-perioperatively allows for a seamless integration into enhanced recovery pathways by optimizing analgesia and overall patient outcomes (Schwenk et al., 2018). Therefore, the role of monitoring also involves the investigation of pain management strategies that contribute to postoperative recovery. Furthermore, the environment of resource-limited settings presents unique challenges and opportunities for surgical monitoring.

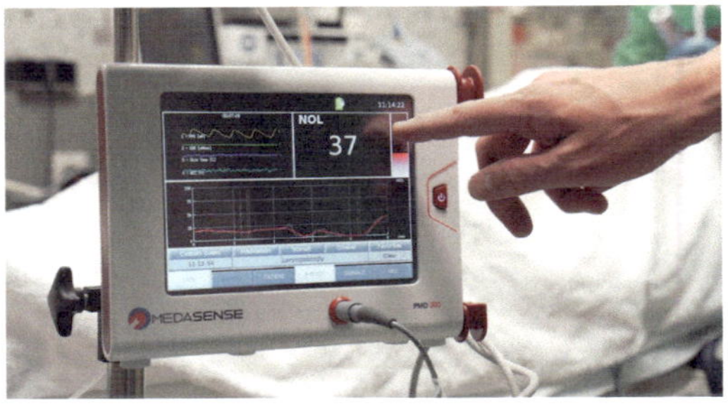

Figure 7.13. Monitoring during surgery is a critical component of anesthetic management.

Source: https://static.israel21c.org/www/uploads/2020/09/medasense-1520x855.png.

In certain regions, primarily where anesthesiologists are scarce, non-physician practitioners such as nurse anesthetists became integral components of anesthesia care. Training programs to equip these providers with the competency to deliver anesthesia safely have been effective in countries like Haiti. These programs not only expand the number of anesthesia providers but also put emphasis on rigorous monitoring policies to guarantee patient safety. The outcomes of training have been promising, and nurse anesthetists have been able to deliver anesthesia safely during urgent surgical interventions (Rosseel et al., 2009). This highlights the importance of ensuring strong monitoring practices across different healthcare systems, demonstrating that excellent anesthesia care is achievable even in resource-limited facilities, if appropriate training and backup are prioritized (Figure 7.13).

7.5.1. Vital Signs and Hemodynamic Monitoring

Hemodynamic monitoring and vital signs form a critical component of anesthesia care in trauma and orthopedic surgery. Monitoring parameters such as blood pressure, heart rate, respiratory rate, and oxygen saturation form a key component in the delivery of valuable information about a patient's physiological status during the preoperative, intraoperative, and postoperative periods. Anesthetic drugs exert significant impacts on hemodynamic stability, and therefore, unwavering attention is necessary in order to detect early alterations. For instance, tachycardia or hypotension may follow vasodilation or loss of fluid as a result of general anesthesia. Their early detection via rigorous monitoring allows anesthesiologists to implement timely interventions, avoid possible complications and minimize patient harm. The use of advanced monitoring techniques, such as intra-arterial pressure monitoring, could potentially give instantaneous feedback on hemodynamic changes, further enhancing the care of patients with major trauma and orthopedic surgery. Furthermore, the severity of monitoring hemodynamics is supplemented by comorbidities that are common among patients who require orthopedic surgery. Most of the patients will have comorbid diseases like cardiovascular disease or diabetes that will make their response to surgery and anesthesia challenging. A tailored method of monitoring is therefore required. Utilization of parameters from comprehensive testing, e.g., cardiopulmonary exercise testing, may provide a preview of a patient's physiological reserve and anesthesia-related risk factors. Continuous monitoring of vital signs, combined with familiarity with the history of a patient and the nature of surgery, allows anesthesiologists to make appropriate fluid replacement, drug management, and other central intervention decisions that maintain hemodynamic stability. The application of a personalized monitoring protocol is critical to enhancing surgical results and minimizing postoperative complications. In trauma and orthopedic surgery, the demand for careful vital sign monitoring lasts longer than in the operating room and continues till the recovery period. Postoperative monitoring is critical for the identification of complications like bleeding or the influence of anesthetic drugs. During this period, fluctuations in significant signs such as an increase in heart rate or hypotension may indicate hemodynamic instability or intraoperative side effects of anesthesia. Continuous monitoring enables early diagnosis and management of such events, particularly important in patients with large fluid shifts or operative trauma. Education of surgical and nursing staff on the importance of monitoring vital signs can also enhance outcomes in such patients. Regular training sessions in which interpreting signs from vital data and recognizing critical changes are highlighted are useful in developing a safety culture within the surgical team. Such a proactive step contributes to improved management strategies for postoperative care and hence reduces the overall risk of morbidity.

7.5.2. Neuromuscular Function Assessment

Assessment of neuromuscular function is important in the context of orthopedic and trauma anesthesia, where both the safe use and reversal of neuromuscular blocking agents are of utmost concern and can be an outcome-determining factor. Neuromuscular blocking agents are common in facilitating surgery by relaxing muscles; however, the return of recovery from their action can be complicated. Assessment of the degree of neuromuscular blockade is required to ensure patients are sufficiently recovered prior to extubation. One proven method is via observation of the train-of-four ratio, which compares muscle response to stimulus and informs anesthesiologists when to administer reversal agents. Proper measurement of neuromuscular function can prevent residual muscle weakness and complications like the requirement for long-term respiratory therapy or intensive care unit stay. In recent times, risk from intermediate-acting neuromuscular blocking agents has been of concern, particularly regarding postoperative respiratory complications. Specifically, research has shown that these agents are associated with higher rates of oxygen desaturation and reintubation following surgery. Specifically, the exposure to these agents was linked with an odds ratio of 1.36 for desaturation below 90% after extubation and with an odds ratio of 1.40 for unplanned ICU admission due to respiratory failure. Importantly, qualitative neuromuscular monitoring was found not to have significantly diminished these risks, highlighting the need for strict evaluation protocols in the perioperative period. Understanding of these relationships is key for anesthesiologists to make informed decisions on drug choice and postoperative care. Perioperative management in elderly patients has additional complexities that necessitate careful neuromuscular function assessment. With a rising average age of surgical patients, particularly those for orthopedic procedures, anesthesiologists must face age-associated physiological alterations impacting neuromuscular blockade. Geriatric patients may exhibit altered responses to neuromuscular agents due to alterations such as decreased renal function, causing impairment in drug metabolism, and sensitivity to muscle relaxants. Research has shown that combined evaluation of neuromuscular function in such patients will aid in safety and postoperative outcomes enhancement. Therefore, patient-specific approaches for observing neuromuscular function in elderly patients undergoing surgery, combined with meticulous observation and tailored anesthetic approaches, are needed to minimize risk and overcome the unique challenges of elderly surgical patients, as specific to assessment of neuromuscular function in each phase of the anesthesia process (Grosse-Sundrup et al., 2012; Krishna & Pathak, 2020) (Figure 7.14).

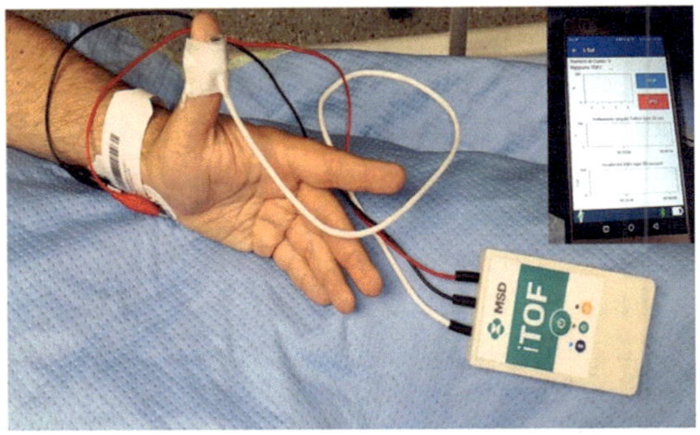

Figure 7.14. The assessment of neuromuscular function.

Source: https://media.springernature.com/full/springer-static/image/art%3A10.1038%2Fs41746-020-00344-w/MediaObjects/41746_2020_344_Fig1_HTML.jpg.

7.5.3. Depth of Anesthesia Monitoring

Depth of anesthesia monitoring is a critical component in patient safety and achieving the optimal surgical results during orthopedic and trauma surgery. Anesthesiologists employ various modalities of monitoring to measure the hypnotic state and physiological effects, preventing too little and too much anesthesia and their ensuing complications. Too little anesthesia can lead to intraoperative awareness, which is distressing to patients and can have unwanted psychological postoperative outcomes. Conversely, excessive anesthesia enhances the risk of hemodynamic instability and respiratory depression. Coupled with advanced monitoring equipment, such as the electroencephalogram bispectral index (BIS), allows anesthesiologists to adjust the degree of hypnosis, within the range of choice BIS 40 to 60, for most operating patients, making anesthesia both safe and effective throughout the procedure. One of the classifying challenges orthopedic and trauma surgeries present is heterogeneity in patient responses to anesthetic medication, particularly in a trauma set. Patients may have pre-existing conditions, e.g., obstructive sleep apnea syndrome (OSAS), such that the normal anesthetic management practice fails to hold. Prevalence of OSAS is especially more frequent among patients undergoing surgery, which heavily raises risks for post-surgical complications, particularly due to anesthesia's impact on the collapsibility of the upper airway. Therefore, depth of anesthesia monitoring not only hinges on routine practice but also has to be personalized in an effort to include every patient's unique health record. Identification of high-risk OSAS patients and complications is important, not only for preoperative optimization but also for anesthesia protocol implementation to enable safer intraoperative management and postoperative outcomes. Following as an expansion of recognition of the cognitive aspects of memory and consciousness in the context of surgery, monitoring depth of anesthesia to prevent cognitive sequelae is increasingly recognized. Studies have demonstrated that ensuring a sufficient hypnosis level can prevent memory from forming throughout surgery. In studies where patients had BIS levels maintained within 40–60, patients showed very little cognitive recall of intraoperative occurrences, providing evidence that proper depth of anesthesia duly protects patients from painful memories. Such a finding is of particular significance in the case of orthopedic and trauma surgery, where psychological and emotional responses to surgical interventions would be the most pronounced. Incorporating such information in clinical practice not only enhances patient outcomes on an individual level but also gives insight into broader strategies of anesthesia management that prioritize overall patient well-being (Kerssens et al., 2001).

Test Your Knowledge

1. Which vital signs are commonly monitored during anesthesia?
2. Why is monitoring the depth of anesthesia important during surgery?

7.6. Postoperative Care

Learning Outcome

1. Pain management strategies
2. Monitoring for complications
3. Transitioning to outpatient care

Postoperative care is a significant process for the general recovery of patients after orthopedic and trauma surgery. Postoperative care management should be executed correctly in this phase to prevent complications and optimize recovery. Venous thromboembolism (VTE) prevention is among the major concerns of postoperative care, as it remains a severe risk among surgical patients. Western Trauma Association (WTA) provides a management algorithm wherein pharmacologic prophylaxis is advised to be started within 24 hours of surgery based on certain risk factors like injury severity score (ISS) and patient history. The advice comes from evidence that the early pharmacologic treatment can significantly reduce the incidence of VTE, thus improving the patient's outcome during a key postoperative period (McCunn et al., 2015). Additionally, proper postoperative monitoring and reevaluation of prophylactic regimens should occur to keep patients on an ideal pathway of care as they transition past the immediate postoperative duration. Also, multimodal analgesia is central to orthopedic and trauma surgery postoperative care. The application of a combination of analgesics like acetaminophen, NSAIDs, and opioids will optimize pain control with minimal opioid consumption and associated side effects. This strategy not only manages acute postoperative pain well but also enables earlier mobilization, which is crucial in recovery and prevention of complications such as pneumonia and VTE. Special care should be taken regarding patients' unique needs, like those with pre-existing diseases that may complicate pain management strategies. The overall assessment of postoperative pain should guide the anesthetic team to modify analgesic strategies so that they are the best current practices grounded in new studies and guidelines (McCunn et al., 2015). Postoperative rehabilitation also restores functional outcomes in orthopedic and trauma patients. The phase consists of therapeutic interventions to support improved mobility, strength, and global physical function. A functional multidisciplinary collaboration among anesthesiologists, surgeons, and rehabilitation specialists is essential in creating individualized goals for rehabilitation, which should be initiated as soon as clinically indicated. Evidence supports the mobilization and formal rehabilitation programs initiated earlier as reducing hospital stay and leading to better long-term outcomes. Patient education regarding the expectation of recovery, potential complications, and adherence to rehabilitation protocols can affect recovery rate and efficacy. Throughout the recovery process, ongoing monitoring and fine-tuning of the rehabilitation process are required to accommodate each patient's unique healing process and enhance overall quality of life during recovery (McCunn et al., 2015) (Figure 7.15).

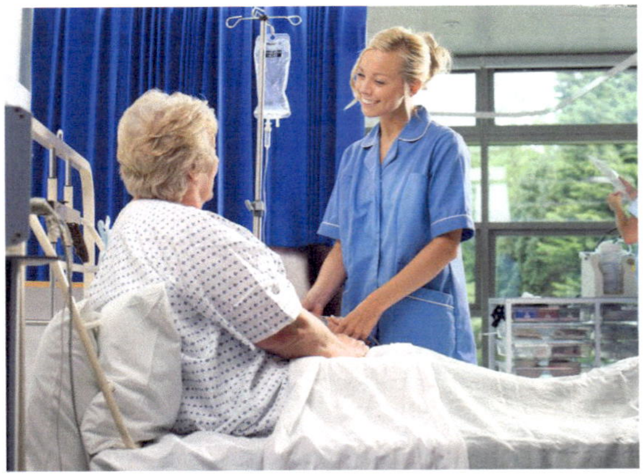

Figure 7.15. Postoperative care plays a pivotal role in the overall recovery process.

Source: https://media.post.rvohealth.io/wp-content/uploads/2020/08/postoperative-care_thumb.jpg.

7.6.1. Pain Management Strategies

Pain management is of prime importance in the specialty of orthopedic and trauma surgery, particularly given the significant variations in patient sensitivity to pain and anesthesia. Multimodal analgesia has emerged as a mainstay for the treatment of postoperative pain, whereby multiple disparate pharmacologic drugs are employed in combination to target diverse pathways of pain. Opioids and NSAIDs may be supplemented with adjuncts such as gabapentinoids or local anesthetics to reduce total opioid consumption and associated side effects. Individualization of pain treatment based on patient factors such as age and comorbidities is the focus of contemporary research. For instance, the old are exposed to certain pain and analgesic drug sensitivities and hence need proper selection of drugs and doses to prevent complications such as postoperative delirium (Urban et al., 2020). Proper utilization of these methods can significantly enhance recovery with decreased patient discomfort from surgical operations. Apart from pharmacologic interventions, regional anesthesia strategies have become fashionable in the effective management of postoperative pain. These methods involve the administration of anesthetic medications to specific groups of nerves and block pain conduction in certain areas with minimal systemic action. Peripheral nerve blocks, for example, may be applied during knee or ankle operations to provide deep analgesia and improve rehabilitation outcomes. Besides, continuous catheter nerve blocks provide a prolonged analgesic effect, allowing early mobilization and reducing the consumption of opioids. By effective pain control with regional modalities, not only is suffering minimized, but also the occurrence of chronic pain developments postoperatively. Pain relief at its peak has been linked with increased recovery times and decreased complication rates of increased immobility, enhancing the effectiveness of surgical procedures overall (Urban et al., 2020). While pharmacologic and regional techniques are integral to postoperative pain management, monitoring and adapting the strategy based on patient reports and clinical acumen is also crucial. Continuous assessment of pain severity, functional mobility, and overall recovery must guide any pain management strategy change. This interactive approach allows clinicians to identify at-risk patients, like those experiencing drug dependency or chronic pain, who may require more specific interventions. Implementing an official protocol for tracking pain outcomes in conjunction with routine assessment can allow clinicians to provide optimal care and improve recovery experiences. In general, adopting complete pain management protocols within the anesthesia model of orthopedic and trauma surgery indicates an observance of optimizing patient comfort and promoting successful surgical procedure outcomes.

7.6.2. Monitoring for Complications

Effective monitoring of complications during anesthesia in orthopedic and trauma surgery is crucial to the maintenance of patient safety and best outcomes. Due to the intrinsic complexities of the procedures, patients can also be carrying pre-existing conditions such as OSAS that significantly predispose them to complications in the postoperative period. To underpin this assertion, evidence indicates that the prevalence of sleep apnea is far greater in the surgical population, with both sedation and anesthesia playing a role in airway collapsibility. It is therefore incumbent upon anesthesiologists to thoroughly screen patients for such risk factors during preoperative evaluations. Failure to identify at-risk individuals may lead to preventable adverse results, making strict intraoperative and postoperative monitoring appropriate. By the implementation of targeted strategies, clinicians can minimize the risk for the complications associated with airway management and sedation in the at-risk group of patients (Vasu et al., 2012). Moreover, the postoperative course necessitates continuous observation for the development of signs of complications arising after anesthesia. One of the major concerns at this point in time is chronic postoperative pain, which has the potential to lead to prolonged opioid use and, consequently, increased risks of adverse effects in the form of dependency. Research finds that several factors lead to this condition, including preoperative opioid use and anxiety disorders. Anesthesiologists must thus be effective in making multimodal analgesia plans that not only reduce opioid use but also optimize overall recovery. Collaborations between anesthesiologists and surgeons in planning postoperative individualized analgesic plans can be instrumental in preventing chronic use of opioids and associated complications. Through careful follow-up on patients' pain status and response to analgesics, healthcare practitioners can intervene promptly, optimizing patient management and healing (Schwenk et al., 2018). In addition to pain and airway control, monitoring for cardiovascular and neurological complications is essential during the perioperative period. Anesthesia itself induces a variety of cardiovascular responses, including hypotension and arrhythmia, particularly in complex orthopedic procedures. Continuous hemodynamic monitoring, along with cautious titration of anesthetic agents, enables clinicians to detect and resolve such issues on time. Moreover, neurological complications, though infrequent, may appear as postoperative nausea and vomiting or changed consciousness and need careful monitoring. The inclusion of advanced monitoring equipment, such as BIS monitors, can provide real-time feedback on the depth of anesthesia and patient responsiveness. Hence, early identification of potential complications makes for a safer operating room and enhances overall quality of anesthesia care in orthopedic and trauma settings, and ultimately results in improved patient outcomes (Figure 7.16).

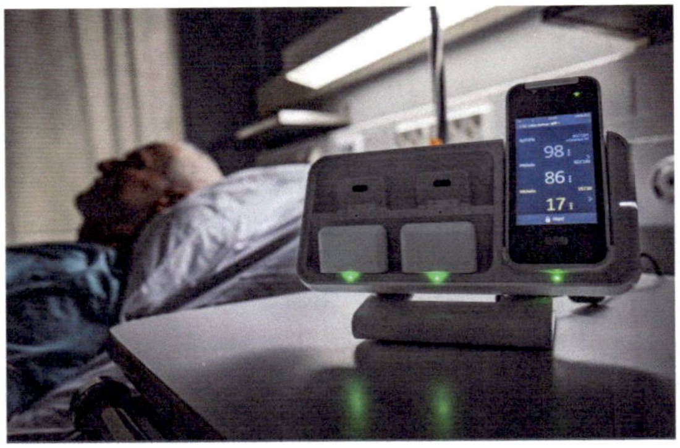

Figure 7.16. The monitoring for complications in anesthesia during orthopedic and trauma surgery.

Source: https://clinicalview.gehealthcare.com/sites/default/files/styles/paragraph_scaled_picture_fallback/public/Syke%2010%20 2020%20Day%201-541.jpg?itok=YC3WDtVn.

7.6.3. Transitioning to Outpatient Care

Transition to outpatient facilities represents a significant shift in orthopedic and trauma surgical anesthesia service delivery. The shift is a sign of the changing healthcare landscape in which providers and consumers alike desire efficiency with improved outcome after surgery. Outpatient care models allow patients to undergo procedures and be discharged home the same day, which is advantageous for patient satisfaction as well as reducing overall costs over inpatient admissions. Success in outpatient anesthesia depends on rigorous preoperative screenings as well as having an intimate familiarity with the individual patient's medical history, including possible comorbidities that present risks under anesthesia. Ensuring that patients are risk-stratified appropriately allows anesthesia practice and postoperative pain control measures to be tailored to meet outpatient needs. Furthermore, postoperative pain control is crucial within the outpatient environment, whereby patients are often discharged several hours postop. To maintain optimal pain control, anesthetic practices such as regional anesthesia or multimodal analgesia are increasingly employed. These methods can lower opioid intake and enhance recovery times, which are in agreement with suggestions of thoroughly established guidelines in pain management (Dowell et al., 2022). Effective pain control not only enhances patient comfort but is also crucial when optimizing orthopedic surgical functional recovery. In this case, the anesthesiologist's clinical experience is particularly pertinent to advise on optimal pain control measures for an uneventful postoperative period and resumption of activities. Of particular importance in the shift to outpatient facilities is an emphasis on patient education and follow-up protocols. Practitioners should make sure that patients acquire and understand their postoperative instructions, including recognition of signs of complications and medication use. Post-discharge follow-up has also been found to have a significant impact on patient outcome, serving as an important safety net for picking up early signs of possible complications (Makita et al., 2022). In addition, the availability of telehealth solutions can enable ongoing monitoring and support, in effect bridging the gap between discharge and traditional postoperative follow-up. This new outpatient care model not only guarantees patient safety but also promotes collaboration between clinicians and patients, ultimately leading to higher post-surgical compliance and quality of life among recovery patients of orthopedic and trauma surgery.

Test Your Knowledge

1. What is the main goal of postoperative care after surgery?
2. Why is effective pain management important for patient recovery?

Summary

The investigation of anesthesia in trauma and orthopedic surgery has shown that an array of options is needed to provide optimal care for patients. The deployment of regional anesthesia methods, in combination with general anesthesia, has been useful in pain management during and after orthopedic surgeries. Regional blocks may decrease opioid use, thus preventing the side effects of excessive opioid intake. This is very relevant in the case of the modern opioid crisis, since it speaks to an immediate need for new modalities of analgesia. Furthermore, the evolution of modalities and equipment, such as advancements in ultrasound-guided regional anesthesia, provides more precise and effective alleviation of pain, resulting in improved overall outcomes for orthopedic patients (Vaglio et al., 2016). The function of ketamine as an adjuvant in orthopedic and trauma surgery for acute and chronic pain cannot be denied. This versatile anesthetic has been shown to provide significant analgesic benefits, especially in high-risk patients, like those tolerant to opioids. For trauma surgery, when pain levels are severe, ketamine offers a unique dissociative state that can be used to break acute pain without the overall depressant effects of traditional opioids (Sarıcaoğlu, 2019). Its utility for decreasing postoperative pain and preventing chronic pain syndromes only further establishes its role in contemporary surgical practice. As the trend in pain management continues to shift, the administration of ketamine will also keep increasing, and further studies on more optimal dosing schedules and its long-term effects on patients are warranted. Finally, the interplay between new anesthetic techniques and medications, such as regional anesthesia and ketamine, is a significant development in orthopedic and trauma surgery. This approach not only maximizes pain management and reduces opioid dependence but also paves the way for enhanced patient recovery and satisfaction. Continued study and education in anesthetic technique will be critical to adapting to changing surgical patient demands. As the practitioners fine-tune their skills in managing pain complexities, the future of anesthetics in trauma and orthopedic surgery is highly promising with the potential for better patient outcomes and a dramatic reduction in the complications arising from inadequate pain control (Vaglio et al., 2016; Sarıcaoğlu, 2019).

The application of anesthesia to trauma and orthopedic operations must be clearly understood in terms of procedural efficacy as well as patient safety. One of the most critical areas is managing venous thromboembolism (VTE), which is a risk factor for surgery patients. Current evidence indicates a need for the application of effective prophylaxis and treatment interventions to decrease the risk. Specifically, American Society of Clinical Oncology (ASCO) guidelines suggest that clinicians should offer thromboprophylaxis to some patients with a high risk of cancer, advocating for medications such as low-molecular-weight heparin (LMWH) and direct oral anticoagulants (DOACs) such as rivaroxaban and edoxaban. Individualized practice not only enhances patient outcomes but also highlights the significance of individualized treatment in anesthesia practice (Nelson et al., 2019). Outside of VTE care, neuroinflammatory reaction to anesthesia and surgery is an emerging issue. Recent evidence indicates that neuroinflammation plays a central role in postoperative neurocognitive dysfunction, such as delirium and cognitive impairment. These complications can be dangerous to the healing process, particularly in the elderly or those with pre-existing cognitive impairment. The recent discovery puts into perspective inflammatory processes and the well-being of neurons and hypothesizes that understanding such processes is crucial for anesthesiologists interested in enhancing patient safety and outcomes after surgery. Management of neuroinflammation can pave the way for new ways of tailoring perioperative care to minimize surgical intervention's cognitive side effects (Subramaniyan & Terrando, 2019). Further, the implementation of multidisciplinary approaches to anesthesia in trauma and orthopedic surgery is important in improving the overall patient care experience. There should be synergy between the surgeons, the anesthesiologists, and the nursing staff that facilitates better coordination and implementation of the perioperative processes. The integrated process not only considers the technical aspects of anesthesia administration but also instills in the practicing clinicians a culture of constant assessment and modification of each patient's unique needs. Patient involvement in preoperative counseling about the potential risks and benefits of anesthesia also empowers patients and their care experience overall. Thus, an integrated approach that combines advanced anesthetic techniques with prudent risk assessment and efficient multidisciplinary planning can significantly enhance the overall quality of care in orthopedic and trauma surgery.

KEY TERMS FROM THIS CHAPTER

- Anesthetic approach
- Anesthetic modalities
- Certain demographics
- Demand rapid anesthetic
- Obstructive sleep apnea syndrome (OSAS)
- Opioid analgesics
- Orthopedic
- Orthopedic patients
- Orthopedic trauma
- Pain management strategies
- Patient health
- Postoperative delirium (POD)
- Total hip arthroplasty (THA)
- Total knee arthroplasty (TKA)
- Trauma surgery

Critical Thinking Questions

1. **Which nerve block is most commonly used for knee surgeries?**
   a. Axillary block
   b. Femoral nerve block
   c. Interscalene block
   d. Sciatic nerve block
2. **What is the most significant anesthetic consideration in patients with long bone fractures?**
   a. Hemodynamic stability
   b. Airway management
   c. Pulmonary embolism risk
   d. Hypothermia
3. **In trauma patients, the "lethal triad" includes all of the following EXCEPT:**
   a. Hypothermia
   b. Acidosis
   c. Hyperkalemia
   d. Coagulopathy
4. **What is the ideal anesthetic approach for a patient undergoing total hip arthroplasty?**
   a. General anesthesia only
   b. Regional anesthesia only
   c. Combined spinal-epidural anesthesia
   d. Total intravenous anesthesia (TIVA)
5. **Which of the following is a common complication of prolonged use of a pneumatic tourniquet?**
   a. Nerve injury
   b. Hypertension
   c. Hypovolemia
   d. Bradycardia

Short Answer Questions

1. What are the unique challenges of providing anesthesia for patients with multiple traumatic injuries?
2. How does the use of regional anesthesia benefit patients undergoing orthopedic procedures compared to general anesthesia?
3. Describe the anesthetic considerations for patients with significant blood loss during major orthopedic surgery.
4. What are the risks associated with using tourniquets during orthopedic surgeries, and how can they be mitigated?
5. How does the presence of cervical spine instability alter the anesthetic approach in patients with trauma?

Answer to Critical Thinking Questions

1. (b); 2. (c); 3. (c); 4. (c); 5. (a)

References

1. Vaglio, S., Prisco, D., Biancofiore, G., Rafanelli, D., Antonioli, P., Lisanti, M., Andreani, L., Basso, L., Velati, C., Grazzini, G., & Liumbruno, G. M. (2016). Recommendations for the implementation of a Patient Blood Management programme. Application to elective major orthopaedic surgery in adults. *Blood transfusion = Trasfusione del sangue, 14*(1), 23–65. https://doi.org/10.2450/2015.0172-15 (accessed on 28th June 2025).
2. Aygören-Pürsün, E., Klingebiel, T., Kreuz, W., Martinez Saguer, I., et al. (2013). Risk of angioedema following invasive or surgical procedures in HAE type I and II: The natural history. https://core.ac.uk/download/17179827.pdf (accessed on 28th June 2025).
3. White, K. K., Jester, A., Bache, C. E., Harmatz, P. R., Shediac, R., Thacker, M. M., & Mackenzie, W. G. (2014). Orthopedic management of the extremities in patients with Morquio A syndrome. *Journal of children's orthopaedics, 8*(4), 295–304. https://doi.org/10.1007/s11832-014-0601-4(accessed on 28th June 2025).
4. Grosse-Sundrup, M., Henneman, J. P., Sandberg, W. S., Bateman, B. T., Uribe, J. V., Nguyen, N. T., Ehrenfeld, J. M., Martinez, E. A., Kurth, T., & Eikermann, M. (2012). Intermediate acting non-depolarizing neuromuscular blocking agents and risk of postoperative respiratory complications: prospective propensity score matched cohort study. *BMJ (Clinical research ed.), 345*, e6329. https://doi.org/10.1136/bmj.e6329(accessed on 28th June 2025).
5. Kerssens, C., Klein, J., van der Woerd, A., & Bonke, B. (2001). Auditory information processing during adequate propofol anesthesia monitored by electroencephalogram bispectral index. *Anesthesia and analgesia, 92*(5), 1210–1214. https://doi.org/10.1097/00000539-200105000-00024 (accessed on 28th June 2025).
6. Gjeltema, J., De Voe, R. S., Minter, L. J., & Trumpatori, B. J. (2017). Intertarsal Joint Stabilization in a Bateleur Eagle *(Terathopius ecaudatus)* Using a Novel Application of a Braided Suture and Titanium Button System. *Case reports in veterinary medicine, 2017*, 7373242. https://doi.org/10.1155/2017/7373242(accessed on 28th June 2025).
7. DiLoreto, M. (2023). Benefits of ketamine versus propofol in acute traumatic brain injuries with elevated intracranial pressure. https://core.ac.uk/download/572705251.pdf (accessed on 28th June 2025).
8. Vasu, T. S., Grewal, R., & Doghramji, K. (2012). Obstructive sleep apnea syndrome and perioperative complications: a systematic review of the literature. *Journal of clinical sleep medicine : JCSM : official publication of the American Academy of Sleep Medicine, 8*(2), 199–207. https://doi.org/10.5664/jcsm.1784(accessed on 28th June 2025).
9. Dowell, D., Ragan, K., Jones, C. M., Baldwin, G., & Chou, R. (2022). CDC clinical practice guideline for prescribing opioids for pain—United States, 2022. *MMWR Recommendations and Reports, 71*, 1–95. https://doi.org/10.15585/mmwr.rr7103a1 (accessed on 28th June 2025).
10. Ford, N. P., Chu, K. M., & Trelles, M. (2011). Providing surgical care in Somalia: A model of task shifting. https://core.ac.uk/download/pdf/41160575.pdf (accessed on 28th June 2025).
11. Wu JJ, Lollo L, Grabinsky A. Regional anesthesia in trauma medicine. *Anesthesiol Res Pract.* 2011;2011:713281. doi:10.1155/2011/713281(accessed on 28th June 2025).
12. James, M. A., Manske, M. C. B., Rios Roque, J. J., Zelaya, C., et al. (2017). Pediatric hand

surgery training in Nicaragua: A sustainable model of surgical education in a resource-poor environment. https://core.ac.uk/download/323069430.pdf (accessed on 28th June 2025).

13. McKune, C. M., Pascoe, P. J., Lascelles, B. D., & Kass, P. H. (2014). The challenge of evaluating pain and a pre-incisional local anesthetic block. *PeerJ*, *2*, e341. https://doi.org/10.7717/peerj.341(accessed on 28th June 2025).

14. Kelly, J. R., Levy, M., Reyes, J., & Anders, J. (2020). Effectiveness of the combat application tourniquet for arterial occlusion in young children. *Journal of Trauma and Acute Care Surgery, 88*, 644–647. https://www.semanticscholar.org/paper/c7c15e0978b22fb81570883d77ea09f43cb32267 (accessed on 28th June 2025).

15. Key, N. S., Khorana, A. A., Kuderer, N. M., Bohlke, K., Lee, A. Y. Y., Arcelus, J. I., Wong, S. L., et al. (2019). Venous thromboembolism prophylaxis and treatment in patients with cancer: ASCO clinical practice guideline update. *Journal of Clinical Oncology, 38*, 496–520. https://doi.org/10.1200/jco.19.01461 (accessed on 28th June 2025).

16. Krishna, B., & Pathak, N. (2020). Perioperative management of geriatric patients for orthopedic surgeries. *International Journal of Research in Orthopaedics*, *6*(2), 427–434. https://doi.org/10.18203/issn.2455-4510.IntJResOrthop20200749(accessed on 28th June 2025).

17. Ley, E. J., Brown, C. V. R., Moore, E. E., Sava, J., Peck, K. A., Ciesla, D. J., Sperry, J. L., et al. (2020). Updated guidelines to reduce venous thromboembolism in trauma patients: A Western Trauma Association critical decisions algorithm. *Journal of Trauma and Acute Care Surgery, 89*, 971–981. https://doi.org/10.1097/ta.0000000000002830 (accessed on 28th June 2025).

18. Lorenz, W., & Rothmund, M. (1989). Theoretical surgery: A new specialty in operative medicine. https://core.ac.uk/download/11550720.pdf (accessed on 28th June 2025).

19. Urban, M. K., Sasaki, M., Schmucker, A. M., & Magid, S. K. (2020). Postoperative delirium after major orthopedic surgery. *World journal of orthopedics*, *11*(2), 90–106. https://doi.org/10.5312/wjo.v11.i2.90(accessed on 28th June 2025).

20. Makita, S., Yasu, T., Akashi, Y. J., Adachi, H., Izawa, H., Ishihara, S., Iso, Y., et al. (2022). JCS/JACR 2021 guideline on rehabilitation in patients with cardiovascular disease. *Circulation Journal, 87*, 155–235. https://doi.org/10.1253/circj.cj-22-0234 (accessed on 28th June 2025).

21. Schwenk, E. S., & Mariano, E. R. (2018). Designing the ideal perioperative pain management plan starts with multimodal analgesia. *Korean journal of anesthesiology*, *71*(5), 345–352. https://doi.org/10.4097/kja.d.18.00217(accessed on 28th June 2025).

22. McCunn, M., Dutton, R. P., Dagal, A., Varon, A. J., Kaslow, O., Kucik, C., Hagberg, C. A., et al. (2015). Trauma, critical care, and emergency care anesthesiology. *Anesthesia & Analgesia, 121*, 1668–1673. https://doi.org/10.1213/ane.0000000000000782 (accessed on 28th June 2025).

23. Van Vynckt, D., Mosselmans, L., Samoy, Y., Van Ryssen, B., et al. (2012). The use of intra-articular anesthesia as a diagnostic tool in canine lameness. https://core.ac.uk/download/55711601.pdf (accessed on 28th June 2025).

24. Mudia, K. A. M., Oktaliansah, E., & Prajitno, I. P. (2016). Anesthesia technique selection pattern in patients undergoing lower extremities surgery at Dr. Hasan Sadikin General Hospital from January–June 2013. https://core.ac.uk/download/296616469.pdf (accessed on 28th June 2025).

25. Rosseel, P., Trelles, M., Guilavogui, S., Ford, N., & Chu, K. (2010). Ten years of experience training non-physician anesthesia providers in Haiti. *World journal of surgery*, *34*(3), 453–458. https://doi.org/10.1007/s00268-009-0192-2(accessed on 28th June 2025).

26. Schwenk, E. S., Pozek, J. J., & Viscusi, E. R. (2018). Managing Prolonged Pain After Surgery: Examining the Role of Opioids. *The Journal of arthroplasty*, *33*(11), 3389–3393. https://doi.org/10.1016/j.arth.2018.08.005 (accessed on 28th June 2025).

27. Sarıcaoğlu, F. (2019). ESRA19-0256 Ketamine for pain: Complications and best practice. *Regional Anesthesia & Pain Medicine, 44*, A52–A53. https://www.semanticscholar.org/paper/de09c4a5ce328386f2efdb34f0e1acfb8a3b9494 (accessed on 28th June 2025).

28. Subramaniyan, S., & Terrando, N. (2019). Neuroinflammation and perioperative neurocognitive disorders. *Anesthesia & Analgesia, 128*, 781–788. https://doi.org/10.1213/ane.0000000000004053 (accessed on 28th June 2025).

29. Department of Anesthesia. University of Iowa. Spring 2011. https://core.ac.uk/download/18608347.pdf

30. Waller, P. G. (2012). Surgical delay for hip fracture clients and the use of clopidogrel: An integrative review. https://core.ac.uk/download/58824498.pdf (accessed on 28th June 2025).

31. Wang, A., Lv, G., Cheng, X., Ma, X., Wang, W., Gui, J., Hu, J., et al. (2020). Guidelines on multidisciplinary approaches for the prevention and management of diabetic foot disease (2020 edition). *Burns & Trauma, 8.* https://doi.org/10.1093/burnst/tkaa017 (accessed on 28th June 2025).

ANESTHESIA IN LIVER AND GASTROINTESTINAL SURGERY

8

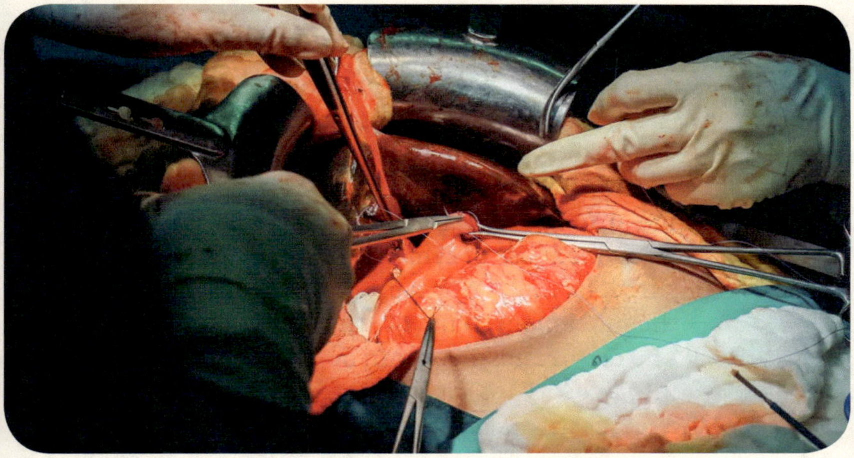

Introduction

In modern medicine, the administration of anesthesia for liver and gastrointestinal surgery is a key factor in ensuring patient comfort and safety. Such high-tech operations often involve fragile anatomical structures, so the demand for precise anesthetic control to counter hemodynamic instability and postoperative morbidity hazards becomes essential. The liver, with its intimate involvement in drug metabolism and detoxification, presents a unique anesthesiologic challenge, particularly in patients with pre-existing liver disease. Sound anesthesia strategies not only enhance the success of surgery but also significantly reduce the rate of postoperative complications, including infection and prolonged recovery times. The intricate relationship between anesthetic agents and liver function warrants patient-specific anesthetic protocols that are formulated on the basis of surgical considerations and the condition of the patient health. In addition, recent advances in anesthetic practices and monitoring devices have enhanced the anesthetic management strategy in liver and gastrointestinal operations.

LEARNING OBJECTIVES

After studying this chapter, you will be able to:

1. Explain the hepatic function and drug metabolism
2. Discuss the anesthesia for hepatic resection
3. Know anesthesia for liver transplantation
4. Focus on gastrointestinal surgery: laparoscopic vs. Open techniques
5. Understand fluid management in gastrointestinal surgery
6. Describe the coagulopathy and anesthesia

Innovations such as regional anesthesia and ERAS pathways have been found effective in the minimization of side effects of opioid therapy with continued optimal pain control. A comprehension of the effect of varying hepatic function on the pharmacokinetics and dynamics of anesthetics is required to provide patients with appropriately dosed anesthetic drugs for their liver function status. Furthermore, careful monitoring of hemodynamic stability, especially in high-risk patients, is of vital importance. The collaboration of anesthesiologists, surgeons, and other healthcare team members creates a holistic approach to patient care based on collaborative decision-making, based on the patient's individual circumstance.

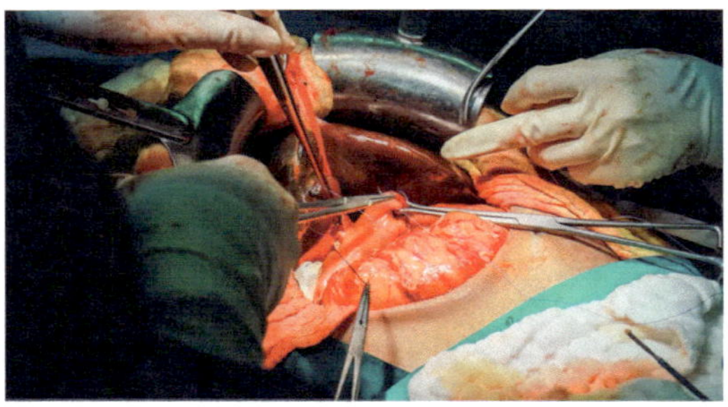

Figure 8.1. The administration of anesthesia during liver and gastrointestinal surgery.

Source: https://i0.wp.com/anaesthesianews.wordpress.com/wp-content/uploads/2023/06/liver_transplant2.webp?fit=1200%2C675&ssl=1.

The value of multidisciplinary collaboration extends beyond the planning of procedures; it is critical to the ongoing monitoring of postoperative outcomes in liver and GI surgery. Evidence-based analyses of complications involving anesthesia guide clinical practice, determining best practices while highlighting areas for further study and innovation. Research emphasizes the requirement for continuous professional education among anesthesiologists to maintain pace with evidence-based best practice. As surgical technique progresses and populations of patients change to encompass an older population with the concomitant presence of complex comorbidities, the anesthetic practice in such cases becomes increasingly sophisticated and critical. Paying attention to the nuances of anesthesia during liver and gastrointestinal procedures ultimately leads to improved patient outcomes, affecting not only short-term surgical results but also far-off trajectories of health (Hilscher et al., 2022; Lee et al., 2023) (Figure 8.1).

Definition of Anesthesia

Anesthesia in liver and gastrointestinal surgery is a crucial component that facilitates surgical operations by ensuring patient safety and comfort. Essentially, anesthesia consists of the provision of drugs for the induction of a controlled loss of sensation or awareness so that surgeons can perform operations without risking the movement, pain, or distress of the patients. The use of anesthesia can be broadly categorized into a few types, i.e., general, regional, and local anesthesia, each appropriate for specific surgery requirements and patient conditions. In complex surgeries, such as those for treating liver disease, a good understanding of anesthesia is crucial as such patients have certain physiological complications that need to be addressed with intensive anesthetic management. One such significant factor in gastrointestinal and liver surgery is the prevalence of comorbidities associated with malnutrition, recognized as a key predictive factor for surgical complications. Recent literature has highlighted the relationship between malnutrition and complications from surgery, with studies indicating that patients with malnutrition have higher rates of major complications (Skeie et al., 2019). This link highlights the role of anesthesia practitioners in assessing not only the surgical requirements of the patients but also their nutritional status and overall health before the surgery. Understanding these aspects, an anesthetic strategy can be devised to combat potential complications arising from malnutrition with the ultimate aim of enhancing recovery and curtailing mortality among high-risk groups. Also, advancements in anesthetic techniques and monitoring equipment have significantly improved safety outcomes in dangerous operations in the liver and gastrointestinal tract. Procedures such as transjugular intrahepatic portosystemic shunt (TIPS) require a multidisciplinary approach among anesthesiologists, interventional radiologists, and hepatologists to ensure optimal management of such complicated procedures in critical care (Boike et al., 2021). Thus, the function of anesthesia extends beyond the administration of sedation and analgesia; it involves an interprofessional collaboration to tailor anesthetic plans according to the complex interplay of several medical conditions to achieve better patient outcomes and minimize surgical risk. This holistic concept of anesthesia is essential in achieving optimal success in the extremely demanding field of liver and gastrointestinal surgery (Figure 8.2).

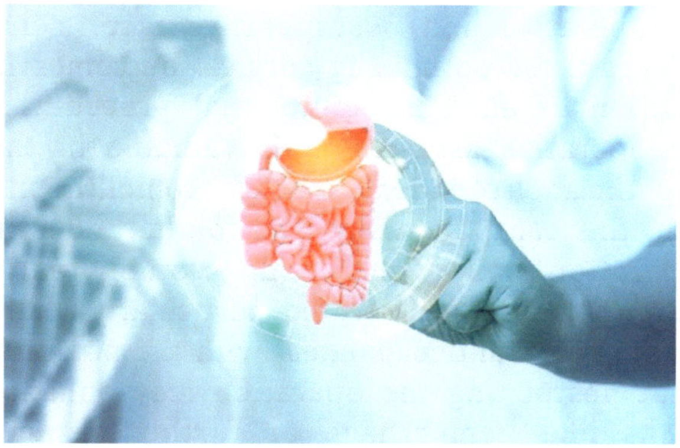

Figure 8.2. The context of liver and gastrointestinal surgery.

Source: https://genesis-hospital.com/wp-content/uploads/2024/03/Gastrointestinal-Surgery1.jpg.

Importance of Anesthesia in Surgical Procedures

In gastrointestinal and liver surgery, smooth anesthesia administration is essential for patient safety and procedural success. Anesthesia is not only pain-relieving but also ensures a quiet working atmosphere that enhances the concentration of the surgical team on complex operating procedures. The anesthetics are tailored to respond to the specific needs of surgical patients, especially those who undergo procedures like laparoscopic anti-reflux surgery or hiatal hernia repair, in which precise measurement of the esophageal hiatus surface area is vital for planning intervention. Techniques like the recently evolved multiplanar multislice computer tomography (MDCT) scan allow for closer inspection of the operative field, and the anesthetic plan is additionally streamlined consequent to it. This versatility underscores the importance of adopting an appropriate anesthetic strategy in minimizing surgery-related stress as well as enhancing postoperative recovery (25th International Congress of the European Association for Endoscopic Surgery (EAES) Frankfurt, 2017).

Moreover, the influence of uncontrolled pain and poor anesthesia during liver and gastrointestinal surgery can significantly affect recovery pathways. Poorly managed pain has been associated with numerous complications, including prolonged hospital stay, impaired gastrointestinal motility, and increased morbidity due to stress response. Not only does anesthesia induce analgesia, but it also plays an important role in hemodynamic stability, particularly in patients with comorbid conditions and autonomic dysfunction due to spinal cord injury. Evidence confirms that arterial hypotension is capable of causing mesenteric dilation in areas with decreased blood flow, hence exacerbating postoperative gastrointestinal disturbances (Besecker et al., 2016). Thus, anesthesia's complete value goes beyond its direct effect, affecting long-term recovery and quality of life after surgery for patients. Additionally, improvements in techniques in anesthesia have significantly enhanced surgical precision and patient outcomes in hepatic and gastrointestinal surgery. The use of advanced monitoring technology and the improvement of multimodal analgesia methods help to minimize risks related to anesthesia. Such breakthroughs allow for the customization of anesthetic plans to the specific health history and procedure difficulty of a given patient. For instance, combining regional anesthetic techniques with general anesthesia can lead to improved postoperative outcomes, such as lower opioid consumption and quicker gastrointestinal recovery. These combined approaches point toward the importance of collaboration between surgical and anesthetic personnel through open communication that eventually benefits the patient and the patient's pain control. The strategic application of anesthesia during liver and gastrointestinal surgery is an indispensable aspect not just of patient ease but also of the overall success of surgical interventions.

Overview of Liver and Gastrointestinal Surgeries

In regard to liver and gastrointestinal surgery, these operations' heterogeneity and intricacy must be underscored, as they often entail therapy of severe digestive tract conditions. Operations on the liver, including tumor resection, liver transplant, and therapy of hepatic trauma, require great levels of operating proficiency owing to the complexity of the organ's anatomy and critical metabolic processes. For instance, hepatic resections carry critical risks in that abnormal bleeding and the reinstitution of hepatic blood flow can compromise liver viability. Gastrointestinal procedures, such as those related to the stomach, intestine, and pancreas, are also complex, often calling for meticulous surgical techniques to evade complications and maintain recovery. Both operations involve much planning and an individually tailored approach, considering the overall health of a patient and individual comorbidities. Anesthesia is an essential element in liver and gastrointestinal surgery, having a fundamental role in intraoperative conditions as well as postoperative outcomes. Anesthesia care for these operations commonly relies on a complicated understanding of the specialist physiological responses involved in liver integrity and the gastrointestinal tract. Anesthesiologists must balance the demands for efficient analgesia and sedation against the risks of interfering with liver metabolism and hemodynamic stability. The perioperative time puts the patient at risk of various factors, including alterations in blood flow, oxygenation, and the liver's metabolic profile, all of which are quite crucial in determining the success or failure of surgery. Pharmacological management of anesthetics therefore, must be modified according to the patient's liver function, particularly in preventing postoperative liver dysfunction, a critical factor in this group of surgery (Talebi et al., 2017). Furthermore, preoperative and postoperative factors are essential for optimizing surgical outcomes in both liver and gastrointestinal procedures. Preoperative assessment is valuable in the identification of patients at risk for complications, and this can potentially lead to alterations in operation timing and mode. Notably, early surgery has been advocated, particularly where patients are anticoagulated, with the potential that postponing the operation may enhance risks like hemorrhage or further hepatic impairment (Waller, 2012). Postoperatively, adequate pain relief and observation of liver function become critical, since interruption of blood supply and overall metabolism may lead to morbidity. Proper care during these times can enhance recovery and reduce complications and thereby emphasizing the importance of surgical techniques and anesthetic intervention in achieving optimal surgical results (Figure 8.3).

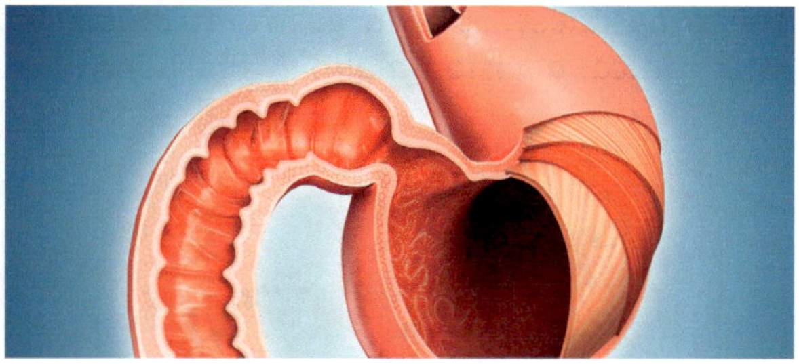

Figure 8.3. When examining liver and gastrointestinal surgeries.

Source: https://s3-us-west-2.amazonaws.com/utsw-patientcare-web-production/original_images/general-gastrointestinal-surgery-1600x732.jpg.

8.1. Hepatic Function and Drug Metabolism

Learning Outcome

1. Role of the liver in drug metabolism
2. Impact of liver function on anesthetic agents
3. Considerations for patients with liver disease

The liver has a central role to play in the metabolism of drugs, significantly impacting pharmacokinetics and pharmacodynamics, particularly in patients who are being administered anesthesia for surgery of the liver and gastrointestinal tract. Liver function is important for the biotransformation of drugs, whereby phase I reactions, viz., oxidation, hydrolysis, and reduction, followed by phase II conjugation reactions, occur. In anesthesia, the ability of the liver to metabolize anesthetic agents may be significantly influenced by underlying liver disease, such as cirrhosis or hepatitis. Thus, drug choice and dosage in patients with compromised liver function are important, since alterations in drug metabolism may result in increased sensitivity or delayed action. Thus, anesthesiologists must evaluate hepatic function before surgery because it is important in determining outcomes for the patient and creating anesthetic regimens that minimize complications during and after liver surgery. Additionally, new advancements concerning enhanced recovery after surgery (ERAS) protocols emphasize the importance of optimizing hepatic function in the treatment of patients undergoing liver surgery during the perioperative period. These guidelines propose implementing prehabilitation protocols, such as smoking and alcohol abstinence before surgery to enhance hepatic function and recovery. Consensus guidelines derived from comprehensive literature reviews indicate that preoperative treatment can lead to reduced rates of complications and enhanced drug metabolism, which has direct implications for anesthetic management approaches. A methodical anesthesia administration strategy is encouraged by recovery protocols emphasizing the function of the liver in the elimination of drugs. Implementing such evidence-based guidelines can significantly benefit patients with standardization of care and prevention of perioperatively and postoperatively occurring adverse drug reactions, particularly for patients with chronic liver disease, as outlined in the latest ERAS guidelines (Gaëtan-Joliat et al., 2022). Finally, the association between liver function and drug metabolism is also not exclusive to anesthetic agents but extends to analgesics and adjunctive drugs utilized both during and following surgery. The enzyme-driven processes within the liver are responsible for metabolizing a wide variety of drugs, and an insufficiency in their functioning can lead to toxic accumulation, particularly in drugs with narrow therapeutic windows. This requires a precise understanding of the pharmacokinetics of drugs commonly employed in patients with liver dysfunction to direct dosing regimens safely. Furthermore, progress in studies of drug metabolism genetics is defining variation in drug response among patients and, in the future, will impact anesthetic care. With advances in the specialty, regular updates of pharmacological guidelines will be essential to the care of patients receiving anesthetics in gastrointestinal and liver surgery, so that current emerging evidence informs clinical decision-making (Pierpont et al., 2018) (Figure 8.4).

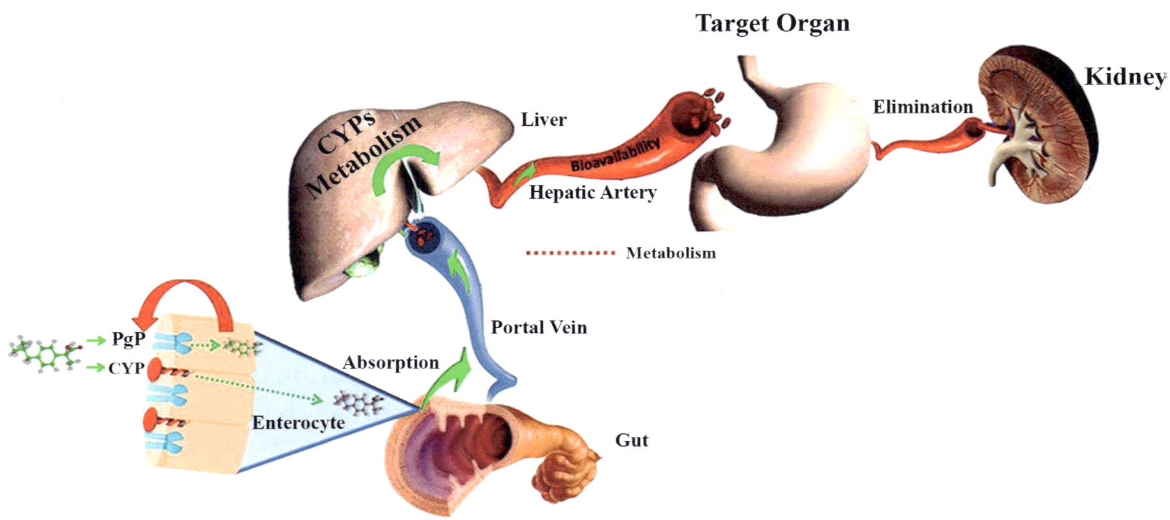

Figure 8.4. Hepatic function and drug metabolism.

Source: https://www.researchgate.net/profile/Rafael-Leon-Cachon/publication/233890192/figure/fig1/AS:421578522533888@1477523560036/Drug-metabolism-After-administration-drugs-1-Interact-and-are-absorbed-by.png.

8.1.1. Role of the Liver in Drug Metabolism

The liver plays a vital role in drug metabolism as the primary organ for the biotransformation of drugs and endogenous substances. The organ uses complex enzymatic processes, mostly through the cytochrome P450 enzyme system, to break down lipophilic chemicals into hydrophilic forms to be eliminated. The effectiveness of the liver in drug metabolism is essential in patients who receive anesthesia for liver and gastrointestinal surgeries. Individual differences in metabolic function, determined by genetic polymorphisms, age, and concomitant drugs, can have a wide influence on the way anesthetic drugs are metabolized. Awareness of these determinants is critical for anesthesiologists when they individualize anesthetic care to maximize effectiveness and avoid potentially harmful reactions, hence promoting patient security during operative procedures that tend to stress the liver's metabolic capacity (Lee et al., 2023). Also, liver function would be considerably impaired in patients with pre-existing liver disease, making drug metabolism a serious issue. Liver diseases such as cirrhosis or hepatitis reduce hepatic blood flow as well as enzyme activity, leading to a shift in the pharmacokinetics of anesthetic drugs. In such patients, the risk is higher for prolonged sedation, increased toxicity, and reduced analgesia, and therefore it is critical for clinicians to closely monitor drug levels and vary dosages accordingly. The relationship between anesthetic drug pharmacodynamics and preoperative liver function underscores the significance of judicious assessment before surgery. The anesthesiologists must remain attuned to the patient's liver status to alter anesthetic plans accordingly and thereby prevent complications from impaired drug metabolism in liver and intestinal surgery (Guo et al., 2022). Moreover, the aging population introduces new challenges to liver metabolism during perioperative times. With advancing age, physiological alterations such as a reduced liver size, reduced blood flow, and altered enzyme expression further retard drug metabolism. These alterations make patients susceptible to the buildup of anesthetic drugs as well as postoperative complications. Prevalence of comorbid conditions, i.e., cardiovascular and metabolic diseases, may also interfere with hepatic metabolism, and therefore deliberate thought in anesthetic management is all the more necessary. Pain relief, sedation, and safety need to be balanced by anesthesiologists in keeping with both the liver's metabolic capacity and the particular challenges of a population aging. Through the implementation of a patient-centered approach, clinicians can optimize outcomes and minimize possible harmful effects related to compromised liver function during anesthesia in operating rooms (Lee et al., 2023).

8.1.2. Impact of Liver Function on Anesthetic Agents

The liver metabolizes anesthetic agents and influences their pharmacokinetics in the surgical patient. Pathophysiologic liver dysfunction can significantly alter the pharmacokinetics and pharmacodynamics of most anesthetics, rendering dosage needs varied and complications likely. Anesthetic agents will exhibit varying rates of hepatic metabolism, which means that patients with impaired liver function will most likely experience extended drug effects and recovery from anesthesia. For instance, reduced liver blood supply and enzymatic activity can inhibit the elimination of such drugs, resulting in heightened sensitivity and susceptibility to side effects during recovery following surgery. Thus, knowledge of the interaction between liver function and anesthetic metabolism is essential for safe anesthetic management in hepatic dysfunction patients. Liver function testing is not only valuable in the choice of anesthetic drugs but also in intraoperative hemodynamic monitoring. Compromised patients generally have coagulopathy and an altered pharmacologic response and therefore, require careful drug selection with minimal liver metabolism and trustworthy results. Agents like remimazolam have been created for their rapid onset and short half-life of action, which makes them the perfect choice for patients with hepatic dysfunction as they are less liver metabolism-dependent than the previous agents. Additionally, the postoperative implications of liver dysfunction cannot be overstated, with patients prone to experiencing setbacks like hepatic encephalopathy and coagulopathy, which hamper recovery protocols.

The integration of liver function testing into anesthetic planning can therefore optimize patient results for gastrointestinal procedures. Preoperative anxiety management also has implications in terms of liver function disorders since the stress response can actually exacerbate hepatic disease. Studies have proven that preoperative administration of anxiolytic medications such as estazolam and remimazolam can reduce anxiety, which subsequently will improve postoperative recovery metrics such as gastrointestinal function and overall patient satisfaction. For patients who are having gastrointestinal surgeries, the provision of good-quality anxiolysis can be especially helpful in augmenting psychological preparedness and physical recovery upon recovery from anesthesia. While the choice of anesthetic regimen must take into account hepatic function, it is also important to adopt anesthetics that enhance recovery parameters, which ultimately leads to a more uneventful postoperative course in patients with varying degrees of liver dysfunction (Dandemmanavar et al., 2025; Mao et al., 2025) (Figure 8.5).

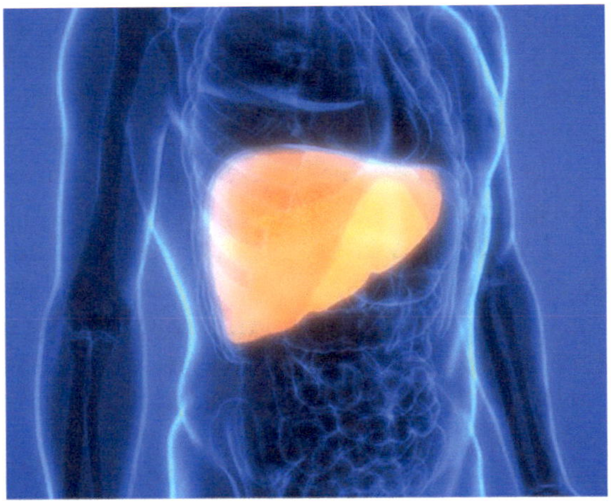

Figure 8.5. The liver plays a crucial role in the metabolism of anesthetic agents.

Source: https://draxe.com/wp-content/uploads/2017/06/LiverFunctionHeader.jpg.

8.1.3. Considerations for Patients with Liver Disease

Liver disease requires a careful approach to anesthesia management due to the vast array of physiological changes that occur in this patient population. Liver disease can significantly influence both pharmacokinetic and pharmacodynamic drug characteristics of anesthetics, perpetuating an increased risk of adverse effects during surgery. For instance, impaired hepatic metabolism can lead to delayed clearance of drugs and consequent drug buildup and enhanced effects of anesthetics that lead to hemodynamic instability or respiratory depression.

Hence, anesthesiologists must adjust their medication dosage based on the patient's status of possessing a healthy liver, frequently requiring the use of other agents less hepatic-dependent in their metabolism, thus highlighting the requirement for a personalized anesthetic approach in such a unique patient population (Besecker et al., 2016). In addition, anesthesia techniques are dictated by the patient's status of liver disease, say between regional and general anesthesia. Severely ill patients with liver disease most commonly have coagulopathy as a consequence of failure of synthesis of coagulation factors, which complicates postoperative recovery after regional blocks and, therefore, warrants detailed evaluation of risks of bleeding before administration of these blocks. Portal hypertension in patients with liver disease also constitutes a risk for perioperative complications such as ascites or gastrointestinal bleeding and, therefore, needs monitoring and intervention during the operation. The anesthesiologists thus need to contrast the benefits and drawbacks of each anesthetic technique to ensure that the anesthesia plan, as well as surgical intervention, is according to the patient's hepatic status (Besecker et al., 2016). Furthermore, perioperative care of the patient with liver disease must take nutritional support and hydration status into account since they play important roles in surgery outcomes. Malnutrition is frequent in patients with liver disease due to impaired absorption and metabolic derangement; hence, preoperative assessment should include screening for malnutrition to attain optimal patient status before anesthetic administration. The utilization of enteral nutrition (EN) when possible sustains gut integrity and improves immune function, both of which are important in surgical patients. Moreover, it is also important to determine the risk of aspiration in such patients because impaired liver function likely predisposes them to increased intra-abdominal pressure and consequent gastric dysmotility. Individualized nutritional therapy can thus be a helpful adjunct that stabilizes such patients, keeping them resistant to surgical stress along with following guideline protocols and recommendations (Besecker et al., 2016).

Test Your Knowledge

1. How does the liver affect drug metabolism?
2. Why must drug doses be adjusted in patients with liver disease?

8.2. Anesthesia for Hepatic Resection

Learning Outcome

1. Preoperative assessment and planning
2. Anesthetic techniques used in hepatic resection
3. Postoperative care and monitoring

Anesthesia management of hepatic resection is crucial given the unique physiological requirements imposed by surgery of the liver. The liver performs numerous essential functions, one of which is metabolism of anesthetic agents that can be altered in patients with prior liver disease. The anesthesiologist must accurately evaluate the liver function pre-operatively with the appropriate scoring systems, e.g., the Child-Pugh score, to determine the patient's tolerance to the planned surgical intervention. Furthermore, an understanding of intraoperative hemodynamic stability is essential, with the reality that hepatic resection can lead to significant blood loss and necessitate advanced monitoring techniques. Continuous blood pressure and cardiac output monitoring provide instant feedback, enabling prompt correction to optimize patient outcomes during surgery. Lastly, an individualized anesthetic plan that takes into consideration the unique challenges of hepatic resection is crucial for the success of liver surgery overall. Intraoperative stability during hepatic resection demands the application of various anesthetic techniques to ensure maximal patient stability. Choice of anesthetic agents will significantly impact the liver's metabolism, thus affecting drug clearance and hemodynamics. More specifically, the use of agents with minimal hepatic metabolism, such as propofol and dexmedetomidine, is invariably preferable for hepatic resection. Opioids are also pivotal in the management of intraoperative analgesia, but their accumulation leads to delayed recovery in patients with impaired liver function. The incorporation of regional methods of anesthesia, such as continuous thoracic epidural analgesia, can also maximize postoperative pain control and potentially minimize systemic opioid administration. An ideally conceived anesthetic strategy, thus, seamlessly weaves together systemic and regional modalities to address the unique challenges of hepatic resections. Postoperative management following hepatic resection is equally critical and warrants conscientious anesthetic management. Anesthesia providers must stay vigilant for complications such as postoperative liver failure, particularly in the setting of pre-existing liver disease. ERAS protocols have been shown to play an important role in improving outcomes through handling standardized care and minimizing complications. Integration of multimodal analgesic measures reduces opioid consumption and hastens recovery, thus facilitating early mobilization and prevention of complications like venous thromboembolism. Moreover, existing evidence argues that attention to monitoring liver function and appropriate intervention in older patients with potential comorbidities that increase surgical risk must be followed. By using a full understanding of these variables, anesthesiologists can make a highly significant impact on long-term recovery trajectories after hepatic resection procedures (Zhang et al., 2018; Zhou et al., 2020) (Figure 8.6).

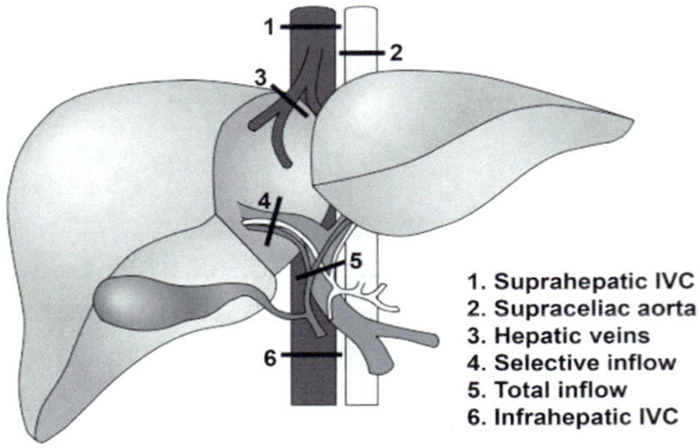

Figure 8.6. The management of anesthesia in hepatic resection.

Source: https://www.anesthesiology.theclinics.com/cms/10.1016/j.anclin.2021.11.004/asset/a46ee407-51f4-428d-940d-028509513c17/main.assets/gr2_lrg.jpg.

8.2.1. Preoperative Assessment and Planning

No aspect of anesthesiology for liver and gastrointestinal tract surgery should be more emphasized than the preoperative evaluation and planning. Careful evaluations are crucial elements in the identification of potential complications, optimization of patients' medical status, and anesthetic protocol individualization. A proper preoperative approach should encompass thorough history taking, physical examination, and pertinent laboratory investigations, aimed at an assessment of the overall condition of the patient and identification of any underlying comorbid conditions. Such evaluation not only guides anesthetic management but also informs surgical teams about forthcoming intraoperative challenges. Furthermore, resources for necessary perioperative interventions can be better allocated, possibly avoiding delays resulting from unforeseen complications during surgery. A reflective process of preoperative assessment thus lays a foundation for better surgical outcomes and patient safety in liver and gastrointestinal surgery. As a reaction to evolving standards of clinical practice, enhanced recovery pathways are more common nowadays, stressing the importance of preoperative assessment techniques even more. These pathways lay specific emphasis on the inclusion of multi-modal multidisciplinary approaches that are meant to enhance patient outcomes while posing minimal risk through surgery. Based on advice developed by organizations such as the ASCRS and SAGES, preoperative nutrition, bowel prep, and patient education are integral components. Patients, particularly those who have had prolonged colorectal surgery, are encouraged to be involved in oral nutritional supplementation and mechanical bowel preparation because these measures have been established to reduce surgical site infection and recovery durations. Additionally, effective preoperative counseling serves to familiarize patients with the surgery process, eliminating myths and discharge conditions, thus optimizing recovery protocol adherence after the surgery. Systematic preoperative planning that involves such improved recovery expertise ultimately translates into better long-term outcomes for patients. Furthermore, the importance of incorporating evidence-based practice as part of preoperative assessment cannot be overstated. Referral guidelines, such as updated guidelines for liver cancer management, underscore the value of multidisciplinary referral and sophisticated imaging modalities for optimal tailoring of interventions. Since liver disorders are common and multidimensional, the incorporation of high-quality evidence in preoperative evaluations prepares providers to provide patient-centered care informed by the unique circumstances of every patient. That is, patients undergoing hepatic resection can have similar anesthetic needs to patients who undergo laparoscopy for gastrointestinal disorders. Thus, employing updated guidelines instills a sense among healthcare professionals to foster team-based practice that enhances the quality of perioperative care. The incorporation of these practices into preoperative planning ultimately enhances patient safety and optimizes surgical outcomes, stressing the value of thorough evaluations before the administration of anesthesia in liver and gastrointestinal surgery (Figure 8.7).

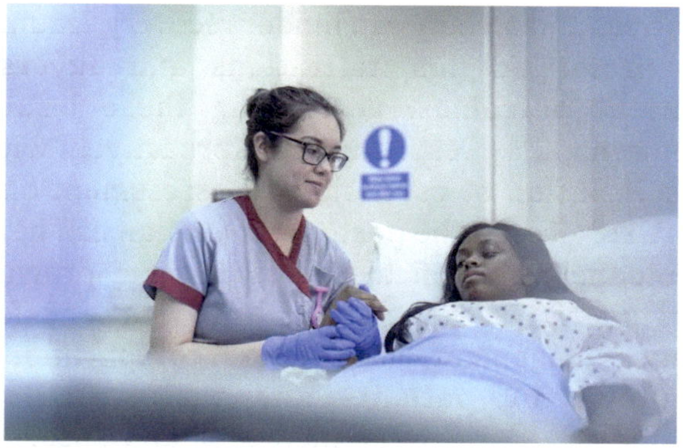

Figure 8.7. Preoperative assessment and planning.

Source: https://www.pasadenauc.com/wp-content/uploads/2024/07/pre-operative-assessment.jpg.

8.2.2. Anesthetic Techniques Used in Hepatic Resection

Patient management for hepatic resection is very precise in relation to anesthetic technique due to the liver's central role in drug metabolism and the intricate anatomy of the liver. Anesthetic strategies should be designed to ensure optimal hepatic perfusion while avoiding liver injury. The most frequently employed techniques are balanced general anesthesia, which entails the use of inhalational anesthetics in combination with intravenous agents. Importantly, agents like sevoflurane are desired for their liver-catalog profiles, which are of great importance in patients with underlying liver disease. Furthermore, monitoring technology, e.g., bispectral index (BIS) monitoring, can assist anesthesiologists in achieving ideal depth of anesthesia without compromising hemodynamic stability. Its use not only maximizes patient safety and recovery but also is in line with evolving trends in surgical techniques, e.g., multimodal analgesia pathways, with the aim of minimizing postoperative pain effectively. Multimodal analgesia increasingly forms an integral component of anesthetic management for hepatic resection, especially in the context of the opioid epidemic. This approach emphasizes the combination of several analgesic modalities, such as regional anesthesia and adjuvant drugs, to prevent opioid dependence. For instance, the addition of neuraxial procedures such as epidural analgesia or peripheral nerve blocks can readily decrease opioid consumption with successful postoperative pain relief. The literature has proven that such procedures are associated with improved recovery times and fewer side effects, such as postoperative nausea and vomiting. Emphasis on opioid-sparing strategies is particularly relevant in the context of ERAS protocols, which are increasingly applied to liver surgery. For optimal outcomes, anesthetic protocols must be specifically fitted to patient factors and the severity of the liver procedure undertaken. Anesthetic implications are more than the control of pain during hepatic resection; they also extend to steps that are intended to counteract intraoperative hemodynamic instability and postoperative liver function. Because of the potential for significant blood loss throughout liver resections, preservation of hemostatic control and perfusion adequacy is of utmost concern. Techniques such as goal-directed fluid therapy and minimized volatile anesthetic use play a pivotal role in attaining hemodynamic stability. Moreover, the anticipation of postoperative hepatic dysfunction necessitates meticulous postoperative observation, particularly of liver function tests and coagulation assays. Mobilization and optimal nutrition are generally promoted in enhanced recovery protocols, and these can be organized through meticulous anesthetic planning. By attention to these sophisticated anesthetic techniques, surgeons can dramatically improve surgical outcomes and patient quality of life after hepatic resection in line with innovations in surgical care and patient management during liver surgery (Lee et al., 2023).

8.2.3. Postoperative Care and Monitoring

Postoperative monitoring and care are critical aspects of anesthesia management in gastrointestinal and liver surgery owing to the unique physiological requirements of these surgeries. These patients have compromised liver function, which directly affects drug metabolism and recovery. A customized postoperative care plan should be aimed at monitoring the vital signs, fluid balance, and any indication of potential complications like bleeding or infections that can arise as a consequence of the invasive intervention. Constant monitoring of the liver function tests and studies of coagulation becomes essential in order to avoid undesirable outcomes. Further, proper management of analgesia is important; with the evolving opioid crisis awareness, multimodal analgesic strategies with inclusion of non-opioid medications to optimize recovery while minimizing opioid harm are increasingly being targeted (Lee et al., 2023). Monitoring also involves neurological assessment, particularly in evaluating postoperative cognitive dysfunction, which occurs in elderly patients who have had significant surgery. Delirium and cognitive decline are ominous complications that need to be closely observed after surgery. Multidisciplinary postoperative care has to be included with anesthesiologists, surgeons, and nurses to facilitate communication and shared decision-making. Postoperative teams need to be educated to recognize early signs of cognitive decline so they can act accordingly for optimal results. ERAS guidelines support early mobilization and nutrition, which are the pillars of preventing such complications as deep vein thrombosis and pneumonia that, in turn, complicate recovery in these patients (Lee et al., 2023). Besides physical rehabilitation, emotional support during the postoperative period is a significant contributor to outcomes in these patients. Psychological distress and anxiety can hinder recovery, leading to prolonged hospitalizations and adverse patient outcomes. Foreseeing these issues beforehand by resolving them proactively with the inclusion of psychological assessment and care services in the postoperative plan can help avoid them. Simplified explanations may provide postoperative expectations, interventions for pain management, and potential complications, empowering patients and their families, adherence to recovery measures and security. Prioritizing global care in the postoperative setting aligns with contemporary ideas around patient-centered care in health care, ultimately enhancing recovery experiences and results among patients undergoing liver and gastrointestinal surgery (Michael et al., 2021) (Figure 8.8).

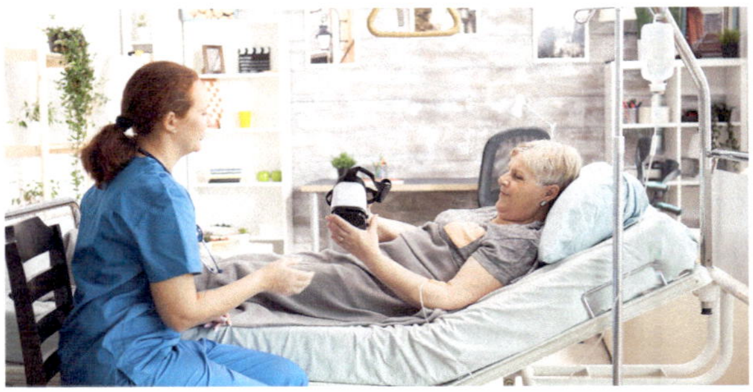

Figure 8.8. Postoperative care and monitoring are critical components of anesthesia management.

Source: https://rustingtonconvalescenthome.co.uk/wp-content/uploads/2023/05/Post-Operative-Care-Types-Benefits-and-Importance.jpg.

Test Your Knowledge

1. Why is maintaining low central venous pressure important during hepatic resection?
2. What is a major anesthetic concern related to liver function in these surgeries?

8.3. Anesthesia for Liver Transplantation

Learning Outcome

1. Unique challenges in liver transplant anesthesia
2. Anesthetic management during transplantation
3. Recovery and complications post-transplant

Liver transplant anesthesia has to be multimodal due to the complexity of surgery and the unique physiological challenges of end-stage liver disease patients. The anesthetic approach needs to stabilize hemodynamics, minimize blood loss, and ensure adequate organ perfusion intraoperatively. As liver transplant recipients often have severe coagulopathy and altered hemodynamic status, careful preoperative assessments and individualized anesthetic strategies are required. Anesthesiologists must remain vigilant for intraoperative systemic monitoring, evaluating hemodynamic parameters, oxygenation delivery, and fluid balance, given the common occurrence of fluid shifts and blood loss inherent to liver surgery. Ideal blood product administration must occur, but choosing the drugs and techniques must also be based on consideration of the deranged hepatic metabolism and responsiveness that these patients might exhibit, allowing for safety as well as efficacy during the process of the anesthetic. Intraoperative management of liver transplant also emphasizes the requirement for advanced anesthetic strategies. The procedure carries a high risk of liver-related complications like coagulopathy, which makes it risky to utilize large amounts of blood products and fluid resuscitation to manage blood loss. A critical aspect of anesthesia in such a situation is the use of extrarenal purification techniques, which have taken center stage in situations where the patients have combined kidney failure. New breakthroughs, such as simultaneous liver-kidney transplantation (SLKT), have made it necessary to adopt optimized anesthetic techniques that ensure hemodynamic stability while managing electrolyte disturbances and fluid overload. Anesthetists must monitor the patient's physiological responses carefully and employ advanced monitoring systems in order to regulate intraoperative fluids appropriately, achieving maximum benefits with a decline in possible complications associated with multi-organ damage as noted in recent studies (Huh et al., 2002; Swindle & Hughes, 2007). Moreover, post-transplantation liver maintenance is equally crucial as the intraoperative period, and anesthetic vigilance remains inevitable. It is not unusual for patients to experience great difficulty in recovering due to altered pharmacokinetics of drugs that are metabolized by the liver, necessitating a reoriented approach in pain management and sedation. Pain management protocols must be adjusted to account for the high risk of complications in this population, but still provide effective relief to enable recovery. Postoperative monitoring is critical, particularly for early hepatic dysfunction or failure, which may manifest as changes in consciousness or hemodynamic instability. The completion of a well-coordinated transition from intraoperative to postoperative care is needed to ensure patient safety and optimize recovery pathways in the complex environment of liver transplantation, thereby reinforcing the central position of anesthetic management to enhance surgical outcomes (Figure 8.9).

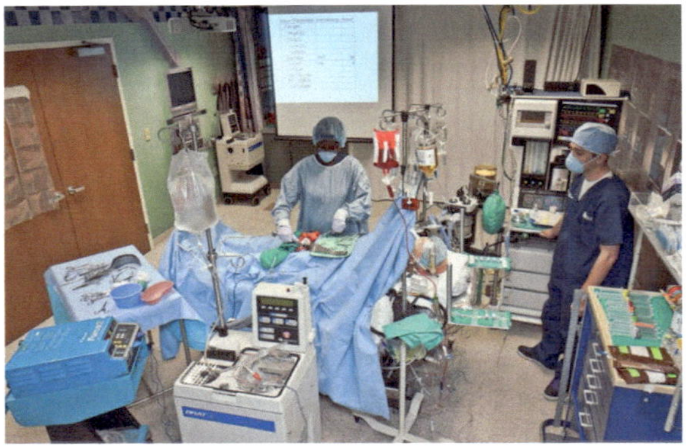

Figure 8.9. Anesthesia for liver transplantation requires a multifaceted approach.

Source: https://aneskey.com/wp-content/uploads/2017/07/A312535_1_En_37_Fig2_HTML.jpg.

8.3.1. Unique Challenges in Liver Transplant Anesthesia

Liver transplant anesthesia is a specialty with several challenges unique to this field, and one of them is a thorough knowledge of liver physiology and liver pathology. Among the most significant challenges is the control of coagulopathy seen in a typical patient with liver disease. Such patients have abnormal coagulation profiles because of the central role of the liver in synthesizing the clotting factors and in maintaining hemostasis. Anesthesiologists must adapt their technique to minimize blood loss during surgery, in addition to preoperative tests for assessing each patient's coagulation level appropriately. Moreover, the use of anticoagulant medications such as heparin also presents management issues, and close monitoring and immediate interventions are needed to provide ideal surgical conditions. The complexity of these variables requires an individualized anesthesia regimen able to meet the specific characteristics of unique liver transplant donors. Secondly, anesthetic management in liver transplant patients is also complicated by the pharmacokinetic and pharmacodynamic changes observed in hepatic impairment. Patients with liver failure typically have impaired drug clearance and metabolism, which makes it significant for anesthesiologists to select agents with certain pharmacological properties. Commonly used anesthetic agents will be altered at doses to prevent toxicity, especially in patients with a history of liver disease. Anesthesiologists also must be cautious in using agents that provide hemodynamic stability, since alterations in blood pressure can jeopardize graft perfusion during the all-important reperfusion phase. The unique demands of liver transplant anesthesia call for a good knowledge of drug interactions and the physiological effects of liver disease so that practitioners may individualize anesthesia plans correctly in each patient's own condition. The sophisticated problems of liver transplant anesthesia are beyond the hemodynamic and pharmacologic; they also encompass the psychological and physiological status of the patients undergoing these high-risk procedures. Patients getting liver transplants are usually stressed and anxious, and this complicates their pre-existing conditions. The anesthesiologist's function in such procedures extends beyond the simple administration of anesthetics; it also involves taking care of patient's emotional well-being. Combining reassurance with effective intraoperative monitoring goes a long way in offering psychological support during surgery. Furthermore, postoperative complications such as acute kidney injury (AKI) have been reported as a common occurrence following liver transplantation, particularly when not very well anticipated and managed. For instance, a research study found much lower incidence of AKI in patients who were administered dexmedetomidine during surgery (Kwon et al., 2024), showing anesthesia protocols have quite some influence on outcomes. Therefore, understanding the intricate interaction between anesthetic care, patient psychology, and physiological response is necessary to optimize patient outcomes using proper care during liver transplant.

8.3.2. Anesthetic Management During Transplantation

The anesthesia care during transplantation, particularly liver and gastrointestinal transplantations, needs a precise measure due to the complex physiological effects involved. Anesthesiologists' role is not limited to mere administration of anesthesia; it extends to preoperative evaluation, intraoperative management, and postoperative care. Preoperatively, thorough examination of the patient's comorbidities, liver function, and the severity of cirrhotic disease is crucial. These evaluations direct the planning of anesthesia, selecting agents that are optimal in drug modifications of hepatic metabolism and risk of coagulopathy. Continuous monitoring of vital signs and organ function parameters during surgery is crucial since acute alterations endanger serious risks.

This plan supports rapid adjustment of anesthesia plans to maintain hemodynamic stability as well as best outcomes. In liver transplant, the application of specific anesthetic maneuvers significantly influences surgical success and patient outcome. Total intravenous anesthesia (TIVA) is especially preferred in this context because it can provide quick recovery with reduced postoperative nausea, one of the most common complications among this population of patients. Opioid-sparing techniques, such as regional anesthesia techniques, such as epidurals or nerve blocks, can be utilized to enhance analgesia while reducing the chance of respiratory depression in patients with compromised liver function. Also, the application of agents that induce hepatic protection during ischemic events, like the remote ischemic preconditioning, has gained more attention. Such procedures are intended to promote liver viability while modifying probable complications of fluid resuscitation as well as bleeding, a special problem in radical transplantation operations. Post-transplantation care also has great demands on anesthetic care because of the greater potential for complications from bleeding and infection. Proper monitoring in the intensive care unit (ICU) is therefore greatly important. Anesthesia staff are a vital part of the detection and management of early post-transplant complications like hemodynamic instability and graft rejection. In the transitional phase, pain management protocols must be titrated to avoid excessive sedation with poor pain control. Multidisciplinary collaboration among anesthesiologists, surgeons, and intensive care staff ensures maximum patient benefit from transplant. Such coordinated efforts emphasize the necessity of a whole-of-the-transplant-procedure anesthetic strategy that addresses the totality of the transplant procedure, with a continuum of care prioritizing the patient's recovery and long-term health (Lee et al., 2023) (Figure 8.10).

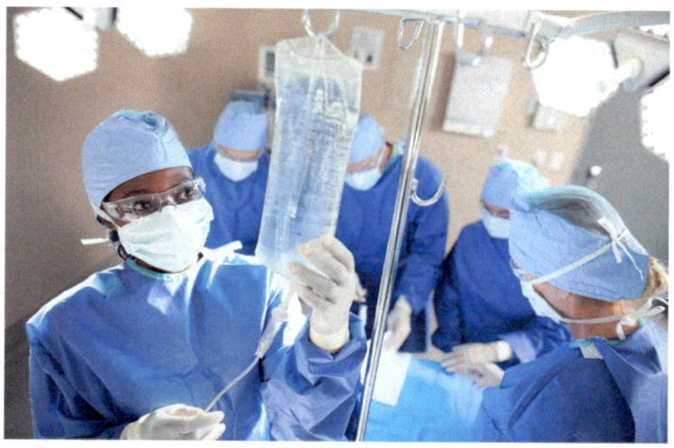

Figure 8.10. The anesthetic management during transplantation.

Source: https://njanesthesiaservices.com/wp-content/uploads/2025/03/anesthesiarenaltransplantation.jpg.

8.3.3. Recovery and Complications Post-Transplant

The recovery after liver transplant is intricate, involving the management of the physiological and the psychological factors that have a bearing on outcomes in patients. The patients are closely monitored in the beginning in an intensive care unit where vital signs, liver function, and the potential complications are assessed rigorously. Complications can range from surgical complications, i.e., bile leakage and bleeding, to systemic responses such as infection and organ rejection. These complications demand an interdisciplinary model of recovery, convening surgical, medical, and anesthetic personnel to deliver integrated care. Involving patients in the process of recovery is also essential, since education on self-care and warning signs for complications is central to their rehabilitation. An agreement of a systematic recovery process protocol for these organs is thus needed to optimize the post-transplant course and, ultimately, enhance survival rates, as has been the case for prior research on liver transplantation (Van Thiel et al., 1982). Anesthesia management in liver transplant recovery patients necessitates special regard due to their status from a physiological standpoint. Immunosuppressive therapy required to prevent organ rejection escalates the risk of infection and makes anesthetic management more complex, necessitating an individualized anesthetic plan based on patient-specific factors. Monitoring of fluid balance, along with replacement of blood products, becomes crucial in the maintenance of hemodynamic stability during surgery and postoperative courses. Moreover, special complications related to liver function, such as coagulopathy and altered drug metabolism, require careful attention and adaptability on the part of anesthesiologists in the perioperative period. Most importantly, a thorough preoperative workup with a focus on graft condition is essential, providing data that guides anesthesia management to minimize risk from surgery and anesthesia in this at-risk patient population (Brusich & Acan, 2018). Post-transplant complications can significantly affect both short-term and long-term recovery and ultimately determine the overall success of the liver transplant procedure. Of these, acute rejection episodes can occur relatively early in the post-transplant period and typically require modification of immunosuppressive treatment. In addition, the risk for chronic rejection is a long-term risk that needs to be managed by ongoing medical monitoring and patient education. Besides rejection, patients will also likely experience complications such as cardiovascular damage, renal damage, and post-transplant diabetes. The health practitioners, therefore, need to be vigilant in detecting and managing the complications through follow-ups and care strategies across disciplines. While managing these complexities, a systematic and vigilant approach in surveillance and maintaining potential complications following transplant goes a long way in facilitating the patient's prognosis and quality of life, illustrating how significant complete recovery protocols are (Van Thiel et al., 1982).

Test Your Knowledge

1. What is a major hemodynamic challenge during liver transplantation?
2. Why is careful monitoring of coagulation important in liver transplant patients?

8.4. Gastrointestinal Surgery: Laparoscopic vs. Open Techniques

Learning Outcome

1. Differences in anesthesia requirements
2. Advantages and disadvantages of each technique
3. Patient outcomes and recovery times

The evolution of surgical techniques in gastrointestinal surgery has ushered in a paradigm shift from open surgery to minimally invasive laparoscopic surgery. Laparoscopy, with its minimal incisions and use of camera-based technology, has gained popularity due to the advantages it offers in terms of reduced postoperative pain, shorter recovery times, and fewer postoperative surgical-site infections. Literature reports how these advantages have been associated with shorter hospital stay lengths and improved patient satisfaction over open surgery. There have then come along enhanced recovery protocols (ERPs) to complement laparoscopic techniques, integrating intensive-care strategies for the optimal postoperative results. ERPs have been demonstrated by research to reduce complications and hospital length of stay regardless of whether the surgical technique employed is laparoscopic or open. Therefore, anesthesiologists should understand the nuances of these techniques in order to condition anesthesia management in gastrointestinal operations (Irani et al., 2022). Despite the appealing characteristics of laparoscopic surgery, whether to apply the laparoscopic or the open approach is often determined by the specific clinical circumstance and patient-related considerations. For instance, those with serious comorbidities or severe illness can present difficulties, which result in open surgery as a safer option. Furthermore, visualization and access that are given through traditional techniques are useful in the setting of significant anatomical variation or a high burden of disease. Reflecting upon these points in relation to anesthesia for gastrointestinal and liver surgery is necessary because anesthetic risk profiles, the extent of anesthesia required, and postoperative pain control measures might be influenced by the surgical technique. Therefore, mutual consultations between surgical and anesthetic teams are the key to defining the most appropriate approach for every patient's special case (Zhou et al., 2020). The use of anesthesia techniques also underlines the importance of the employed surgical technique. Laparoscopic procedures tend to leverage advanced anesthetic techniques to reduce the use of opioids, enable rapid recovery, and enable faster postoperative mobilization. For example, multimodal pain relief techniques, including regional anesthesia, can be used to successfully alleviate pain without the widespread use of narcotics.

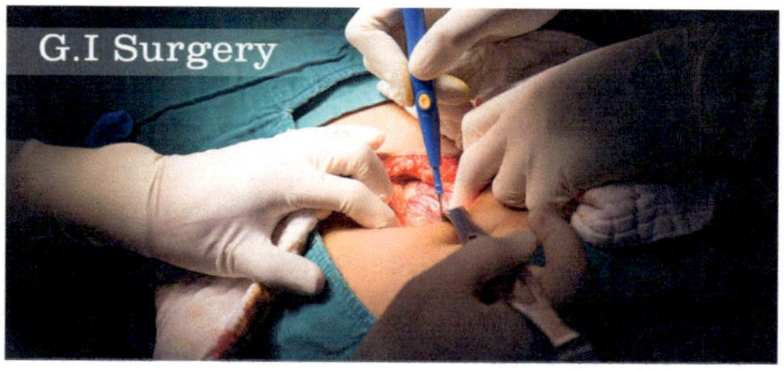

Figure 8.11. The evolution of surgical techniques in gastrointestinal surgery has presented a pivotal shift from traditional open surgery to minimally invasive laparoscopic approaches.

Source: https://www.kksurology.com/images/treatments/GI-Surgery.jpg.

This minimizes opioid-induced risks such as respiratory depression and prolonged recovery times. Patients operated upon openly, on the other hand, may require another form of anesthesia, usually one that involves deeper sedation and more powerful analgesics due to increased incisional pain. The anesthetic team plays a critical role to play in balancing paradigms of pain control with the surgery technique being undertaken, hence improving patient outcomes in the context of gastrointestinal surgery (Irani et al., 2022) (Figure 8.11).

8.4.1. Differences in Anesthesia Requirements

Anesthetic administration in liver and gastrointestinal surgery involves a delicate understanding of the diverse physiological and pathological factors unique to such procedures. The liver, its unique blood supply and metabolic behavior, influence anesthetic requirements profoundly. Patients with hepatic impairment present challenges such as drug metabolism and clearance changes; therefore, anesthetic choice needs to be well addressed. General anesthesia is generally utilized in more extensive liver resections, where deep relaxation and sedation are paramount. Furthermore, the coagulopathy and fluid status variability in these patients might necessitate the individualization of anesthetic technique and dosing, emphasizing the importance of the anesthesiology team to ensure minimal patient complications during the operation. Gastrointestinal surgeries, while sharing some anesthetic principles with liver surgery, have a tendency to demand modifications due to their unique anatomical and functional intricacies. Uniformity in surgical method, i.e., open vs. laparoscopic technique, decides the depth of anesthesia required. Laparoscopic procedures, for instance, normally require lighter anesthesia since they entail less incisional pain and earlier postoperative recovery. Additionally, the comorbidities such as obesity or diabetes that are common in patients undergoing gastrointestinal procedures might enhance anesthesia risk and necessitate extensive preoperative evaluation and intraoperative monitoring. Anesthetic management must also address the risk of postoperative nausea and vomiting, which is also plausible in this patient population and affects recovery. In addition, the incorporation of updated clinical guidelines is required in order to ensure that anesthetic care is aligned with the novel evidence-based practices. For instance, the updated guidelines for liver cancer management provide insight into how anesthesia is modified to adapt to evolving clinical standards. These are recommendations from the experience of most practitioners in the field and are particularly relevant to understanding differences in anesthesia requirements between cohorts of patients requiring liver resection. As observed in recent studies, increased emphasis on patient-tailored anesthesia strategies emphasizes the need for thorough assessment of factors considering the patient's uniqueness, complexity of surgery, and overall health condition to optimize perioperative care and improve surgical outcomes in liver and gastrointestinal surgeries (Zhou et al., 2020; Lee et al., 2023) (Figure 8.12).

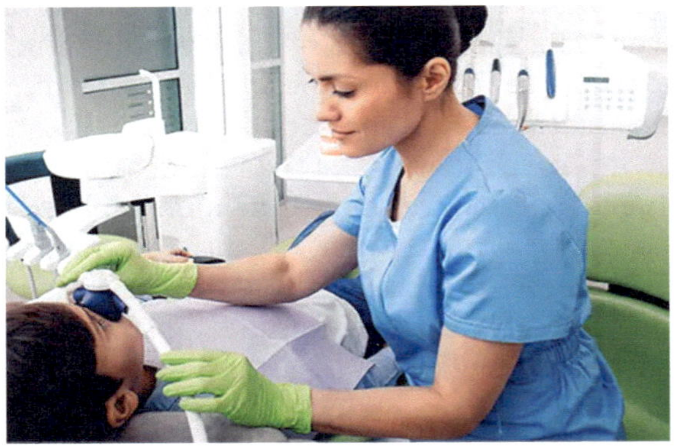

Figure 8.12. Differences in anesthesia requirements.

Source: https://images.emedicinehealth.com/images/article/main_image/sedation-dentist.jpg?output-quality=75.

8.4.2. Advantages and Disadvantages of Each Technique

Among the methods utilized in anesthesia during gastrointestinal and liver surgery, there are various pros and cons that can influence patient outcome and operation success significantly.

General anesthesia is highly utilized because of its ability to cause deep sedation, muscle relaxation, and airway patency. The technique has the advantage of causing postoperative analgesia, which is essential in enabling patient comfort following major operations. However, in comorbid conditions such as liver failure, the risks of general anesthesia in such patients are also high, e.g., respiratory and cardiovascular instability. Therefore, while general anesthesia can provide good pain relief and conduct complex surgery, the clinician will have to balance these benefits for every patient against patient-specific risks during selecting an anesthetic strategy (Lee et al., 2023). Conversely, regional anesthesia using neuraxial blocks has emerged as an alternative strategy that can be particularly valuable in liver and gastrointestinal surgery. Regional anesthesia provides effective pain relief with fewer systemic side effects, which is particularly valuable in patients with decreased hepatic function. It provides the potential for faster recovery times along with reduced need for systemic opiates, thus preventing some of the undesirable postoperative outcomes. However, the technique has its limitations. Anticoagulant therapy or those with certain anatomical issues cannot be ideal subjects for the technique, and it carries some risk of hematoma or inadequate analgesia. Therefore, while the advantages of regional anesthesia are compelling, its use is most likely to be constrained by some patient-related factors and clinical situations (Walter et al., 2016). Another method well worth exploring is monitored anesthesia care (MAC), a combination of sedation and local anesthesia that affords a more personalized degree of patient care. One of the most significant advantages of MAC is its ability to leave patients conscious, which can result in faster recovery and discharge times. MAC's less invasive nature also reduces the risk of certain complications associated with general anesthesia, such as airway management difficulties. On the downside, this technique may not provide a sufficient degree of analgesia for more extensive operations and therefore demands close observation of patients' comfort level. As a general rule, MAC is a well-adjusted system with major benefits but requires proficiency in monitoring to ensure safety and efficacy in liver and gastrointestinal surgery (Lee et al., 2023).

8.4.3. Patient Outcomes and Recovery Times

Overlap of post-operative patient outcomes and anesthesia methods in liver and gastrointestinal surgery is a relevant area of research, with emphasis on recovery times and postoperative wellness. Management of anesthesia needs to be done correctly, as it can directly influence the way patients respond physiologically to complex procedures. To illustrate, administration of anesthetic medication, as well as procedures such as regional versus general anesthesia, can have a considerable influence on pain relief and recovery patterns. Extensive pain management guidelines are significant, especially in light of evidence illustrating the need for careful prescription of opioids to reverse post-operative pain without complications ensuing from opioid use, including dependency and overdosing, as illustrated by guidelines to advance pain treatment (Dowell et al., 2022). In the end, anesthesia success not only determines short-term surgical outcome but also governs longer-term healing, impacting overall patient quality of life. Recovery times following liver and gastrointestinal surgery can vary significantly based upon surgical complexity, patient physical status, and anesthetic type employed. Studies have indicated that minimally invasive surgical techniques, often coupled with ERAS protocols, can lead to reduced recovery times and hospital stays. Pre-op assessment and tailor-made anesthesia plans are important, enabling clinicians to modify anesthetic techniques to meet the individual needs of each patient. This personalized approach has been seen to hold the promise of better recovery times, with patients often experiencing less postoperative pain and quicker mobilization, being key drivers of successful recovery in gastrointestinal surgery (Zhou et al., 2020). Such a nuanced understanding of how anesthesia may be employed to facilitate ultimate recovery is therefore a necessity to optimize patient outcomes within this field. Furthermore, patient outcomes are measured in terms of more than just recovery times and involve more general metrics of quality of life. Integration of patient-reported outcomes in measuring the efficacy of various approaches to anesthesia is increasingly recognized as being vital in liver and gastrointestinal surgery. By monitoring factors such as psychological well-being, functional status, and amounts of pain, healthcare providers are better able to understand the overall effectiveness of anesthetic interventions. Optimal postoperative recovery is not only linked to anesthetic practice but also with integral perioperative care such as pain relief, mobilization regimens, and nutritional optimization. Lastly, optimizing outcomes for the patient through well-designed anesthetic regimens and coordinated postoperative care is important, with emphasis placed on the complementarity between anesthetic choices and the patient's path to recovery (Zhou et al., 2020; Dowell et al., 2022) (Figure 8.13).

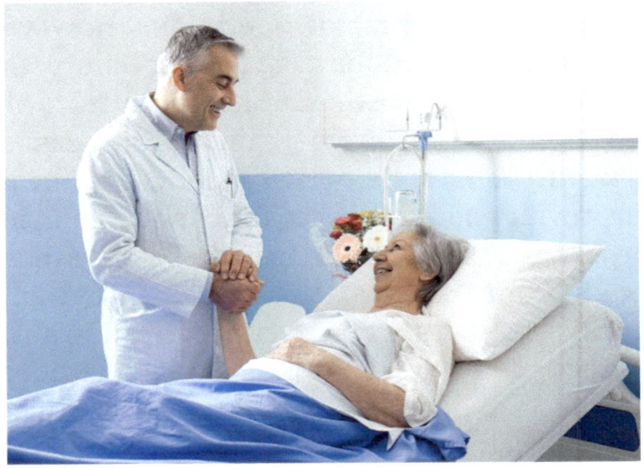

Figure 8.13. The intersection of anesthesia practices and patient outcomes in liver and gastrointestinal surgery.

Source: https://www.rightpatient.com/wp-content/uploads/2023/11/The-Importance-of-Patient-Comfort-and-How-Biometrics-Can-Help-1030x772.jpg.

Test Your Knowledge

1. What is one key difference between laparoscopic and open surgery?
2. How does laparoscopic surgery benefit patient recovery?

8.5. Fluid Management in Gastrointestinal Surgery

Learning Outcome

1. Importance of fluid balance during surgery
2. Strategies for fluid management
3. Monitoring and adjusting fluid therapy

Optimal fluid management is a critical aspect of gastrointestinal surgery and has implications for patient outcome as well as anesthetic care. Virtually all surgical interventions cause significant fluid shifts due to tissue trauma, surgical manipulation, and hemodynamic changes. The goal of fluid management under these circumstances is to maintain intravascular volume and perfusion of vital organs in their best state. It is a fine balance because hypovolemia and hypervolemia can result in significant complications such as cardiovascular instability and wound healing impairment. A variety of monitoring techniques have to be employed by anesthesiologists to measure fluid status, such as measurement of urine output and central venous pressure, as well as the volume and nature of fluid administered during the procedure. Thus, personalized practice according to the unique needs of the patients and the operating environment is essential to provide maximum intravenous fluid management during gastrointestinal surgery. Fluid selection is also necessary because different fluids expand intravascular volume and help achieve electrolyte balance differently. Crystalloid fluid, such as lactated Ringer's or normal saline, is commonly used in the operating room due to its cost-effectiveness and efficiency. However, they have been in controversy regarding their optimal use, most notably whether it poses risk for perioperative complications such as acute kidney injury or disturbances of electrolytes. In addition, the choice of colloid solutions may be more effective for volume expansion in certain cases, although with varying cost and associated risk. Understanding the pharmacokinetics and pharmacodynamics of these fluids is critical for anesthesiologists as well as surgeons, as it will enable precise decision-making in relation to the patient's individual clinical setting. Fluid choice cannot be exaggerated upon, as this has immediate implications for surgical and postoperative outcomes. Postoperative fluid management must then follow to accommodate the dynamic changes in recovery from gastrointestinal surgery. Patients may also develop gastrointestinal function changes, which will produce fluctuations in fluid intake and output, making fluid management difficult. The risk of developing complications such as ileus will also affect a patient's fluid status. In this regard, constant monitoring is needed to guide fluid replacement, including the monitoring of vital signs, laboratory investigations, and urine output. Effective communication between surgical and anesthetic teams is of utmost importance in an effort to present a unified fluid management plan that adapts to evolving patient needs in the postoperative period. Moreover, optimization of fluid management guidance in response to emerging evidence and clinical practice recommendations remains key to enhancing safety and outcomes in patients undergoing gastrointestinal procedures, with emphasis on the role of interprofessional collaboration in such a setting.

8.5.1. Importance of Fluid Balance During Surgery

Ideal fluid management during surgery is crucial to minimize complications and ensure optimal patient outcomes, particularly in risky surgeries such as liver and gastrointestinal surgery. They often involve excessive fluid loss due to extensive tissue manipulation and potential blood loss, leading to hypovolemia and decreased organ perfusion. The anesthesiologist's role in such a situation is to monitor fluid status and administer intravenous fluids to maintain hemodynamic stability. Fluid management planning is particularly important in gastrointestinal tract surgery, where deranged absorption and movement of fluids may aggravate postoperative complications. From the observation through studies of patients with high-risk surgical procedures, volume resuscitation, as well as meticulous management of electrolytes, have significant roles to play in influencing recovery courses and lengths of stay, thus emphasizing the importance of comprehensive preoperative assessment and customized perioperative planning to safeguard patient safety during and after surgical intervention. Physiologic adaptation to fluid shifts is a critical issue in the context of anesthesia and surgical practice. Patients undergoing operations such as pancreatic surgeries are at great risk of fluid overload or insufficiency, which may trigger unwanted sequelae such as acute respiratory distress syndrome and infection complications. Prompt and conservative fluid management is essential, especially in the first 48 hours post-surgery, as hinted in high crystalloid consumption and blood product transfusion reports in patients. Best fluid management not only minimizes complications but is also essential to hemodynamic stability return, as deviation can generate postoperative morbidities that slow recovery and increase intensive care unit stays. Hence, an active and responsive fluid management policy is priceless in avoiding harmful postoperative consequences, particularly among risky patients undergoing complex gastrointestinal surgery (Canter et al., 2003). Furthermore, interspecialist communication among anesthesiologists and surgeons optimizes fluid management policies to guarantee an increased strategy of patient treatment throughout complex surgical procedures.

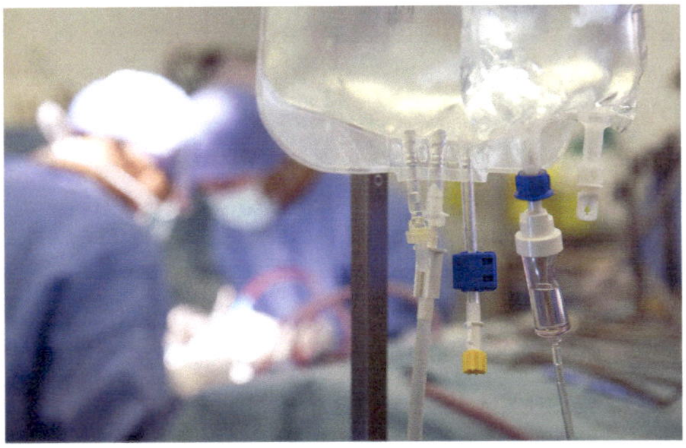

Figure 8.14. Achieving optimal fluid balance during surgery.

Source: https://www.verywellhealth.com/thmb/apITY3xSF_vAiX8X6onq47xcVek=/1500x0/filters:no_upscale():max_bytes(150000):strip_icc()/118609582-56a9125e5f9b58b7d0f7da80.JPG.

The multidisciplinary team framework is particularly beneficial in circumstances calling for an in-depth understanding of fluid dynamics, for example, intraperitoneal photodynamic therapy patients who undergo complex surgical procedures, such as this, wherein aggressive surgical techniques can lead to significant capillary leak syndrome. This calls for not only vigilant observation but even prophylactic fluid resuscitation protocol, with significant volumes of fluid intra-operatively. Through coordination of aligned practice among anesthesia and surgical providers, care procedures can be standardized to achieve maximum patient outcomes while reducing the incidence of postoperative complications (De Pietri et al., 2014). Effective fluid management is hence not only important but indispensable to advancing overall surgical performance and patient safety during major liver and gastrointestinal surgery (Figure 8.14).

8.5.2. Strategies for Fluid Management

Effective anesthesia fluid management during liver and gastrointestinal surgery is a critical determinant for decreasing perioperative complications. Excessive administration of fluids leads to volume overload and postoperative edema, while in its absence, hypovolemia and subsequent organ dysfunction may ensue. Modern guidelines suggest individualized fluid therapy based on patient factors, surgical status, and ongoing hemodynamic monitoring. For example, the maintenance infusions with balanced chloride-restricted crystalloids have been demonstrated to be useful in colorectal surgery in order to prevent postoperative renal disturbances. Furthermore, goal-directed hemodynamic therapy ensures a more personalized intervention, particularly in patients who are at risk because they are subject to significant intravascular loss during surgery (Irani et al., 2022). The application of ERAS pathways offers a structured approach to fluid management during the perioperative period in gastrointestinal surgery. ERAS protocols are usually composed of preoperative, intraoperative, and postoperative interventions that are intended to optimize fluid status and enhance recovery. Preoperative optimization can involve patient education and counseling regarding fluid intake, while intraoperative fluid therapy can be achieved through careful observation of blood loss and urine output. Evidence has established that the use of ERAS guidelines has been linked to reduced morbidity, reduced hospital stay, and patient satisfaction (Chen et al., 2020). Standardization of fluid management guidelines will enable clinicians to minimize practice variability and ultimately improve patient outcomes from liver and gastrointestinal surgery. In the postoperative period, adequate fluid management is crucial in order to allow recovery and prevent complications. Fluid resuscitation monitoring in accordance with the patient's clinical status, urine output, and laboratory findings, such as electrolyte levels, is important.

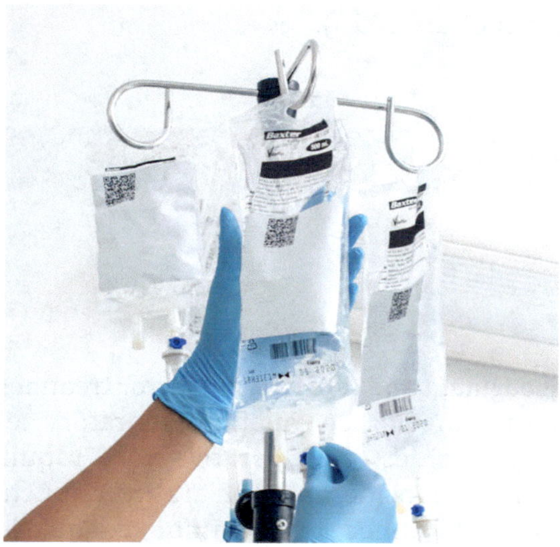

Figure 8.15. Strategies for fluid management.

Source: https://emeamedicationdelivery.baxter.com/sites/g/files/ebysai3906/files/styles/profile_card/public/2022-09/02_FluidManagementTherapySuite_CTA_1200x1200_CUT.jpg?h=cd2a7045&itok=-lwrSvH0.

The procedure of early oral fluid replacement after surgery has been promoted as a beneficial method in reducing ileus after surgery and hospital stay. Apart from this, the use of multimodal analgesia techniques helps to decrease opioid intake, which can further dampen the gastrointestinal side effects classically associated with narcotic drugs. Recent evidence supports that the best management of fluids and adherence to ERAS protocols on an individual basis lead to improved surgical outcomes, including postoperative recovery and readmission rate decrease (Irani et al., 2022) (Figure 8.15).

8.5.3. Monitoring and Adjusting Fluid Therapy

In gastrointestinal and liver surgery, fluid therapy monitoring and management are key components of maximizing patient outcomes. Fluid therapy is necessary for sustaining hemodynamic stability and ensuring sufficient organ perfusion during a significant procedure. The liver has a role at the center in fluid balance and metabolism, and therefore meticulous management of fluid therapy must be done in patients with hepatic dysfunction. Anesthesiologists must continually assess fluid status in relation to various parameters, such as blood pressure, heart rate, central venous pressure, and urine output, to determine volume status and adequacy of continuing fluid replacement. Incorporation of individualized fluid management protocols can reduce risks of fluid overload and deficit and have a quantifiable effect on patient recovery and surgical success. Monitoring must be dynamic and responsive to the second-to-second changes in patient status, necessitating a close understanding of fluid dynamics and patient physiology (Dowell et al., 2016). In addition to conventional monitoring techniques, novel cardiovascular monitoring modalities like pulse contour analysis and transthoracic echocardiography can fine-tune the assessment of fluid responsiveness in anesthetized patients. These technologies provide anesthesiologists with feedback regarding stroke volume variations and cardiac output, allowing for more precise fluid management during extensive liver and gastrointestinal surgery. Application of such advanced monitoring equipment allows for more judicious fluid replacement choices by anesthesiologists, thereby decreasing the risk of hypovolemia- and fluid overload-related complications. Hence, fluid therapy based on continuous data monitoring can lead to improved hemodynamic stability and enhance the recovery trajectory, particularly for high-risk surgical patients. This individualized approach emphasizes the importance of personalized fluid therapy for each patient's individual physiological demands and surgical context (Taylor et al., 2016). Fluid therapy protocols must be able to maintain adaptability to the dynamic shifts in the patient throughout the process of surgery. In gastrointestinal and liver surgery, postoperative complications such as fluid overload or hypotension are more likely because patients are in various hemodynamic states and can lose significant amounts of blood. So, anesthesiologists are faced with reorganizing fluid treatment programs based on intraoperative data and estimated postoperative fluid requirements. Providers. They should be vigilant for signs of fluid imbalance, depending on clinical judgment and monitoring devices to guide interventions. The general goal is to ensure that fluid resuscitation interventions promote optimal circulation without producing untoward effects of overly aggressive fluid therapy. This proactive and systemic fluid management is essential to achieve favorable surgical results and enhance the safety profile of anesthesia in complex liver and gastrointestinal surgery (Dowell et al., 2016).

Test Your Knowledge

1. Why is fluid balance important during gastrointestinal surgery?
2. What can happen if fluid management is inadequate during surgery?

8.6. Coagulopathy and Anesthesia

Learning Outcome

1. Understanding coagulopathy in surgical patients
2. Anesthetic implications of coagulopathy
3. Management strategies for coagulopathy during surgery

Coagulopathy is a significant challenge during anesthesia for liver and GI surgeries. Liver disease patients often have complex coagulopathic conditions due to impaired clotting factor production, leading to a heightened risk of bleeding during surgery. This is a challenge during anesthesia since clinicians must weigh anticoagulant and replacement factor treatments while monitoring coagulation laboratory tests closely. Besides, perioperative care requires thoughtful consideration of the liver function of patients since even minor coagulation disturbances can result in catastrophic events like massive bleeding and resultant hemodynamic instability. Coping with such issues must be a multi-pronged effort involving preoperative assessment, intraoperative monitoring, and postoperative management strategies. Cooperation between anesthesiologists and hepatologists is particularly crucial in handling acute liver failure patients. Fulminant hepatitis and other diseases induce coagulopathy that can rapidly evolve, complicating surgery. In surgery on such patients, the risk of complications such as uncontrollable bleeding and graft failure becomes real. Special precautions to safeguard against consideration of the unique physiological derangements that occur in liver disease should be part of careful anesthesia management. These include understanding the impact of liver failure on the pharmacodynamics and pharmacokinetics of drugs employed in anesthesia, which can be altered, resulting in augmented drug sensitivity. Patient selection and preparation are key in preventing complications at this delicate phase of treatment, hence enhancing surgical outcomes and ensuring patient safety. Postoperative care after liver transplantation is another equally important area where coagulopathy needs to be understood. The initial postoperative time is also plagued by complications such as hemorrhage, hemodynamic instability, and primary graft non-function, all of which are dependent on patients pre-existing coagulopathy (Bates & Martin, 2017).

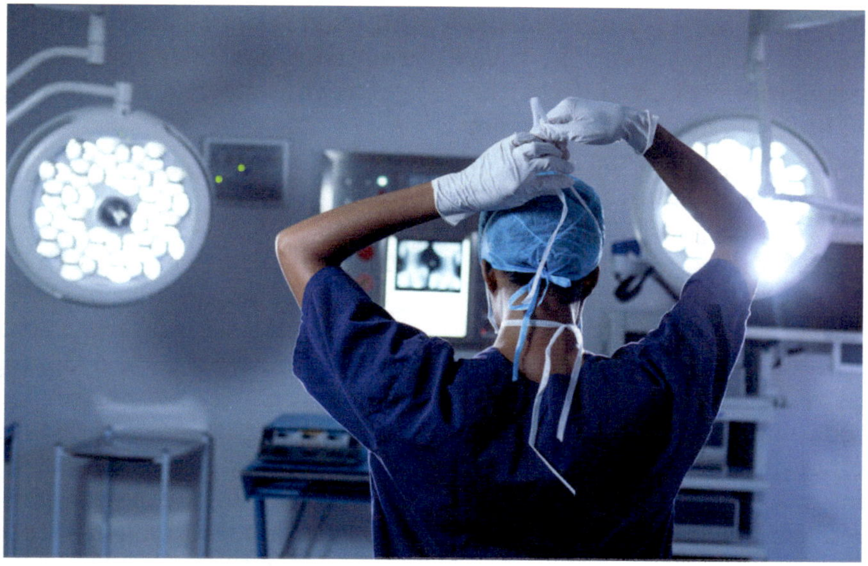

Figure 8.16. Coagulopathy presents a significant challenge in the context of anesthesia for liver and gastrointestinal surgeries.

Source: https://external-content.duckduckgo.com/iu/?u=https%3A%2F%2Fradiusanesthesia.com%2Fwp-content%2Fuploads%2F2020%2F01%2FiStock-1162543608-1024x683.jpg&f=1&nofb=1&ipt=3f706e95ff649930d3b7bb094369d2e65650c848f3599a1bd2b96398ee36a09e.

Hemostatic care must be given priority since superficial hemorrhages can soon spiral out of control and pose a life-threatening risk. Continuous monitoring of coagulation status, along with emergency intervention plans, is warranted to avert these complications. The intricacy of managing these patients necessitates a model of collaborative care that includes the expertise of surgical teams, anesthesiologists, and critical care specialists, which ultimately translates into optimized outcomes and reduced morbidity in this vulnerable population. Understanding the intricate relationship between coagulopathy and anesthesia is key to optimizing the prognosis for liver procedures, especially in the patient with acute liver failure (Stieber et al., 1988) (Figure 8.16).

8.6.1. Understanding Coagulopathy in Surgical Patients

Surgical coagulopathy is a complex entity that poses major challenges, particularly with liver and intestinal surgery. It is crucial that the pathophysiology of coagulopathy be appreciated because such operations may trigger latent coagulopathies or even induce de novo ones. The functioning of the liver, medication, and even the operating room environment, per se, can upset the delicate equilibrium of hemostasis. For instance, patients with liver disease typically present with coagulopathy secondary to impaired synthesis of coagulation factors, not just raising the risk of intraoperative bleeding but also complicating postoperative recovery (Lee et al., 2023). Anesthesia management must therefore include strategies for the tight monitoring of coagulation status and for the prediction of complications that can result from both the surgery as well as from the inherent nature of the patient's coagulopathy. Assessment of surgical patients with coagulopathy involves a multimodal process that integrates clinical evaluation with objective laboratory testing. Standard laboratory tests, such as prothrombin time (PT) and activated partial thromboplastin time (aPTT), provide useful information regarding the coagulation pathways. The standard tests do not provide a comprehensive picture of the hemostatic function of a patient, particularly in liver surgery patients. Point-of-care testing and thromboelastography (TEG) offer immediate feedback on the coagulation process, allowing anesthesia professionals to modify their management plan accordingly. In addition, clinicians must consider the contribution of an array of comorbid illnesses, such as cardiovascular disease characterized by right-sided heart failure, adding further complexity to the patient's coagulation profile. Management of these dynamics becomes pivotal to optimizing patient outcomes under the surgical process (Marvin et al., 2018). It is essential in liver and gastrointestinal surgery to define and apply personalized coagulation management plans. These plans need to account for the patient's unique genetic coagulopathic conditions, the nature of the surgery, and potential anesthetic issues. Multidisciplinary collaboration is paramount, including feedback from surgeons, anesthesiologists, and hematologists to develop an integrated management strategy that considers the surgical and hemostatic challenges posed by the patient. Furthermore, postoperative monitoring for signs of bleeding and thrombosis also plays a similar, equally vital role in patient safety. An aggressive practice—founded on adequate preoperative assessment, intraoperative monitoring, and postoperative management—prevents surgical patient coagulopathy complications, thereby improving the outcome of surgery and reducing complications from anesthesia in gastroenterological and liver operations.

8.6.2. Anesthetic Implications of Coagulopathy

Management of coagulopathy is critical in the practice of anesthetics, particularly in liver and gastrointestinal surgery. Patients undergoing such operations have a deranged hemostatic profile due to liver disease or those that negatively influence coagulation pathways. The anesthetist must thoroughly assess the coagulation of the patients prior to surgery, with the laboratory INR value, platelet count, and history of recent bleeding being utilized to guide the choice of anesthesia and perioperative care. The anticipation of intraoperative and postoperative bleeding is important, as the risk of hemorrhage is greatly increased in the setting of hepatic insufficiency and may lead to greater morbidity and mortality. Therefore, customized anesthetic regimens that incorporate these particular coagulopathic factors are essential to patient safety and surgical success. Monitoring the correct methods during surgery is essential in coagulopathic patient care. Continuous monitoring of fluid resuscitation needs, blood loss, and coagulation factors may enable timely intervention and correction of any abnormalities that occur during surgery. Newer technologies, such as TEG or rotational thromboelastometry (ROTEM), can provide real-time information on hemostatic function, and thus allow the anesthesiologist to make an informed judgment on whether or not to replace products such as fresh frozen plasma, platelets, or cryoprecipitate. This active management of coagulopathy is particularly pertinent in liver and gastrointestinal surgery, where a profound range in coagulation factors can be seen due to the liver's ability to synthesize these proteins. Thus, careful observation and dynamic management can have a major impact on surgical outcomes in these patients. Moreover, the extent of coagulopathy is not only intraoperative but also extends into the postoperative phase, and sound appreciation of risk potential for thromboembolic complications needs to be known. Liver disease patients or patients who have had extensive GI manipulation might be at risk for both bleeding as well as thrombotic complications, including VTE. As highlighted by current literature, adjunct therapy for prevention of such outcomes, particularly in COVID-19 infection, needs advanced strategies, like the use of anticoagulation protocols following the surgery (Sakr et al., 2020). The balance between the need for thromboprophylaxis and provoking aggravation of bleeding complications is the crux of the anesthetic protocol in coagulopathic patients. Thus, establishment of an individualized plan that addresses both the risk of bleeding and the thromboembolic complications is critical for optimizing recovery and reducing postoperative complications in this high-risk patient population (Figure 8.17).

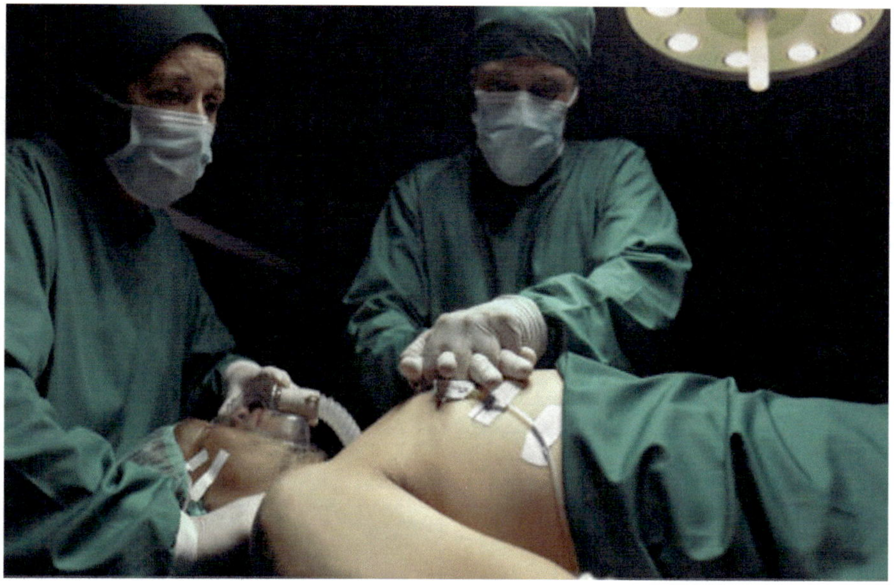

Figure 8.17. The management of coagulopathy is crucial in the realm of anesthetic practice.

Source: https://www.istockphoto.com/photo/cardiac-arrest-and-cardiopulmonary-resuscitation-in-the-operating-room-gm1470404574-501269393?searchscope=image%2Cfilm.

8.6.3. Management Strategies for Coagulopathy During Surgery

During surgical procedures, especially gastrointestinal and liver surgery, coagulopathy management is critical due to the central role of the liver in hemostasis. The liver synthesizes most of the coagulation factors and thus any derangement leads to significant bleeding complications intraoperatively. Preoperative assessment is critical, including careful coagulation studies to assess the patient's baseline hemostatic status. Strategies included can be the use of blood products such as fresh frozen plasma or platelet transfusions for the correction of coagulopathy before incision. Moreover, aggressive use of antifibrinolytics such as tranexamic acid may minimize excessive bleeding in high-risk surgeries. Achieving optimal hemostasis is crucial not only for the success of surgery but also for preventing postoperative complications and hence optimizing overall patient outcomes for these difficult surgeries. Anesthesiologists, intraoperatively, have an integral role in the management of coagulopathy by observing the status of coagulation and making real-time decisions. Treatment tends to involve ongoing monitoring of hemostatic balance through point-of-care testing, reflecting the rapid availability of information about clotting factors and platelet function. Where coagulopathy is recognized, prompt delivery of corrective intervention is vital. This may include the intravenous infusion of clotting factor concentrates or repeated administration of antifibrinolytics, depending on the severity and type of coagulopathy identified. Furthermore, the capability to utilize viscoelastic tools such as TEG allows the anesthesiology team to individualize fluid and transfusion care to the patient's coagulation needs, significantly enhancing hemostatic care in the dynamic operating room environment. Postoperatively, the management challenge of coagulopathy continues as the patient recovers from surgery. Close observation for bleeding, hematoma formation, and other difficulties in the early postoperative period is needed. Prophylactic measures may include continuous transfusion of blood products and having the patient as optimized as possible from a hemostatic function basis before discharge to the operating room. Education of the healthcare team on the recognition and treatment of coagulopathy will enhance overall care. Application of evidence-based recommendations, as described in recent articles, can also restrict coagulopathy-related practices in and after liver and gastrointestinal surgery. Synergy between guidelines, as described in Van der Merwe et al. (2021) and Lee et al. (2023), and clinical practice can also enhance the safety of patients and surgical success rates in this high-risk population.

Test Your Knowledge

1. Why is coagulopathy a concern during anesthesia?
2. How can anesthesia management be modified in patients with bleeding disorders?

SUMMARY

In a review of the imperative role of anesthesia in gastrointestinal and liver surgery, it is evident that excellent anesthetic care plays an important part in optimizing surgical outcomes and enhancing patient recovery. Anesthesia not only supports surgery through patient safety and comfort, but it also has significant implications for minimizing postoperative recovery time and postoperative complications. The implementation of ERAS protocols has demonstrated positive outcomes, minimizing hospital stays and associated healthcare costs substantially. These guidelines emphasize the importance of a multidisciplinary regimen in perioperative care, and this is in line with the evolving environment of anesthetic practice in surgical care, including liver and gastrointestinal surgery. Successful adoption of these guidelines has the potential to improve substantially the predictability and safety of patient outcomes in such high-risk surgeries, which suggests further innovation in anesthetic approaches and strategies (Ljungqvist et al., 2017). Moreover, the importance of professional training and skill in anesthetic technique for difficult procedures such as ERCP cannot be overstressed. As ERCP is becoming a procedure that is not only diagnostic but also therapeutically intricate, the requirement for proper anesthesia management becomes that much greater. According to the American Society for Gastrointestinal Endoscopy, not only do endoscopists need to be technically capable, but even the anesthetic team needs to deliver ideal levels of sedation and monitor potential adverse events occurring during the process (Adler et al., 2014). All these factors are crucial to avoid complications, like pancreatitis or cardiopulmonary events, that may arise during ERCP. Thus, there is a need for a collaborative partnership among surgical teams and anesthesia providers to provide enhanced general safety and effectiveness of gastrointestinal procedures. Finally, the ongoing need for research and quality improvement in anesthesia services with regard to liver and gastrointestinal surgery is a significant finding. Ongoing surveillance of performance measures and the implementation of known quality measures can offer valuable feedback on where improvement is required. For instance, trends in adverse event rates against anesthetic choice can be used to support best practice and improve guidelines. The collaborative effort of the anesthesia and surgical teams towards adopting evidence-based protocols, such as those presented by ERAS, is the foundation for continuing to improve patient outcomes. Through focusing on training, education, and continuous assessment, the anesthetic community is in a position to facilitate the enhancement of care levels within liver and gastrointestinal surgery, hence resulting in a better surgical experience and postoperative recovery for patients (Adler et al., 2014; Ljungqvist et al., 2017).

The anesthetic procedure in liver and gastrointestinal surgery is particularly demanding based on the intricacy of the procedures and the physiological implications for the patient. Anesthesiologists must account for the compromised function of the liver in patients with liver disorders who have been exposed to surgery, especially conditions like hepatocellular carcinoma, which causes the majority of primary liver cancers in China and globally. It is essential to learn the pharmacokinetics of anesthetic agents in the liver-compromised patient to avoid postoperative morbidity and to maximize the patient's recovery. For example, those drugs that are metabolized by the liver must be carefully selected and administered, as impaired hepatic function can significantly alter their clearance and thereby the patient's reaction to the anesthetic. This requires extensive testing of liver function preoperatively. In addition to assessment of liver function, anesthetic management must include provisions to deal with the risk for large intraoperative blood loss, as is common in liver and gastrointestinal resections. The risk for hemorrhage does not only arise from the liver's vascular nature but also due to the technique employed in resections or transplantation. Preoperative optimization, including the use of blood products and fluid resuscitation strategies, is vital to hemodynamic stability during the course of the procedure. Anesthesiologists should also be prepared for the possibility of massive transfusion protocols and be attentive to monitoring coagulation factors. This multidisciplinary approach is essential to the prevention of morbidity and mortality from these high-risk surgeries, pointing out the interprofessional function of the anesthesiologist as part of the surgical team. Recent guidelines have stressed the importance of personalized anesthetic approaches for patients presenting for surgery to correct liver and gastrointestinal illness. Notably, Guidelines for Diagnosis and Treatment of Primary Liver Cancer (2017 Edition) and its 2019 update reflect the evolving context of hepatocellular carcinoma treatment in China, asserting the need for evidence-based care practice. The recommendations, penned by over 70 contributors to the field, emphasize the significance of employing high-quality evidence in assessing surgical plans and anesthetic techniques. These recommendations emphasize the significance of current guidelines in maximizing patient outcomes and optimizing a multidisciplinary management strategy targeting anesthetic and surgical concerns in liver and gastrointestinal surgery. In conclusion, the highlights present here underscore the intricacy and requirement of personalized anesthetic care in this type of surgery, and in turn, result in enhanced safety and performance for patients undergoing these significant surgeries (Lee et al., 2023; Zhou et al., 2020).

KEY TERMS FROM THIS CHAPTER

- Anesthesiologists
- Drug metabolism
- Gastrointestinal surgery
- Hepatic function
- Modern medicine
- Opioid-related side effects
- Complexity
- Fluctuations
- Hemodynamic
- Infection
- Necessitating precise
- Procedure complexity

CRITICAL THINKING QUESTIONS

1. **What is the primary anesthetic concern during liver resection surgery?**
   a. Hyperkalemia
   b. Coagulopathy
   c. Hypervolemia
   d. Hypoglycemia
2. **During laparoscopic gastrointestinal surgery, insufflation of the abdomen with CO_2 can cause:**
   a. Hypocapnia
   b. Hypercapnia
   c. Decreased intracranial pressure
   d. Increased cardiac output
3. **Which of the following is an absolute contraindication for neuraxial anesthesia in liver surgery?**
   a. Hepatic encephalopathy
   b. Ascites
   c. Coagulopathy
   d. Hypovolemia
4. **Which intravenous fluid is preferred for patients undergoing liver surgery?**
   a. Normal saline
   b. Lactated Ringer's
   c. 5% Dextrose
   d. Albumin
5. **What is the most common cause of hemodynamic instability during major liver surgery?**
   a. Hyperkalemia
   b. Blood loss
   c. Arrhythmias
   d. Hypocalcemia

Short Answer Questions

1. What are the anesthetic considerations for patients with liver cirrhosis undergoing gastrointestinal surgery?
2. How does portal hypertension affect perioperative management in patients undergoing liver surgery?
3. What are the implications of coagulopathy in patients with liver disease on anesthesia and surgical planning?
4. Discuss the role of hemodynamic monitoring in liver transplantation and major liver resections.
5. How does hepatic metabolism influence drug selection and dosing during anesthesia for liver surgery?
6. Explain the role of total intravenous anesthesia (TIVA) compared to inhalational anesthesia in liver surgery.

Answer to Critical Thinking Questions

1. (b); 2. (b); 3. (c); 4. (d); 5.(b)

REFERENCES

1. Brusich KT, Acan I. Anesthetic Considerations in Transplant Recipients for Nontransplant Surgery [Internet]. Organ Donation and Transplantation - Current Status and Future Challenges. InTech; 2018. Available from: http://dx.doi.org/10.5772/intechopen.74329(accessed on 28th June 2025).
2. Adler, D. G., Lieb, J., Cohen, J., Pike, I. M., Park, W. G., Rizk, M., Sawhney, M. S., et al. (2014). Quality indicators for ERCP. *The American Journal of Gastroenterology, 110*, 91–101. https://doi.org/10.1038/ajg.2014.386 (accessed on 28th June 2025).
3. Bates, E., & Martin, D. (2017). Immediate postoperative management and complications on the intensive care unit. https://core.ac.uk/download/111010646.pdf (accessed on 28th June 2025).
4. De Pietri L, Montalti R, Begliomini B. Anaesthetic perioperative management of patients with pancreatic cancer. *World J Gastroenterol*. 2014;20(9):2304-2320. doi:10.3748/wjg.v20.i9.2304(accessed on 28th June 2025).
5. Besecker, E. M., Deiter, G. M., Pironi, N., Cooper, T. K., & Holmes, G. M. (2017). Mesenteric vascular dysregulation and intestinal inflammation accompanies experimental spinal cord injury. *American journal of physiology. Regulatory, integrative and comparative physiology, 312*(1), R146–R156. https://doi.org/10.1152/ajpregu.00347.2016 (accessed on 28th June 2025).
6. Boike, J., Thornburg, B., Asrani, S. K., Fallon, M. B., Fortune, B. E., Izzy, M., Verna, E. C., et al. (2021). North American practice-based recommendations for trans jugular intrahepatic portosystemic shunts in portal hypertension. *Clinical Gastroenterology and Hepatology, 20*, 1636–1662.e36. https://doi.org/10.1016/j.cgh.2021.07.018 (accessed on 28th June 2025).
7. 25th International Congress of the European Association for Endoscopic Surgery (EAES) Frankfurt, Germany, 14-17 June 2017 : Oral Presentations. (2017). *Surgical endoscopy, 31*(Suppl 2), 1–59. https://doi.org/10.1007/s00464-017-5540-y(accessed on 28th June 2025).
8. Canter, R. J., Mick, R., Kesmodel, S. B., Raz, D. J., Spitz, F. R., Metz, J. M., Glatstein, E. J., Hahn, S. M., & Fraker, D. L. (2003). Intraperitoneal photodynamic therapy causes a capillary-leak syndrome. *Annals of surgical oncology, 10*(5), 514–524. https://doi.org/10.1245/aso.2003.11.005(accessed on 28th June 2025).
9. Chen, C., Gao, G., Xu, Y., Pu, L., Wang, Q., Wang, L., Wang, W., et al. (2020). SARS-CoV-2–positive sputum and feces after conversion of pharyngeal samples in patients with COVID-19. *Annals of Internal Medicine, 172*, 832–834. https://doi.org/10.7326/m20-0991 (accessed on 28th June 2025).
10. Talebi Z, Peyvandi H, Dabbagh A. Cellular and Molecular Mechanisms in Perioperative Hepatic Protection: A Review of Current Interventions.J Cell Mol Anesth.2017;2(2):e149530.https://doi.org/10.22037/jcma.v2i2.14839.(accessed on 28th June 2025).
11. Dandemmanavar, V., Kn, V., R, V., Bandyopadhyay, S., Gakhar, H., & Dey, A. (2025). The impact of anesthetic agents on neurocognitive outcomes in pediatric patients. *Journal of Neonatal Surgery*. https://www.semanticscholar.org/paper/56a8165418161a15d7018b8d1f4e7fdc66d25666 (accessed on 28th June 2025).
12. Dowell, D., Haegerich, T. M., & Chou, R. (2016). CDC guideline for prescribing opioids for chronic pain—United States, 2016. *MMWR Recommendations and Reports, 65*, 1–49. https://doi.org/10.15585/mmwr.rr6501e1 (accessed on 28th June 2025).

13. Dowell, D., Ragan, K., Jones, C. M., Baldwin, G., & Chou, R. (2022). CDC clinical practice guideline for prescribing opioids for pain—United States, 2022. *MMWR Recommendations and Reports, 71*, 1–95. https://doi.org/10.15585/mmwr.rr7103a1 (accessed on 28th June 2025).

14. Van Thiel, D. H., Schade, R. R., Starzl, T. E., Iwatsuki, S., Shaw, B. W., Jr, Gavaler, J. S., & Dugas, M. (1982). Liver transplantation in adults. *Hepatology (Baltimore, Md.), 2*(5), 637–640. https://doi.org/10.1002/hep.1840020517(accessed on 28th June 2025).

15. Grant, M. C., Suffredini, G., & Cho, B. C. (2021). Is it time to eliminate the use of opioids in cardiac surgery? *JTCVS Open, 7*, 247–252. https://doi.org/10.1016/j.xjon.2021.03.022 (accessed on 28th June 2025).

16. Guo, J., Huang, X., Dou, L., Yan, M., Shen, T., Tang, W., & Li, J. (2022). Aging and aging-related diseases: From molecular mechanisms to interventions and treatments. *Signal Transduction and Targeted Therapy, 7*. https://doi.org/10.1038/s41392-022-01251-0 (accessed on 28th June 2025).

17. Hilscher, M., Wells, M., Venkatesh, S. K., Cetta, F., & Kamath, P. S. (2022). Fontan-associated liver disease. *Hepatology, 75*, 1300–1321. https://doi.org/10.1002/hep.32406 (accessed on 28th June 2025).

18. Huh, I. S., Cho, K., & Choi, K. T. (2002). Anesthesia for synchronous liver-kidney transplantation. *Korean Journal of Anesthesiology, 42*, 414–421. https://www.semanticscholar.org/paper/946bad352f093c2e6cf9d4480f1266106ab8ce7e (accessed on 28th June 2025).

19. Irani, J., Hedrick, T. L., Miller, T. E., Lee, L., Steinhagen, E., Shogan, B. D., Goldberg, J. E., et al. (2022). Clinical practice guidelines for enhanced recovery after colon and rectal surgery from the American Society of Colon and Rectal Surgeons and the Society of American Gastrointestinal and Endoscopic Surgeons. *Diseases of the Colon & Rectum, 66*, 15–40. https://doi.org/10.1097/dcr.0000000000002650 (accessed on 28th June 2025).

20. Stieber, A. C., Ambrosino, G., Van Thiel, D., Iwatsuki, S., & Starzl, T. E. (1988). Orthotopic liver transplantation for fulminant and subacute hepatic failure. *Gastroenterology clinics of North America, 17*(1), 157–165.(accessed on 28th June 2025).

21. Joglar, J. A., Chung, M. K., Armbruster, A. L., Benjamin, E. J., Chyou, J. Y., Cronin, E. M., Deswal, A., et al. (2023). 2023 ACC/AHA/ACCP/HRS guideline for the diagnosis and management of atrial fibrillation: A report of the American College of Cardiology/American Heart Association Joint Committee on Clinical Practice Guidelines. *Circulation, 149*. https://doi.org/10.1161/cir.0000000000001193 (accessed on 28th June 2025).

22. Joliat, G. R., Kobayashi, K., Hasegawa, K., Thomson, J. E., Padbury, R., Scott, M. J., Brustia, R., et al. (2022). Guidelines for perioperative care for liver surgery: Enhanced Recovery After Surgery (ERAS) Society recommendations 2022. *World Journal of Surgery, 47*, 11–34. https://doi.org/10.1007/s00268-022-06732-5 (accessed on 28th June 2025).

23. Kahaly, G. J., Bartalena, L., Hegedüs, L., Leenhardt, L., Poppe, K., & Pearce, S. H. S. (2018). 2018 European Thyroid Association guideline for the management of Graves' hyperthyroidism. *European Thyroid Journal, 7*, 167–186. https://doi.org/10.1159/000490384 (accessed on 28th June 2025).

24. Konstam, M. A., Kiernan, M. S., Bernstein, D., Bozkurt, B., Jacob, M., Kapur, N. K., Kociol, R. D., et al. (2018). Evaluation and management of right-sided heart failure: A scientific

statement from the American Heart Association. *Circulation, 137*. https://doi.org/10.1161/cir.0000000000000560 (accessed on 28th June 2025).

25. Kwon, H. M., Kang, S. J., Han, S. B., Kim, J. H., Kim, S. H., Jun, I. G., Song, J. G., et al. (2024). Effect of dexmedetomidine on the incidence of postoperative acute kidney injury in living donor liver transplantation recipients: A randomized controlled trial. *International Journal of Surgery (London, England), 110*, 4161–4169. https://www.semanticscholar.org/paper/a194e1e28df99e97653fce921260400db71d398b (accessed on 28th June 2025).
26. Lee, E., Eghtesad, B., García-Tsao, G., Haskal, Z. J., Hernández-Gea, V., Jalaeian, H., Kalva, S. P., et al. (2023). AASLD practice guidance on the use of TIPS, variceal embolization, and retrograde transvenous obliteration in the management of variceal hemorrhage. *Hepatology, 79*, 224–250. https://doi.org/10.1097/hep.0000000000000530 (accessed on 28th June 2025).
27. Ljungqvist, O., Scott, M. J., & Fearon, K. C. H. (2017). Enhanced recovery after surgery. *JAMA Surgery, 152*, 292–292. https://doi.org/10.1001/jamasurg.2016.4952 (accessed on 28th June 2025).
28. Maluccio, M. A., & Covey, A. M. (2012). Recent progress in understanding, diagnosing, and treating hepatocellular carcinoma. *CA: A Cancer Journal for Clinicians, 62*, 394–399. https://doi.org/10.3322/caac.21161 (accessed on 28th June 2025).
29. Mao, S., Gao, R., Huang, Y., He, H., Yao, J., & Feng, J. (2025). Effect of remimazolam combined with estazolam on anxiety levels and postoperative gastrointestinal function recovery in patients undergoing laparoscopic cholecystectomy surgery. *European Journal of Medical Research, 30*. https://www.semanticscholar.org/paper/48efb44ca75fb6825d8a040c82e42d9a256145c2 (accessed on 28th June 2025).
30. McClave, S. A., Taylor, B., Martindale, R. G., Warren, M., Johnson, D. R., Braunschweig, C., McCarthy, M. S., et al. (2016). Guidelines for the provision and assessment of nutrition support therapy in the adult critically ill patient. *Journal of Parenteral and Enteral Nutrition, 40*, 159–211. https://doi.org/10.1177/0148607115621863 (accessed on 28th June 2025).
31. Pierpont, M. E., Brueckner, M., Chung, W. K., Garg, V., Lacro, R. V., McGuire, A. L., Mital, S., et al. (2018). Genetic basis for congenital heart disease: Revisited: A scientific statement from the American Heart Association. *Circulation, 138*. https://doi.org/10.1161/cir.0000000000000606 (accessed on 28th June 2025).
32. Sakr, Y., Giovini, M., Léone, M., Pizzilli, G., Kortgen, A., Bauer, M., Tonetti, T., et al. (2020). Pulmonary embolism in patients with coronavirus disease-2019 (COVID-19) pneumonia: A narrative review. *Annals of Intensive Care, 10*. https://doi.org/10.1186/s13613-020-00741-0 (accessed on 28th June 2025).
33. Shah, Y. R., Cezar, C., Khan, H., Inamdar, S., Garcia Saenz De Sicilia, M., Deneke, M., & Rude, M. K. (2024). Metastatic jejunal adenocarcinoma in the hepatobiliary limb post-liver transplant: Diagnostic challenges in a patient with Roux-en-Y gastric bypass. *Gastrointestinal Disorders*. https://www.semanticscholar.org/paper/ced94000dbe8dd8a285fda53f8b9ad996a6f4ab0 (accessed on 28th June 2025).
34. Skeie, E., Tangvik, R. J., Såve Nymo, L., Harthug, S., Lassen, K., & Viste, A. (2019). Weight loss and BMI criteria in GLIM's definition of malnutrition is associated with postoperative complications following abdominal resections–Results from a national quality registry. *Clinical Nutrition, 39*, 1593–1599. https://doi.org/10.1016/j.clnu.2019.07.003 (accessed on 28th June 2025).

35. Swarm, R. A., Paice, J. A., Anghelescu, D. L., Are, M., Bruce, J. Y., Buga, S., Chwistek, M., et al. (2019). Adult cancer pain, version 3.2019, NCCN clinical practice guidelines in oncology. *Journal of the National Comprehensive Cancer Network, 17*, 977–1007. https://doi.org/10.6004/jnccn.2019.0038 (accessed on 28th June 2025).

36. Swindle, M., & Hughes, R. (2007). *Swine in the Laboratory: Surgery, Anesthesia, Imaging, and Experimental Techniques.* https://www.semanticscholar.org/paper/5823c68e22b7cc4fe8fdd1cb1263dcd434669da6 (accessed on 28th June 2025).

37. Taylor, B., McClave, S. A., Martindale, R. G., Warren, M., Johnson, D. R., Braunschweig, C., McCarthy, M. S., et al. (2016). Guidelines for the provision and assessment of nutrition support therapy in the adult critically ill patient. *Critical Care Medicine, 44*, 390–438. https://doi.org/10.1097/ccm.0000000000001525 (accessed on 28th June 2025).

38. Van der Merwe, R. L. J., van Wanrooij, M., Bronswijk, M., Everett, S., Lakhtakia, S., Rimbaş, M., Hucl, T., et al. (2021). Therapeutic endoscopic ultrasound: European Society of Gastrointestinal Endoscopy (ESGE) guideline. *Endoscopy, 54*, 185–205. https://doi.org/10.1055/a-1717-1391 (accessed on 28th June 2025).

39. Waller, P. G. (2012). Surgical delay for hip fracture clients and the use of clopidogrel: An integrative review. https://core.ac.uk/download/58824498.pdf (accessed on 28th June 2025).

40. Wick, E. C., Grant, M. C., & Wu, C. L. (2017). Postoperative multimodal analgesia pain management with nonopioid analgesics and techniques. *JAMA Surgery, 152*, 691–691. https://doi.org/10.1001/jamasurg.2017.0898 (accessed on 28th June 2025).

41. Wilson, W. R., Bower, T. C., Creager, M. A., Amin-Hanjani, S., O'Gara, P. T., Lockhart, P. B., Darouiche, R. O., et al. (2016). Vascular graft infections, mycotic aneurysms, and endovascular infections: A scientific statement from the American Heart Association. *Circulation, 134.* https://doi.org/10.1161/cir.0000000000000457 (accessed on 28th June 2025).

42. Zhang, Z., Dong, J., Lin, F., Wang, Q., Xu, Z., He, X., Zhang, C., et al. (2018). Current status of surgical treatment of biliary diseases in elderly patients in China. *Chinese Medical Journal, 131*, 1873–1876. https://doi.org/10.4103/0366-6999.237405 (accessed on 28th June 2025).

43. Zhou, J., Sun, H. C., Wang, Z., Cong, W. M., Wang, J., Zeng, M., Zhou, W., et al. (2020). Guidelines for the diagnosis and treatment of hepatocellular carcinoma (2019 edition). *Liver Cancer, 9*, 682–720. https://doi.org/10.1159/000509424 (accessed on 28th June 2025).

ANESTHESIA OUTSIDE THE OPERATING ROOM (NON-OR ANESTHESIA)

9

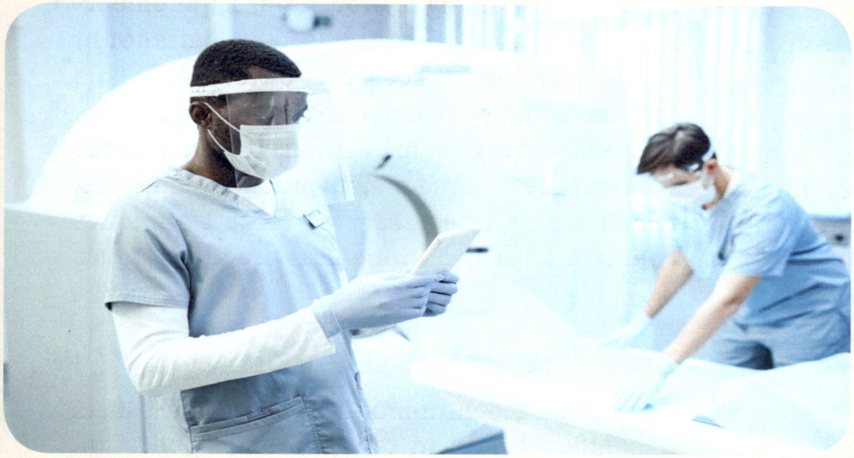

LEARNING OBJECTIVES

After studying this chapter, you will be able to:

1. Discuss the types of non-OR anesthesia
2. Focus on indications for non-OR anesthesia
3. Understand techniques used in non-OR anesthesia
4. Evaluate safety considerations
5 Know the training and qualifications of anesthesia providers
6. Focus on challenges and limitations

Introduction

The evolution of anesthesia has now taken a radical leap from the conventional operating room to usher in Non-OR Anesthesia. This evolution allows for a broad range of medical procedures in a wide range of settings, such as outpatient centers, emergency departments, and even intensive care units. Non-OR Anesthesia allows medical practitioners to deliver analgesia and sedation in spaces where patient comfort is important without compromising procedural efficiency. The application of general, local, and topical anesthetics in numerous operations underscores the adaptability and efficacy of the anesthetic techniques in non-surgical therapy, proving their right to a place in modern medicine. Use of anesthesia outside the operating room becomes ever more prized not only for its clinical value but also for its value in enhancing patient satisfaction and the optimization of healthcare resource utilization, bringing with it the potential for a broader focus on pain management and procedural sedation. The primary purpose of Non-OR Anesthesia is to achieve patient comfort and safety while providing effective treatment, especially in cases that do not require a full surgical procedure. Varying anesthetic medications employed in such centers, such as benzocaine, prilocaine, and lidocaine, are well established to be effective in the development of localized analgesia. These local anesthetics facilitate minimally invasive therapy by inhibiting pain and anxiety and allowing medical professionals to perform necessary interventions more smoothly and with lower degrees of discomfort to patients. Mechanisms by which these drugs function are reversible sodium channel blockade, inhibiting the conduction of pain signals, which is necessary in procedures requiring accuracy, i.e., dermatological procedures or dental procedures. Understanding the pharmacologic foundation of such anesthetics is essential to practitioners who seek to implement Non-OR Anesthesia effectively.

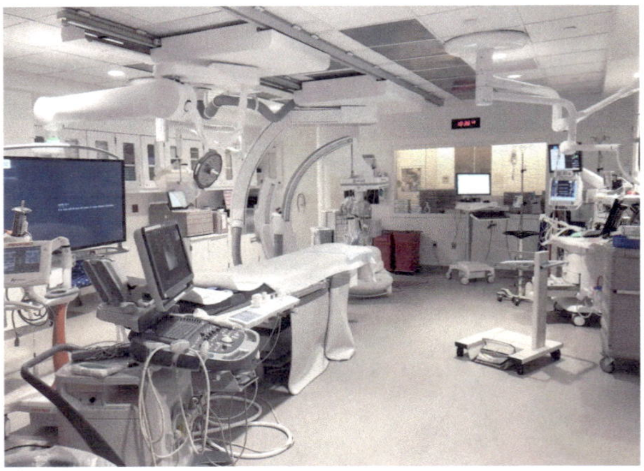

Figure 9.1. The evolution of anesthesia has significantly expanded beyond the traditional confines of the operating room.

Source: https://i0.wp.com/sambanew.dream.press/wp-content/uploads/2019/06/NORA-Interventional-Radiology-Suite-C-arm.jpg?fit=1030%2C773&ssl=1.

Moreover, the evolving literature on Non-OR Anesthesia is not merely highlighting its clinical advantages but also a few disadvantages encountered by practitioners. While advances in anesthetic techniques and the development of safer drugs have greatly helped improve outcomes, the inherent risk and adversity of non-operating rooms cannot be overlooked. Among the issues are patient monitoring, variability of response to anesthetics, and emergency preparedness in case of adverse effects. Therefore, ongoing training and education in anesthetic management, along with a full understanding of procedural requirements in various clinical settings, are paramount to optimizing successful outcomes. This interdisciplinary reaction to anesthesia outside of the operating room eventually mandates the continuance of research and practice guidelines, which are still necessary as these techniques continue to evolve in medical practice (Figure 9.1).

Definition of Non-OR Anesthesia

Increased recognition of Non-OR Anesthesia is a significant shift in the field and application of anesthesia practice. Non-OR Anesthesia is frequently practiced in diverse clinical settings outside of traditional operating rooms, such as outpatient operating rooms, dental offices, and interventional radiology suites. It is important in managing patient safety and comfort in cases that do not need the full-blown environment of an operating room. Application of Non-OR Anesthesia increases the scope of those procedures that can be performed safely and maximizes the utilization of resources at health facilities. By providing sedation for treatment and diagnostic procedures, it enables clinicians to continue providing a high standard of care, thus ensuring minimally invasive procedures are performed, focusing on patient-centered practices. The Non-OR Anesthesia is a set of various methods of sedation that concentrate on the patient's experience under treatment. Non-OR Anesthesia may be categorized as minimal, moderate, and deep sedation based on the level of consciousness and responsiveness achieved. In the majority of instances, anxiolytics and sedatives is significant, as can be seen through the widespread problem of dental anxiety (DA) among many patients. It is critical to understand how to handle DA since it is linked with medical emergencies that could be experienced outside the operating rooms. Thus, anesthesia professionals must assess each patient's requirements carefully in order to apply the most effective techniques, like iatrosedation and hypnosis combined with classical pharmacological agents, thereby establishing trust and reducing complications under their procedures (Facco & Zanette, 2017).

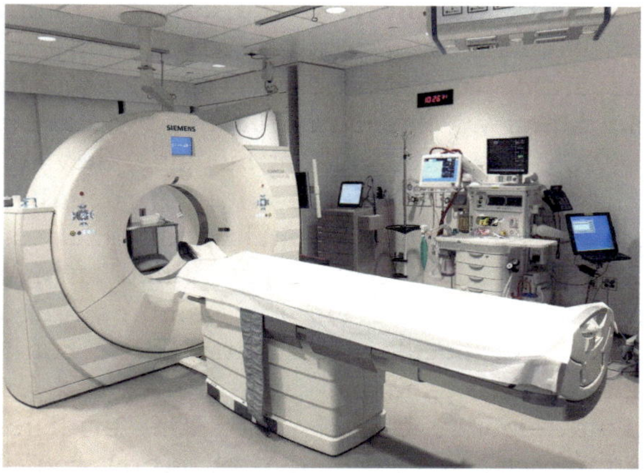

Figure 9.2. Increased recognition of non-OR anesthesia.

Source: https://i0.wp.com/sambanew.dream.press/wp-content/uploads/2019/06/NORA-Interventional-Radiology-Suite-CT.jpg?fit=1030%2C773&ssl=1.

Beyond adding to the levels of anxiety and patient satisfaction, Non-OR Anesthesia has far-reaching implications for the management of healthcare resources. With the added focus on outpatient procedures and minimally invasive surgery, the inclusion of Non-OR Anesthesia provides effective management of medical staff and equipment in a more flexible setup. Additional understanding of patient flows and the interdepartmental interactions within a hospital points to the necessity of coordinating anesthesia services. As noted in the latest literature, the integrated character of patient care pathways obliges anesthesia practitioners to consider how their own practice influences hospital operations as a whole (Vanberkel et al., 2010). This integrated vision eventually leads to enhanced patient outcomes and recognition of the vital role of Non-OR Anesthesia within the hectic environment of health care delivery (Figure 9.2).

Importance of Non-OR Anesthesia in Modern Medicine

The significance of Non-OR Anesthesia in modern medicine is brought to light by the fact that it can facilitate numerous procedures outside of standard surgical settings. By doing so, healthcare practitioners can perform diagnostic as well as treatment interventions comfortably and efficiently, usually within the outpatient department or emergency rooms. The ability to use anesthesia effectively beyond the operating room has revolutionized patient care practice by reducing the need for more involved surgical procedures and allowing patients to recover in a more cozy and familiar environment. With improvements in anesthetic drugs and monitoring devices, practitioners can now provide patient safety and comfort even in unconventional environments, greatly improving the patient experience and satisfaction. Besides, the development of Non-OR Anesthesia has also made a huge impact on resource planning among healthcare systems. With the utilization of non-OR locations, operating rooms in hospitals can be alleviated, which are normally in limited quantities. This trend not only processes the operation in a simplified fashion but also facilitates resource utilization in hospitals efficiently, ultimately leading to increased efficiency in patient handling. Because outpatient and same-day discharge surgeries are becoming increasingly popular, the administration of safe and efficient anesthesia in a setting other than the traditional operating room is paramount. Therefore, such a strategy ensures the maximization of the operational capability of healthcare centers without impairing patients' access to maximum care in a timely manner. Besides maximizing efficiency, Non-OR Anesthesia also ensures the solution of focused patient populations that can be maximally improved through anesthetic interventions outside surgery.

For instance, pediatric patient populations and those with certain comorbidities can find the surgery and operating room environment anxiety to be compounded. Non-OR Anesthesia provides for a less stressful and more welcoming alternative, allowing such at-risk populations to experience a positive health encounter. Moreover, this modality allows for the performance of endoscopies, radiology interventions, and pain management interventions that require sedation and analgesia but not complete surgical intervention. The inclusion of Non-OR Anesthesia in these practices is an indication of the dynamic nature of medical practice, the need for patient-centered practice, and the ongoing need for innovation in the healthcare sector (Vanberkel et al., 2010) (Figure 9.3).

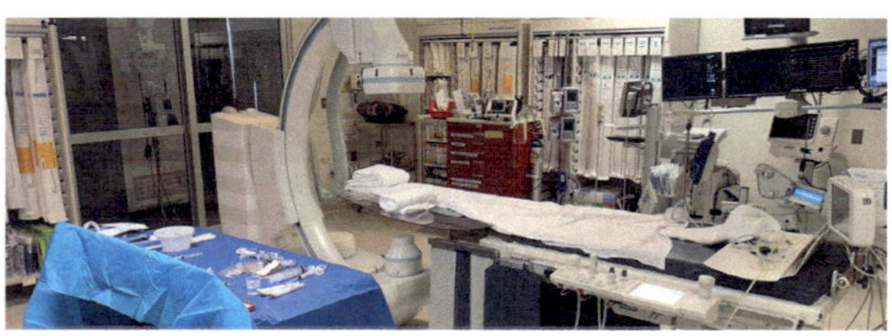

Figure 9.3. The significance of non-OR anesthesia in modern medicine.

Source: https://www.apsf.org/wp-content/uploads/newsletters/2019/3401/interventional-radiology-suite-2.jpg.

9.1. Types of Non-OR Anesthesia

Learning Outcome

1. Sedation for diagnostic procedures
2. Anesthesia in pain management clinics
3. Anesthesia for dental procedures

Non-operating room anesthesia practice comprises series of procedures intended to function in various medical environments, such as in outpatient facilities, imaging centers, and interventional procedures. A predominant type of non-OR anesthesia is the use of sedation on procedures that otherwise would be unbearable to patients, such as endoscopies and dental work. Sedation in these situations not only alleviates anxiety but also alleviates pain, producing more fluid procedural processes. In particular, multimodal analgesia techniques have increasingly gained favor in such settings, wherein the combination of several pharmacological agents is beneficial in that it offers enhanced pain control and less opioid dependence. As per existing evidence, multimodal regimens in non-OR settings consist of several classes of analgesics, which treat pain with success without the concurrent side effects of single opioid therapy (Schwenk & Mariano, 2018). Regional anesthetic techniques, including nerve blocks and spinal blocks, are paramount in non-OR environments, particularly in the management of pain cases. Regional anesthesia provides goal-directed analgesia, allowing patients to be provided with minimally invasive or outpatient procedures with fewer systemic effects than general anesthetics. For example, spinal anesthesia has been applied in operations such as inguinal hernia repair, whereby patient outcomes have been dramatically improved when elective operations are conducted under spinal or local anesthesia. Studies have revealed that elective herniorrhaphy under spinal anesthesia might yield decreased complication rates and recovery times versus general anesthesia (Kingsnorth et al., 2012). Furthermore, the technique of regional anesthesia reflects an increase in more patient-centered care, enabling faster rehabilitation and shorter hospitalization. Moreover, non-OR anesthesia has also expanded to include advanced techniques such as intravenous sedation and monitored anesthesia care (MAC). They provide more flexibility and higher safety for patients who undergo procedures in locations outside normal operating rooms. IV sedation allows professionals to administer anesthetics in a managed manner, addressing various levels of patient comfort and anxiety management. With observation, professionals can offer assurance for the safety of their patients while allowing procedures to proceed uninterrupted.

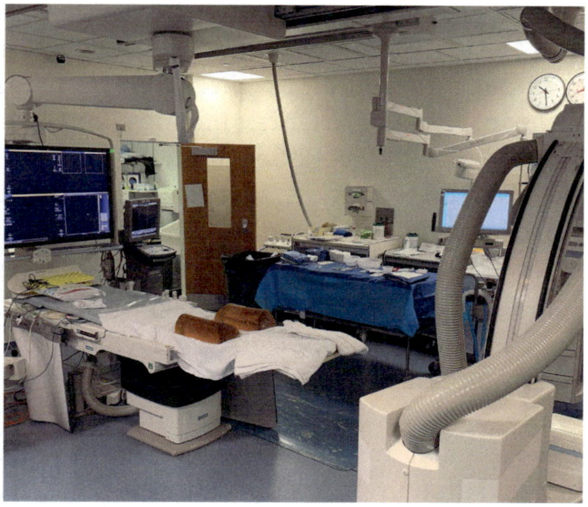

Figure 9.4. The practice of non-operating room anesthesia.

Source: https://www.apsf.org/wp-content/uploads/newsletters/2019/3401/interventional-radiology-suite.jpg.

This is especially important in outpatient clinics where high-volume patient flow is the standard. The integration of IV sedation and MAC puts non-OR anesthesia at the center of current medical practice, supporting many different kinds of surgery and diagnosis while providing maximum levels of care and comfort to patients (Figure 9.4).

9.1.1. Sedation for Diagnostic Procedures

Sedation of diagnostic interventions is a key area of Non-OR Anesthesia, facilitating patient comfort and procedural success. Several strategies of sedation are being used to manage anxiety and pain associated with invasive diagnostic tests such as endoscopies and radiologic imaging. Deep sedation, for instance, enables doctors to perform complex procedures with fewer opportunities for patient movement, which may compromise the quality of the diagnostic test. Comparison among different sedation regimens illustrates their efficacy; i.e., intermittent bolus (IB) sedation versus continuous infusion (CG) of propofol has been shown to achieve acceptable levels of sedation, with both regimens resulting in comparable safety outcomes and physiological stability in patients undergoing auditory brainstem response testing and nuclear medicine scans (Ahmed et al., 2017). In assessing sedation practice efficiency, research identifies differences in recovery and discharge rates in relation to different methods of delivery. Patients on continuous propofol infusion were found to recover faster, thus allowing for smoother patient flow in diagnostic settings. Results are an affirmation of the necessity to optimize sedation approaches for enhanced patient experience while ensuring diagnostic accuracy. Furthermore, shorter procedure times using the IB technique illustrate a potential advantage in outpatient procedures, in which saving sedation time is essential for timely discharge and enhanced access to care (Ahmed et al., 2017). Therefore, tailored sedation protocols truly have a significant impact on not just patient comfort but overall healthcare delivery in non-OR environments. In addition, the role of specialist anesthesia providers, i.e., dentist anesthesiologists, in providing sedation for diagnostic and therapeutic purposes is ever better documented. This group generally treats a younger demographic that requires complete dental assessments and stress alleviation from treatment. The efficacy of care provided by dentist anesthesiologists is particularly notable; office-based anesthesia for complete dental rehabilitation significantly reduces overall treatment time compared to more traditional hospital settings. In this way, as these experts codify sedation practices, they develop a body of evidence testifying to the efficacy and safety of Non-OR Anesthesia for a wide variety of diagnostic tests. The evolution of sedation expertise in this environment ultimately appears to generate improved patient outcomes, forming an evidentiary argument for implementing robust sedation protocols in multiple non-operating room venues.

9.1.2. Anesthesia in Pain Management Clinics

Anesthesia care in pain management clinics is a key component of improving the quality of life of patients when they experience chronic pain. Pain management clinics have developed as core non-operating room units in which multiple interventions, such as nerve blocks and epidural steroid injections, are performed to alleviate pain. Unlike an ordinary operating room, pain management clinics aim at maximizing patients' comfort and reducing discomfort during procedures. Anesthesiologists in such clinics are tasked with applying safe anesthetic techniques tailored to outpatient surgery while facilitating proper pain relief. This multifaceted process not only increases patient satisfaction but also reduces the use of general anesthetics, hence reducing complications due to more invasive surgery. In a combined environment, anesthesiologists and pain specialists can optimize patient outcomes through pre-arranged anesthetic management. In pain clinics, the choice of anesthetic medication is based on the type of pain, comorbidities of the patient, and the procedure to be performed. Regional anesthesia techniques, such as local anesthetics or sedation, are also frequently utilized based on their safety and efficacy. This method is particularly valuable since it allows for shortened recovery times and promotes outpatient therapy, which can generally return patients to normal functioning relatively soon after they have undergone their procedures. Ultrasound-guided methods have changed the method of delivering regional anesthesia, further improving its precision and efficacy. Studies indicate that the implementation of such methodologies in the management of pain not only improves anesthetic outcomes but also mitigates complications' occurrence, hence aligning with non-OR anesthesia goals (Sturges et al., 2013).

Pain management clinics also emphasize multidisciplinary coordination, which is paramount in handling the overall needs of chronic pain patients. In such settings, anesthesiologists collaborate with physical therapists, psychologists, and rehab specialists to provide an integrated treatment of pain. This collaborative philosophy enables them to develop personalized care plans that take into account the emotional, psychological, and physical aspects of pain. Through such a philosophical approach, pain management clinics are able to provide patients with more than anesthetic relief; they aim to restore the well-being of patients. Besides, communication among the healthcare team is essential in monitoring the success of anesthesia and adjusting treatment plans accordingly. This integrated approach prioritizes improved health outcomes, demanding that anesthesia beyond OR sites, such as pain management clinics, has a far larger mission than sedation or pain relief (Department of Anesthesia, University of Iowa, 2011) (Figure 9.5).

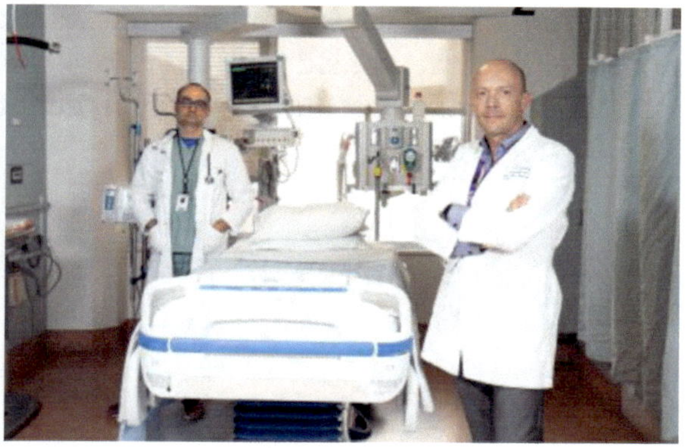

Figure 9.5. The provision of anesthesia in pain management clinics.

Source: https://unityhealth.to/wp-content/uploads/2021/03/unity_pain-e1616594895952-400x266.jpg.

9.1.3. Anesthesia for Dental Procedures

Dental treatment anesthesia is a significant aspect of modern dentistry to provide an improvement in patient comfort and pain mitigation during procedures. Various anesthesia procedures are used, especially for localized procedures such as endodontics, extractions, and implant placement, which occur outside the operating room (Non-OR Anesthesia). Regional anesthesia, such as the maxillary nerve block (MNB), is one of the techniques with a primary role to provide effective analgesia. Current Opinion, for instance, comparing high tuberosity and greater palatine canal approaches, shows that each approach has significant patient comfort and satisfaction. Such findings demonstrate how anesthesia not only functions to alleviate pain in some regions but also is crucial for enhancing the overall patient experience and compliance in dental procedures (Bacci et al., 2018). The application of general anesthesia to dentistry, particularly in children or special needs patients, raises the importance of tailoring anesthesia techniques to patient types. For instance, studies comparing treatment sessions between healthy children and medically compromised or developmentally disabled children uncover significant differences in treatment time and complexity of procedure under general anesthesia. Healthier children were more likely to require more extensive dental treatments, involving longer intervention durations, compared to their medically unstable counterparts, illustrating the way that anesthesia is tailored on the basis of patient status of health and unique individual clinical circumstances (Loyola-Rodriguez et al., 2009). This special treatment not only enhances the efficacy of dental treatment but also attempts to prevent potential complications associated with inoperative settings.

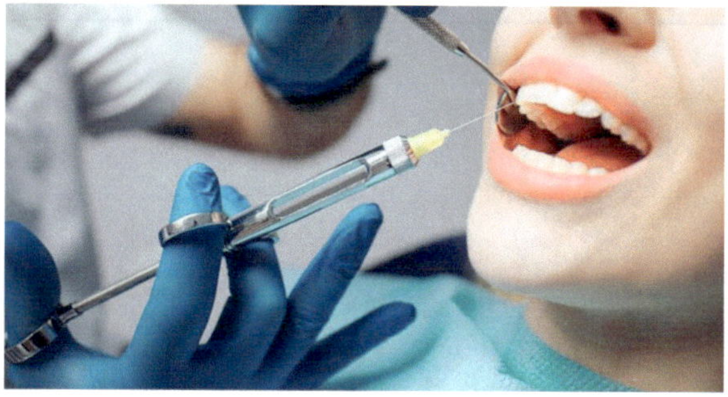

Figure 9.6. Anesthesia for dental procedures.

Source: https://euro-dent.be/wp-content/uploads/elementor/thumbs/Dental-Anesthesia-Types-Uses-Side-effects-qbrjlqtryqarfvz8lnjhwak86hk83vb5huj0cia5jc.jpg.

Moreover, the evolution of non-OR anesthesia has helped improve patient outcomes and satisfaction. Techniques that promote patient safety without compromising comfort, such as the combination of anxiolytics with local anesthetics, demonstrate the dynamic nature of dental anesthetic practice. The preventive approach to anesthetic administration with increasing vigilance for susceptible patients is essential to provide a satisfactory dental experience. The low complication rates and high patient satisfaction levels found in a number of studies are a testament to the value of considerate application of anesthesia techniques in dentistry. This considerate attention to anesthesia techniques, as seen through techniques like regional blocks and the considerate application of general anesthesia, shows the interactive harmony of patient care and procedural success in dental medicine (Bacci et al., 2018; Loyola-Rodriguez et al., 2009) (Figure 9.6).

Test Your Knowledge

1. What are common settings where non-OR anesthesia is used?
2. Name one type of anesthesia commonly administered outside the operating room.

9.2. Indications for Non-OR Anesthesia

Learning Outcome

1. Patient anxiety and comfort
2. Minimally invasive procedures
3. Chronic pain management

Non-operating room (Non-OR) anesthesia is increasingly used due to the increasing need for a variety of procedures needing anesthetic care outside the conventional surgical setting. Procedural sedation is among the important indications for Non-OR anesthesia and has gained extensive application in settings such as endoscopy, interventional radiology, and dentistry. These interventions often involve a level of sedation that can minimize patient discomfort and anxiety while facilitating good pain control, hence enhancing the patient's overall experience. Accurate use of local anesthetics and sedatives gives clinicians a means of performing complicated procedures with acceptable risks associated with general anesthesia, particularly in patients who may have contraindications to more invasive forms of anesthesia. Hence, awareness regarding the nuances of Non-OR anesthesia use is crucial for improving the success of procedures and patient safety in numerous specialties. Other than procedural sedation, Non-OR anesthesia can effectively administer the anesthetic needs of patients who are undergoing certain diagnostic procedures. A good example would be patients who are undergoing magnetic resonance imaging (MRI), which makes them anxious due to the enclosed space and long scanning process. In these cases, mild sedation administration can assist in keeping patients quiet and comfortable during examination, thereby enhancing the quality of diagnostic results. Research indicates that adjunctive anesthesia assists in sufficiently reducing anxiety, pain, and discomfort in procedures, thereby leading to greater patient compliance. Non-OR anesthetic techniques are beneficial to both patients and healthcare professionals since they make procedures simpler and less complicated, reducing the need for further diagnostic imaging due to motion artifacts. Identification of the indications maximizes healthcare resource use within healthcare systems and enhances patient satisfaction. Another important indication for Non-OR anesthesia includes its application in managing pain during obstetric procedures, particularly labor and delivery. Methods, like perineural blocks and epidural anesthesia, have become the focal point for pain relief administration, allowing women in labor to give birth in more comfort. These methods offer a wide range of maternal and fetal monitoring without compromising the mother's ability to remain actively engaged in the birthing process.

Besides, Non-OR anesthesia has progressively embraced newer methods and medications that offer better analgesia with fewer side effects, further expanding its practice in obstetrics. With this continued development in the specialty, clinicians must remain updated with new techniques and standards of practice to effectively manage pain in non-OR settings. This ongoing growth emphasizes the central role of anesthesia in enhancing patient care across many medical specialties and underscores the importance of continued research and education in this essential area of healthcare.

9.2.1. Patient Anxiety and Comfort

Patient anxiety stands at the core of the patient experience of patients undergoing non-OR anesthesia, with significant effects on surgical outcomes and, ultimately, patient comfort. The clinical environment, which is normally noisy and disorganized, fosters significant fear when patients have to stay awake for a procedure. Research has underscored that patients become anxious because of aspects such as the knowledge that they are awake, having the feeling that surgery is taking place, and the fear of pain, all of which enhance pain in what otherwise is a less stressful, localized surgery (Mitchell, 2008). Accordingly, medical experts need to know these causative factors for anxiety and act in advance to reverse them. Through the creation of an understanding environment and clear communication to de-mystify the experience, practitioners can successfully reduce patient anxiety, enhancing the overall experience and satisfaction. One of the important tools in patient anxiety management regarding non-OR anesthesia has also been identified as communication. A clear explanation of the procedure, how anesthesia works, and what can be expected by patients can effectively calm the fears that they face before surgery. Insufficient information, however, will likely lead to heightened anxiety because patients feel threatened or fearful about their condition (Mitchell , 2008). Communication, listening to the patient's fears, and offering reassurance are basic interventions that can be utilized by medical staff to alleviate anxiety. Free-flowing communication not only breeds confidence but also empowers the patients, making them active agents in their own health care. Through a consideration of these psychological and emotional factors, practitioners can offer a more supportive environment for patients undergoing procedures outside of the typical operating rooms.

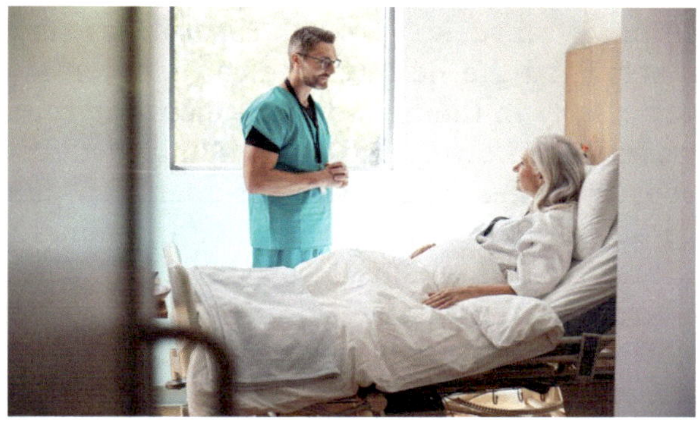

Figure 9.7. Patient anxiety plays a critical role in the overall experience of those undergoing non-OR anesthesia.

Source: https://b764203.smushcdn.com/764203/wp-content/uploads/BaxterAssociatesLLC-279543-Reassure-Anxious-Patients-blogbanner1-825x510.jpg?lossy=0&strip=1&webp=1.

The ethical dimensions of patient comfort and anxiety should not be overlooked, particularly with vulnerable populations such as children. In pediatric settings, holding or restraining procedures are typically a decision that provokes moral distress among parents and healthcare providers equally, considering the natural conflict between procedural expediency and the child's autonomy. This underscores the importance of acknowledging children's rights and the importance of promoting their comfort, which is sacrificed when coercive interventions are used during clinical encounters. Therefore, establishing guidelines that respect children's voices and decisions is essential in both reducing anxiety and enhancing their overall experience. By making sure that doctors consider these moral standards when providing non-OR anesthesia, patient satisfaction and comfort can be significantly increased, and eventually develop a kinder and patient-centered healthcare system (Figure 9.7).

9.2.2. Minimally Invasive Procedures

Minimally invasive procedures (MIPs) have transformed the field of medical intervention, particularly in the field of non-operating room anesthesia. Lower patient trauma, reduced recovery times, and less post-operative pain are all possible with the smaller incisions or natural orifices of such procedures compared to traditional interventions. As a result, anesthesia practice in such settings has been altered to accommodate the patients as well as practitioners themselves, with increased emphasis on safety and comfort. For instance, local anesthetics applied topically, such as lidocaine and prilocaine, are utilized to minimize pain when there are endoscopies or biopsies, and patient consciousness is effectively preserved by analgesia. The position of local anesthesia as a main part in MIPs has a significant impact on patient outcome, as evidenced by research acknowledging the decreased complication rate because of decreased surgical trauma and effective anesthesia control (Cantisani et al., 2014). Furthermore, the application of newer monitoring technology has enhanced anesthesia care in minimally invasive procedures. With no requirement for invasive lines, continuous measurement of cardiac output and other vital signs with non-invasive devices, such as the qCO monitor, allows for real-time management decision-making in anesthesia. With these breakthroughs, practitioners can more effectively optimize hemodynamics and ensure patient safety and comfort during the procedure. Calibration of these devices establishes their ability to provide accurate readings that guide anesthesia delivery and support patient management (Escrivá et al., 2016). As a result, innovation in monitoring technologies is important in enhancing the anesthetic practice involved with MIPs towards the end of reducing perioperative adverse effects and promoting recovery. Minimally invasive procedures are numerous in their benefits but also present unique challenges in the field of anesthesia. The anesthetic method selected must balance the severity of the intervention against the effectiveness of the analgesia and the compliance of the patient. Proceduralists in specific cases may opt for sedation in addition to local anesthesia, which must be handled with caution to avoid over-sedation or interference with the airway. Practitioners must also be competent at recognizing patient-specific variables affecting the choice of an anesthetic, such as comorbidities or the degree of anxiety. The work of anesthesiologists in such settings is more than dispensing medication; they must also conduct thorough preoperative assessments and provide consultation on the procedure to ensure the optimal outcome. In that respect, enhancing inter-disciplinary coordination between surgery teams and anesthesiologists ensures the efficacy of procedures and the safety of patients as MIPs gain prominence in current clinical practices.

9.2.3. Chronic Pain Management

Management of chronic pain is a complex process that needs a multi-modal strategy, particularly in the setting of non-operating room (non-OR) anesthesia techniques. Inclusion of various therapeutic modalities like pharmacological agents, physical therapy, and psychotherapy is a complex strategy to treat the complex nature of chronic pain. Use of non-OR anesthesia can enhance the quality of life in patients with chronic pain by providing an acceptable pain relief experience at outpatient settings. It allows the patients to conduct their normal activities with decreased pain, thus promoting better general health results. Secondly, the offering of non-OR anesthesia care can also help to avoid the rampant issue of opioid dependency, providing a useful substitute for those seeking relief for chronic pain. Non-OR anesthesia is also a highly significant element in pediatric pain management procedures. Techniques such as distraction through cognitive interventions, i.e., the presence of Clown Doctors, have been found to be more than mere anesthetic procedures. Although the evidence indicates minimal impact on the anxiety of children before surgery, the results, caregivers paint a different picture. Reduced caregiver anxiety is linked to reduced functional health problems along with the presence of supportive interventions such as Clown Doctors, showing the importance of addressing emotional health in addition to physical pain management (Arriaga & Pacheco, 2016). This highlights the importance of innovative solutions in non-OR environments that target both child and caregiver experience. Besides, education and communication are also central to chronic pain treatment, particularly with the use of non-OR anesthesia. Educating the patients and families fully about the process and available alternatives is an important determinant for the alleviation of pain- and anxiety-related issues. This proactive involvement empowers the patient, facilitating ease in understanding the treatment procedures and adherence to prescribed therapy. The University of Iowa Anesthesia Department has recognized the necessity for such educational programs, noting efforts to integrate comprehensive pain management protocols into outpatient clinical practices (Department of Anesthesia, University of Iowa, 2011). With collaboration between healthcare professionals and patients, non-OR anesthesia practices have the greatest opportunity to maximize the effectiveness of chronic pain management methods and enhance patient satisfaction and outcomes (Figure 9.8).

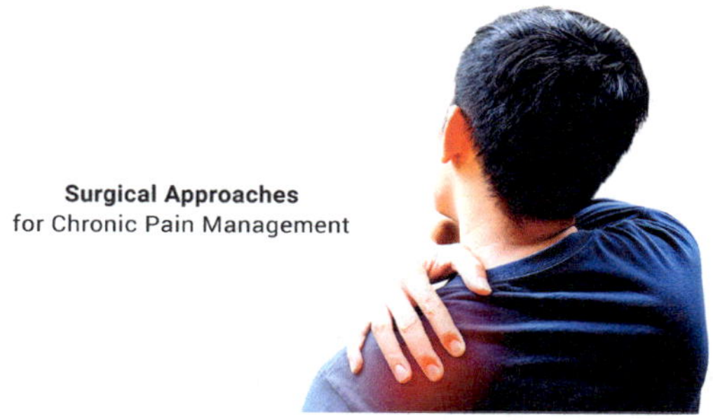

Figure 9.8. Chronic pain management is a complex endeavor that necessitates a multifaceted approach.

Source: https://www.eternalhospital.com/uploadedfiles/gallery/1689326006_1300-x-700-Surgical-Approaches-for-Chronic-Pain-Management.jpg.

Test Your Knowledge

1. What are typical procedures that require non-OR anesthesia?
2. Why might a patient need anesthesia outside the operating room?

9.3. Techniques Used in Non-OR Anesthesia

Learning Outcome

1. Intravenous sedation
2. Local anesthesia
3. Regional anesthesia

Non-OR anesthesia has been established with a number of techniques that are appropriate to the individual patient's requirements outside of the hospital operating room setting. The most popular method is the use of local anesthesia, which allows localized pain relief for minor procedures. It is especially successful in dental procedures, as it is utilized by specialty anesthesiologists for dentists. Their unique role to provide general anesthesia in office settings has revealed a deep impact compared to hospital-based routines, particularly for the treatment of child patients with long dental procedures for disorders such as early childhood caries (Saxen et al., 2017). Using localized anesthetics or sedation methods, practitioners can reduce the invasiveness of the procedures, minimize recovery periods, and enhance patient comfort, hence local anesthesia is an integral technique in Non-OR applications. Sedation is also a critical technique employed in Non-OR anesthesia aimed at decreasing anxiety while ensuring patient responsiveness. Sedation can range from light to deep depending on the procedural requirements and patient needs. This modality is commonplace in many outpatient centers, including endoscopy or interventional radiology, where fast patient turnover is necessary. Real-time monitoring and adjustment of the amount of sedation provides flexibility and responsivity in practice for clinicians. Moreover, new technology developments, such as telemedicine decision support systems, have begun to play a role in enhancing the safety and effectiveness of such sedation procedures (Saxen et al., 2017). With smoother communication and patient management methods, these technologies provide improved outcomes for Non-OR anesthesia procedures, with superior levels of care. Lastly, regional anesthesia has been found to have a diverse application in Non-OR settings because it achieves pain control with fewer systemic side effects. Nerve blocks are increasingly becoming popular for outpatient surgeries because they achieve deep analgesia while minimizing general anesthetic use. The application of this technique is particularly valuable in managing postoperative pain and hence achieves faster recovery times as well as less hospitalization. The flexibility of the method applies in many procedural environments, from orthopedic procedures to pain clinic settings, where specific nerves are entered to provide relief from discomfort. Despite research being mentioned on the success and unique nature of such anesthesia methods, the fact is that non-OR methods are crucial in ensuring patient comfort and procedural success, which ultimately enhances the experience for both patients and practitioners (Saxen et al., 2017).

9.3.1. Intravenous Sedation

Intravenous sedation has emerged as a critical component of the practice of anesthesia outside the operating suite, particularly in dental and outpatient surgery. With the administration of drugs like propofol and midazolam, physicians can achieve levels of sedation that are appropriate to patient demand. The controlled administration of these sedative medications allows physicians to provide for patient comfort while also facilitating required diagnostic and therapeutic maneuvers. Notably, intravenous sedation is particularly useful in populations that can be more anxious or require prolonged therapy since it can frequently minimize the psychological load of medical procedures. By carefully controlling the levels of sedation, practitioners are able to achieve a subtle interplay between patient safety and procedure efficiency, an important consideration in non-OR settings where rapid turnaround and effectiveness are often paramount. The methodology of administration in itself plays a significant role in the success of intravenous sedation. Continuous infusion and intermittent bolus administration are found to be two popular methods with advantages and disadvantages. A recent study comparing the two modalities reflected no significant differences between patient demographics, as well as cardiovascular and respiratory parameters, which suggested that both modalities can be utilized successfully in a wide population of patients. But the constant infusion method required longer procedure time at the cost of no compromise in the quality of sedation as perceived by the patient, evidenced by an increased mean total dose of propofol in the group. This information tells us that while practitioners will have longer procedural times, the enhanced depth of sedation control with constant infusion can lead to improved patient outcomes in non-OR settings (Ahmed et al., 2017). Moreover, intravenous sedation usage has been discovered to vary significantly with the demographics of patients, particularly between individuals who are healthy and patients with medical or developmental conditions. One study assessing dental treatment under general anesthesia discovered huge variations in the amount and duration of treatment completed for these two groups of patients. Healthy children required more interventions and longer periods of working time compared to their medically impaired counterparts, which highlights the need for condition-specific sedation protocols. These findings demonstrate the importance of thorough pre-procedure assessment in determining the most appropriate sedation protocols. In light of continued advancements in non-OR anesthetic practices, these differences are crucial to recognize to improve patient care and optimize sedation protocols (Loyola-Rodriguez et al., 2009) (Figure 9.9).

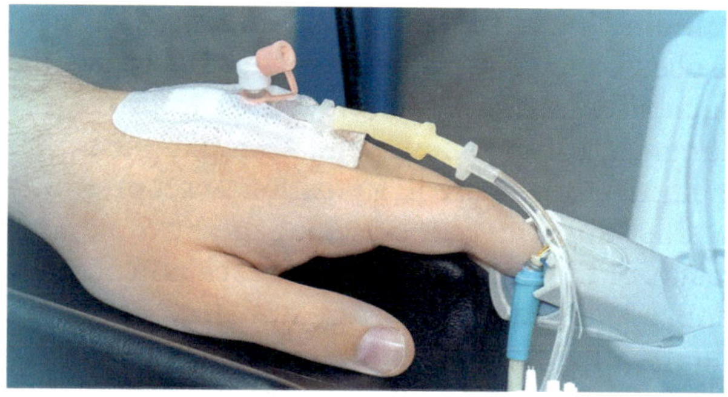

Figure 9.9. Intravenous sedation has emerged as a critical component in the realm of anesthesia outside the operating room.

Source: https://windycityanesthesia.com/wp-content/uploads/2022/08/4-Great-Benefits-of-Intravenous-Sedation-IV-blog-min.jpg.

9.3.2. Local Anesthesia

In non-operating room anesthesia, local anesthesia plays an important role, particularly in outpatient and minimally invasive procedures. Local anesthesia refers to the administration of anesthetic drugs to a specific body region, theoretically eliminating the sensation within the local area without affecting the overall awareness of the patients. This approach is highly useful in non-OR settings since it allows rapid recovery and circumvents the need for prolonged monitoring that normally follows general anesthesia. By providing relief of pain to the intervention site, local anesthesia facilitates a wide array of procedures, such as dental work, dermatological procedures, and even some orthopedic examinations, whereby patients are able to go about their normal activities very quickly with less pain. Evidence of the efficacy and use of local anesthesia in non-OR settings is provided by improved monitoring and tracking systems that supplement patient care in these types of procedures. For example, platforms such as INCOMING! provide real-time monitoring of patient status from the time a patient is given local anesthesia until recovery. These platforms use manual timestamps and are designed to combine data streams from multiple clinical processes to gain context-sensitive information. Such integration is employed to improve the handling of workflows and to make sure that medical workers are in a position to act promptly against any emergencies that might arise as a result of the administration of local anesthesia. Improved patient tracking not only enhances safety but also maximizes the efficiency of outpatient healthcare services so that clinics can treat more people with less equipment. Additionally, the subject of local anesthesia is also its effect on healthcare administration and policy. With ongoing pursuits towards low-cost and efficient care, local anesthesia presents itself as a reasonable choice in decreasing resource utilization while maintaining maximum levels of patient safety and satisfaction. The inclusion of advanced monitoring systems also aids providers in providing an efficient mechanism towards patient care, as seen with the development of integrated perioperative systems to maximize access to real-time data related to patient readiness and physiological data. As explicated in the broader debate about the efficacy and accessibility of healthcare organizations, understanding and implementation of effective local anesthesia strategies in non-OR settings positions healthcare practitioners in a positive position to meet increasing demands of modern medical practice while simultaneously enhancing patient outcomes and satisfaction (Meyer, 2006; Bonica, 2017).

9.3.3. Regional Anesthesia

Regional anesthesia use has gained popularity as a significant modality in anesthesiology practice, particularly in settings other than the conventional operating room. Regional anesthesia is characterized as techniques that suggest injection of an anesthetic drug along a group of nerves that causes momentary insensibility in a localized region of the body. It is being used more in the outpatient setting, as well as pain management centers or in association with surgical procedures in emergency rooms. The process not only contributes to patient comfort but also reduces recovery and the need for systemic narcotics, which can reduce the risk of opioid dependence. Thus, regional anesthesia can make a difference in patient care by virtue of strategic utilization in providing appropriate analgesia along with optimizing surgical technique and mitigating the cumulative burden on hospital resources, especially in the context of an evolving healthcare milieu where efficiency is the catchword. Additionally, the utilization of regional anesthesia in non-OR settings necessitate strict training and awareness of its techniques and complications attendant thereto. Clinicians must be well-versed in a variety of regional anesthesia methods, such as nerve blocks or epidurals, and their appropriate usages based on patient needs and procedural considerations. These are skillful techniques, and inappropriate performance has adverse effects such as nerve injury or systemic toxicity. With recent studies, optimizing equipment and monitoring equipment for regional anesthesia has also enhanced its safety and effectiveness. For instance, advanced monitoring systems provide immediate feedback regarding hemodynamic stability under regional block procedures, thereby enabling practitioners to make rational decisions based on dynamic cardiac parameters such as cardiac output and systemic blood flow, as evident in recent research on non-invasive monitoring devices that enhance patient safety during anesthesia care (Escrivá et al., 2016). The expansion of regional anesthesia outside the operating room also fits with greater efforts to improve the results and satisfaction of patients. Research has indicated that adequate pain control with regional techniques may reduce postoperative complications and reduce recovery time, which are prime issues in the contemporary health system focused on value-based care. By adopting regional anesthesia, clinicians are able to deliver tailored pain management strategies that can be tailored to the individual's profile, thus driving personalized medicine. Moreover, the evidence-based introduction of regional anesthesia protocols across specialties has the potential to alleviate operating room pressures and enable more cases to be managed outside of the operating room. These advancements underscore the pivotal position of regional anesthesia within the broader context of non-OR anesthesia, fueling innovation and raising the general level of care in highly complex healthcare environments (Hulshof et al., 2012) (Figure 9.10).

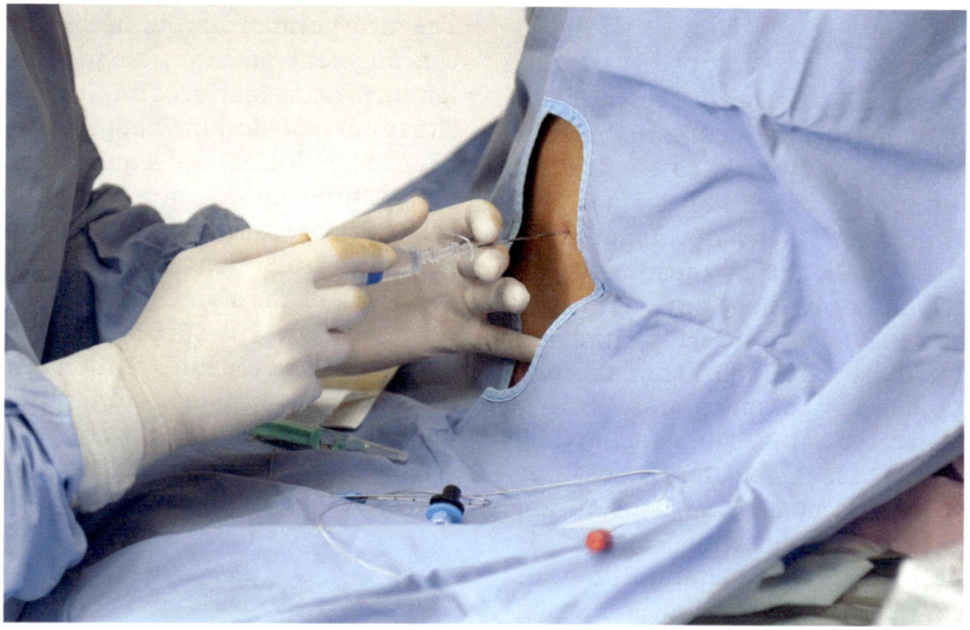

Figure 9.10. The use of regional anesthesia.

Source: https://www.verywellhealth.com/thmb/YwoG7Rb7TaAEUUS1pxNEMCUEcvQ=/1500x0/filters:no_upscale():max_bytes(150000):strip_icc()/GettyImages-154725435-59a034a50d327a001006171b.jpg.

Test Your Knowledge

1. What anesthetic techniques are commonly used in non-OR settings?
2. Why is sedation often preferred over general anesthesia in non-OR procedures?

9.4. Safety Considerations

Learning Outcome

1. Monitoring and equipment requirements
2. Risk assessment and patient selection
3. Emergency protocols and preparedness

Safety in non-OR anesthesia is a top concern, given the expanding role of anesthesia outside of the operating room. With cases finding their way out of the operating room, solid safety protocols need to be developed that will address the challenge of these settings. Unlike traditional operating environments, non-OR settings may lack essential monitoring equipment and improved support staff, thereby representing risks for complications. Having standards comparable to those implemented by accreditation agencies for ambulatory procedures can enhance safety outcomes. Clinician-clinician and clinician-expert-accreditation committees can help determine safety standards that support patient well-being without overly taxing practitioners, with the complexity of delivering care across various settings increasing (Berglas & Roberts, 2018). Demographic shifts towards an older population also complicate considerations of safety for non-OR anesthesia. Geriatric patients are more likely to have specialized vulnerabilities that need to be dealt with by raising vigilance in anesthesia management. Postoperative residual neuromuscular blockade, which is a state with the ability to produce severe complications like airway obstruction or respiratory failure, occurs more frequently among this group (Carron et al., 2017). As such, personal measures in neuromuscular blockade must be taken, including the cautious use of reversal agents and careful monitoring during the procedure. Anesthesiologists are required to balance the risks in managing elderly patients with the requirements of providing effective anesthesia and taking all precautions in advance to formulate the safest possible strategies in non-OR settings. To ensure optimal patient safety, continuous training and education of anesthesia professionals are essential. The unique environments in the non-OR settings require practitioners' extensive knowledge of the potential complications and emergency protocols that may apply across a range of practice settings. The incorporation of routine simulation training can augment anesthesiologists' preparedness for surprise scenarios, bridging gaps in non-OR situation-specific knowledge. Also, the use of new technologies and equipment utilized for the monitoring of patients in other settings can mitigate safety outcomes significantly. Regulation of open communication between members of the non-OR procedure healthcare team that governs support for a collaborative approach to safety intervention ultimately ends in achieving a vigilance culture that focuses on patients' safety and health, receiving anesthesia outside the traditional operating room (Berglas & Roberts, 2018) (Figure 9.11).

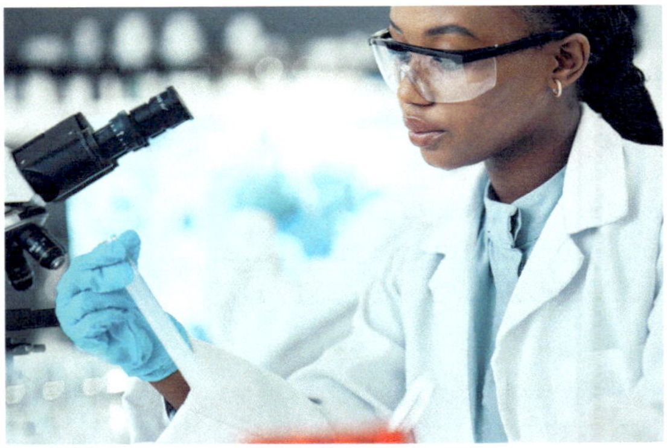

Figure 9.11. Safety considerations in non-OR anesthesia are paramount.

Source: https://www.cdc.gov/candida-auris/media/images/2024/03/GettyImages-1729701915.jpg.

9.4.1. Monitoring and Equipment Requirements

Non-OR Anesthesia setting entails a difficult environment requiring close monitoring and equipment parameters to deliver safe patient care. Most importantly, utilization of procedural sedation has increased, with an in-depth examination of current monitoring procedures. A recent study indicates there are discrepancies in state regulation and personnel training participating in the administration of sedation, causing potential knowledge gaps and practice variation, threatening the well-being of patients. These complications underscore the importance of adhering to set guidelines, such as the AORN's guidelines, which require comprehensive monitoring procedures under sedation. Use of capnography for monitoring ventilation in real-time, along with the use of standardized recovery assessment measures, are some of the best practices required in minimizing risks in Non-OR facilities (Martin, 2016). Effective monitoring has to extend beyond just basic vital signs, involving a more sophisticated model that considers both the physical and psychological status of patients undergoing sedation. This involves pre-procedure patient education and the creation of objective criteria to determine recovery readiness. The inclusion of the Aldrete discharge readiness assessment tool, for instance, is imperative in determining when it will be safe to discharge a patient from a monitored setting. Institutional policies should comply with these instruments to create an environment that supports patient safety. Additionally, increased training initiatives to enhance nurses' knowledge of sedation medications and practices are essential in closing current gaps and providing adherence to a shared standard of care in Non-OR anesthesia procedures (Gozal & Mason, 2010). As the pediatric sedation case illustrates, Non-OR Anesthesia's nuances are compounded by variations between local and national guidelines for the dispensation of sedatives. Where varying specialties vary in credentialing and training standards, the solution lies in an overarching set of standards. Inconsistencies like these can yield inconsistent practice, necessitating a concerted effort from sedation practitioners to standardize guidelines and adapt them to fit specific cases. This collaboration addresses not just the issue of equipment requirements but also tries to create an integrated system that tries to put patient safety first, irrespective of the sedation context. Standardization of monitoring and equipment standards across specialties in the 21st century remains an ongoing process in need of active participation from the wider sedation community to develop guidelines universally applicable (Gozal & Mason, 2010).

9.4.2. Risk Assessment and Patient Selection

Risk evaluation and patient selection throughout the process of anesthesia outside the operating room (Non-OR Anesthesia) are critical to ensuring patient safety and optimal outcomes. Anesthesia delivered in non-traditional settings necessitates a comprehensive understanding of patient-specific concerns, including comorbidities, history of anesthesia, and type of surgical procedure or intervention. Effective risk assessment assists anesthesiologists in identifying patients who will be susceptible to side effects and complications, allowing for personalized practice of anesthesia and minimizing risk. With this dynamic arrangement, interprofessional collaboration is also essential. Anesthesiologists must perform interprofessional communication in order to mitigate potential risks and come up with a collaborative plan that adheres to best practice in patient safety. The postoperative pain management has a direct relation with the elements of risk assessment and selection of the patient. Studies demonstrate that unrelieved pain could lead to severe complications, particularly in those patients who have opioid use histories, as these are more likely to be more sensitive to pain and at increased risk of chronic pain development (Wenzel et al., 2016). The challenge with such patients is to strike a balance between the need for adequate analgesia and the avoidance of adverse effects of opioid use. Anesthesiology professionals must critically evaluate each patient's unique circumstances and develop an all-encompassing perioperative analgesic plan using multimodal strategies. The strategy not only enhances patient satisfaction but also markedly decreases factors associated with inadequate pain control. Furthermore, the evolving nature of healthcare calls for risk assessment models to capture the multidimensionality of heterogeneous patient populations that often present in non-OR settings. The patients with comorbidities require a sophisticated understanding of how their diseases influence outcomes for anesthesia delivery and recovery in general. As quoted in recent interdisciplinary education training programs, students in health management are being taught to analyze and manage healthcare organizations effectively (Bonica, 2017). This educational emphasis highlights the importance of having a team approach to anesthetic care, ensuring that patient selection considers all relevant health information. Through continuous education and risk assessment process utilization, anesthesia professionals can enhance both the safety and efficiency of non-OR anesthesia care.

9.4.3. Emergency Protocols and Preparedness

In Non-OR Anesthesia, smooth emergency protocols should be established properly to ensure patient safety and optimal outcomes. These protocols must have a properly defined response to unanticipated complications that may arise during procedures outside the normal operating room setup. Emergency preparation of the anesthesia practitioners for situations involving airway management and techniques for rapid resuscitation is necessary. For instance, professionals need to learn how to apply emergency drugs and devices that are present in non-OR environments. With the simulation of various clinical cases, including those on extreme adverse incidents, clinical practitioners become ready and confident enough to act in time. The lessons learned from prior emergencies, i.e., mass casualty events, have a tendency to emphasize the necessity for adaptable and scalable procedures that can be integrated into operational procedures so that teams are able to work in coordination when emergencies arise (Tobias et al., 2020). Approaches to preparedness will need to consider the unique challenges of anesthesia outside the operating room, including diverse environments and populations of patients. Having enough resources, such as personal protective equipment and necessary supplies, is vital to reducing risk under procedures. Constant checking of their stock is essential for hospitals to implement systems that guarantee the supply of all necessary materials, especially during unprecedented circumstances, such as the COVID-19 pandemic. For instance, effective triage protocols can enable surgical teams to set priorities while conserving manpower and retaining essential resources, as has been witnessed in recent experiences where operating room volumes were significantly reduced from overwhelming levels (Lancaster et al., 2020). Improved interdepartmental communication and coordination enable healthcare facilities to enhance overall preparedness for emergencies, ultimately leading to high-quality care of patients in unexpected occurrences. The success of emergency procedures hinges not only on official plans but also on a culture of preparedness and safety within the field of anesthesia professionals. Such a culture encourages continuous learning and engagement with responsive protocols based on experience and case histories. Encouraging interdisciplinarity may also assist in streamlining such protocols and overall patient safety. Practice runs and simulations of high-stress emergency situations prepare anesthesia practitioners to better manage the complexities of practice outside the operating room. Furthermore, critical reviews of past emergency performances assist in identifying areas of insufficient preparation and provoke ongoing improvement of response strategies. By embracing a proactive role in emergency preparedness, healthcare groups can ensure they are responsive and adaptable, thereby safeguarding patient well-being in diverse settings where anesthesia is administered, upholding the core concepts of quality care and safety throughout the continuum of anesthesia practice (Figure 9.12).

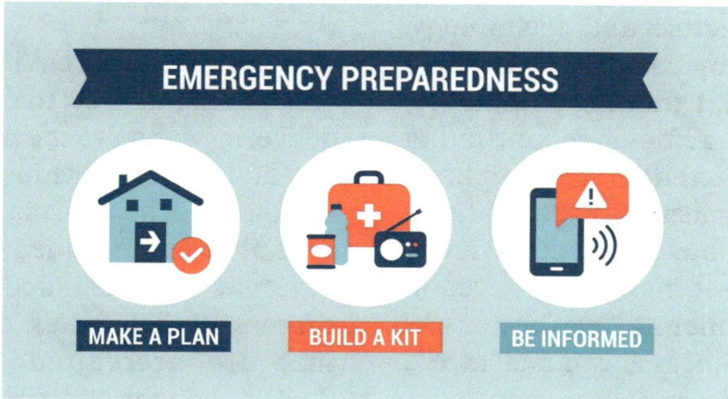

Figure 9.12. The establishment of effective emergency protocols is paramount to ensuring patient safety and optimal outcomes.

Source: https://cityofslt.us/ImageRepository/Document?documentId=17644.

Test Your Knowledge

1. What key factors should be evaluated when selecting a patient for anesthesia outside the operating room?
2. Why must emergency preparedness and contingency plans be in place during nonOR anesthesia procedures?

9.5. Training and Qualifications of Anesthesia Providers

Learning Outcome

1. Education and certification requirements
2. Role of anesthesiologists vs. nurse anesthetists
3. Continuing education and skills development

Anesthesia practitioners' training and education are critical in ensuring patient safety and quality care, particularly outside the operating room environment. Anesthesia practitioners include anesthesiologists, nurse anesthetists, and anesthesia assistants, who all pursue specialized educational routes. Anesthesiologists typically pursue four years of undergraduate education, four years of medical school, and a minimum of three years of anesthesiology residency training. This extensive training equips them with the expertise and knowledge to handle complex medical cases, preparing them to handle the complexities of non-OR anesthesia scenarios more effectively. Certified registered nurse anesthetists (CRNAs), on the other hand, are expected to possess a master's or doctoral degree in nurse anesthesia with additional advanced clinical training and board certification, elevating the level of care they can provide outside of conventional settings. Each provider's intensive training ultimately enhances the overall quality of anesthesia care that is delivered outside the typical surgical suites. Maybe just as beneficial to their training is continuous professional development that anesthesia providers must undertake to maintain pace with evolving practice and technology. Certification and licensing requirements make continuous education and training mandatory, typically by means of achieving continuing medical education (CME) credits. Such emphasis on continuing education ensures that anesthesia professionals not only have core knowledge but also are competent in newer advances in anesthesia and patient monitoring. In non-OR environments, where clinicians can face mixed clinical cases—ranging from pain management procedures to diagnostic imaging sedation—the ability to utilize the latest best practices is of paramount concern. This commitment to ongoing education enhances the anesthesia provider's capacity to deliver effective and safe anesthesia beyond operating rooms, thereby directly on patient outcomes and safety. Finally, the team-oriented nature of anesthesia practice beyond operating rooms demands that providers possess high levels of communication and interpersonal skills as well as technical proficiency. Anesthesia providers often serve as members of multidisciplinary teams comprising surgeons, nurses, and other healthcare professionals. The ability to collaborate and communicate effectively is important to ensure that all team members agree as far as the needs of the patient and procedural requirements are concerned. In addition, knowledge of the protocols to use in case of emergent situations that may arise in the course of the procedure is important. The training of anesthesia providers, therefore, encompasses not only technical and pharmacologic knowledge but also soft skills for effective teamwork and patient encounters. Lastly, education and qualifications of anesthesia professionals play a critical role in ensuring safe and quality care of anesthesia in various non-operating room settings, thus further supporting their key place in the healthcare system as reflected in controversy surrounding anesthesia practice (Chatterton, 2013; Bonica, 2017).

9.5.1. Education and Certification Requirements

Non-OR anesthesia environments need stringent educational and certification requirements for delivering safety to the patient and best practice. The anesthesia providers should possess a good background in pharmacology, physiology, and specialized techniques that can be utilized in different settings, such as outpatient surgery centers, dental clinics, or pain clinics. Schemes that are accredited by the Accreditation Commission for Midwifery Education (ACME) or the Council on Accreditation of Nurse Anesthesia Educational Programs (COA) facilitate this required training. Apart from the fundamental knowledge, these schemes must offer practice hours in the clinical field, equipping anesthetists to manage the unique needs presented in non-OR environments well. Certification is crucial in establishing proof of expertise and accountability in non-OR anesthesia practice. CRNAs are the cornerstone of delivering anesthesia care in office-based surgery centers, multispecialty clinics, and other settings, requiring the attainment of a master's or doctoral degree in nurse anesthesia and national certification. This process keeps CRNAs proficient in traditional anesthesia practice as well as educated to administer sedation safely in the ambulatory setting. The test for certification evaluates essential skills required for effective practice in such diverse clinical environments, ensuring practitioners are properly prepared to address patient safety concerns and specific procedural requirements unique to non-OR anesthesia cases. Aside from formal education and certification, ongoing professional development is necessary in non-operating room anesthesia practice. The ever-evolving nature of healthcare requires practitioners to be current with the latest anesthesia techniques, technology, and regulatory guidelines. Continuing education units (CEUs) and specialized workshops are necessary in maintaining a high level of care. According to a baseline study conducted by the MacArthur Foundation on maternal health programs, systematic training and competency assessments implemented in professional practices can significantly improve patient outcomes. Fostering lifelong learning is important for CRNAs and other anesthesiology providers so that they can stay current with the ever-changing demands of non-OR anesthesia without compromising the standards of patient safety and quality of care (Figure 9.13).

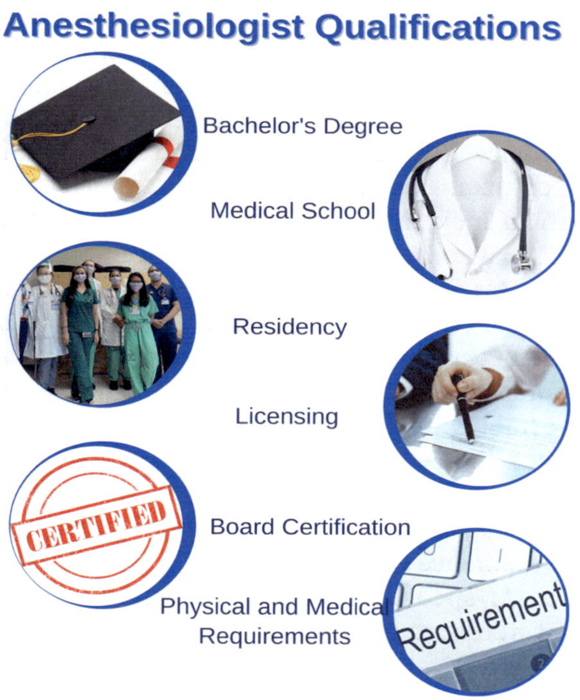
Anesthesiologist Qualifications
Bachelor's Degree
Medical School
Residency
Licensing
CERTIFIED
Board Certification
Physical and Medical Requirements
Requirement

Figure 9.13. The landscape of anesthesia outside the operating room (non-OR anesthesia) necessitates rigorous educational and certification requirements to ensure patient safety and effective practice.

Source: https://d3tlrw2g95xqiz.cloudfront.net/media/public/attachment/2023_09_08_17_28_07_How_to_Become_an_Anesthesiologist_1.png.

9.5.2. Role of Anesthesiologists vs. Nurse Anesthetists

The role of anesthesiologists and nurse anesthetists has undergone a revolution, especially when it comes to non-operating room anesthesia, i.e., sedation for diagnostic work such as endoscopies and interventions for pain management. Anesthesiologists, trained in medication administration, physiology of the patient, and technical aspects of the delivery of anesthesia, have a very important role to fulfill when dealing with complex and high-risk cases where close supervision is called for. Their education allows them to address the complex needs of patients, ensure safety in diverse settings, and deal with critical situations efficiently. CRNAs are particularly well-equipped to provide anesthesia services in non-OR settings, where they function independently. Their training allows them to offer anesthesia safely while, at the same time, allowing them to observe the patient and assist in post-anesthesia recovery, further enhancing access to anesthesia services in settings that otherwise have no competent providers. The anesthesiologist-nurse anesthetist difference assumes special importance in non-OR settings, in which team role and dynamics may impact patient outcome. For instance, nurse anesthetists tend to practice to a very high degree of autonomy, particularly in rural or underserved areas where the anesthesiologist may not be as readily available. This independence is an ongoing trend in anesthesia practice, which allows CRNAs to adapt depending on the unique requirements of the procedure and the patients' conditions. However, there should be active collaboration between anesthesiologists and nurse anesthetists so that there will be uniformity among all clinical decisions and guidelines for best practice and patient safety. Communication among members of the anesthesia team, as highlighted in recent research, significantly improves the quality of care with a focus on the need for respect and understanding of each other's role in the team dynamics (Britz, 2022). Furthermore, the pathways of training and practice fields of anesthesiologists and nurse anesthetists differentiate their roles within the non-OR setting. Anesthesiologists typically experience vast education and residency training, culminating in expertise in a variety of anesthesia-related conditions as well as treatment methods. On the other hand, CRNAs gain intensive education in administering anesthesia and patient care with a focus on practical experiences, such as simulated conditions (Heyes et al., 2018). From this special education, both professional groups extend anesthesia services beyond the scope of hospital operations. With the increasing advancement of healthcare, it is important to comprehend and demarcate the roles of anesthesiologists and nurse anesthetists to provide patient-centered care, maximize resource utilization, and improve the administration of anesthesia in varied clinical settings (Figure 9.14).

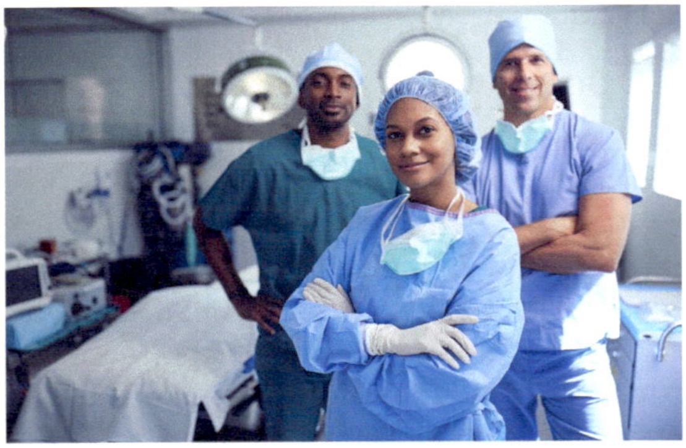

Figure 9.14. The role of anesthesiologists and nurse anesthetists has evolved significantly.

Source: https://www.tagmedstaffing.com/wp-content/uploads/2024/02/Nurse-Anesthetist.jpg.

9.5.3. Continuing Education and Skills Development

In Non-OR Anesthesia, Continuing Skills Development and Education are of significant value in promoting maximum levels of patient care and ensuring practitioner competence. Anesthesia practitioners like CRNAs are frequently confronted with intricate problems involving basic and advanced skills. Integration of continuous learning in their professional development is needed to counteract evolving practices, technologies, and populations. Effective Continuing Education programs not only enhance individual competence but also overall team performance, culminating in better patient outcomes. This dynamic educational setting fosters critical thinking and decision-making skills required for managing situations beyond the confines of traditional operating rooms, where practitioners face special challenges and high-stakes situations. Moreover, professional skill development among anesthesia practitioners can be enhanced by customized training courses aimed at mitigating recognized needs pertaining to experiencing critical incidents. A pilot program to support CRNAs who have experienced critical incidents and is tailored to enhance recovery and rebuild confidence to facilitate the resumption of patient care by clinicians in a prompt fashion would serve as an example. Through the use of established models such as the Scott Three-Tiered Interventional Model of Second Victim Support, this project highlights the significance of psychological and emotional support in fostering the resilience of anesthesia professionals. Such success speaks volumes about the value of continuous education programs that cover not only technical competence but also emotional wellness, enhancing overall practitioner performance beyond OR environments (Slivinski & Hickey, 2019). Lastly, bridging the education gap between special populations for Non-OR Anesthesia is necessary to facilitate practitioners with the full set of skills needed for disparate patient encounters. The lack of explicit coverage of sexual and gender minorities (SGM) in postgraduate anesthesia training is a significant development opportunity. Although most program directors appreciated the educational importance of SGM content, few indicated its inclusion in their curricula. The overall impression is that there is a high educational interest in adding this important module because it directly affects the quality of care delivered to vulnerable populations. In the future, taking feedback from trainees and patients will provide a stronger foundation for the development of curricula in response to the realities of present-day practice of anesthesia, leading to enhanced preparedness of practitioners in Non-OR Anesthesia settings (MacCormick & George, 2020).

Test Your Knowledge

1. What formal training is required to become a qualified anesthesia provider?
2. Why is continuing education important for anesthesia professionals?

9.6. Challenges and Limitations

Learning Outcome

1. Regulatory and legal issues
2. Patient access and availability of services
3. Public perception and awareness

The practice of non-operating room anesthesia (NORA) is associated with numerous challenges that can significantly influence its safety and efficacy. Anesthesia care outside the conventional operating room involves serious planning and coordination of care among medical staff. One major limitation is the potential for suboptimal clinical areas where procedures are conducted, e.g., procedural suites or intensive care units. These settings may not be as well equipped with monitoring equipment and emergency backup systems as an OR is, and hence, risks for complications during the administration of anesthesia are increased. Secondly, Non-OR environments have inconsistencies in levels of training and experience among the operating room personnel engaged, which can lower the level of care being provided, considering the absence of exposure of some practitioners to certain procedures carried out in such facilities (Liang, 2022). Hence, these problems need to be resolved to ensure patient safety and optimize anesthesia delivery in non-OR settings. Communication and inter-disciplinary cooperation among healthcare teams may also prove to be an additional problem for NORA. Because procedures are likely to occur in diverse settings, coordination between anesthesia personnel, surgeons, and nursing staff is essential to achieve the best outcomes. Recurrent alterations in team membership can lead to confusion in preoperative assessment, anesthesia techniques, or postoperative care, and thus affect patient management. Moreover, the noise that is present in clinics, particularly during anesthesia emergence, can reduce effective communication between participants involved in the procedure (Liang, 2022). As studies have indicated, higher noise levels can decrease the cognitive efficiency of anesthesiology specialists, rendering clinical decisions more complicated. Therefore, establishing effective communication modes and minimizing intrusive environmental factors are crucial in overcoming such obstacles regarding NORA. Another significant challenge in the NORA model is managing surgical duration variation, which can be difficult to schedule and allocate resources for. The unpredictability of surgical cases requires anesthesiologists to be adaptable, adjusting plans in the course of work as situations evolve. The unpredictability also creates inefficiency in scheduling for operating rooms, as current models may be insufficient to accommodate the uniqueness of NORA scenarios. For example, an NORA policy discussed in recent studies can increase overall efficiency in operating rooms, but its efficiency may be dependent upon the power of various factors like patient wait times, OR overtime, and slack time due to extended recovery times (Liang, 2022). Hence, recognizing and controlling the built-in variability of surgical durations is vital to enhancing NORA practice in a bid to ensure enhanced efficacy as well as safety in non-OR anesthesia procedures (Figure 9.15).

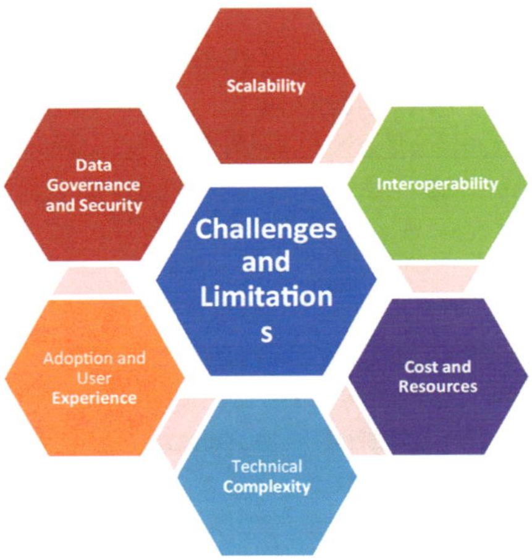

Figure 9.15. The implementation of non-operating room anesthesia (NORA) presents several challenges.

Source: https://www.researchgate.net/profile/Baraa-Alsamarai/publication/375612620/figure/fig1/AS:11431281206072712@1700551321091/Navigating-Challenges-and-Limitations-in-Educational-Blockchain-Integration-Scalability.png.

9.6.1. Regulatory and Legal Issues

Regulatory and legal issues with non-OR anesthesia are a multi-pronged challenge that is challenging for practitioners. As the health system becomes more patient-focused, regulations regarding anesthesia in non-traditional operating room settings must change as practice evolves. Change is not often a homogeneous process; however, as states develop unique standards that can be both beneficial or limiting to the provision of anesthesia in various settings, such as outpatient facilities or mobile operations. The dynamic interplay of market forces and regulation demands practitioners to confront a patchwork quilt of legal requirements that, when inadequately governed, risk subjecting them to liability or sanctions. The lack of national consistency adds inconsistencies to patient safety protocols that raise ethical concerns about patient accessibility and the quality of service provided outside the confines of conventional surgical environments, directly impacting patient outcomes and practitioner accountability. Regulatory frameworks that cover anesthesia in areas other than the operating room are often influenced by historical debates and experiences along the spectrum of medical specialties. The regulatory environment in the context of abortion facilities is an example of the way that politically charged situations can establish standards and practices in health care. The states generally regulate abortion facilities closely in most cases, more due to political motivations than evidence-based practice. If standards for non-OR anesthesia were developed under a more equitable model—similar to those developed for other ambulatory procedures—physicians' perspectives would have a key role to play in ensuring that standards are both effective and implementable. This joint procedure among doctors free from undeserved political influence can be in aid of patient safety in conjunction with a care facilitative environment for innovative care delivery, as seen in procedures in recent research studies on facility standards development (Berglas & Roberts, 2018). Further, regulatory and legal compliance in non-OR anesthesia is also crucial in building public trust in healthcare processes conducted outside the standard setting. Since increasingly more patients are opting for less invasive treatments as opposed to surgery, clear regulation can minimize risks associated with sedation and anesthesia administration. Regulating bodies must work hard to establish guidelines reflecting modern clinical knowledge and best practices so that providers adopt a culture of safety and accountability. This also protects patients, in addition to building professional reputations of anesthesia providers. Moreover, with increasingly advanced health care, inter-cooperation between stakeholders—healthcare providers, regulatory agencies, and policy-makers—will be vital in ensuring that the legal frameworks support safe, effective, and accessible anesthetic practice. Creating such concerted standards will eventually drive better patient care while maintaining the integrity of medical practice in this important field of medicine (Department of Anesthesia, University of Iowa, 2011).

9.6.2. Patient Access and Availability of Services

Patient access and service access are key components in effective non-OR anesthesia delivery since they have a direct effect on patient satisfaction and outcome. With the evolving healthcare systems, there has been increased demand for anesthesia services outside the operating room. This evolution calls for reevaluation of resource allocation and capacity planning within healthcare facilities such that timely and pertinent care is attainable by the patient. By the application of structured planning methods, managers can better forecast the demands of several departments so that workflow is better optimized and patient access is enhanced. In this regard, health care managers must be aware of the intricate nature of patient care pathways and implement measures permitting seamless transitions between the various stages of treatment so that delays in accessing anesthesia services are minimized and an unbroken patient experience is ensured (Hulshof et al., 2012). Furthermore, an understanding of the interdependencies among hospital departments also becomes essential in enabling seamless patient access to anesthesia services. Anesthesia provided outside the operating room, e.g., during interventional radiology or within pain management clinics, relies on efficient coordination among various medical teams. The multi-departmental interactions inducing complexity within may complicate patient flow and scheduling, and therefore potentially lengthen wait times for anesthesia services. Systems thinking, borrowing ideas from clinical pathways literature, can enable healthcare professionals to analyze flows for patients and optimize overall availability of non-OR anesthesia care. Defining these routes and understanding how departments are interconnected, healthcare professionals can make better plans for patient access and realize that resources are utilized properly as per demand (Vanberkel et al., 2010). Lastly, ensuring equal access to anesthesia services is challenging, particularly for those who are underserved or resource-poor.

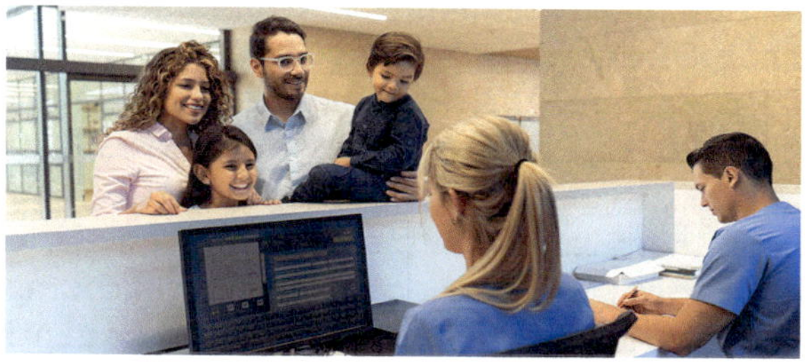

Figure 9.16. Patient access and the availability of services.

Source: https://www.experian.com/blogs/healthcare/wp-content/uploads/2023/05/what-is-patient-access-exploring-key-benefits-and-challenges.png.

The success of health systems to provide anesthesia outside of traditional settings primarily relies on their capability to eliminate barriers to care in the form of economic, geographical, and systemic barriers. Effective resource capacity planning, as the literature documents, has the potential to allow healthcare managers to identify such issues and implement targeted interventions to improve access to services. Furthermore, education of stakeholders within the community and health system awareness raising regarding available non-OR anesthesia options has the potential to decrease disparities in access. Lastly, considering patient access and service availability, healthcare systems can deliver enhanced outcomes and enhance the quality of care to patients in need of anesthesia services outside the operating room (Hulshof et al., 2012) (Figure 9.16).

9.6.3. Public Perception and Awareness

Public perception and comprehension of non-OR anesthesia are important to patient choice and to healthcare delivery. As anesthesia moves outside the conventional operating rooms, the public generally questions the safety and efficacy of procedures in alternative locations. Education and training are fundamental to eliminating fear of non-OR anesthesia, particularly in outpatient and procedural environments. Increased public education can demystify the practices so that patients are able to make an informed decision about their care. Healthcare professionals, by encouraging better understanding, can encourage more patient participation and consequently improved compliance, which equals improved overall health outcomes. The incorporation of effective communication skills in anesthesia education can help bridge the knowledge gap and enhance the safety perception of non-OR anesthesia practices. Moreover, the role of nursing professionals is crucial in educating patients and ensuring that they understand their anesthesia care. Evidence demonstrates that preoperative education greatly influences patient outcomes, particularly in OR environments, but the same concept can be utilized in non-OR settings as well. Nurses are often the first line of caregivers who are required to relay essential information about the anesthesia procedure, related risks, and post-procedure management. Nevertheless, barriers exist in the form of language differences and time constraints, which can interfere with the exchange of information (Ablan, 2016). A breaking of these barriers is critical because it aids in improving public understanding and confidence in non-OR anesthesiology practice. With nurses being able to share detailed knowledge and communicate with patients well, the overall perception of safety and efficacy of non-OR anesthesia improves significantly. Apart from this, systemic initiatives to improve patient safety and the quality of care also contribute to shaping opinion concerning non-OR anesthesia. The introduction of elaborate safety programs, just like those applied in other health care settings, substantiates the endeavors towards minimizing risks associated with anesthesia outside the operating room. Such initiatives, as are witnessed in the VA's National Center for Patient Safety case, not only result in better clinical outcomes but also result in a culture of transparency and accountability (McCarthy & Chase, 2011). Public campaigns highlighting these activities can also reassure patients further regarding the safety of non-OR anesthesia by highlighting continued improvement in procedures and patient outcomes. Consequently, with the public psyche shifting towards more acceptance and understanding of non-OR anesthesia, medical practitioners will have more support in taking up such new trends, with resulting increased acceptance within the medical world.

Test Your Knowledge

1. What factors can affect a patient's access to anesthesia services?
2. Why is the availability of trained anesthesia providers important for surgical care?

SUMMARY

Anesthesia in the non-OR environment is now a central element in modern surgical practice, emphasizing the adaptability and security of non-OR anesthesia. As health systems evolve, procedures traditionally performed within the surgical environment are increasingly being carried out in many settings such as outpatient facilities, emergency departments, and even in remote areas. This shift not only promotes greater patient access to interventions but also decreases the burden on operating room facilities. Furthermore, integrating advanced anesthetic techniques and patient monitoring systems guarantees that procedures carried out outside of the OR have high safety and efficacy standards. As anesthesia practitioners become more accustomed to this paradigm, ongoing education and research will be essential to address the unique challenges and demands of non-OR anesthesia. Clinical and financial implications of incorporating non-OR anesthesia are considerable. For instance, research indicates that certain anesthetic practices not only enhance patient outcomes but also result in significant cost savings over traditional methods. A notable example is seen in the review of rocuronium-neostigmine-sugammadex protocols, which showed a 36% reduction in mean neuromuscular block management costs while also improving patient recovery times (Carron et al., 2016). Effective anesthesia management across various facilities allows healthcare organizations to process more efficiently, reduce waiting times, and ultimately provide more comprehensive care. Consequently, an understanding of the economic value of non-OR anesthesia is required for hospital administrators and policymakers intending to maximize healthcare delivery. Further, the safety profile of non-OR anesthesia continues to be established through comprehensive research. Research on parameters such as sensory regression times in different patient populations, including the obese, illustrates how practices in anesthesia can be optimized to yield the same outcomes among different population groups (Hilton, 1989). These findings imply the use of individualized anesthetic approaches in unconventional settings to reduce complications and enhance recovery. With the growing development of non-OR anesthesia, there must be a collaborative effort instituted to ensure that the practitioners are informed about optimal practices, newer technologies, and techniques of patient management. All these combined together increase the significance of the role that will be played by anesthesia outside the operating room in offering the most optimal patient-centric care and affirming its place in the future of medicine.

In today's dynamic healthcare era, Non-OR Anesthesia has become an integral component of the medical practice. Its fundamental objective is ensuring patient safety and comfort during many procedures conducted outside traditional operating room environments. These include operations in outpatient departments, diagnostic imaging, and other treatment rooms. The need for effective analgesia and sedation in such environments highlights the value of specialist training among anesthesia personnel to meet the unique risks involved in such environments. The use of rigid protocols for patient assessment, monitoring, and emergency preparedness is critical in minimizing risk and enhancing patient outcomes. A clear understanding of the practice of Non-OR Anesthesia is thus a requirement for medical practitioners to ensure the highest quality of care is maintained, demonstrating a clear devotion to patient safety and satisfaction, a critical measure for every medical facility, particularly in competitive market environments (Lloyd et al., 2001). Moreover, the expanding list of Non-OR Anesthesia modalities has consequences of significant magnitude for surgical pathways and management of patients. Techniques such as regional anesthesia not only contribute to pain management but also influence postoperative recovery and ultimate outcomes.

It has been discovered that regional anesthesia may potentially reduce cancer recurrence after surgery through numerous mechanisms, including preservation of immune function (Xuan et al., 2016). This discovery encourages anesthesiologists to consider more significant impacts of their methods beyond simple intra-procedural comfort. Their translation to non-traditional settings illustrates the necessity of ongoing education and research in the specialty. By keeping current with emerging studies and how they can be adapted, practitioners are better able to tailor anesthesia care to the unique needs of diverse patient populations undergoing an array of procedures outside the operating room. In addition, the financial implications of Non-OR Anesthesia practices cannot be overlooked. Pricing systems for services delivered in alternative settings require strict analysis and a close understanding of market forces. Competitor pricing, customers' perceived value, and the method applied to set prices at healthcare centers are a few factors influencing price. As the example of the Veterinary Teaching Hospital at Michigan State University indicates, competitor pricing still plays a crucial role in achieving financial success under a clinical setting (Lloyd et al., 2001). As anesthesia practitioners adapt their practice, they must also ensure that cost issues are reconcilable with the delivery of quality care. Balancing patient satisfaction with the fiscal realities of healthcare will be a paradigm challenge because optimizing patient outcomes, operational efficiency, and financial viability is at the heart of the Non-OR Anesthesia practice's future.

KEY TERMS FROM THIS CHAPTER

- Chronic pain
- Continuous infusion (CG)
- Diagnostic modalities
- Healthcare
- Holistic approach
- Medical procedures
- Consciousness
- Dental anxiety (DA)
- Flexibility
- Healthcare resource management
- Intermittent bolus (IB)
- Monitored anesthesia care (MAC)

CRITICAL THINKING QUESTIONS

1. **What is the most common anesthetic complication in non-operating room anesthesia (NORA)?**
   a. Respiratory depression
   b. Hemodynamic instability
   c. Allergic reaction
   d. Equipment malfunction
2. **Which of the following is critical when providing anesthesia in MRI suites?**
   a. Avoidance of metal-containing equipment
   b. Use of nitrous oxide for sedation
   c. Strict fasting protocols
   d. Avoidance of neuromuscular blockers
3. **What is the most significant risk during sedation for endoscopy procedures?**
   a. Hemorrhage
   b. Hypotension
   c. Aspiration
   d. Tachycardia
4. **In which non-OR setting is the use of total intravenous anesthesia (TIVA) most common?**
   a. Interventional cardiology
   b. Radiology/MRI
   c. Radiation oncology
   d. Dental procedures
5. **What monitoring standard must always be maintained during anesthesia in non-OR settings?**
   a. BIS monitoring
   b. Continuous EKG and pulse oximetry
   c. Capnography for spontaneous breathing
   d. Non-invasive blood pressure every 15 minutes

Short Answer Questions

1. What are the unique challenges associated with providing anesthesia in non-operating room locations such as endoscopy suites or radiology departments?
2. Discuss the indications and anesthetic considerations for performing sedation during magnetic resonance imaging (MRI).
3. How do the risks of airway management differ in non-OR anesthesia settings compared to traditional operating rooms?
4. What specific safety measures should be implemented when providing anesthesia in remote locations without full surgical support?
5. Describe the role of capnography in monitoring patients undergoing procedural sedation outside the OR.
6. What is the significance of pre-procedural evaluation in patients undergoing anesthesia for interventional cardiology procedures?

Answer to Critical Thinking Questions

1. (a); 2. (a); 3. (c); 4.(b); 5. (b)

REFERENCES

1. Ablan, R. (2016). Barriers to preoperative teaching in a culturally diverse healthcare environment. https://core.ac.uk/download/129532351.pdf (accessed on 28th June 2025).
2. Facco, E., & Zanette, G. (2017). The Odyssey of Dental Anxiety: From Prehistory to the Present. A Narrative Review. *Frontiers in psychology*, *8*, 1155. https://doi.org/10.3389/fpsyg.2017.01155(accessed on 28th June 2025).
3. ACTFAST Study Group, Avidan, M. S., Ben Abdallah, A., Fritz, B., et al. (2018). Study protocol for the Anesthesiology Control Tower—Feedback Alerts to Supplement Treatments (ACTFAST-3) trial: A pilot randomized controlled trial in intraoperative telemedicine [version 1; referees: 2 approved]. https://core.ac.uk/download/212865789.pdf (accessed on 28th June 2025).
4. Ahmed, S. S., Hicks, S., Slaven, J. E., & Nitu, M. (2017). Intermittent Bolus versus Continuous Infusion of Propofol for Deep Sedation during ABR/Nuclear Medicine Studies. *Journal of pediatric intensive care*, *6*(3), 176–181. https://doi.org/10.1055/s-0036-1597628 (accessed on 28th June 2025).
5. Ali, A., DeMonaco, H. J., & von Hippel, E. A. (2005). The major role of clinicians in the discovery of off-label drug therapies. https://core.ac.uk/download/4394523.pdf (accessed on 28th June 2025).
6. Arriaga, P., & Pacheco, C. (2016). Effects of clown doctors on child and caregiver anxiety at the entrance to the surgery care unit and separation from caregivers. https://core.ac.uk/download/46603912.pdf (accessed on 28th June 2025).
7. Bacci, C., Bartorelli, L. M. G., Ferrario, S., Grossi, E., et al. (2018). Maxillary nerve block: A comparison between the greater palatine canal and high tuberosity approaches. https://core.ac.uk/download/168403724.pdf (accessed on 28th June 2025).
8. Wenzel, J. T., Schwenk, E. S., Baratta, J. L., & Viscusi, E. R. (2016). Managing Opioid-Tolerant Patients in the Perioperative Surgical Home. *Anesthesiology clinics*, *34*(2), 287–301. https://doi.org/10.1016/j.anclin.2016.01.005(accessed on 28th June 2025).
9. Carron, M., Baratto, F., Zarantonello, F., & Ori, C. (2016). Sugammadex for reversal of neuromuscular blockade: a retrospective analysis of clinical outcomes and cost-effectiveness in a single center. *ClinicoEconomics and outcomes research : CEOR*, *8*, 43–52. https://doi.org/10.2147/CEOR.S100921(accessed on 28th June 2025).
10. Mitchell M. (2008). Conscious surgery: influence of the environment on patient anxiety. *Journal of advanced nursing*, *64*(3), 261–271. https://doi.org/10.1111/j.1365-2648.2008.04769.x(accessed on 28th June 2025).
11. Berglas, N. F., & Roberts, S. C. M. (2018). The development of facility standards for common outpatient procedures and implications for the context of abortion. *BMC health services research*, *18*(1), 212. https://doi.org/10.1186/s12913-018-3048-3 (accessed on 28th June 2025).
12. Carron, M., Bertoncello, F., & Ieppariello, G. (2017). Profile of sugammadex for reversal of neuromuscular blockade in the elderly: current perspectives. *Clinical interventions in aging*, *13*, 13–24. https://doi.org/10.2147/CIA.S134108(accessed on 28th June 2025).
13. Bonica, M., Students of Health Management 721.01 (2017). *Healthcare Management Primer*. University of New Hampshire. https://core.ac.uk/download/215509297.pdf (accessed on 28th June 2025).

14. Hulshof, P., Kortbeek, N., Boucherie, R. *et al.* Taxonomic classification of planning decisions in health care: a structured review of the state of the art in OR/MS. *Health Syst* **1**, 129–175 (2012). https://doi.org/10.1057/hs.2012.18 (accessed on 28th June 2025).
15. Vanberkel, P. T., Boucherie, R. J., Hans, E. W., Hurink, J. L., & Litvak, N. (2010). A survey of health care models that encompass multiple departments. International journal of health management and information (IJHMI), 1(1), 37-69. (accessed on 28th June 2025).
16. Britz, J. L. (2022). A novel tool to promote surgical team awareness of nurse anesthesia students' level of training. https://core.ac.uk/download/552577714.pdf (accessed on 28th June 2025).
17. Cantisani, C., Macaluso, L., Frascani, F., Paolino, G., D'Andrea, V., Richetta, A. G., & Calvieri, S. (2014). New patents on topical anesthetics. *Recent patents on inflammation & allergy drug discovery*, *8*(2), 125–131. https://doi.org/10.2174/1872213x08666140515152837(accessed on 28th June 2025).
18. Lloyd, J. W., Leeper, D., Donovan, D., Camara, Y., Smith, S. G., Lloyd, J. W., Leeper, D., Donovan, D., Camara, Y., & Smith, S. G. (2001). PRICES AND PRICING POLICIES FOR SMALL ANIMAL AND EQUINE VETERINARY SERVICES: A STUDY OF TEACHING HOSPITALS AND MICHIGAN PRIVATE PRACTICES DURING 2000. Unknown. https://doi.org/10.22004/AG.ECON.11552(accessed on 28th June 2025).
19. D. McCarthy and D. Chase, Advancing Patient Safety in the U.S. Department of Veterans Affairs, The Commonwealth Fund, March 2011.(accessed on 28th June 2025).
20. Chatterton, C. (2013). "An unsuitable job for a woman? Gender and mental health nursing." https://core.ac.uk/download/18306482.pdf (accessed on 28th June 2025).
21. Xuan, W., Zhao, H., Hankin, J., Chen, L., Yao, S., & Ma, D. (2016). Local anesthetic bupivacaine induced ovarian and prostate cancer apoptotic cell death and underlying mechanisms in vitro. *Scientific reports*, *6*, 26277. https://doi.org/10.1038/srep26277 (accessed on 28th June 2025).
22. Lancaster, E. M., Sosa, J. A., Sammann, A., Pierce, L., Shen, W., Conte, M. C., & Wick, E. C. (2020). Rapid Response of an Academic Surgical Department to the COVID-19 Pandemic: Implications for Patients, Surgeons, and the Community. *Journal of the American College of Surgeons*, *230*(6), 1064–1073. https://doi.org/10.1016/j.jamcollsurg.2020.04.007(accessed on 28th June 2025).
23. Schwarzkopf, R., Gross, S. C., Coopersmith, A., & Gidumal, R. (2013). Ankle fracture surgery on a pregnant patient complicated by intraoperative emergency caesarian section. *Case reports in orthopedics*, *2013*, 962794. https://doi.org/10.1155/2013/962794(accessed on 28th June 2025).
24. De Keyser, R., & Ionescu, C. M. (2016). Model based control strategies for a class of nonlinear mechanical sub-systems. https://core.ac.uk/download/55822951.pdf (accessed on 28th June 2025).
25. Escrivá, J., Fort, P., Gabarrón, E., Liao, Y., et al. (2016). Comparison of two cardiac output monitors, qCO and LiDCO, during general anesthesia. https://core.ac.uk/download/81578536.pdf (accessed on 28th June 2025).
26. Saxen, M. A., Urman, R. D., Yepes, J. F., Gabriel, R. A., & Jones, J. E. (2017). Comparison of Anesthesia for Dental/Oral Surgery by Office-based Dentist Anesthesiologists versus Operating

Room-based Physician Anesthesiologists. *Anesthesia progress*, *64*(4), 212–220. https://doi.org/10.2344/anpr-65-01-04 (accessed on 28th June 2025).

27. MacCormick, H., & George, R. B. (2020). Sexual and gender minorities educational content within obstetric anesthesia fellowship programs: a survey. Contenu éducatif traitant des minorités sexuelles et de genre au sein des programmes de fellowship en anesthésie obstétricale : un sondage. *Canadian journal of anaesthesia = Journal canadien d'anesthesie*, *67*(5), 532–540. https://doi.org/10.1007/s12630-019-01562-x(accessed on 28th June 2025).
28. Loyola-Rodriguez, J. P., Zavala-Alonso, V., Gonzalez-Alvarez, C. L., Juarez-Lopez, L. A., Patiño-Marin, N., & Gonzalez, C. D. (2009). Dental treatment under general anesthesia in healthy and medically compromised developmentally disabled children: a comparative study. *The Journal of clinical pediatric dentistry*, *34*(2), 177–182. https://doi.org/10.17796/jcpd.34.2.u665328k4g467pg2(accessed on 28th June 2025).
29. Gozal, D., & Mason, K. P. (2010). Pediatric sedation: a global challenge. *International journal of pediatrics*, *2010*, 701257. https://doi.org/10.1155/2010/701257(accessed on 28th June 2025).
30. Heyes, M. E., Muckler, V. C., Schnitzen, L., Starr, K., et al. (2018). Recertification and reentry to practice for nurse anesthetists: Determining core competencies and evaluating performance via high-fidelity simulation technology. https://core.ac.uk/download/213088562.pdf (accessed on 28th June 2025).
31. Slivinski, P. C., & Hickey, J. V. (2019). Implementation of a Critical Incident Stress Management Program for Nurse Anesthetists.. Journal of Nursing & Interprofessional Leadership in Quality & Safety, 2 (2). Retrieved from https://digitalcommons.library.tmc.edu/uthoustonjqualsafe/vol2/iss2/3(accessed on 28th June 2025).
32. Hilton, G. L. (1989). Sensory regression time from subarachnoid block with hyperbaric 0.75% bupivacaine in the obese patient. https://core.ac.uk/download/130355392.pdf (accessed on 28th June 2025).
33. Kingsnorth, A. N., Adesunkanmi, A. R., Schutz, C., Maggiore, D., Watkin, D., Lewis, D. C., Crawford, D. L., et al. (2012). Surgical management of inguinal hernias at Bugando Medical Centre in Northwestern Tanzania: Our experiences in a resource-limited setting. https://core.ac.uk/download/pdf/11307796.pdf (accessed on 28th June 2025).
34. Liang, Y. (2022). Implications of non-operating room anesthesia policy for operating room efficiency. https://core.ac.uk/download/513486986.pdf (accessed on 28th June 2025).
35. Schwenk, E. S., & Mariano, E. R. (2018). Designing the ideal perioperative pain management plan starts with multimodal analgesia. *Korean journal of anesthesiology*, *71*(5), 345–352. https://doi.org/10.4097/kja.d.18.00217(accessed on 28th June 2025).
36. Martin, J. A. (2016). Procedural sedation: Policy, practice & knowledge. https://core.ac.uk/download/153202186.pdf (accessed on 28th June 2025).
37. Meyer, M. A. (2006). Use of location data for the surveillance, analysis, and optimization of clinical processes. https://core.ac.uk/download/4400477.pdf (accessed on 28th June 2025).
38. Tobias, A. Z., Roth, R. N., Weiss, L. S., Murray, K., & Yealy, D. M. (2020). Tree of Life Synagogue Shooting in Pittsburgh: Preparedness, Prehospital Care, and Lessons Learned. *The western journal of emergency medicine*, *21*(2), 374–381. https://doi.org/10.5811/westjem.2019.11.42809(accessed on 28th June 2025).

INTENSIVE CARE AND CRITICAL CARE ANESTHESIA

10

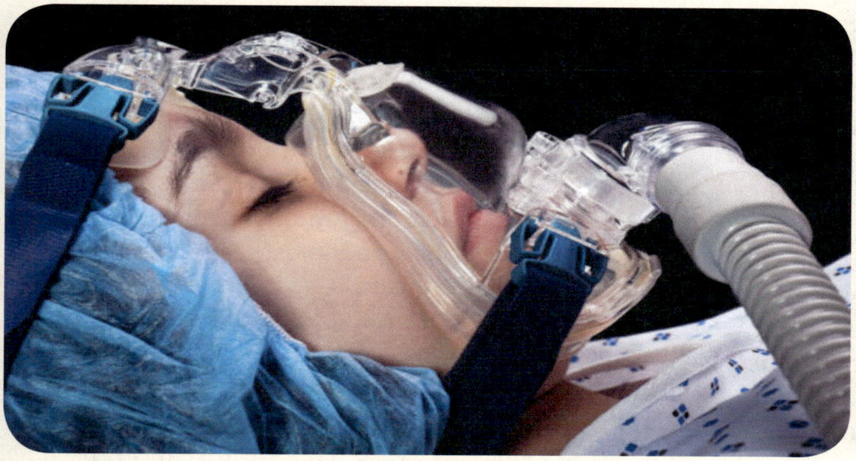

LEARNING OBJECTIVES

After studying this chapter, you will be able to:

1. Give an overview of intensive care units (ICUs)
2. Discuss the principles of critical care anesthesia
3. Know patient assessment in critical care
4. Explain the anesthetic techniques in intensive care
5. Understand complications and challenges in critical care anesthesia
6. Focus on advances in critical care anesthesia

Introduction

The field of intensive care and critical care anesthesiology is one such valuable intersection of leading medical technology and the need for specialized patient care. As healthcare systems across the world seek to provide the optimal care for critically ill patients, the need arises to have a emphasis on innovative approaches. Intensive care units (ICUs) are designed to treat patients with severe and potentially life-endangering illnesses, where timely input can make a huge difference in outcome. Anesthesia is the key to it all in this environment, allowing procedural sedation and proper management of pain to occur. Anesthesiologists in ICUs don't just provide comfort, but rather also work to make their patients safe, navigate the subtleties of pharmacology, and anticipate complications. The marriage between anesthesia and critical care really does offer a model by which health professionals can provide a high level of care during some of their patients' most desperate times. The last couple of decades have seen critical care dramatically change the way patients are treated in ICUs. The inclusion of technologies such as AI and telemedicine has completely overhauled patient monitoring and decision-making, and more targeted and streamlined care is now a reality. From the anesthetic perspective, techniques such as regional anesthesia and continuous infusion of local anesthetics have emerged as powerful pain management modalities in critically ill patients, presenting alternatives to traditional opioid-based approaches. Not only do these technologies lower the side effects of systemic analgesics, but they also enhance patient safety and comfort during postoperative periods. The mounting body of literature surrounding these advancements signals an intent to improve critical care outcomes, citing a need for ongoing study and education within this highly specialized care setting (Padte et al., 2024). Further, it is also important to address challenges in pain and sedation management in ICUs. The patient's state dynamics—e.g., renal failure, sepsis, or anticoagulant therapy—must be weighed with consideration in employing anesthetic techniques and pharmacologic protocols.

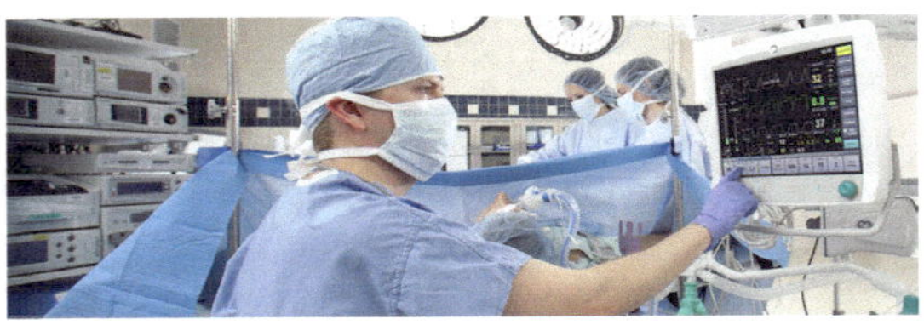

Figure 10.1. The field of intensive care and critical care anesthesia.

Source: https://glenfieldmallareddybrainhearthospital.com/images/inner_imagese/Anesthesia%20and%20Critical%20Care1.webp.

Anesthesia providers must remain alert and clever, optimizing pain management processes with minimal effect on already compromised patients. The harmony between critical care practitioners and anesthesiologists is crucial in the development of guidelines that will facilitate the efficient use of regional anesthesia and other new forms of pain relief (Lazar & Farczádi, 2024). As the healthcare sector continues to explore these details, interdisciplinary cooperation will be the core to improving practices that prioritize patient safety and satisfaction in intensive care units (Figure 10.1).

Definition of Intensive Care

The intensive care concept extends beyond clinical observation itself; it is a specialized way of managing critically ill patients requiring constant watching and high-level therapeutic interventions. ICUs offer facilities to house high-acuity patients, such as those with life-threatening conditions requiring close monitoring. Such units employ an interdisciplinary team of health care providers, including intensivists, nurses, respiratory therapists, and anesthesiologists, to deliver synchronized care based on the intricate physiologic needs of these patients. The general purpose of intensive care is to stabilize the patients through continuous assessment and timely intervention, thereby enhancing the possibility of recovery. The union of high-tech monitoring modalities and therapeutic interventions is pivotal in achieving these goals, as it allows for timely detection of menacing physiological changes in patient stability. Intensive care closely overlaps with anesthesia, particularly at critical points requiring immediate interventions. Anesthesiologists, as part of the intensive care team, possess specialized skills that are vital in managing airway complications and providing hemodynamic stability in critically ill patients. Their role extends well beyond the confines of the operating room, with responsibilities encompassing initial triage during emergencies and ongoing care of ventilated patients. In high-stress situations, like mass casualty events, anesthesiologists add the essential skill of pharmacologic sedation and critical care management that is central to both procedural intervention and triage. As per (Simjanovska, 2025), the use of anesthesiologists in high-acuity settings shows the necessity of instant coordination and inter-professional collaboration, emphasizing their extensive skillset within a wide variety of clinical settings. Effective pain management is a part of the care offered in ICUs, wherein patients are frequently quite uncomfortable due to their acute illness or postoperative state. Pain treatment in these environments often requires a subtle understanding of both drug options and patient factors since failure to control pain may exacerbate morbidity and extend the length of stay. Use of local anesthetics has emerged as an improved choice for the conventional opioids, which usually come with side effects that can hinder the recovery process. As stated by Lazar & Farczádi (2024), anesthesiology experts can apply local anesthetics effectively to manage pain in critically ill patients, emphasizing the need for continuous analgesia techniques. The evolving context of pain management in intensive care not only seeks to reduce distress but also wants to have a positive impact on patient outcomes, thus reaffirming the importance of anesthesiologists in this special domain of care (Figure 10.2).

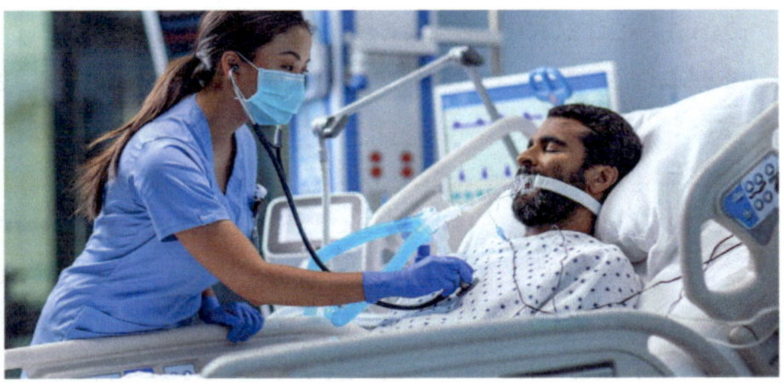

Figure 10.2. The concept of intensive care extends beyond mere clinical observation.

Source: https://external-content.duckduckgo.com/iu/?u=https%3A%2F%2Fassets.hillrom.com%2Fis%2Fimage%2Fhillrom%2FHero%2520Banner%2520-%2520Solutions%2520-%2520Desktop%2520-%25202880%2520x%25201400_b%3F%24heroBannerFocusAreaDesktop%24&f=1&nofb=1&ipt=3aada25955663b39bb9953affb43621c5eb0b48d17d1b73feca19c7351d0ec27.

Definition of Critical Care Anesthesia

In modern medicine, critical care anesthesia is a specialized anesthesia practice for critically ill patients with life-threatening illnesses. Critical care anesthesia attempts to provide full perioperative care for critically ill patients, where often a multidisciplinary team approach may be essential to maximize outcomes. Anesthesiologists not only provide anesthesia but also handle complex medical conditions seen in critically ill patients. This role demands extensive pharmacology, physiology, and intricate critical care environment dynamics knowledge. The inclusion of novel monitoring techniques and point-of-care ultrasound application, as discussed in more recent literature, significantly enhance the anesthesiologists' ability to achieve sound decisions in timely and effective ways under high-pressure situations (Kleinpell et al., 2021). Furthermore, critical care anesthesia is characterized by its team nature, with several health professionals in the ICU. Close interprofessional collaboration between intensivists, nurses, pharmacists, and respiratory therapists is needed, particularly when dealing with the complex needs of critically ill patients requiring close monitoring and more complex interventions. The value of effective communication and collaboration has been highlighted by numerous studies that have demonstrated that structured collaboration can lead to improved patient outcomes (Kleinpell et al., 2021). Anesthesiologists play a significant role in this inter-professional setting by ensuring best practices and making decisions related to anesthesia based on the overall management of critically ill patients. This collaborative model is the very definition of critical care anesthesia, where healthcare providers benefit from synergy to improve the quality of care offered. The extent of critical care anesthesia is also being developed and improved upon continually, with new developments in medical technology and shifts in patient populations. New methods, including novel airway management and regional anesthesia protocols, have become integral parts of perioperative care in the ICU. The incorporation of point-of-care ultrasound, particularly in vascular access and cardiac evaluation, is a testament to the growing focus on educating anesthesiologists in multimodal patient care (Mahmood et al., 2016). To meet these developments, continuing education and proficiency training in the latest anesthetic practices are necessary for anesthesiologists wishing to deliver safe, efficient care for patients. As the specialty evolves, critical care anesthesia's definition will probably broaden, continuing to highlight the need for flexible, highly competent practitioners able to navigate the nuances of contemporary critical care settings.

Importance of the Topic in Modern Medicine

In the realm of modern medicine, the requirement for complex sedation methods in critical care and intensive care anesthesiology cannot be overstated. Sedatives are pivotal in the management of critical illnesses, especially in the critically ill patient requiring mechanical ventilation, by relieving anxiety and easing required medical procedures. The existence of agents like dexmedetomidine has revolutionized the administration of sedation practice, providing practitioners with options for alternatives that reduce psychological and physiological stress induced in patients. Appropriate usage of such agents is vital, as not only do they maximize patient outcomes, but also contribute to the overall success of the surgical and anesthetic processes.

However, particularly in elderly patients, careful attention to sedation use risks and benefits is the most important consideration. There is greater evidence now for the need for careful selection of anesthetic agents based on patient-specific profiles to ensure maximum efficacy and safety (Paschoal et al., 2025). The use of artificial intelligence (AI) in intensive care units is also a revolutionary new approach to clinical decision-making that addresses the inadequacies of traditional methods. AI models, particularly those simplifying data collection during the process of critical care episodes, are being increasingly incorporated to improve prediction as well as diagnostic performance. The development of such models as CoAI demonstrates the capability of AI in effectively utilizing a small set of inexpensive patient features to enhance prediction while concurrently discharging workload on healthcare professionals. This shift not only improves resource management but also influences the priority of care in high-risk environments. As AI continues to develop, its use with intensive care and critical care anesthesia should provide greater clinical value, which should result in more prompt interventions and improved patient outcomes (Erion et al., 2021).

Taking these shifts into account, the general utility of continuous education and the adaptability of healthcare practices emerge. Ongoing education of medical professionals in both sedation techniques and the use of AI ensures practitioners can implement the latest evidence-based practices of care daily. Increased education regarding the complexities of sedation in vulnerable populations, such as the elderly, defends the necessity for individualized treatment plans that consider personalized medical histories and present situations. Moreover, the interaction of AI technology with critical care guidelines insists on interdisciplinary collaboration that encourages environments in which evidence-based practice is routinely implemented to realize maximum patient care. In this rapidly evolving discipline, the synthesis of innovative practices and traditional approaches is fundamental to the optimization of patient safety and satisfaction in modern medical settings (Figure 10.3).

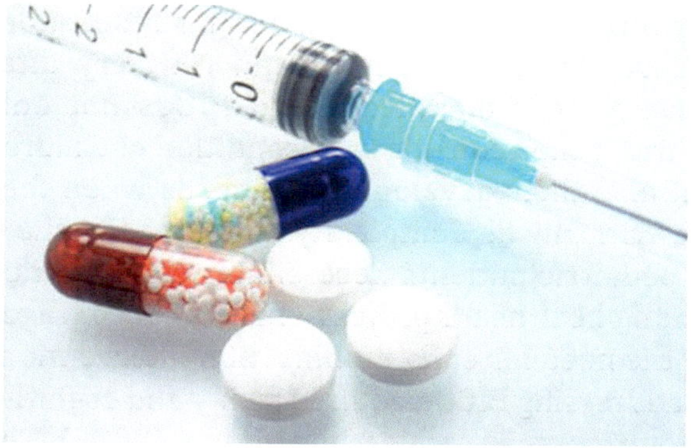

Figure 10.3. The realm of modern medicine.

Source: https://external-content.duckduckgo.com/iu/?u=https%3A%2F%2Fmiro.medium.com%2Fmax%2F450%2F1*0TDov6r0ustrZPkng7slfg.jpeg&f=1&nofb=1&ipt=307b5bc2431402d1ceb362fa395516473497126aeac6b9a99d4e0a323e17be09.

10.1. Overview of Intensive Care Units (ICUs)

Learning Outcome

1. Types of ICUs (e.g., Medical, Surgical, Pediatric)
2. Role of healthcare professionals in ICUs
3. common conditions treated in ICUs

Intensive care units (ICUs) are intensive care centers that provide comprehensive and continuous care to critically ill patients. ICUs are technologically advanced and staffed with highly trained healthcare professionals such as intensivists, nurses, and respiratory therapists. The primary function of an ICU is to monitor and manage patients suffering from life-threatening complications such as severe infections, respiratory insufficiency, and surgical complications. The ICU setting is one of heightened alert, with patients requiring close observation for shifts in their clinical status. The complexity of the cases entering the ICU also underscores the importance of interdisciplinary cooperation, as various aspects of patient management are optimized to yield enhanced results. Critically ill patient pain management, particularly in the ICU, has been brought into the limelight due to its critical impact on patient recovery and satisfaction. Effective pain management not only reduces pain but also offsets stress response, which tends to decrease morbidity and mortality. Current research indicates that inadequate pain control is frequently associated with inadequate education and continuation of fears regarding the use of opioids and their adverse effects. Alternatives, such as local anesthetics, have been a better substitute for pain management with fewer side effects. As explained in research, local anesthetics have the potential to meet individual ICU patients' needs, particularly when administered continuously; long-lasting pain relief is achieved when the administration is continuous during critical recovery times (Lazar & Farczádi, 2024).

The effect of nurse-to-patient ratios within ICUs on patient outcomes, including hospital-acquired pneumonia (HAP), has been the subject of studies in the past couple of years. A study conducted with surgical patients in South Korea identified a direct correlation between the ratio of nurse staffing and the incidence of HAP, where decreased staffing levels were found to have increased complication rates. The findings identify a stark disparity in risk levels based on the nurse-to-bed ratio, demonstrating the necessity of nurses in infection prevention and overall patient care. Higher staffing levels enhanced monitoring and timely responses to patient needs, thus reducing the risk associated with critical illnesses. Finally, adequate nurse staffing not only improves immediate patient outcomes but also highlights the importance of formal ICU management to maximize recovery patterns in critically ill patients (Park et al., 2024).

10.1.1. Types of ICUs (e.g., Medical, Surgical, Pediatric)

The ICU landscape is diverse, suited to address a variety of medical requirements faced among severely ill patient populations. Among the different types of ICUs, MICUs stand out, handling primarily critical cases of medical conditions such as respiratory failure, sepsis, or acute renal failure. MICUs are adequately technology-backed and staffed with skilled doctors who conduct detailed monitoring and management of complex medical conditions. Apart from life support, MICUs could also incorporate specialized treatment strategies to address complicated pathologies. According to Lisitsa et al. (2025), nutrition management in MICUs could potentially have a significant impact on patient outcomes, which emphasizes the importance of personalized care in high-stakes environments. Surgical intensive care units (SICUs) offer special treatment for post-operative patients who require close monitoring following extensive surgeries. SICU patients may be patients recovering from complex surgery, such as cardiac surgery, major trauma, or neurosurgery. The focus in these units is on careful management of postoperative complications, pain control, and stabilization of vital parameters. Because of the nature of surgery recovery, SICUs are endowed with advanced monitoring facilities and technologies to detect any deterioration early. Additionally, research shows that early mobilization in SICUs can potentially increase recovery times and patient outcomes significantly. As explained in a research paper, rehabilitation policy improvement in such settings has been more embraced, illustrating the necessity for an integrative care approach to caring for patients in surgical settings, as seen through dialogue by Al-Harbi (2024). Pediatric intensive care units (PICUs) are intensive care units specifically developed to address the unique medical needs of critically ill children. The PICUs provide complete care to infant and child patients with various acute illnesses, including respiratory failure, severe infections, and recovery after surgery. It is significant that PICUs not only consider the acute physical condition of children but also their developmental needs when they are critically ill. Complexity in the management of pediatric patients necessitates collaboration among healthcare professionals, as encouraged by the need for early mobilization interventions in addressing PICU-acquired frailty and cognitive impairment, as tackled in Al-Harbi (2024). The nuances of the pediatric patient population, including proper nutritional supplementation and psychological support, also highlight the importance of specialized facilities to address the varied degrees of pediatric critical illness and thereby optimize outcomes among this vulnerable population of patients (Figure 10.4).

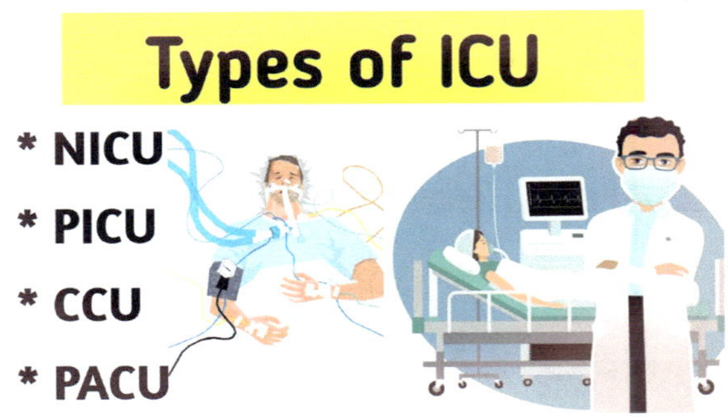

Figure 10.4. The landscape of intensive care units (ICUs).

Source: https://external-content.duckduckgo.com/iu/?u=https%3A%2F%2Fi.ytimg.com%2Fvi%2FDofQX6_NrxU%2Fmaxresdefault.jpg&f=1&nofb=1&ipt=7d630017d9b16bfb12db15e675418d8d69e9cbdf840767efe2da4793eb2a31a3.

10.1.2. Role of Healthcare Professionals in ICUs

The role of the healthcare practitioners in ICUs is two-pronged, with both clinical and operational functions being essential to effective patient management. Anesthesiologists are central to the role played in the setting through their expertise in airway management and hemodynamic stabilization, which is also critical in the high-acuity situations that are typically encountered within the ICU context. Their domain of specialty specifically encompasses the initial patient triage, provision of procedural emergency care, and ongoing care of ventilated and intensively monitored patients. While this goes to the clinical significance of their role, it also serves to identify the applicability of interdisciplinary cooperation paradigms that play a key role in ensuring optimal patient outcomes in critical care situations. The participation of the anesthesiologists becomes even more essential as health systems continue to grapple with mass casualty incidents, further identifying their place within the entire gamut of patient care within critical environments (Simjanovska, 2025). Also, the increasing trend of healthcare-associated infections (HAIs) among ICU settings is yet another area of greater concern for the work of healthcare professionals. One of the more resistant-to-treat infections is carbapenem-resistant Enterobacteriaceae (CRE), with New Delhi Metallo-β-lactamase 1 (NDM-1) strains being predominantly resistant to conventional treatments. Management of such infections necessitates in-depth knowledge of antibiotic resistance and forward-looking measures for infection control. Medical practitioners, especially those in intensive care, engage in continuous assessment and application of optimal antibiotic therapy, as evidenced by recent studies that attempted to capture their attitude and behaviors regarding the management of such resistant infections. Their active engagement not only guarantees prevailing conditions are effectively treated but also promotes a prevention strategy towards preventing HAIs in the ICU (Pandit et al., 2024). Furthermore, the role of healthcare professionals' work in ICUs extends beyond immediate patient care to education and policy-making with an impact on best practices in critical care. Ongoing participation in professional development allows healthcare teams to effectively address the unfolding issues in the ICU, such as acute crises due to mass casualty incidents or emerging infectious diseases. The organization of disaster planning, crisis standards of care activation, and ICU surge capacity management are responsibilities that showcase the importance of an organized healthcare workforce. By infusing the clinical, functional, and ethical aspects of treatment, health practitioners have a critical responsibility in the provision of high-quality treatment of patients, with leadership roles played by anesthesiologists in such efforts. Together, their collective action is paramount in bolstering the strength and ability of ICUs to deal with the demands of intensive and critical care (Simjanovska, 2025) (Figure 10.5).

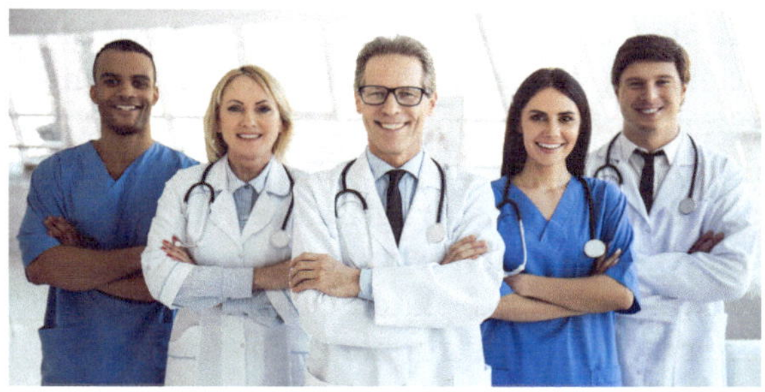

Figure 10.5. The role of healthcare professionals in intensive care units (ICUs).

Source: https://external-content.duckduckgo.com/iu/?u=https%3A%2F%2Fwww.studentdoctor.net%2Fwp-content%2Fuploads%2F2019%2F03%2Fshutterstock_582888679.png&f=1&nofb=1&ipt=21975d0e1c0329c63bcc03ffad03c6c3f6553597e342b2650e0f2469b67cd065.

10.1.3. Common Conditions Treated in ICUs

The ICU is an intensive care environment for the management of a wide range of complex and severe medical conditions. The most frequent condition managed in ICUs is respiratory failure, in which there is a failure to exchange oxygen and carbon dioxide adequately. Sepsis, pneumonia, chronic obstructive pulmonary disease (COPD), and acute respiratory distress syndrome (ARDS) all need intensive and emergent treatment. Patients may require aggressive ventilatory support in the form of invasive mechanical ventilation to facilitate adequate gas exchange. This is an important intervention since respiratory failure can evolve quickly to systemic complications and increased mortality. A multidisciplinary approach, including anesthesiologists with critical care anesthesia experience, must be employed to optimize patient outcomes in such crises, particularly airway management and sedation practices unique to the critically ill patient. The other common ICU condition is thrombocytopenia, a clinically extremely low platelet count with multiple etiologies. It is commonly encountered in critically ill patients and is an independent predictor of poor prognosis. Thrombocytopenia can be caused by sepsis, hematological disorders, or as a drug side effect, which all make the clinical scenario very complicated. The more reduced platelet counts represent a more dangerous risk of bleeding, and thus, close monitoring and intervention are called for. The treatment policy is generally founded on platelet transfusions to neutralize the risk of bleeding; nonetheless, the lack of concrete evidence regarding individual transfusion thresholds points to further studies into optimal practices of care in the ICU setting (Pène et al., 2025). Complicating these cases, the pathophysiology of thrombocytopenia necessitates an individualized therapeutic approach based on each patient's unique medical scenario. Pain control in the ICU is always a priority and often a challenging component of care, particularly with the diverse conditions treated within such settings. Regional anesthesia techniques have emerged as valuable adjuncts to pain control in critically ill patients, providing advantages beyond simple analgesia. For example, such techniques can be employed to manage potentially life-threatening complications like cerebral vasospasm or ventricular storm and thus improve overall clinical outcomes (Campbell et al., 2024). The introduction of ultrasound-guided regional anesthesia revolutionized such pain management techniques by facilitating safer and more effective interventions. Evidence shows that effective pain control not only reduces hospital stays and prevents unnecessary ICU admission but can also enhance long-term outcomes of recovery. Thus, the addition of regional anesthesia to the care of critically ill patients highlights the technologically varied therapeutic modalities at clinicians' disposal in intensive care settings.

Test Your Knowledge

1. What is the primary goal of intensive or critical care?
2. Why is continuous monitoring essential in critical care settings?

10.2. Principles of Critical Care Anesthesia

Learning Outcome

1. Differences between general and critical care anesthesia
2. Pharmacological considerations in critical care
3. Monitoring techniques in critical care anesthesia

In intensive care, critical care anesthesia practice is the mainstay of optimizing outcomes and ensuring patient safety. Part of the basis for this practice is very close monitoring of anesthetic depth and responsiveness intraoperatively. Advances such as Bispectral Index (BIS) monitoring have revolutionized anesthesiologists' assessment of patient response to anesthetic drugs. This technology quantifies the hypnotic effects of anesthesia with electroencephalogram (EEG) analysis, giving real-time feedback that dramatically enhances perioperative management. By providing an objective measurement of the patient's neurological state, BIS integration into anesthesia machines both enhances patient safety and aids in precise titration of anesthetic drug doses. This is a critically important method in eluding the twin dangers of over-sedation and under-anesthesia, thus minimizing the occurrence of anesthesia awareness, a situation with high ethical and psychological morbidity for patients (Zahid et al., 2024). Besides, critically ill patient care demands complex choices based on multi-dimensional physiological determinants. In this regard, digital twin technology is a groundbreaking breakthrough in critical care anesthesia. By creating a virtual patient model that simulates various respiratory pathophysiologies, clinicians can evaluate the potential result of therapeutic intervention without placing actual patients at risk. Consensus statement development by an expert panel with a multidisciplinary background also contributes to knowledge about the pathophysiology of respiratory failure, which is of utmost importance in deciding appropriate anesthetic and treatment strategies. The ability to simulate and test these approaches virtually makes it feasible to provide individualized patient care, supporting the need to personalize anesthesia practices to meet the diversity of intensive care unit patients (Almottowa et al., 2025).

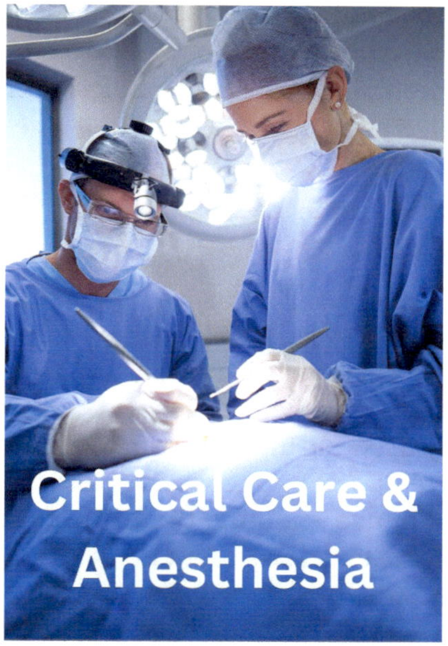

Figure 10.6. The principles of critical care anesthesia are pivotal for optimizing surgical outcomes and ensuring patient safety.

Source: https://external-content.duckduckgo.com/iu/?u=https%3A%2F%2Fi.pinimg.com%2F736x%2Fde%2F48%2Fa6%2Fde48a6cc49bc968e97673c903488462a.jpg&f=1&nofb=1&ipt=10507f719e448577600b1cc0250afb6023667185acf5e06ae0c3fcf0339a0294.

The use of advanced monitoring technology and virtual modeling in critical care anesthesia emphasizes the ongoing evolution of this specialty. With continued advances in anesthetic technology, technology such as BIS monitoring combined with digital twin patient modeling will become standard practice for intensive care units. These developments emphasize the need for widespread training and ongoing professional development on the part of anesthesia providers, so they remain competent in traditional as well as emerging technologies. The confluence of these principles promotes enhanced patient comfort and safety and a culture for continued quality improvement in anesthesia care, which responds to the ethical, clinical, and financial considerations that are vital to successful results within critical care environments (Zahid et al., 2024; Almottowa et al., 2025) (Figure 10.6).

10.2.1. Differences Between General and Critical Care Anesthesia

Anesthesia plays a vital role in handling the patients in critical care units, where general versus critical care anesthesia becomes increasingly significant. General anesthesia is primarily used during operations, rendering the patients temporarily unconscious and insensitive to pain, hence making them susceptible to invasive procedures without their awareness. In contrast to the other specialization, critical care anesthesia is more comprehensive in scope and deals with the maintenance and monitoring of the physiological status of critically ill patients who can be exposed to sedative therapy for a myriad of medical conditions, such as mechanical ventilation or emergency intervention. The specialty requires finesse in knowledge of drug agents since critical patient response to anesthesia is potentially variable based on their underlying conditions and comorbidities, and subsequently influences overall outcomes. The evolving practice of anesthesia techniques has raised issues regarding the efficacy and safety of different types of anesthesia in patient subgroups. Recent evidence points to the superiority of neuraxial anesthesia in comparison to general anesthesia in certain populations, namely in elective surgeries like total hip and knee replacements. Specifically, research indicates that patients who receive neuraxial anesthesia have fewer opportunities for negative outcomes, such as pulmonary complications and acute renal failure, according to research from the period of 2006–2021 (Illescas et al., 2024). These findings are of utmost importance in the case of critical care anesthesia, as anesthesia professionals must take care when they opt for anesthetic strategies that, on the one hand, optimize operating efficiency and, on the other hand, maximize recovery and minimize complications in vulnerable patients. Besides, the inflammatory response after diverse anesthesia protocols can also impact patient outcomes in operative and critical care settings. A study highlighted that cesarean section under general anesthesia is linked with a greater inflammatory reaction compared to spinal anesthesia and normal delivery methods (Almottowa et al., 2025). This variation highlights the importance of preference in anesthetic procedures, particularly among patients with ongoing inflammatory or respiratory illnesses, as it may exacerbate their clinical status. Understanding how these differences in anesthesia affect the body's response allows anesthesiologists and intensive care clinicians to better tailor their practices, thereby improving patient safety, decreasing complications, and optimizing recovery markers in intensive care.

10.2.2. Pharmacological Considerations in Critical Care

In intensive care, the choice of pharmacological agents is paramount due to the unique physiological complexities presented by ICU patients. Sedation and analgesia drugs must be carefully selected to meet the particular needs of the patient, particularly those with hemodynamic instability or multi-organ failure. Remimazolam is an ultra-short-acting benzodiazepine that represents a new and fascinating choice for critically ill patient sedation. Its short onset and short duration of action make it appropriate for procedures with short recovery, and its safety profile, especially in vulnerable groups such as the elderly and liver or kidney function-impaired patients, makes it valuable in the ICU setting. Adding Remimazolam to sedation protocols may revolutionize patient comfort, and, by inference, the quality of care overall in critical situations (Elmati et al., 2024). Dexmedetomidine, another drug gaining popularity for critical care anesthesiology, offers a new way of sedation due to its anesthetic and sedative effects. The drug has been established to be neuroprotective in action, with effects seen in a variety of preclinical models of ischemic and hemorrhagic brain damage. The evidence is such that dexmedetomidine not only causes sedation but also optimizes the outcome of ICU patients by attenuating stress responses to sedation. Apart from that, its non-opioid analgesic characteristic provides an essential alternative in cases where minimizing opioid-induced side effects is crucial. All of these notwithstanding, caution in monitoring for potential adverse effects such as hypotension and bradycardia is required, as they complicate the critical clinical management of critically ill patients (Bozorgi et al., 2021). Pharmacologic factors in critical care extend far beyond the choice of sedation agents to encompass broader factors of safety and outcomes of the patient. The addition of novel agents like Remimazolam and dexmedetomidine to sedation strategies is indicative of a trend toward more personalized approaches, based on the individual requirements of each patient. By minimizing sedative burdens and optimizing drug choice based upon pharmacokinetic and pharmacodynamic profiles, clinicians can maximize patient satisfaction with fewer complications. Further study of these drugs, including long-term safety and efficacy across a broad range of patient populations, is necessary to establish best practice in the rapidly evolving specialty of critical care anesthesia. Future studies should not only focus on efficacy but also on attempts to establish these medications as a standard component of clinical practice, thus maximizing the overall management of critically ill patients in the ICU (Figure 10.7).

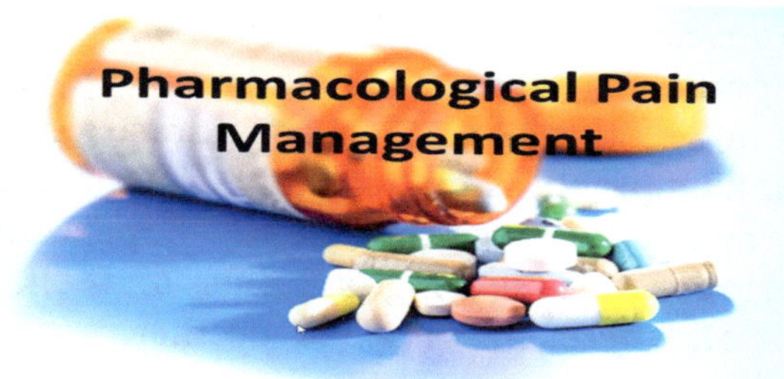

Figure 10.7. Pharmacological considerations in critical care.

Source: https://external-content.duckduckgo.com/iu/?u=https%3A%2F%2Fi.ytimg.com%2Fvi%2Fk3TqRFQGbbM%2Fmaxresdefault.jpg&f=1&nofb=1&ipt=2605c978ae6ec0416df56dd513020443c63662c99cc930eedfccd281cd146393.

10.2.3. Monitoring Techniques in Critical Care Anesthesia

Monitoring techniques in critical care anesthesia are important to ensure the comfort and safety of patients who are subjected to complex surgical operations and postoperative care. Advances in monitoring technology have significantly improved patient outcomes, particularly under high-risk scenarios like ICUs. Continual monitoring of physiological metrics such as heart rate, blood pressure, and oxygen saturation allows anesthesiologists to make rapid decisions. Advanced surveillance systems now incorporate parameters like BIS monitoring, which measures anesthetic depth more accurately, and hemodynamic monitoring devices that monitor cardiac output and fluid status, allowing for interventions in a timely manner. These advancements are of great importance in managing potential complications, emphasizing the responsibility of anesthesiologists to remain proficient in managing these technologies for patient stability and reduced perioperative risks, as emphasized in the literature examining the impact of surgical manipulations and their systemic effects (De Gasperi et al., 2024). The management of postoperative complications, including posthepatectomy liver failure (PHLF), imposes the merit of rigorous monitoring. After major liver resections in the operating room, anesthesiologists must embrace forward-thinking practices that extend beyond the door of the operating room to the ICU. Sophisticated perioperative scoring systems and clinical criteria increasingly make predictive ability and management of the differing grades of PHLF possible. Anesthesiologists are tasked with playing an important role in this chain of care, being asked to have close consultation with surgical teams and intensivists. This cross-disciplinary approach guarantees optimal intensive care according to the patient's status, eventually improving survival rates following complex surgeries. Enhanced Monitoring methods thus not only serve as a device for guaranteeing patient safety in the near future but also as a platform for diagnosing and preventing postoperative complications (De Gasperi et al., 2024). In addition to the technological advancement, anesthetic care for older, frail patients has unique challenges that require individual monitoring approaches. As the population of older patients increases, the demand for anesthesia and pain management in vulnerable patients becomes more urgent, requiring a fine balance between efficacy and safety. Modern anesthetic therapy aims to utilize drug regimens more appropriate for this cohort, with an emphasis on accuracy to accommodate each patient's unique care. Regular monitoring, particularly in specialized settings like geriatric intensive therapy units, is a necessity to identify adverse reactions early and accordingly adjust the treatment protocols. Admittance of evidence-based best practices into monitoring techniques significantly enhances patient safety and postoperative recovery among frail older adults. This indicates that the function of anesthesiologists must extend to the need to adapt their monitoring techniques according to the nuances of diverse patient populations.

Test Your Knowledge

1. What is a key principle of critical care anesthesia in managing unstable patients?
2. Why is airway and hemodynamic management crucial in critical care anesthesia?

10.3. Patient Assessment in Critical Care

Learning Outcome

1. Preoperative evaluation of critical patients
2. Risk stratification and management
3. Importance of multidisciplinary collaboration

In critical care settings, patient evaluation is a paramount component that has an immediate influence on management strategies and clinical outcomes. The single physiological derangements evident in critically ill patients necessitate a comprehensive evaluation in multiple areas of vital signs, lab reports, and overall clinical condition. Active detection of potential complications such as malnutrition is an invaluable function in implementing optimal intervention and the greatest chances of recovery courses. Studies have suggested that the application of tools like the Nutrition Risk in the Critically Ill (mNUTRIC) Score within the first 24 hours of admission is effective to stratify patients by risk of malnutrition to enable targeted nutritional therapy for preventing muscle loss and facilitating recovery (Sharon et al., 2024). Thus, the careful and systematic process of evaluation is essential to critical care environments. Sedative management is also an area of patient evaluation in critical care, with evaluation of both safety and efficacy of various pharmacologic agents. An instance of this is ketamine, which was investigated as a potential analgesic-sedative for mechanically ventilated patients and demonstrated considerable uncertainty about its use compared to traditional sedatives. Research highlights the need to examine the evaluation of ketamine as an independent intervention as well as combined with current sedation practices in order to determine its net benefit (Amer et al., 2024). These evaluations are vital in informing best practice for sedation strategy since improper management may lead to unfavorable outcomes, including increased duration of mechanical ventilation or delirium rates. Hence, the implementation of evidence-based recommendations is vital in optimizing sedation regimens for the individual needs of critically ill patients. Moreover, patient assessment is a holistic process that involves continuous reassessment to address the dynamic nature of critical illness. According to changes in a patient's clinical condition, close monitoring allows timely readjustments in treatment regimes that involve modifications in sedation depth, nutrition therapy, and fluid resuscitation. The use of advanced monitoring equipment facilitates constant observation of vital signs and other physiological parameters, allowing for prompt reaction to deviations from the normal norms. Multidisciplinary team assessments standardized into standard formats promote joint decision-making that incorporates multiple views, further enhancing the quality of patient care. In general, an effective critical care patient assessment process is multifaceted and involves ongoing attention to detail, multidisciplinary coordination, and application of evidence-based practice to optimize therapeutic interventions with this vulnerable population of patients (Figure 10.8).

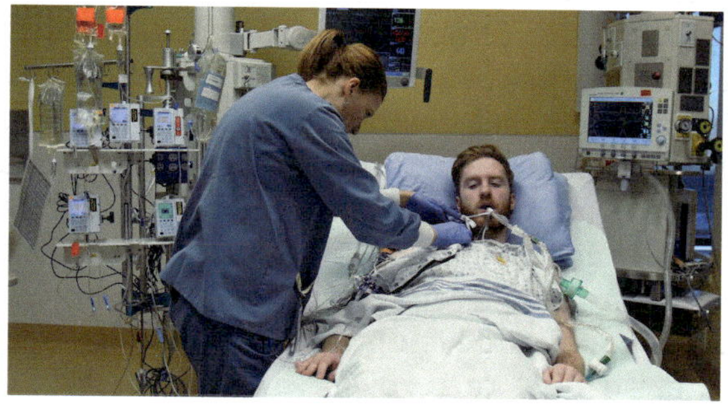

Figure 10.8. The assessment of patients is an integral component that directly influences management strategies and clinical outcomes.

Source: https://external-content.duckduckgo.com/iu/?u=https%3A%2F%2Fi.ytimg.com%2Fvi%2FJF-94zLg2QQ%2Fmaxresdefault.jpg&f=1&nofb=1&ipt=98b3853dcbdcbd1fd193b8e2aaf7813e3b312ce4b399a3b46666cde0b4788eb5.

10.3.1. Preoperative Evaluation of Critical Patients

Preoperative evaluation of critical patients forms a central role in the context of intensive care and critical care anesthesiology. Because of their complexity, it is necessary to perform a thorough evaluation so as to identify any potential risks and schedule an extensive surgical procedure. The evaluation typically consists of a patient's overview of history, such as previous illnesses, American Society of Anesthesiologists (ASA) risk class, and current physiological status. Moreover, laboratory tests, including biochemical and hematological studies, are needed to establish baseline organ function and the presence of major comorbidities like chronic kidney disease that play significant roles in surgery and anesthetic outcomes. Understanding these clinical issues allows anesthesiologists to predict complication development during and after surgery, guiding changes in anesthetic plans or interventions that can be made to enhance patient safety and maximize overall outcomes in postoperative care. Control of specific hazards attributed to the preoperative period is particularly critical in the scenario of acute kidney injury (AKI), which has been observed with unmatched frequency among surgical critical patients. Scientific studies reveal that surgical patients with significant risk factors like higher Charlson Comorbidity Index (CCI) scores and abnormal preoperative laboratory test results tend to develop AKI following surgery and contribute to recovery and mortality. The evaluation must also consider the urgency of the operation and the potential impact of intraoperative interventions. For instance, the amount and type of fluid infused can have a direct impact on renal function after the operation. This communication underlines the importance of stratifying the patients not only demographically but also according to individual assessment of their fluid management in such a manner that risk for AKI is minimized and overall operative outcomes are enhanced as per the latest perioperative care research studies among critical populations (Hajili et al., 2024).

In addition, preoperative assessment needs to go beyond physiological reasons to encompass logistical issues faced in austere environments, where traditional facilities may be unavailable. The guidelines set by the Italian Society of Anesthesia, Analgesia, Resuscitation and Intensive Care (SIAARTI) underscore the importance of tailoring assessment practice to overcome the singular challenges experienced in such environments. A focus on core care skills—especially those concerning airway management, bleeding control, and proper analgesia—has a substantial impact on survival rates. By setting priorities in immediate interventions and implementing effective pain protocols, practitioners are able to manage the complexity involved in critical patient care. Hence, establishing a preoperative evaluation protocol overall is essential as regards optimizing the surgical procedure of critically ill patients so that short-term and long-term outcomes are of satisfactory quality under diverse situations (Bixio et al., 2024).

10.3.2. Risk Stratification and Management

The concept of risk stratification is at the heart of intensive care and critical care anesthetic practice since it gives clinicians a method of assessing the likelihood of complications in critically ill patients. Through thorough investigation of various clinical parameters, risk stratification allows for tailored management plans aimed at optimizing patient outcomes. This approach is particularly relevant regarding delirium, a pervasive but complex neuropsychiatric syndrome experienced by the critically ill population. Delirium is currently being researched with a focus on its multi-dimensionality, and practitioners are urged to move beyond the traditional treatment paradigms like haloperidol. The emphasis on stratifying delirium into subtypes and etiology is a reflection of the requirement for greater clarity in understanding the condition, which may play a role in more-targeted interventions and, in the long run, better patient care in the intensive care unit, as set out in Jiang et al. (2025). Parallel to this, risk stratification plays a crucial role in the treatment of invasive fungal infections, such as invasive candidiasis (IC), that are serious challenges to the intensive care environment. The most prevalent etiologic agent of severe fungal infection, Candida species, may cause high mortality and morbidity, necessitating prompt and effective therapeutic interventions. Risk factor identification, including breaches of protective barriers routinely present in ICUs, is a significant piece of the puzzle in understanding who may be at higher risk for developing IC. Risk stratification tools, along with prompt diagnosis and treatment recommendations, are valuable for avoiding the potential healthcare costs of such infections. Such strategies have been highly sought within expert forums on discussions regarding them, which mirrors the urgent need to tap into individualized management plans in an endeavor to maximally improve patient outcomes compared to current challenges resulting from emerging new fungal ecologies, as shown in Sharon et al. (2024).

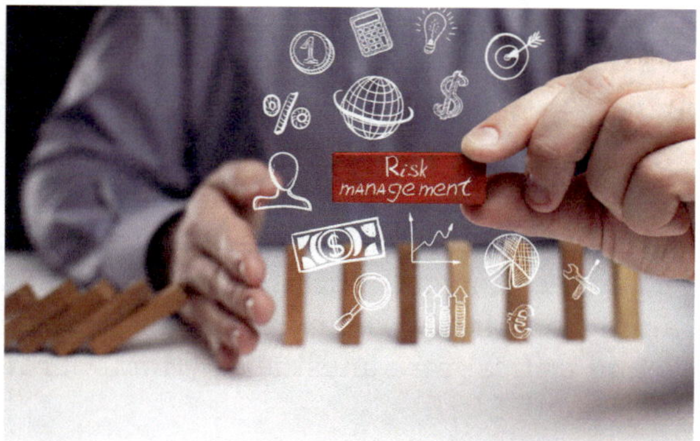

Figure 10.9. The concept of risk stratification is pivotal within the domain of intensive care and critical care anesthesia.

Source: https://external-content.duckduckgo.com/iu/?u=https%3A%2F%2Fblog.curemd.com%2Fwp-content%2Fuploads%2F2021%2F10%2FRisk-Stratification-Combining-Objective-And-Subjective-Insights-for-Risk-Stratified-Care-Management.jpg&f=1&nofb=1&ipt=14d20f7bae e5f20ae9242815cbb24f5921e73b35fe85b6017 9087893a162cc43.

Furthermore, the integration of risk stratification with management cannot be limited to short-term clinical intervention but must involve a multi-disciplinary strategy within critical care environments. Coordination of various specialists, including infectious disease specialists and pharmacists, enables a comprehensive approach to the management of complicated cases, particularly delirium or invasive fungal infection. It appears increasingly clear that successful management is not only a function of individual treatment strategies but also of coordinated action in managing the overall neuropsychiatric manifestation or the evolving pattern of fungal infection. By the use of psychological testing tools and emerging diagnostic techniques, critical care teams can more precisely stratify risk, which will improve management strategies. In the end, embracing a more holistic strategy to patient care in intensive care units will result in further advances in clinical outcomes and patient satisfaction, further affirming the importance of interdisciplinary collaboration in maintaining improved quality care for critically ill patients (Figure 10.9).

10.3.3. Importance of Multidisciplinary Collaboration

Optimal multidisciplinary collaboration is at the heart of improving intensive care and critical care anesthesia outcomes. In complex clinical situations, i.e., in the management of patients with acute respiratory distress syndrome, the convergence of various disciplines ensures a proper approach in the management of the patient. For example, in cases of bad pre-eclampsia and acute lung oedema, an effective intervention relies not only on anesthetists' proficiency in airway management but also on the obstetrician's expertise to keep the mother and child under close observation. Such collaboration enables improved clinical decision-making and accommodates rapid changes in treatment modalities, thereby reducing mortality and morbidity. As highlighted by current studies, the integration of several medical specialties maximizes the avenues for innovative solutions, leading to more effective protocols in critical care areas (Carenzo et al., 2025). Furthermore, establishing well-defined channels of communication among several healthcare experts serves as the basis for effective collaboration. Within an intensive care setting, there is a need for timely sharing of patient information between nurses, anesthesiologists, surgeons, and other team members in order to adopt care practices that are both effective and safe. Multidisciplinary rounds where team members work together in reviewing patient cases are a valuable practice that not only ensures knowledge sharing but also supports and accountability among practitioners. Additionally, the application of standardized practices, observed in protocols developed through multidisciplinary collaboration, provides adherence to best practices within critical care settings. Compliance with regulatory requirements, which are quintessential in maintaining patient care quality and safety, is also supported by collaborative models (Carenzo et al., 2025). A collaborative model's value transcends clinical performance because it also enhances professional development among healthcare professionals. Collaborating with other colleagues from various specialties allows the exchange of information and skills, promoting a culture of continuous improvement in practice through continuous learning. It promotes critical thinking as well as enhances the skills of the team members, preparing them to address complex patient needs in a high-stress environment. Further, if multidisciplinary teams are frequently undergoing training simulations and interprofessional education, it enhances relationships and builds mutual respect among professionals. This increased synergy serves not only individual practitioner competence but ultimately aids in better patient care pathways, hence affirming the importance of multidisciplinary collaboration for intensive care and critical care anesthesia (Hotabilardus & Anggraeni, 2025).

Test Your Knowledge

1. What are the main components of patient assessment in critical care?
2. Why is frequent reassessment important for critically ill patients?

10.4. Anesthetic Techniques in Intensive Care

Learning Outcome

1. Induction and maintenance of anesthesia
2. Use of regional anesthesia in critical care
3. Postoperative pain management strategies

Anesthetic methods utilized within intensive care are critical in the management of critically ill patients with the need for advanced monitoring and support. Such patients tend to have complex medical illnesses, whose anesthetic management must be individualized, focusing on hemodynamic stability and fast recovery. Regional anesthesia has become increasingly popular among used techniques because it can offer good pain relief without systemic side effects. This is especially worthwhile in critical care settings where patients are at an increased risk for the development of complications. For instance, the use of nerve blocks can help with recovery after surgery, reduce opioid consumption, and enhance patient comfort, all of which cumulatively result in improved critically ill outcomes. By applying such techniques wisely, clinicians can provide appropriate control of pain without significantly affecting the functioning of major organs for maximum recovery profiles and patient satisfaction as a whole (Michard et al., 2025). In combination with regional anesthesia, improvements in monitoring devices have transformed anesthetic care in intensive care units. With the addition of sophisticated cardiovascular imaging devices, real-time hemodynamic monitoring of values significantly enhances decision-making processes. For example, echocardiographic techniques such as speckle tracking have arrived for non-invasive evaluation of myocardial function so that the cardiovascular condition of a patient can be comprehended more subtly. These innovations are critical in managing fluid resuscitation and pharmacological treatment, particularly if patients have compromised hemodynamics.

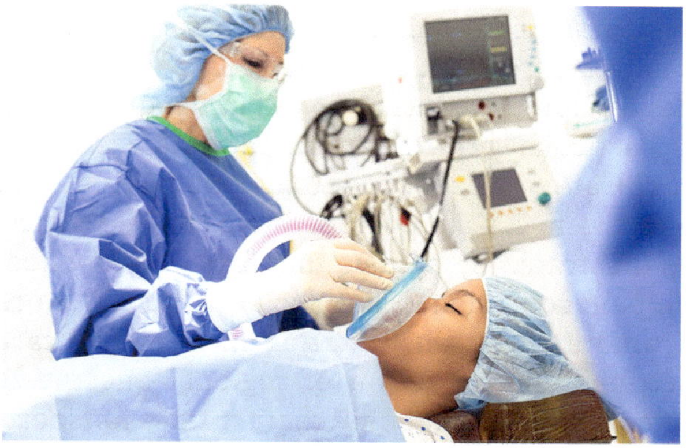

Figure 10.10. Anesthetic techniques employed in intensive care.

Source: https://external-content.duckduckgo.com/iu/?u=https%3A%2F%2Fhealthjade.com%2Fwp-content%2Fuploads%2F2017%2F11%2Fgeneral-anesthesia.jpg&f=1&nofb=1&ipt=6328d2f3080d6f568baeb1bb650a99d033b9850f2f50149951ae8435ffb4f112.

In addition, microcirculation visualization using handheld devices provides insight into tissue perfusion, which is fundamental in guiding therapeutic intervention during critical illness. Anesthetic practice in intensive care is therefore not just the administration of anesthetics but a comprehensive approach to monitoring and patient care (Michard et al., 2025). Furthermore, the incidence of technical errors in intensive care anesthesia underscores the importance of simulation training among clinical teams. Research has indicated that mistakes such as device failure significantly affect patient management and outcomes, thus the need to implement an active approach in enhancing team response to crises. In a study involving a high-fidelity simulation, airway management critical incident response times were measured and were delayed in instances of technical malfunctions involved. This finding highlights the value of regular simulation training for high-risk situations among critical care personnel, ultimately leading to improved preparedness for real challenges. These learning activities are the core of enhancing procedure responses and developing teamwork and thus overall intensive care unit patient care (Figure 10.10).

10.4.1. Induction and Maintenance of Anesthesia

Induction and maintenance of anesthesia are key elements both in intensive care and critical care environments, to make surgical and procedural treatments safe and comfortable for patients. Induction is generally characterized by the quick infusion of anesthetic drugs, which enable quick induction into unconsciousness. These drugs have extremely variable pharmacokinetics and pharmacodynamics, for which careful consideration by anesthesiologists must be given in order to tailor the approach to the individual clinical situation for each patient. In patients who are critically ill, the choice of induction agents is particularly challenging, as they may have abnormal physiology or more than one comorbidity that will affect drug metabolism and action. Moreover, the selection process may be complex, with hemodynamic stability, respiratory function, and potential interactions with existing pharmacologic interventions among various factors that are taken into account, emphasizing the complexity of anesthesia care in such vulnerable populations. Maintenance once anesthesia has been effectively induced maintains the patient in an appropriate condition of unconsciousness and analgesia throughout the duration of a procedure. This stage may involve ongoing monitoring and adjustment of anesthetic depth and adjunct drugs to best maximize patient outcomes. Importantly, monitoring methods have improved dramatically to provide higher technologies of anesthetic depth measurement and physiologic stability, improving patient safety. Opioid-based analgesia, as well as multimodal analgesic techniques, are commonly employed by anesthesiologists to avoid causing pain while lowering the total anesthetic demand. In addition, recent advances in local anesthetic techniques, including the use of ultrasound for blocks, have been promising in the successful treatment of pain in critically ill patients, which could translate to shorter postoperative recovery times and a reduced period of intensive care stay (Campbell et al., 2024). In addition to proper anesthesia being ensured, induction and maintenance also have to be properly monitored and managed to avoid intraoperative complications. These may include hemodynamic changes, respiratory impairment, or unforeseen anesthetic reactions, all of which need to be addressed immediately by the anesthesia practitioner. With advancements in technology, e.g., real-time hemodynamic monitoring and computerized decision support systems, practitioners are facilitated to deliver quick hemodynamic reactions to evolving situations in the operating room. The integration of such equipment can maximize decision-making and results, particularly in intensive care units where the stakes are so much greater (Michard et al., 2025). Lastly, the initiation and maintenance of anesthesia in intensive and critical care require not only meticulous planning and implementation but also ongoing dedication to improving techniques and technologies that provide optimal patient care during some of the most challenging medical procedures.

10.4.2. Use of Regional Anesthesia in Critical Care

The application of regional anesthesia to intensive care units is a significant advancement in pain treatment and the improvement of patients' outcomes during the intensive and critical care phases. As opposed to standard general anesthesia, regional forms of anesthesia, such as nerve blocks and epidurals, target specific areas to provide analgesia without losing patient consciousness. This judicious utilization is particularly useful in critically ill patients who can have contraindications to general anesthesia or can benefit from reduced systemic opioid utilization. Regional anesthesia can avert frequent side effects like respiratory depression by reducing opioid utilization, which is particularly important in patients with poor respiratory reserve. Furthermore, regional anesthesia can aid postoperative convalescence, as illustrated by studies that focus on its effect on pain control and mobilization and therefore promote early rehabilitation in intensive care settings. Incorporation of regional anesthesia into critical care not only compensates for short-term analgesic needs but also is favorable to long-term patient benefit. For instance, the introduction of continuous regional anesthetic techniques has been associated with lower rates of chronic postoperative pain as well as fewer instances of post-surgical complications. Continuous infusion of local anesthetics can achieve effective pain relief even beyond the duration of immediate recovery from surgery, which allows for increased mobilization and physiological stability. Further, regional anesthesia enhances the overall patient experience by providing a tailored approach to pain control, which is paramount in the high-stakes environment of an intensive care unit. The tailored approach can lead to an overall model of care that emphasizes comfort and satisfaction for the patient while meeting the complexity of critical illness. Despite the clear benefits of regional anesthesia for application in critical care, there remain a number of issues that must be solved by practitioners in order to obtain optimal results. The need for trained anesthesiologists skilled in the administration of regional procedures could limit extensive use of these methods in some clinical settings. Furthermore, patient preference, potential complications, and effective monitoring of anesthesia remain pivotal. With emerging fields, ongoing research is essential to make certain methods and technologies, such as the new continuous cardiac output monitors, such as the qCO monitor, become more effective and safe in regional anesthesia administrations (Escrivá et al., 2016). Lastly, integration of regional anesthetic methods into critical care models will need a multi-disciplinary approach to guarantee harmonious integration of pain management as an integral part of the comprehensive goal of patient care and overcoming the particular difficulties related to these high-acuity environments (Prosser et al., 1998) (Figure 10.11).

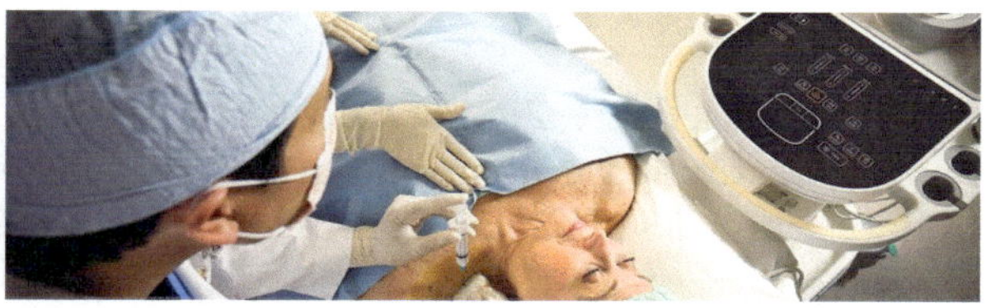

Figure 10.11. Use of regional anesthesia in critical care.

Source: https://external-content.duckduckgo.com/iu/?u=https%3A%2F%2Fassets.website-files.com%2F57c8447991c61fe936e83cfb%2F586c07c7fcd66fc24dbfa537_Regional%2520Anesthesia-p-800x247.jpeg&f=1&nofb=1&ipt=20d319015134edffa0a47488e94c9660ccfd42c8705109d88480890d9060dcdc.

10.4.3. Postoperative Pain Management Strategies

Effective postoperative pain control is crucial in critical care anesthesia and intensive care, with inadequate pain control undermining recovery and causing chronic pain syndromes, significantly affecting patient quality of life. This necessitates a multidisciplinary approach to pain management using both regional and multimodal techniques of anesthesia. Multimodal analgesia is the use of various pharmacologic agents, including NSAIDs and local anesthetics, together to achieve better pain relief with less opiate consumption and side effects. For instance, local nerve blocks and neuraxial analgesia are effective in the prevention of the development of persistent postoperative pain by allowing early mobilization and functional recovery. Integration of these strategies within enhanced recovery after surgery (ERAS) protocols emphasizes patient-centered care, ultimately leading to improved outcomes and satisfaction post-surgery (Kim, 2025). Within the intensive care unit (ICU), the nuances of pain management are compounded by the need to address heterogeneous medical problems and patient populations. Strategies employed within this unique environment must consider both pharmacologic and non-pharmacologic strategies. Based on the patient's condition and pain tolerance, universal analgesics like opioids can be used effectively in combination with NSAIDs to maximize pain management. In addition, novel non-pharmacologic therapies—such as music therapy, relaxation therapy, and massage—are becoming increasingly popular for their utility in practical use in critically ill patients. These strategies are not only valuable as adjuncts to medication therapy but also can be reasonable substitutes for analgesic medication, highlighting the necessity of a multidisciplinary model in the ICU setting, wherein clinician-to-patient ratios could be such that pain evaluation and management become compromised (Zakeri et al., 2024). Continued research is essential to the establishment of postoperative pain management strategies. While existing evidence supports the integration of multimodal analgesia and regional techniques into practice, less is known regarding the best protocols under various settings of surgery and among various groups of patients. Closing these knowledge gaps demands concerted effort to evaluate the effectiveness of pain management modalities and their consistent implementation within the clinical setting. Future studies must prioritize individualized medicine approaches to tailor pain management to the unique needs of the patient. In addition, collaboration among anesthesiologists, surgeons, and pain experts is paramount to overcoming systemic obstacles in providing evidence-based care. Collaboration not only enhances patient recovery but also minimizes the long-term psychosocial outcomes of poorly managed postoperative pain, illustrating an overall enhancement of patient care and outcomes (Kim, 2025) (Figure 10.12).

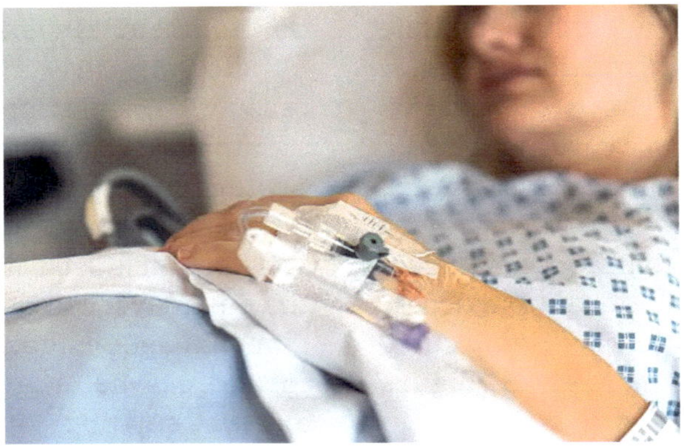

Figure 10.12. Postoperative pain management strategies.

Source: https://external-content.duckduckgo.com/iu/?u=https%3A%2F%2Fpharmaceutical-journal.com%2Fwp-content%2Fuploads%2F2022%2F09%2Fpostoperative-pain-hospital-patient-recovery-650x433.jpg&f=1&nofb=1&ipt=56f9d13a17d1060a00adae3afbe2f6312b2e55f4c1e5c99f798625e3214d0da9.

Test Your Knowledge

1. What types of anesthetic techniques are commonly used in the ICU?
2. Why is careful titration of anesthetic drugs important in critically ill patients?

10.5. Complications and Challenges in Critical Care Anesthesia

Learning Outcome

1. Common anesthetic complications
2. Management of complications in the ICU setting
3. Ethical considerations in critical care anesthesia

Complications from critical care anesthesia are most commonly a result of the complex nature of patients' illnesses, particularly in groups of multiple co-morbidities. Intensive care unit patients often have heterogeneous pathophysiologic states such as cardiovascular illness, respiratory failure, or renal failure, making anesthetic care complicated. Each condition has various challenges related to affecting drug metabolism, dosing accuracy, and consequently leading to enhanced perioperative complications. Aside from this, the intricate relationship between anesthesia and ongoing health conditions requires anesthesiologists to demonstrate a sound understanding of pharmacodynamics and pharmacokinetics when designing individualized anesthetic regimens. A case in point is the administration of anesthetics to patients with dysfunctional livers, which requires careful consideration to prevent toxic accumulation and subsequent complications, reinforcing the essential role of individualized methods in such vulnerable populations. One of the specific challenges in critical care anesthesia is airway complication control, which can have adverse effects on patient outcomes. Securing and maintaining the airway typically falls to anesthesiologists, particularly in patients with complicated anatomy or those who have experienced trauma. Failure to intubate can lead to severe complications such as hypoxia or aspiration pneumonia, particularly in emergency cases where timing is critical. Techniques such as video laryngoscopy have been developed to enhance visualization and the chances of successful intubation. Although these new devices are not necessarily available in every clinical context, there is indeed a particular requirement for a wide range of training and simulation sessions to prepare practitioners for unexpected airway management challenges. The implementation of new technologies must be balanced with hands-on training to develop competency in high-stress contexts. Furthermore, the late onset of complications, such as perioperative bronchospasm, further complicates critical care anesthesia. Asthmatic patients, for instance, may be stable with induction but experience sudden severe bronchospasm upon recovery, as indicated in the case of a 77-year-old female patient who experienced bronchospasm during recovery from tumor resection. Her situation was not altered by initial measures, indicating that standard protocols are not sufficient. This situation emphasizes the need for anesthesiologists to develop responsive management strategies to counter such unexpected situations. The case also points to leading-edge equipment, such as the MAD Nasal™, which provides for quick intervention in case of a crisis. Besides, structured simulations can enhance the education of healthcare professionals through addressing the necessity for preparedness and quick decision-making in the event of perioperative complications like bronchospasm, thus enhancing patient outcomes for critical care (Ji et al., 2025) (Figure 10.13).

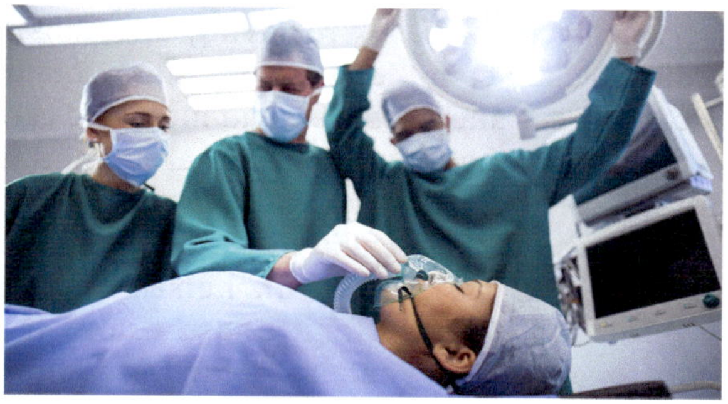

Figure 10.13. Complications in critical care anesthesia often stem from the complex nature of patients' medical histories.

Source: https://external-content.duckduckgo.com/iu/?u=https%3A%2F%2Fmediparkhospital.in%2Fmedia%2F2023%2F04%2Fanesthesia-and-critical-care-medipark.jpg&f=1&nofb=1&ipt=a454e33e1dc5a3fc8cca445420107d80f0f5832bcf496c09075ff72c5acaf861.

10.5.1. Common Anesthetic Complications

The administration of anesthesia during critical procedures is an intricate process fraught with potential complications, necessitating rigorous training and awareness among medical practitioners. Among the most common complications encountered are respiratory issues, which can manifest as hypoxemia or hypercapnia, particularly during intubation or mechanical ventilation. In intensive care cases, the management of respiratory complications is imperative, and this is what makes productive sedation practices important to ensure effective weaning from mechanical ventilation. A review of the practice of sedations indicated that the use of anesthetic medication like dexmedetomidine may improve extubation success and reduce the state of delirium among critical illness patients, which would translate to better outcomes post-surgery and during recovery (Majed et al., 2025). Nonetheless, respiratory depression is still at risk, which calls for clinical surveillance and appropriate intervention to prevent such risks in critically ill patients receiving anesthesia. Cardiovascular complications are also a major concern under anesthesia care in intensive care unit (ICU) settings. Hypotension, arrhythmias, and in severe cases, cardiac arrest, can occur with anesthesia, especially in cardiac patients. The impact of anesthesia on hemodynamics is wide-ranging; therefore, anesthesiologists have to regularly observe cardiovascular parameters and be ready to take action rapidly. Research has demonstrated that the anesthetic strategy employed can dramatically affect the prevalence of these complications, emphasizing the importance of individualized anesthetic methods for the improvement of patient safety. Moreover, regional anesthesia methods such as epidural analgesia have been linked with improved cardiovascular stability, offering a complement to systemic opioids that exacerbate cardiac conditions. The judicious selection and administration of anesthetics can therefore become critical in avoiding cardiovascular complications in critically ill patients (Lazar & Farczádi, 2024). Neurological complications, although less frequent, carry serious risks in anesthesia practice, particularly intensive care. Anesthetics can cause postoperative cognitive dysfunction, delirium, or severe complications such as stroke in vulnerable populations. The balance between the patient's pre-existing comorbidities and anesthetic type determines the risk of neurological adverse effects to a significant degree. Furthermore, there has been growing concern regarding the administration of long-duration anesthetics and sedatives, which cause prolonged recovery time and cognitive impairment. The development of monitoring tactics and neuroprotective therapies is paramount in the ICU, especially as the population served becomes more commonly older individuals at higher risk of such complications. Some evidence has arisen to indicate the efficacy of local anesthetic use for pain management in critical illness as a potential method of reducing the need for systemic anesthetics and improving neurological outcomes (Lazar & Farczádi, 2024). This underscores the need for a holistic strategy to anesthesia that considers both short-term and long-term well-being of the patient.

10.5.2. Management of Complications in the ICU Setting

Effective complication management within the ICU setting is paramount to good patient outcomes, particularly following major surgery. Complexity calls for multidisciplinary management, especially in the case of postoperative complications, which are the leading cause of death following elective major abdominal surgery. Critical care teams must be proficient in expedited assessment and intervention to manage complications such as hemodynamic instability, infection, and respiratory failure that typically arise in the postoperative period. Individualized steps, determined on the basis of careful preoperative risk assessment with validated scoring systems, are necessary to optimize resource use. This proactive effort decreases instances of unplanned ICU admissions, thereby enhancing patient care and resource use in the ICU (Lavezzo et al., 2025). Identification of surgical and patient-specific risk factors allows medical staff to anticipate and prevent complications more effectively. Intubation and airway management in the ICU is yet another such challenging area requiring careful attention to avoid complications and ensure patient safety. The choice of method of intubation, particularly in critically ill patients, can significantly impact the success of airway control. The introduction of newer, advanced devices such as the SANYAR video laryngoscope has been found to have enormous benefits over traditional direct laryngoscopy methods, particularly in challenging airway scenarios. Evidence indicates that the use of video laryngoscopy improves glottic visualization and first-pass successful intubation rates, both of which are key to minimizing risks for airway complications. Through enabling quicker and more accurate intubation techniques, the care team can dramatically reduce undesirable outcomes, enhancing the quality of care provided in the ICU setting (Khajavi et al., 2023). Secondly, continuous monitoring and reassessment after the operation are also included in successfully managing complications in the ICU. After surgery, patients can have dynamic clinical statuses that need to be closely monitored, particularly those admitted following abdominal surgery when the risk for complications is greatest. A structured protocol involving high-dependency unit usage and continuous monitoring of vital cardiovascular and respiratory indices allows for early intervention when complications arise. Preoperative assessments using instruments like the Clinical Frailty Scale can inform care plans and predict patient needs, so healthcare teams are prepared for complications. With an integration of state-of-the-art technologies, targeted assessments, and vigilant monitoring, critical care professionals are able to enhance patient outcomes and effectively navigate the complexities of ICU management after major surgeries (Lavezzo et al., 2025) (Figure 10.14).

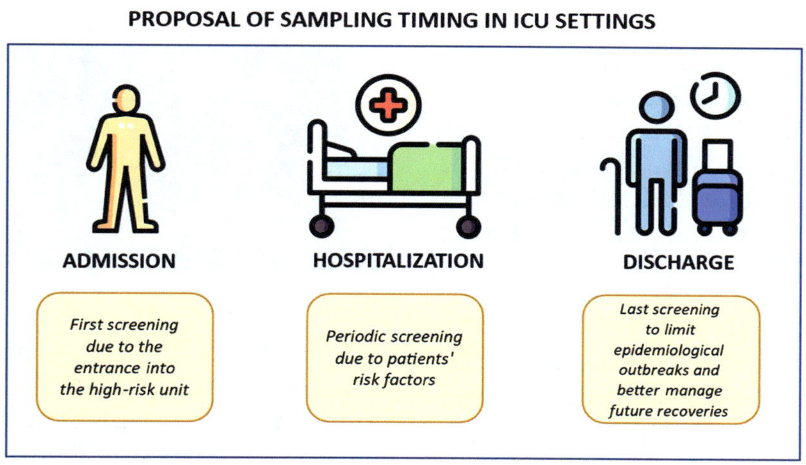

Figure 10.14. The management of complications in the intensive care unit (ICU) setting.

Source: https://www.mdpi.com/antibiotics/antibiotics-13-00238/article_deploy/html/images/antibiotics-13-00238-g001.png.

10.5.3. Ethical Considerations in Critical Care Anesthesia

For critical care anesthesia, ethical issues are foremost, most prominently patient autonomy and informed consent. Anesthetic technique could require spontaneous decision-making, especially where the patient's ability to consent is compromised in emergency, life-threatening situations. Physicians need to walk the thin tightrope between deciding in the patient's best interest and holding back from interfering with their autonomy as much as possible. This also raises a severe ethical issue, especially in cases where family members or surrogates need to make decisions without the consent of patients. The ethical obligation to provide care that adheres to a patient values and preferences indicates the complexity associated with regard to anesthesiologists making choices in acute cases in intensive and critical care units. The use of physical restraints during critical care conditions adds another level of ethical concern to anesthesiologists. Deployed primarily to limit self-harm or interference with life-supporting medical devices, restraint is very ethically challenging, possibly infringing on a patient's dignity and autonomy. While their use may be justified in specific conditions, the negative psychological impacts of restraining patients always give rise to criticism regarding the effectiveness and necessity of such actions. The ethical and legal considerations necessitate the implementation of restraints to be made thoughtfully, balancing short-term needs for safety with long-term effects on patient welfare. Moreover, discussion of restraint substitutes such as augmented communication and patient engagement are positive strides in solving ethical problems in critical care anesthesia (Benzakour et al., 2025).

In addition, the ethical basis of critical care anesthesia extends even to pediatric-specific considerations where cultural, economic, and resource determinants significantly impact the provision of care. Parental preference and issues of budgets are typical for pediatric critical care units that complicate decision-making in treatment. The ethical obligation to provide equal and effective care is hindered by the availability of limited resources in low- and middle-income contexts. Ethical issues are encountered when treatment family choices must be balanced with requirements for resource utilization and potential impact on outcomes. Multi-dimensional ethical problems are resolved by collaborating with stakeholders, including health practitioners and global organizations, to offer all children optimal care regardless of context-based challenges (Olatunji et al., 2024) (Figure 10.15).

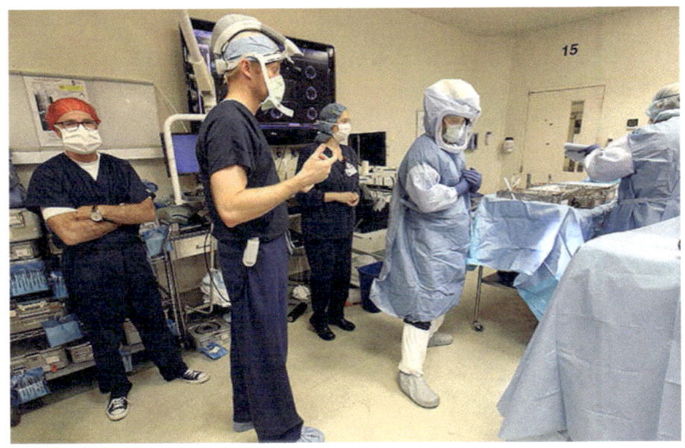

Figure 10.15. Ethical considerations in critical care anesthesia.

Source: https://external-content.duckduckgo.com/iu/?u=https%3A%2F%2Fmedicine.musc.edu%2F-%2Fsm%2Fmedicine%2Fdepartments%2Fanesthesia%2Fi%2Fclinical-division-649x433.ashx&f=1&nofb=1&ipt=c3b6532bdba0640afdaf2e6924f97fb7804621d4f224b0ba59fe6708b367de1d.

Test Your Knowledge

1. What is a common complication associated with anesthesia in critically ill patients?
2. Why is managing hemodynamic instability a major challenge in critical care anesthesia?

10.6. Advances in Critical Care Anesthesia

Learning Outcome

1. Technological innovations in monitoring
2. Research and evidence-based practices
3. Future trends in critical care anesthesia

The history of critical care anesthesia has seen great advancements in introducing better patient outcomes in intensive care units. Among the major developments has been the introduction of dexmedetomidine (DEX), an anesthetic sedative whose invention enhances the management of pain and anxiety in critically ill patients. Unlike other anesthetics, DEX also possesses unique neuroprotective characteristics whose effectiveness has been shown through clinical trials and is especially useful for patients with ischemic and hemorrhagic brain injuries. Its ability to reduce opioid requirements and concomitant side effects works to emphasize further its value in critical care anesthetics. Nonetheless, practitioners should be careful to watch for the potential side effects of DEX, such as hypotension and bradycardia, which will interfere with recovery from the patient.

This sensitive balance between the benefits and the harms of DEX highlights the fine art performed by advanced pharmacotherapy in providing successful care to critical illness patients and thus becoming the basis of modern critical care practice (Bozorgi et al., 2021). Advances in mechanical thrombectomy techniques in acute ischemic stroke are another crucial field of critical care anesthesia. With the introduction of pre-reperfusion computed tomographic angiography, patient selection has become better and the timing of intervention has been reduced, significantly enhancing outcomes for the patient. In this context, the anesthesiologist's role becomes increasingly crucial. Anesthesiologists must tailor their approach—selecting between monitored anesthesia care and general anesthesia—to optimize patient stability for the intervention. Besides, peri- and postinterventional management strategies are relevant, ranging from blood pressure optimization to agitation management. These advancements in anesthesia methods not only facilitate successful procedures but also ensure improved neurological outcomes by minimizing intra- and post-procedure complications. The delicacy of application of advanced techniques highlights the growing value of critical care anesthesia as a multidisciplinary process with direct implications for recovery pathways in neurologically impaired patients (Al-Mufti et al., 2016). In conjunction with pharmacologic improvements and procedural techniques, critically ill intensive care unit patients require a multidisciplinary approach to their care. Postoperative care pathways are significantly influenced by advances in them and must be optimized through a multidisciplinary approach that includes optimizing blood pressure and glucose levels, temperature control, and optimal nutrition. Enhanced recovery pathways, like early rehabilitation, have grown in popularity as cornerstones of critical care. Evidence-based practice allows for a comprehensive plan that addresses not only the patients' medical needs but functional recovery. By incorporating advanced technology and models of shared care, critical care anesthesia is evolving to meet the multi-component needs of the patients, reflecting an evolution toward more patient-centered care in intensive care units. The ongoing development of such strategies indicates a bright future for enhancement in critical care anesthesia that focuses on both acute care and long-term recovery (Al-Mufti et al., 2016; Bozorgi et al., 2021) (Figure 10.16).

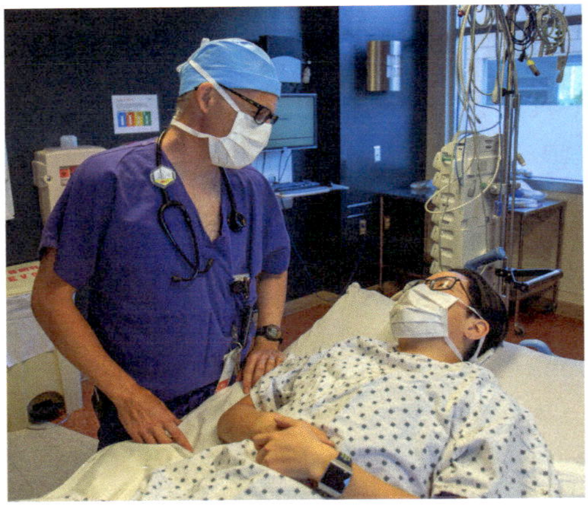

Figure 10.16. The evolution of critical care anesthesia.

Source: https://external-content.duckduckgo.com/iu/?u=https%3A%2F%2Fhsc.unm.edu%2Fmedicine%2Fdepartments%2Fanesthesiology%2F_media%2Fbanner-home.jpg&f=1&nofb=1&ipt=c48eef0b4df8a511b6911633391ec1977409c8abb84d4f9184609801762bd23d.

10.6.1. Technological Innovations in Monitoring

The critical care and intensive care anesthesia environment has been revolutionized with the advancement in monitoring technologies. Advanced monitoring systems have become the cornerstone in providing live continuous feedback of patients' vital signs and physiological conditions. These technologies allow for early complication identification, enabling timely responses from healthcare providers to adjustments in a patient's status. Multi-parameter monitors can display vital signs such as heart rate, blood pressure, oxygen saturation, and respiratory rate simultaneously, providing a complete picture of a patient's status. This comprehensive evaluation is not just a benefit in patient safety but also in the potential for anesthesiologists to make well-educated decisions regarding the application of anesthesia and pain management. Therefore, the integration of cutting-edge monitoring devices is crucial in facilitating overall clinical outcomes in critically ill patients, evidencing a direction towards more directed and responsive treatment. One of the most important advancements in monitoring technology is the integration of artificial intelligence (AI) within predictive analytics. Artificial intelligence systems can understand huge volumes of data collected by monitoring devices and identify trends that can portend deteriorating patient statuses before clinicians recognize manual observations. AI enhances pain management procedures, for example, by pre-estimating a patient's level of pain and adapting the administration of painkillers accordingly, thereby optimizing treatment protocols. The integration of patient-controlled analgesia systems has also been representative of this in assuming active functions for patients in controlling their pain. These technologies not only target the patient-by-patient requirements but also stave off opioid dependency, which is particularly crucial in the present scenario of opioid abuse in medicine. Therefore, maximizing the power of AI in monitoring can amount to a paradigm shift in the practice of anesthesiology and critical care. Besides, more advanced technologies are also being developed to ensure patient comfort while undergoing monitoring, minimizing the psychological and emotional load on critically ill patients. For instance, virtual reality and other psychosocial interventions are being investigated to reduce anxiety in intensive care unit environments. Enhanced monitoring equipment with features that enable remote communication enhances patient and healthcare practitioner interaction, generating a patient engagement culture in which the patients themselves have a role in their own care decision-making. These advancements not only increase the patient's experience and perception but can also reduce intensive care unit length of stay, which is financially advantageous for the healthcare system. Ongoing research into these monitoring innovations justifies the merit of holistic, patient-focused care, as reflected in current literature, which underlies the intensifying demand for interprofessional collaboration. Focusing on technological developments, the potential for enhanced patient outcomes and satisfaction is significantly enhanced, thus revolutionizing intensive care delivery (Figure 10.17).

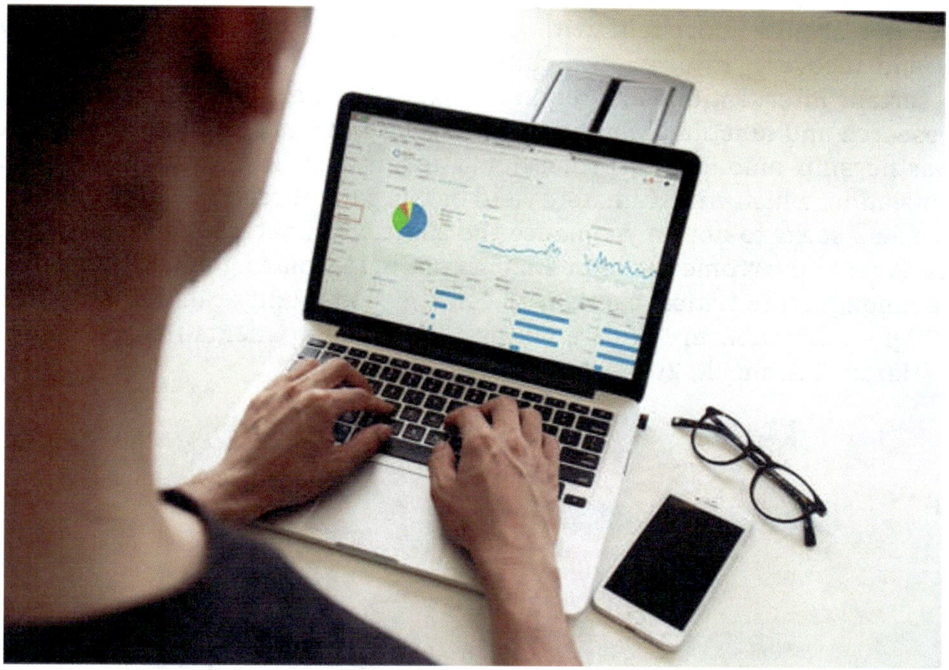

Figure 10.17. The landscape of intensive care and critical care anesthesia has been radically transformed by technological innovations in monitoring.

Source: https://external-content.duckduckgo.com/iu/?u=https%3A%2F%2Fimg-s-msn-com.akamaized.net%2Ftenant%2Famp%2Fentityid%2FAA1B0YoT.img%3Fw%3D800%26h%3D415%26q%3D60%26m%3D2%26f%3Djpg&f=1&nofb=1&ipt=ea1c80e2d785128d5369f921404451fe27c475a06e45e9a2c3736cd94b9d9491.

10.6.2. Research and Evidence-Based Practices

In critical care and intensive care anesthesia, the synthesis of research and evidence-based practice (EBP) is most crucial in the maximization of patient outcomes. Evidence-based practice emphasizes the application of the best existing current evidence to clinical decision-making and its blending with patient preferences and clinical judgment. In intensive care, where patients present with multi-dimensional complex health issues, the need for rigid clinical evidence is magnified. Healthcare professionals are relying on rigorously conducted research, such as the recent Rapid Practice Guideline on using ketamine for analgo-sedation, to design interventions that are precise and aim to improve the quality of care in general and minimize the harms of procedures such as invasive mechanical ventilation, which is crucial for patients with critical illness (Amer et al., 2024). While the value of EBP has been well established, it is typically hindered in its implementation in intensive care units (ICUs) by several barriers. Empirical studies indicate that ICU nurses primarily deal with structural and cultural barriers that prevent embedding new knowledge in practice, as based on qualitative studies that investigate their workplace experiences. Lack of resources, inadequate management support, and outdated protocols can collectively undermine nurses' consistency in evidence-based interventions (Almottowa et al., 2025). Moreover, workplace culture, described as gaps in teamwork and negative attitudes, typically underlies these gaps, which then contribute to care that is not always consistent with established best practice, eventually undermining patient safety and recovery. To develop a culture of evidence-based practice in the critical care environment, certain interventions are required. Educating healthcare professionals on findings of the latest research and functional implementations can enhance evidence-based practice usage. Facilitating partnership among interprofessional teams can also guarantee enhanced patient knowledge translation, which will ultimately yield better patient care (Almottowa et al., 2025). This collective effort also seeks to not only enhance the clinical competence of health professionals but also to prepare them to overcome the impediments of EBP. By placing research and evidence-based practice in the limelight, the critical care anesthesiology community can work towards safer, more effective, and high-quality delivery of care within ICUs so that patients receive the best treatment in acute care (Hazar & Altinişik, 2024) (Figure 10.18).

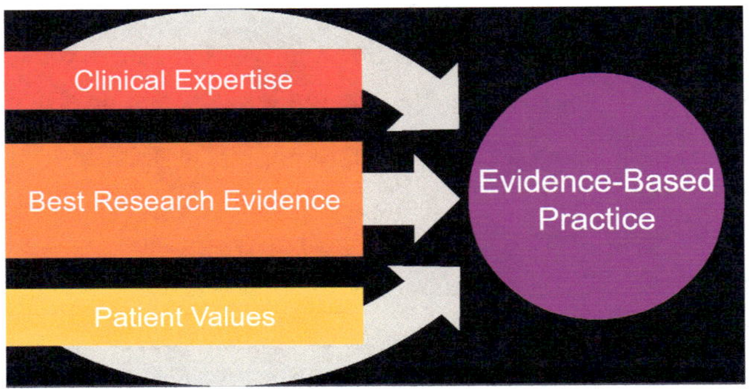

Figure 10.18. The integration of research and evidence-based practices (EBP) is paramount for optimizing patient outcomes.

Source: https://external-content.duckduckgo.com/iu/?u=https%3A%2F%2Flibapps-au.s3-ap-southeast-2.amazonaws.com%2Fcustomers%2F720%2Fimages%2FEBP-diagram.png&f=1&nofb=1&ipt=25d94b4d0e977ec5f049bcecd4de2776d72b5d4aef073e5edefcee476c410067.

10.6.3. Future Trends in Critical Care Anesthesia

The future of anesthetic care in critical conditions will radically transform with technological advancements and increasing emphasis on patient care. The most vivid trend is the integration of point-of-care ultrasound (POCUS) into daily practice within anesthesiology. It enhances procedural safety and diagnostic accuracy, particularly in emergency situations. As highlighted, ultrasound protocols such as POCUS and FAST are becoming increasingly popular to facilitate simplified diagnosis and management of life-threatening conditions. Such protocols not only improve the quality of invasive procedures, such as central venous catheterization and regional nerve blocks, but also render in-real-time monitoring for acute respiratory and cardiac illnesses, thereby opening avenues to more knowledgeable decision-making in the critical care environment (Krishtafor et al., 2025). Personalized medicine is also revolutionizing the background of critical care anesthesia. With more data-driven choices now being made available, anesthesiologists can assess patient-specific risk and tailor anesthetic strategies according to it. Recent bibliometric analyses indicate increased activity within the field of research on critical care echocardiography (CCE), linking this technology with improved outcomes from anesthesia, particularly in ICUs (Wang et al., 2025). This growing body of evidence underlines the need for trained practitioners who can use these new techniques properly, with the direct consequence of lowering complication rates and better treatment of high-risk groups. These interventions will not only improve patient safety but also speed up the recovery times, highlighting the role of innovation in modern anesthetic practice. Finally, digital health technologies have the potential to revolutionize telemedicine and ongoing monitoring in the critical care setting. Technologies such as tele-anesthesia platforms and wearable technologies will enhance anesthesiologists' capabilities to remotely monitor patients' post-surgery and adjust care plans in real time. The application of artificial intelligence (AI) in critical care anesthesia, particularly complications prediction and management, is also poised to increase significantly. With AI systems scanning large patient data sets, healthcare providers will be in a better position to make informed decisions and thus improve outcomes for patients. These innovations are a stepping stone towards a more proactive style of care that is centered on timely intervention and good patient engagement, as aligned with the overall objectives of enhancing efficiency and safety in anesthetic practice (Krishtafor et al., 2025).

Test Your Knowledge

1. What is one recent technological advancement in critical care anesthesia?
2. How have new monitoring techniques improved patient safety in critical care?

SUMMARY

In examining the complexities of Intensive Care and Critical Care Anesthesia, one understands that the integration of robust data systems is essential in optimizing patient outcomes during situations of health emergencies, as has been tested by the COVID-19 pandemic. The very magnitude of challenge brought about by SARS-CoV-2 necessitated sharing real-time information and interoperability among healthcare systems. Regulatory settings must be redesigned to ensure that electronic health records facilitate data analysis and aggregation capable of impacting treatment plans within institutions. Interoperability problems are still unresolved if they are not impacting the ability of healthcare providers to respond well to patients' changing and urgent care requirements in critical care settings. As defined in previous literature, the availability of data and standardization can lead to improved decision-making processes as well as patient care in intensive care units (Campbell et al., 2024). Moreover, experiences advanced in the scenario of the pandemic show an important necessity for healthcare professionals, such as anesthesiologists, to urge for institutional changes permitting easy sharing of data. The call for health informatics modernization is strong among physicians who appreciate the value of integrated data in delivering maximum anesthesia care. Through a concerted effort to transform health policies and practices—like embracing the use of common formats for data and increasing EHR capabilities—critical care teams can maximize their coordinated efforts. This team approach is essential not only for addressing emergent problems but also for preparing for future potential health emergencies where timely and accurate information will be essential to guiding treatment regimens and resource allocation in intensive care environments (Nelson et al., 2019). As the landscape of healthcare evolves, lessons from the present pandemic must inform intensive care and critical care anesthetic practices in the future. A sustained commitment to constructing the infrastructure of health data will be instrumental in ensuring that healthcare providers are positioned to address emerging threats with speed and agility. Patients, caregivers, and families must engage in a discussion about the quality of care and patient safety in the future. By taking the initiative to advance interoperability and data-sharing standards, the medical community can position itself to more effectively respond to crises and minimize risks of disjointed care. Finally, developing a system for sustained improvement in data-sharing capability holds the potential to not only enhance critical care outcomes but to create resilience in the health system itself as it will be exposed to the challenges of upcoming public health emergencies (Campbell et al., 2024).

In critical care and intensive care anesthesia, management of endotracheal intubation (ETI) is a crucial aspect of respiratory care for patients who are critically ill. One of the most important aspects of the procedure is the correct positioning of the endotracheal tube (ETT) to ensure maximum ventilation as well as to prevent adverse outcomes as lung collapse or hyperinflation. Deep learning-based convolutional neural networks (CNNs) have become available with new technology as a method to precisely place the ETT tip on chest radiographs. Research evidence demonstrates that the method has the capacity to improve the sensitivity, specificity, and overall accuracy of verification of correct ETT placement, thus the potential to reduce patient morbidity and mortality from incorrectly placed tubes. By integrating this new approach into practice, healthcare practitioners can even improve the quality of care being provided in intensive settings and, thereby, contribute to mitigating certain of the inbuilt risks in intensive care (Tsai et al., 2022). The high prevalence of obesity necessitates a tailored approach in the intensive care unit, particularly in the approach of anesthesia and mechanical ventilation. Obese patients usually possess unique physiological problems that complicate respiratory management, and as such, evidence-based practices are important. Literature on the subject shows that effective management entails the understanding of the altered mechanics of the respiratory system in obese patients, where they undergo an increased risk of acute respiratory failure. As discussed in current studies, practices such as patient position optimization and application of adequate ventilation modes are essential in determining clinical outcomes among this category of patients. These practices need constant optimization, as they assist in cultivating best practices yielding improved critical care interventions, safety and effectiveness in obese patients (Heil et al., 2018). In addition to correcting isolated issues such as obesity, a general understanding of the broader gaps in knowledge regarding critical care anesthesia remains paramount. Current evidence demonstrates a significant lack of large-scale, randomized controlled trials that specifically address protective ventilation strategies that are tailored to this heterogeneous group of patients. An absence of robust clinical evidence severely limits the guidebooks that professionals practicing within the critically ill patient population can utilize. Specifically, the recognition of knowledge gaps directs research directions that can have the power to create significant advancements in effectively managing respiratory disease in the ICU. There has to be interaction among researchers, physicians, and educators to carry on investigating and developing evidence-based guidelines, being responsive to the heterogeneity of unique patient contexts and maximizing care within critical care settings (Heil et al., 2018).

KEY TERMS FROM THIS CHAPTER

- Artificial intelligence (AI)
- Critical care anesthesia
- Healthcare-associated infections (HAIs)
- Patient demographics
- Pediatric intensive care units (PICUs)
- Post-surgical recovery
- Carbapenem-resistant Enterobacteriaceae (CRE)
- Evidence-based approaches
- Intensive care units (ICUs)
- Patient management
- Pharmacists
- Respiratory therapists

CRITICAL THINKING QUESTIONS

1. **Which of the following is a reliable marker for assessing the adequacy of fluid resuscitation in critically ill patients?**
   a. Blood urea nitrogen (BUN)
   b. Lactate levels
   c. Serum creatinine
   d. Hematocrit
2. **What is the primary goal of mechanical ventilation in acute respiratory distress syndrome (ARDS)?**
   a. High tidal volume to improve oxygenation
   b. Low tidal volume to prevent barotrauma
   c. High respiratory rate to reduce $PaCO_2$
   d. Use of 100% FiO_2 to achieve SpO_2 > 95%
3. **Which sedative agent is most appropriate for long-term sedation in the ICU?**
   a. Midazolam
   b. Propofol
   c. Dexmedetomidine
   d. Ketamine
4. **What is the primary concern when using succinylcholine for intubation in critically ill patients?**
   a. Bradycardia
   b. Hyperkalemia
   c. Hypotension
   d. Increased intracranial pressure
5. **In a patient with septic shock, the primary goal of fluid resuscitation is to:**
   a. Normalize blood pressure to >140/90 mmHg
   b. Restore organ perfusion
   c. Decrease heart rate below 60 bpm
   d. Increase hematocrit levels

Short Answer Questions

1. What are the key parameters used to assess the adequacy of fluid resuscitation in critically ill patients, and how do they guide management?
2. Describe the role of low tidal volume ventilation in preventing ventilator-associated lung injury (VALI) in patients with acute respiratory distress syndrome (ARDS).
3. What are the indications for using dexmedetomidine for sedation in critically ill patients, and what are its potential advantages?
4. Explain the risks associated with succinylcholine in critically ill patients and the alternative options available for rapid-sequence induction.
5. How is vasopressor therapy tailored in septic shock, and why is norepinephrine considered the first-line agent?
6. Discuss the indications and contraindications for extracorporeal membrane oxygenation (ECMO) in critical care.

Answer to Critical Thinking Questions

1. (b); 2. (b); 3. (c); 4. (b); 5.(b)

REFERENCES

1. Al-Harbi, S. (2024). Early mobilization in pediatric critical care: Exploring the gap between theory and practice in Saudi Arabia. *Medical Science Monitor: International Medical Journal of Experimental and Clinical Research, 30*, e942467-1–e942467-13. https://www.semanticscholar.org/paper/55efb44129e4df36d07d6ae866abcf483b14fa80 (accessed on 28th June 2025).
2. Almottowa, H. A., Seraj, A. S., Darwish, H. J., Khubyah, S. Y., Jan, R. H., Hanbashi, A. I., Almutair, R. K., et al. (2025). Patient-centric innovations in pain management for postoperative care. *International Journal of Community Medicine and Public Health*. https://www.semanticscholar.org/paper/55f3792df5e9c5ae0e46734efbf65113a6197619 (accessed on 28th June 2025).
3. Al-Mufti, F., Dancour, E., Amuluru, K., Prestigiacomo, C. J., Mayer, S. A., Connolly, E. S., Claassen, J., et al. (2016). Neurocritical care of emergent large-vessel occlusion: The era of a new standard of care. *Journal of Intensive Care Medicine, 32*, 373–386. https://doi.org/10.1177/0885066616656361 (accessed on 28th June 2025).
4. Amer, M., Møller, M. H., Alshahrani, M. S., Shehabi, Y., Arabi, Y., Alshamsi, F., Sigurðsson, M. I., et al. (2024). Ketamine analgo-sedation for mechanically ventilated critically ill adults: A rapid practice guideline from the Saudi Critical Care Society and the Scandinavian Society of Anesthesiology and Intensive Care Medicine. *Anesthesia and Analgesia*. https://www.semanticscholar.org/paper/e627b0c179c769bd6d36913ce14ef4e245169923 (accessed on 28th June 2025).
5. Beltran Paschoal, J. F., Santos, I. P., Malaquias, D. M., de Freitas, K. C., Barbosa Leão, M. E., Carvalho Silva, A., da Silva, K. L., et al. (2025). Comparative analysis of the best drug of choice for sedation in a surgical procedure in elderly patients: Pros and side effects of sedatives. *Journal of Anesthesia*. https://www.semanticscholar.org/paper/04fed51def341c6feb9a4c7efec75f092c6236ea (accessed on 28th June 2025).
6. Benzakour, M., Mabchour, M., Wafqui, T., Chabbar, S., Mounir, A., & Kettani, C. (2025). The use of physical restraints in critical care units: Physicians and nurses' perspectives and ethical considerations. *International Journal of Advanced Research*. https://www.semanticscholar.org/paper/0b9e66b3bcc9ac00e53e248c80c9c7ddca34d7f5 (accessed on 28th June 2025).
7. Biot, C., Sanoussi, I., & Marechal, Y. (2024). Assessment of the impact of technical incidents in critical situations using high-fidelity simulation techniques in pediatric intensive care. *Cureus, 16*. https://www.semanticscholar.org/paper/0310eb39626037ad8f474218995e45d1fe7ba605 (accessed on 28th June 2025).
8. Bixio, M., Carenzo, L., Accurso, G., Balagna, R., Bazurro, S., Chiarini, G., Cortegiani, A., et al. (2024). Management of critically ill patients in austere environments: Good clinical practice by the Italian Society of Anesthesia, Analgesia, Resuscitation and Intensive Care (SIAARTI). *Journal of Anesthesia, Analgesia and Critical Care, 4*. https://www.semanticscholar.org/paper/9b202bcd64f43d07e5241da96b9324a623dc37f8 (accessed on 28th June 2025).
9. Bozorgi, H., Zamani, M., Motaghi, E., & Eslami, M. (2021). Dexmedetomidine as an analgesic agent with neuroprotective properties: Experimental and clinical aspects. *Journal of Pain & Palliative Care Pharmacotherapy, 35*, 215–225. https://doi.org/10.1080/15360288.2021.1914280 (accessed on 28th June 2025).

10. Bray, D. P., Stricsek, G., Malcolm, J. G., Gutierrez, J., Greven, A., Barrow, D. L., Rodts, G. E., et al. (2020). Letter: Maintaining neurosurgical resident education and safety during the COVID-19 pandemic. *Neurosurgery, 87*, E189–E191. https://doi.org/10.1093/neuros/nyaa164 (accessed on 28th June 2025).

11. Campbell, A., Jacoby, M., & Hernandez, N. (2024). Critical care innovations: Navigating pain relief in intensive care: The role of regional anesthesia. *Current Opinion in Anesthesiology, 37*, 547–552. https://www.semanticscholar.org/paper/786cb27d76a33ea74b3b5256eb626ab7621b4657 (accessed on 28th June 2025).

12. Carenzo, L., Brogi, E., Agostini, V., Armani, S., Balagna, R., Bocci, M., Cascio, A., et al. (2025). Blood product administration in the prehospital setting: A multisociety consensus statement. *Journal of Anesthesia, Analgesia and Critical Care, 5*. https://www.semanticscholar.org/paper/beca67330e97c3a565da9201318101a42892ece3 (accessed on 28th June 2025).

13. De Gasperi, A., Petrò, L., Amici, O., Scaffidi, I., Molinari, P., Barbaglio, C., Cibelli, E., Penzo, B., Roselli, E., Brunetti, A., Neganov, M., Giacomoni, A., Aseni, P., & Guffanti, E. (2024). Major liver resections, perioperative issues and posthepatectomy liver failure: A comprehensive update for the anesthesiologist. *World journal of critical care medicine, 13*(2), 92751. https://doi.org/10.5492/wjccm.v13.i2.92751(accessed on 28th June 2025).

14. Elmati, P., Nagaradona, T., Jagirdhar, G., & Surani, S. (2024). Remimazolam in intensive care unit: Potential applications and considerations. *World Journal of Critical Care Medicine, 13*. https://www.semanticscholar.org/paper/e0b2596bf3c3d86aa3eab24c6c71a5cf7ef9192d (accessed on 28th June 2025).

15. Erion, G., Janizek, J. D., Hudelson, C., Utarnachitt, R., McCoy, A. M., Sayre, M., White, N., et al. (2021). CoAI: Cost-aware artificial intelligence for health care. *medRxiv*. https://www.semanticscholar.org/paper/02f380325741a0c9419df5c0a202e4acbdbf35b5 (accessed on 28th June 2025).

16. Escrivá, J., Fort, P., Gabarrón, E., Liao, Y., et al. (2016). Comparison of two cardiac output monitors, qCO and LiDCO, during general anesthesia. https://core.ac.uk/download/81578536.pdf (accessed on 28th June 2025).

17. Hajili, F., Hancı, V., Özbilgin, Ş., Ayvat, P., Arça, D. Ö., & Gökel, E. (2024). Evaluation of the frequency of kidney injury in the postoperative critical care unit (PACU): A prospective observational study. *Dokuz Eylül Üniversitesi Tıp Fakültesi Dergisi*. https://www.semanticscholar.org/paper/09d610c882e26e840a6066ff53f86fcc94b7f049 (accessed on 28th June 2025).

18. Hazar, E. Ü., & Altinişik, H. B. (2024). Comparison of the effects of normal and cesarean delivery methods and general and spinal anesthesia techniques on the inflammatory response. *Anesthesia, Pain & Intensive Care*. https://www.semanticscholar.org/paper/94b82a11de8bcfb5b69e649514274910336fbcbe (accessed on 28th June 2025).

19. Heil, L. B., Rocco, P., Silva, P., & Pelosi, P. (2018). Mechanical ventilation in the critically ill obese patient. *Anesthesia & Analgesia*. https://www.semanticscholar.org/paper/ce76316245de069d09bf4310c7265169a4331a37 (accessed on 28th June 2025).

20. Hotabilardus, N., & Anggraeni, N. (2025). Acute lung oedema in severe pre-eclampsia: Advanced management and anesthetic interventions. *Indonesian Journal of Anesthesiology and Reanimation*. https://www.semanticscholar.org/paper/290cbfb67054be94c646288b2b80ade369707c16 (accessed on 28th June 2025).

21. Illescas, C., Cozowicz, C., Zhong, H., Reisinger, L., Liu, J., Poeran, J., & Memtsoudis, S. G. (2024). Comparative effectiveness of neuraxial versus general anesthesia in total joint replacement surgery: An updated retrospective analysis using more recent data. *Regional Anesthesia & Pain Medicine*. https://www.semanticscholar.org/paper/b1c45e6222aa2eda117306095de96e5d5a8109df (accessed on 28th June 2025).

22. Ji, S., Song, J., Kwon, M. A., & Yoon, Y. S. (2025). Intraoperative severe bronchospasm treatment with epinephrine puffing by using the MAD Nasal™ intranasal mucosal atomization device: A case report. *Signa Vitae*. https://www.semanticscholar.org/paper/64341e835ce512e4c039eeb4771715ccd740d5c4 (accessed on 28th June 2025).

23. Jiang, S., & Gunther, M. (2025). A critical reappraisal of haloperidol for delirium management in the intensive care unit: Perspective from psychiatry. *Journal of Clinical Medicine, 14*. https://www.semanticscholar.org/paper/f715082b9f2371f725d32665f10c2915abff9bfc (accessed on 28th June 2025).

24. Kgadima, I. M. R., Coetzee, M., Heyns, T., & Coetzee, I. M. (2024). Factors influencing knowledge translation into critical care practice: The reality facing intensive care nurses in Limpopo Province. *Southern African Journal of Critical Care, 40*. https://www.semanticscholar.org/paper/1838077dc806edc82ff04afc8f1813a0464ceb49 (accessed on 28th June 2025).

25. Khajavi, M., Ramezani, R., Sharifnia, H. R., Najafi, A., & Barkhordari, K. (2023). Sanyar video laryngoscope improved time and first pass success of tracheal intubation in intensive care unit compared to direct laryngoscopy. *Archives of Anesthesia and Critical Care*. https://www.semanticscholar.org/paper/8f3c94e3b913b1693d0414030e807566a0279f60 (accessed on 28th June 2025).

26. Kim, Y. D. (2025). Association between postoperative pain management and long-term patient outcomes. *Journal of the Korean Medical Association*. https://www.semanticscholar.org/paper/bb46f1c64120a483ad1dcee92e42e1a36acdd0fe (accessed on 28th June 2025).

27. Kleinpell, R., Grabenkort, W. R., Boyle, W. A., Vines, D., & Olsen, K. M. (2021). The Society of Critical Care Medicine at 50 years: Interprofessional practice in critical care: Looking back and forging ahead. *Critical Care Medicine, 49*, 2017–2032. https://doi.org/10.1097/ccm.0000000000005276 (accessed on 28th June 2025).

28. Krishtafor, A., Krishtafor, D., Kravets, O., & Pylypenko, O. (2025). The importance of using mobile ultrasound devices in improving the quality and safety of emergency care, anesthesia and intensive care. *Modern Medical Technology*. https://www.semanticscholar.org/paper/8d0da15f7b61ab43884c0cd61d9f453a81c6c496 (accessed on 28th June 2025).

29. Lavezzo, B., Biancofiore, G., Luca, E., Balagna, R., Bignami, E., Boggi, U., Cataldo, R., et al. (2025). Planning intensive care unit admission after elective major abdominal surgery: Good clinical practice document by SIAARTI-SIC-ANIARTI. *Journal of Anesthesia, Analgesia and Critical Care, 5*. https://www.semanticscholar.org/paper/8703404d3dbf314457cf26f518dad608da9a5288 (accessed on 28th June 2025).

30. Lazar, M. B., & Farczádi, L. (2024). Challenges of the regional anesthetic techniques in intensive care units–A narrative review. *The Journal of Critical Care Medicine, 10*, 198–208. https://www.semanticscholar.org/paper/bed1b026757e420bf3965e56a2b1f403b7f1953f (accessed on 28th June 2025).

31. Lee, I. K., Lee, K. H., Han, H., Choi, J., Kim, N., & Kim, K. (2025). Different axis approaches for ultrasound-guided centrally inserted central catheterization in children: A systematic review and meta-analysis of randomized controlled trials. *Frontiers in Surgery, 12*. https://www.semanticscholar.org/paper/d74375865bfd78d462abef7871edd9f0d2801440 (accessed on 28th June 2025).

32. Lisitsa, V. L., Gritsinskaya, A. N., Zavyalova, Y., Aleksandrovich, Y., & Lisovskii, O. V. (2025). Clinical and metabolic aspects of protein-energy malnutrition in patients in pediatric intensive care units. *Meditsinskiy sovet = Medical Council*. https://www.semanticscholar.org/paper/d98609925fdc50e9bfa5a075d32da793562e4e7e (accessed on 28th June 2025).

33. Madkhali, M. M., Alfaifi, M. M., Safhi, A. Y., Shmakhi, Y. M., Alammari, A. H., Qaysi, M. M., Hamdi, A. A., et al. (2025). The role of anesthesia in sedation and weaning from mechanical ventilation: A systematic review. *Cureus, 17*. https://www.semanticscholar.org/paper/d9938b5d2623e097872185b83624245394eac5a7 (accessed on 28th June 2025).

34. Mahmood, F., Matyal, R., Skubas, N. J., Montealegre-Gallegos, M., Swaminathan, M., Denault, A., Sniecinski, R. M., et al. (2016). Perioperative ultrasound training in anesthesiology: A call to action. *Anesthesia & Analgesia, 122*, 1794–1804. https://doi.org/10.1213/ane.0000000000001134 (accessed on 28th June 2025).

35. Michard, F., Wong, A., & Kanoore Edul, V. (2025). Visualizing hemodynamics: Innovative graphical displays and imaging techniques in anesthesia and critical care. *Critical Care, 29*. https://www.semanticscholar.org/paper/02671c65a0cc2fe17a8ea48fd8057fe149c6fafc (accessed on 28th June 2025).

36. Montgomery, A. J., Litell, J. M., Dang, J., Flurin, L., Gajic, O., Lal, A., & Digital Twin Platform for Education, et al. (2023). Gaining consensus on expert rule statements for acute respiratory failure digital twin patient model in intensive care unit using a Delphi method. *Biomolecules and Biomedicine, 23*, 1108–1117. https://www.semanticscholar.org/paper/fbb8df8537777fac20d6f0fe913f871d4cc3a313 (accessed on 28th June 2025).

37. Noppè, E., Eloff, J. R. P., Keane, S., & Martín-Loeches, I. (2024). A narrative review of invasive candidiasis in the intensive care unit. *Therapeutic Advances in Pulmonary and Critical Care Medicine, 19*. https://www.semanticscholar.org/paper/4203c5c449d3751e6d99ba9a7a36d29efb6f09f3 (accessed on 28th June 2025).

38. O'Reilly-Shah, V. N., Gentry, K. R., Van Cleve, W., Kendale, S., Jabaley, C. S., & Long, D. R. (2020). The COVID-19 pandemic highlights shortcomings in US health care informatics infrastructure: A call to action. *Anesthesia & Analgesia, 131*, 340–344. https://doi.org/10.1213/ane.0000000000004945 (accessed on 28th June 2025).

39. Olatunji, G., Kokori, E., Aderinto, N., Abdul, A., Tsoi, V., Mohamed, L., & Alsabri, M. H. H. (2024). Challenges and strategies in pediatric critical care: Insights from low-resource settings. *Global Pediatric Health, 11*. https://www.semanticscholar.org/paper/7799e08e449ecc89e3db326867908ff7a8735b24 (accessed on 28th June 2025).

40. Padte, S., Samala Venkata, V., Mehta, P., Tawfeeq, S., Kashyap, R., & Surani, S. R. (2024). 21st century critical care medicine: An overview. *World Journal of Critical Care Medicine, 13*. https://www.semanticscholar.org/paper/8127b1ae8a3d3a3f136c365fc8a5cabe18c3e11f (accessed on 28th June 2025).

41. Pandit, R. A., Vijayakumar, P. C., Shah, M., Jha, S., Patil, B., Dwivedy, A., Patil, K., et al.

(2024). Insights and opinions of critical care healthcare professionals in the management of carbapenem-resistant Enterobacteriaceae cases and antibiotic-resistant infections in the intensive care unit setting: A survey-based approach. *The Journal of the Association of Physicians of India, 72*(1), 43–46. https://www.semanticscholar.org/paper/29c08ef4f73c5ce643e099dfb0d8f6ffb7695d89 (accessed on 28th June 2025).

42. Park, Y., Yun, I., Jang, S. Y., Park, E., & Jang, S. (2024). Association between nurse staffing level in intensive care settings and hospital-acquired pneumonia among surgery patients: Result from the Korea National Health Insurance cohort. *Epidemiology and Infection, 152*. https://www.semanticscholar.org/paper/6130dcacc9cf424658c12f85951b19b4e0ffb02d (accessed on 28th June 2025).

43. Pène, F., Russell, L., & Aubron, C. (2025). Thrombocytopenia in the intensive care unit: Diagnosis and management. *Annals of Intensive Care, 15*. https://www.semanticscholar.org/paper/cb67cf63d89d75654c1eb693da2e16586496454e (accessed on 28th June 2025).

44. Priya, V., Sen, J., & Ninave, S. (2024). A comprehensive review of prone ventilation in the intensive care unit: Challenges and solutions. *Cureus, 16*. https://www.semanticscholar.org/paper/7fcb93258db2e1be68cb9e7f5328a34f34daa065 (accessed on 28th June 2025).

45. Prosser, D., Friesen, M., Allman, P., Grassby, P., & Streisand, J. (1998). Oral transmucosal fentanyl. https://core.ac.uk/download/17353596.pdf (accessed on 28th June 2025).

46. Sharon, T., Nayak, S. G., Shanbhag, V., & Hebbar, S. (2024). An observational study of nutritional assessment, prescription, practices, and its outcome among critically ill patients admitted to an intensive care unit. *Indian Journal of Critical Care Medicine: Peer-reviewed, Official Publication of Indian Society of Critical Care Medicine, 28*, 364–368. https://www.semanticscholar.org/paper/31de3ae814dc18ebd189c794afef54ffd38b642b (accessed on 28th June 2025).

47. Simjanovska, V. O. (2025). Mass casualty event preparedness and anesthesia management in the emergency department and intensive care unit. *Macedonian Journal of Anesthesia*. https://www.semanticscholar.org/paper/21028f96e428808f5394d1d982a5affb17127773 (accessed on 28th June 2025).

48. Tsai, L., Yuan, K., Hou, S. K., Wu, W. L., Hsu, C. H., Liu, T. L., Lee, K. M., et al. (2022). Determining carina and clavicular distance-dependent positioning of endotracheal tube in critically ill patients: An artificial intelligence-based approach. *Biology, 11*. https://www.semanticscholar.org/paper/de5ef4e53b34eb78c2eeb4f5f8e94f62596ac91a (accessed on 28th June 2025).

49. Van Zundert, T. V., Gatt, S. P., & Van Zundert, A. (2023). Anesthesia and perioperative pain relief in the frail elderly patient. *Saudi Journal of Anesthesia, 17*, 566–574. https://www.semanticscholar.org/paper/91c3b6409b95cecafc2f8d07c1b3b9b8008d4095 (accessed on 28th June 2025).

50. Wang, W., Liu, B., & Wang, L. (2025). Critical care echocardiography: A bibliometric analysis of knowledge structure and evolution of development trends from 2005 to 2024. *Echocardiography, 42*(6), e70204. https://www.semanticscholar.org/paper/71aa8d834a6814bfea8eb94ebbfaeac60d2064e1 (accessed on 28th June 2025).

51. Zahid, M. A., Kumar, V., Wadhwani, J., Kumar, A., Hasan, M. F., & Saleh, M. (2024). Enhancing anesthesia precision: Integration of BIS monitoring in anesthesia machines. *Anesthesia, Pain & Intensive Care*. https://www.semanticscholar.org/paper/b85d3976ff10b6d1ea1c9ccb0d534a5eb024ca72 (accessed on 28th June 2025).

CHRONIC PAIN AND PALLIATIVE CARE

11

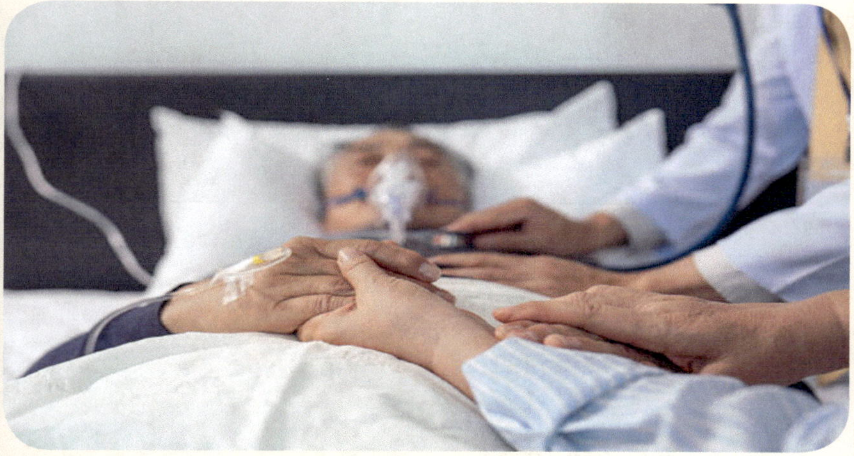

LEARNING OBJECTIVES

After studying this chapter, you will be able to:

1. Understand chronic pain
2. Discuss the role of palliative care
3. Know assessment of chronic pain
4. Focus on treatment options for chronic pain
5 Explain the psychological aspects of chronic pain
6. Focus on ethical considerations in palliative care

Introduction

Chronic pain is a significant public health issue, pervasively impacting the lives of the suffering individuals with numerous various disorders. Prolonged into recent years by terminology coined as pain lasting longer than healing time, chronic pain possesses numerous potential etiologies, including injury, aging, and conditions like arthritis. This constant agony not only exacerbates physical disability but also serves to evoke psychological distress, making it a cycle of despair and disability. The need for effective management practices becomes apparent, particularly in palliative care, where enhancing patients' quality of life in the presence of life-limiting illness is the paramount goal. More recent mechanisms of therapy, such as the administration of medical cannabis, have been shown to be effective in symptom relief of chronic pain as well as in presenting a holistic view of treatments at hand for palliative care patients (Barton et al., 2021). The medical cannabis integration into chronic pain management represents a paradigm shift in how healthcare professionals are treating pain relief, particularly in patients with complex conditions. According to various studies, the effectiveness of treatments involving cannabis has been investigated for diverse symptoms experienced by populations under palliative care, demonstrating that there is an overall approach to care. These interventions have potential benefits in symptom management, providing alternatives to conventional opioids, which are often burdened with significant side effects and risk profiles for addiction. Thus, the integration of such interventions would need to proceed through a scrutinized evaluation of regulatory, clinical, and societal factors, which would necessitate open debate between healthcare providers, patients, and policymakers.

The integration of evidence-based interventions could thereby lead to more holistic and patient-specific palliative care strategies. Chronic pain management issues extend far beyond treatment modalities and into the fabric of healthcare systems globally. As eloquently stated by academics, inequalities in pain relief access persist, with certain groups being disproportionately short-changed by a lack of effective therapies. The opioid epidemic also contributes to issues of managing chronic pain, stigmatizing legitimate pain management, while simultaneously restricting access to vital pain relief medication. These complexities underscore the urgent need for an integrated approach to balance the evolving paradigm of pain education and public policy and maximize the clinical expertise of health practitioners. By increasing the agenda of a comprehensive framework that addresses both the medical and the psychosocial dimensions of chronic pain, the medical field can begin to rechart strategies that are as much about controlling symptoms as dignity and quality of life for the chronically ill within the continuum of palliative care (Barton et al., 2021) (Figure 11.1).

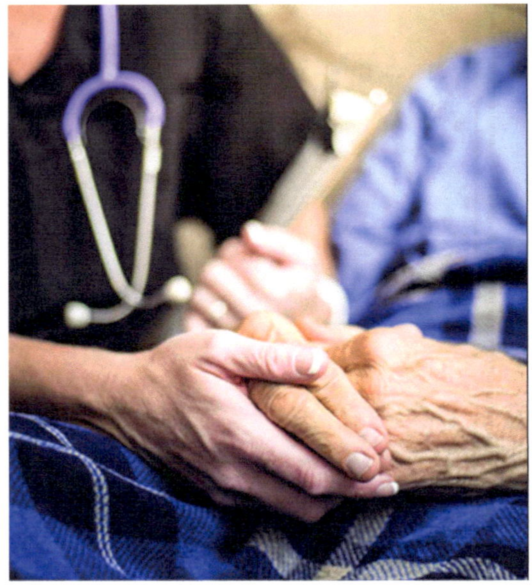

Figure 11.1. Chronic pain represents a significant public health challenge.

Source: https://nscri.in/admin_assets/img/service/palliative_care-min_(2).jpg.

Definition of Chronic Pain

The definition of chronic pain is multifaceted and is more than just physical suffering. Chronic pain is typically used to describe the existence of pain that persists for over three months, typically disrupting normal activities for an individual and compromising overall well-being. Chronic pain can be caused by conditions such as arthritis, neuropathy, or cancer, among others. Significantly, chronic disease pain is not just a symptom but a disabling disease that entails psychological, social, and economic consequences for the patient. Thus, managing chronic pain requires an interdisciplinary plan incorporating physical therapy, drugs, and psychological counseling, which becomes virtually critical in the context of palliative care. Efficacious treatment plans aim to reduce pain and enhance patients' quality of life, calling for extensive knowledge of chronic pain mechanisms in clinical practice. The consequences of chronic pain are far-reaching, impacting patients' psychological and emotional well-being and their response to medication. The majority of patients are depressed, anxious, and experience a reduced sense of control, which all contribute to increased awareness of pain and difficulty in treatment. For instance, chronic pain patients build an avoidance pattern that manifests in a re-injury fear, which leads to decreased activity levels and additional worsening of disability patterns. In the context of palliative care, where maximizing quality of life is the therapeutic objective, familiarity with the complexities linked with chronic pain becomes the primary organizational aspect.

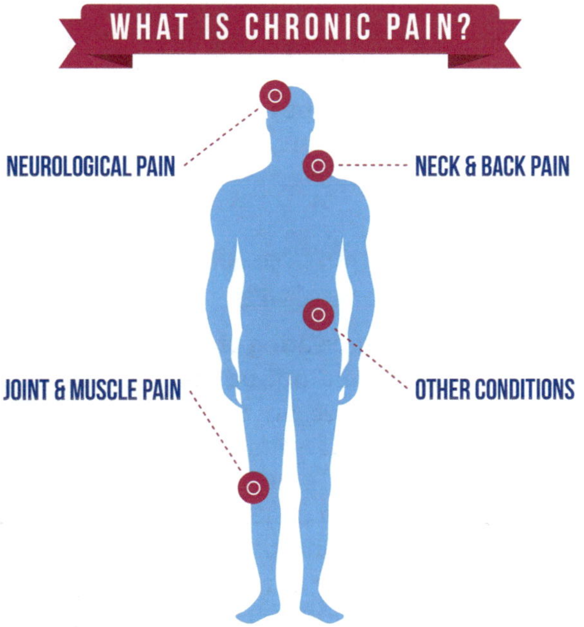

Figure 11.2. The definition of chronic pain.

Source: https://external-content.duckduckgo.com/iu/?u=https%3A%2F%2Fwww.carolinaspaincenter.com%2Fwp-content%2Fuploads%2F2013%2F11%2FChronic-pain-image.jpg&f=1&nofb=1&ipt=1104424fa5c602ab9484a487d75140f075ecf8b5eff730339c13e85dce0fdb74.

As highlighted in research, efficient pain control relies on treating the many-sided dimensions of pain—biological, psychological, and social factors. Practitioners, therefore, must adopt an integrative practice that resonates with the individual's appreciation of pain, each patient has (Schofield et al., 2007). Furthermore, chronic pain classification as both a symptom of underlying medical diseases and an independent condition has immediate implications on palliative care models of treatment. Effective management not only addresses the pain itself but also provides total care that covers mental health and social well-being. Interventions in palliative care usually include the use of medications, such as opioids, with supplementary treatment to reduce pain in line with individual choices and tolerances. Evidence shows routine monitoring and periodic revision of treatment plans as necessary to make sure that management strategies remain aligned with evolving patient needs (Juba et al., 2017). As treatment practice for chronic pain keeps evolving, ongoing education and research will continue to enlighten healthcare professionals on what is necessary to enhance delivery of care to those afflicted by chronic pain (Figure 11.2).

Overview of Palliative Care

Palliative care is an overall approach to enhancing the lives of people who have serious, normally life-threatening illnesses. This kind of care in itself emphasizes symptom control, like relief from chronic pain, coupled with handling patients' and families' emotional, social, and spiritual needs. Evidence suggests that the prevalence of chronic pain can have a major impact on the quality of life of patients, especially in the presence of advanced illness. It is here that palliative care has its essential place, using an all-encompassing approach that combines various forms of pain management with psychosocial support. Through the facilitation of open communication about goals of care and treatment preferences, palliative care practitioners are in a better position to provide interventions that resonate with patients' values and desires and enhance their overall quality of life. Perhaps the most significant aspect of palliative care is its emphasis on interdisciplinary coordination, which unites the skills of various healthcare professionals. Such team effort can include doctors, nurses, social workers, and chaplains, all working in concord together to collectively address the complexities of a patient's situation. A recent study has demonstrated how palliative care that is started in emergency departments is able to improve patient-outcomes among the elderly with serious illnesses, proof of the healing effectiveness of targeted interventions in acute care (Cho et al., 2019).

This multidimensional approach not only enhances management of chronic pain but also reduces healthcare utilization and caregiver burden. When palliative care is integrated into the entire healthcare system, patients can receive comprehensive care that not only alleviates physical symptomatology but also alleviates emotional distress and improves the quality of life. Moreover, the palliative care principles are more expansive than the treatment of acute symptoms. Education and advocacy are the tools that allow families and patients to make informed decisions regarding their care. Incorporation of a model of palliative care is beneficial for individuals with chronic pain due to an underlying disease, such as cancer. A multimodal intervention for managing pain is emphasized by studies, with rational use of opioids as part of other therapeutic modalities being a strong strategy for achieving maximum relief (Ščiupokas et al., 2019). To this purpose, not only is palliative care a symptom supportive intervention but also a vital resource that assists in the working out of difficult medical decisions, ensuring that patients are provided with care that is not only compassionate in nature but also as per their expressed wishes (Figure 11.3).

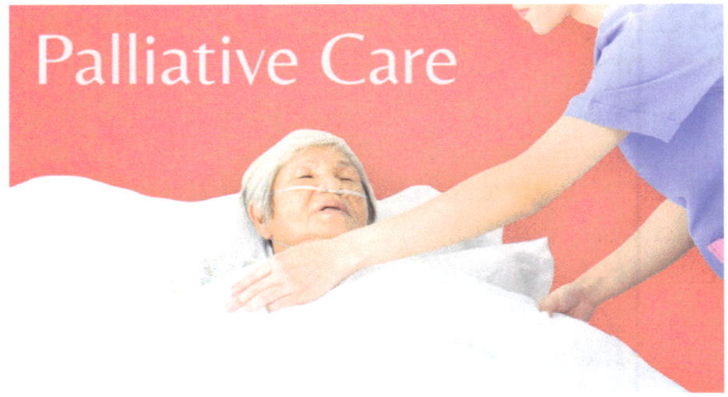

Figure 11.3. Palliative care serves as a holistic approach to enhancing the quality of life for patients facing serious.

Source: https://external-content.duckduckgo.com/iu/?u=https%3A%2F%2Fausmed-images.s3.ap-southeast-2.amazonaws.com%2Fausmed.com%2Fausmed-articles%2F20200603_cover_v2.jpg&f=1&nofb=1&ipt=27bd6422e6d8517478abad4879996e71e6bfc28a5d53a49f2ac019b14b0b35bc.

Importance of Addressing Chronic Pain in Palliative Care

The significance of treating chronic pain during palliative care should not be taken lightly, as it has a direct influence on the patients' quality of life while facing life-limiting illness. Chronic pain tends to make emotional distress more complicated, resulting in heightened anxiety and depression among patients. Pain management under palliative care is more than a physical concern; it needs to be addressed with a refined strategy that can consider the intricate elements of suffering. Effective pain management has the potential to increase activity in activities of daily living and engagement with family members, re-establishing a semblance of normalcy in a challenging situation. Furthermore, empathetic pain management is an ethical manifestation of the values of beneficence and respect for patient autonomy, and it reflects the responsibility of healthcare workers to relieve pain as a vital part of whole-person care. Moreover, the incorporation of psychosocial elements in chronic pain treatment in palliative care remains crucial. The recognition of spirituality as a fundamental component of disease coping has been more and more common in contemporary literature, showing the importance of taking the existential concerns of patients into account (Inbadas, 2016). Spiritual care can provide comfort and meaning in addition to pain relief, increasing overall well-being and quality of life that is acceptable. In conjunction with patient health improvement, the psychosocial elements typically intersect with chronic pain, such that it becomes a requirement for medical providers to establish holistically oriented interventions that address emotional and spiritual care.

In so doing, the practitioners not only address the bodily manifestations of suffering but also legitimize the patients' total experience, ultimately adopting a more noble approach to end-of-life management. Second, the social justice concept is a significant catalyst for equitable accessibility to palliative care for those suffering from chronic pain. Health disparities may intensify the distress and agony of marginalized groups, which underscores the importance of public policy responses that redress these inequalities (Jennings et al., 2003). As palliative care progresses, it is more critical than ever to promote a model with inclusivity, ensuring that all patients, irrespective of their socioeconomic position or culture, are provided with extensive pain relief.

egislative directives that address the expansion of the definition of hospice and the integration of palliative care earlier in the course of the disease will not only alleviate suffering but also create a more equitable healthcare system. By addressing such programs initially, the medical community can step closer towards a utopia where chronic pain in palliative care is treated to its fullest potential, thereby enhancing dignity and quality of care provided for all patients.

11.1. Understanding Chronic Pain

Learning Outcome

1. Types of chronic pain
2. Causes and risk factors
3. Impact on quality of life

Chronic pain is a multifaceted condition that significantly affects the quality of life of millions of individuals worldwide. It has been largely defined as pain that lasts longer than three months, beyond the expected healing process. Chronic pain could be caused by a variety of sources, including injury, disease, or even psychosocial origins and is commonly characterized by incapacitating physical and emotional distress. To understand chronic pain, one has to dig deeper into its psychological, social, and biological aspects because it often entails something more than the physical feeling itself. Medical practitioners must address the condition holistically so that it can be successfully treated, which can translate to incorporating palliative care principles that aim to maximize quality of life and suffering for long-term pain patients. Amongst the most crucial aspects of chronic pain management is the imperative of including patient-reported outcome measures (PROMs) and experience measures (PREMs) into practice. They offer ways in which healthcare providers can gain insights into the patient's experience of pain and care, promoting a patient-centered method of treatment. Research has established that the incorporation of PROMs and PREMs will enhance the understanding of the impact of chronic pain on patients on physical and emotional dimensions, leading to more focused and optimal treatments. However, the application of these measures is likely to unveil practice tensions in relation to standardization and quantification. The qualitative practitioner experience is that clinicians must navigate these issues without sacrificing patient needs as the governing concern in care, as in research, which emphasizes addressing these difficulties when treating chronic pain (Krawczyk et al., 2019). When it comes to palliative care, chronic pain management is a priority because this type of practice is not only meant to alleviate suffering but also improve care for the patients' overall well-being. Palliative care centers on ensuring accessibility, equity, and cultural sensitivity as vital components of its practice, with a focus on seeing to it that care is tailored to the patient's situation and background. In the majority of the world, though, barriers to accessing such intensive palliative care are still elevated, disproportionately affecting vulnerable individuals. In Australia, for instance, investigators have identified that while palliative care is required by all, the reality quite often falls short of expectations, causing inequalities based on age, income, or socio-economic status (Department of Anesthesia, University of Iowa, 2011). This highlights an imperative need for systemic change to provide patients with chronic pain with the comprehensive care they require and ultimately better outcomes and a quality of life for these patients (Figure 11.4).

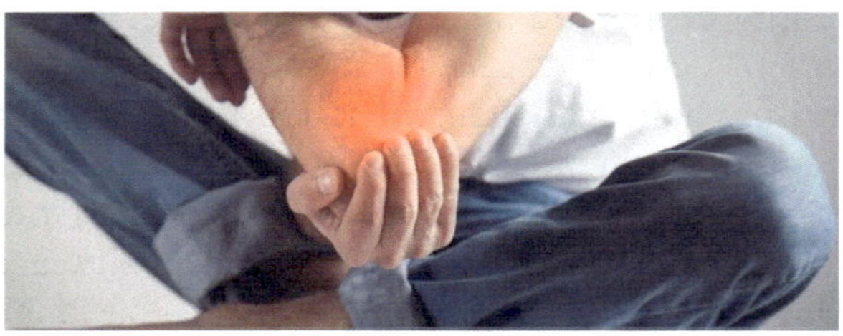

Figure 11.4. Chronic pain is a multifaceted condition.

Source: https://external-content.duckduckgo.com/iu/?u=https%3A%2F%2Fdelmarvapt.com%2Fwp-content%2Fuploads%2F2024%2F04%2FUnderstanding_Chronic_Pain_Types_Causes_and_Management-1024x400.jpeg.webp&f=1&nofb=1&ipt=179feee39e86cd53daa7fe138284a8e6f6f755aa6bba990aaedba19145505cce.

11.1.1. Types of Chronic Pain

Chronic pain comes in numerous different forms, and the primary distinction is between nociceptive and neuropathic pain, which are caused by various physiological mechanisms. Nociceptive pain is further subdivided into somatic and visceral pain. Somatic pain typically results as a result of damage to specific tissues and tends to manifest as sharp or dull pain limited to the skin, muscles, or bones. In contrast, visceral pain is associated with abdominal organs and tends to be a deep, aching pressure sensation and is commonly hard to localize. Both forms can be present at the same time in patients with chronic pain and clinical presentation complicated, necessitating careful evaluation. An understanding of this classification is critical in individualizing effective pain relief interventions in palliative care settings in order to ensure that interventions are effective but also attuned to the unique complexity of each patient's experience of pain (Vahanian et al., 2021). Another extremely prevalent type of chronic pain is neuropathic pain, which results from peripheral or central nervous system damage or malformation. It is typically burning, shooting, or tingling pain and can result from disorders such as diabetic neuropathy, postherpetic neuralgia, or cancer treatment-induced nerve damage. The complexity of neuropathic pain does not end at the sensory level; it is accompanied by significant psychological distress that, in itself, adds to the general disability burden of chronic pain. Hence, effective neuropathic pain management is often a call for multimodal treatment—extending pharmacologic therapy, such as antidepressants and anticonvulsants, to psychological intervention and physical rehabilitation. This calls for professional evaluation that looks into the precise reasons and backgrounds of each patient and in which the importance of person-centered and holistic care in palliative care is utilized (Fallon et al., 2018). Given the diversity of chronic pain syndromes, a key problem in palliative care is the appropriate assessment and management of pain to improve the quality of life of patients. Appropriate knowledge regarding the assessment of pain, including the self-reporting techniques and observation methods, is vital, particularly in cases where patients cannot express their pain. Regular review of pain intensity and character ensures that treatment protocols remain effective and reactive to changing requirements. Furthermore, dedicated methodologies, such as using established pain scales and sophisticated assessment planning, can enhance the specificity of pain management. The combination of these assessment measures allows health care providers to better adapt interventions, ultimately resulting in improved outcomes in chronic pain management within palliative care contexts (Vahanian et al., 2021) (Figure 11.5).

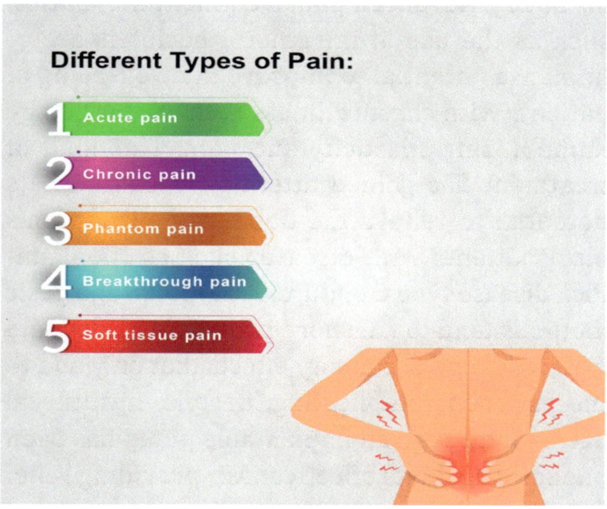

Figure 11.5. Chronic pain manifests in various forms.

Source: https://external-content.duckduckgo.com/iu/?u=https%3A%2F%2Fmangoclinic.com%2Fwp-content%2Fuploads%2F2020%2F07%2F1-1.jpg&f=1&nofb=1&ipt=5488845afe89cfbf31d6018dd02b66c01af04e3907aed58a60576311702e7d5f.

11.1.2. Causes and Risk Factors

Chronic pain is an intricate condition often exacerbated by several causative factors and risk factors. A few of the prominent causes are internal diseases, such as arthritis, fibromyalgia, and neuropathy. All these illnesses may not be responsible for a single persistent discomfort, but they also cause a cascading effect on the health of the patients. Furthermore, psychological factors such as anxiety and depression may sensitize pain, leading to a vicious cycle, making management a challenge. Recognizing these connections is essential for health care professionals employed within palliative care systems, since the treatment of the physical and psychological aspects of pain will contribute substantially to the quality of life of the patient. Recognizing that chronic pain is not usually the result of one specific cause is essential in order to create comprehensive treatment plans that are tailored to the individual patient and holistic in their approach. Lifestyle factors also significantly contribute to an individual's risk of developing chronic pain. For instance, the onset of musculoskeletal pain has been linked with physical inactivity, and obesity serves to worsen such conditions through added stress on the joints. Further, drug abuse, particularly opioids, can trigger complications in the form of addiction or opioid-induced hyperalgesia, rendering pain control unsatisfactory. In fact, studies have yielded findings revealing that patients placed on long-term oral liquid morphine (OLM) develop debilitating adverse drug reactions, even including addiction. These findings underscore the necessity of careful prescribing practices and rigorous education of healthcare workers on balancing effective pain relief against the dangers of opioid therapy, particularly in palliative care settings (Duncan et al., 2025). Moreover, socio-economic status and demographic factors both heavily influence the experience of chronic pain and the use of necessary palliative care services. There are differences in access to healthcare that may result in unmanaged or under-managed pain, especially among vulnerable populations. Cultural beliefs about illness and pain may discourage individuals from accessing treatment or actively participating in treatment regimens. In cancer patients, as in the instance of lung cancer, the need for intensive palliative care is more critical since the control of symptoms is necessary to provide an acceptable quality of life despite continued treatments such as chemotherapy (Ingle et al., 2025). These diverse causes and risk factors need to be identified in developing effective, integrated palliative care and chronic pain management strategies that meet the needs of all patients.

11.1.3. Impact on Quality of Life

Chronic pain significantly lowers the standard of living of millions of individuals, having a drastic impact on their emotional and physical well-being. Chronic pain disrupts daily activities, prevents social interactions, and causes despair and depression. When chronic pain lasts long time, individuals can struggle with relationships, enjoying activities, or working activities. This functional impairment imbalance is not only a physical limitation but also one that affects one's overall sense of identity and purpose. Alleviation of chronic pain is therefore the key to improving quality of life, with an intricate intervention that involves successful pain management skills, psychological therapy, and a compassionate healthcare environment. A well-planned palliative care has the ultimate aim of reducing pain while at the same time addressing the psychological and social dimensions of the patient's illness, emphasizing the need for an interdisciplinary approach to the management of chronic pain.

The interaction between moral empathy and ethical decision-making among healthcare providers significantly impacts the quality of care for patients with chronic pain. Effective moral empathy at high levels among nurses, compounded by recent evidence, is directly linked to effective ethical decision-making that enables them to navigate the delicacies of pain management with sensitivity and compassion. When healthcare providers practice in facilitating ethical environments, they are more inclined to address their moral distress and make decisions supporting the well-being and comfort of patients. However, placed in morally demanding circumstances without proper support, even nurses themselves may experience more moral distress, hindering them even further from delivering quality care.

This speaks volumes for the inclusion of ethics education and crafting moral empathy into the curriculum for nursing, thereby raising not only the providers' quality but the overall quality of life for palliative care patients (Ibrahim et al., 2025). Advanced pain treatment modalities, such as the use of intrathecal baclofen, are of immense potential to improve the well-being of patients with chronic illnesses characterized by immobilizing spasticity and pain. This kind of treatment has gained attention because of its potential to relieve the debilitating symptoms most patients with diseases such as Niemann-Pick disease type C endure. Traditional analgesic methods tend to fall short, providing inadequate pain relief and secondary effects that only add to the patient's complicating lifestyle. Intrathecal baclofen through an implantable pump has been phenomenal in its effectiveness, providing relief from intractable pain and facilitating enhanced functional capacity even with neurodegenerative disease in pediatric patients. This case illustrates the central role of individualized palliative interventions in alleviating suffering, emphasizing the importance of innovative strategies to pain control measures to optimize quality of life outcomes among patients with chronic pain complaints (Tikkanen et al., 2019) (Figure 11.6).

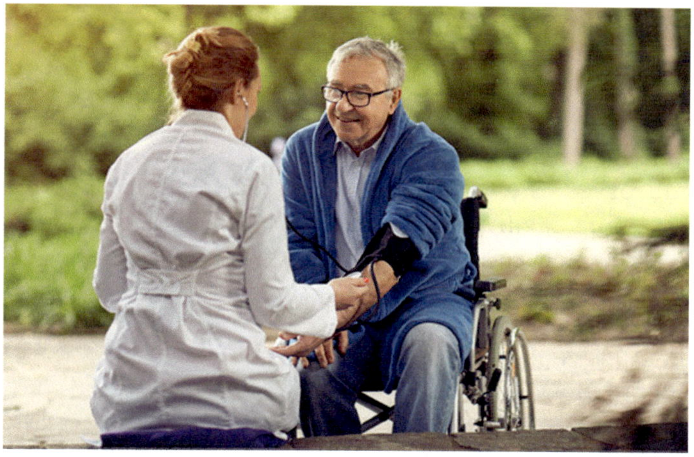

Figure 11.6. Impact on quality of life.

Source: https://external-content.duckduckgo.com/iu/?u=https%3A%2F%2Freversemagazine.us%2Fwp-content%2Fuploads%2F2023%2F12%2FQuality-of-LTC.jpeg&f=1&nofb=1&ipt=278a811bd2ce7e1b84bb38f16dde3d2cecc527fc7ce13aec42aa199f92e8fec6.

Test Your Knowledge

1. How can anesthesia techniques help manage chronic pain?
2. What is the role of regional anesthesia in treating chronic pain?

11.2. The Role of Palliative Care

Learning Outcome

1. Definition and goals of palliative care
2. Differences between palliative care and hospice care
3. Multidisciplinary approach in palliative care

Within the context of chronic pain care, palliative care plays a central position by placing equal emphasis on the patient's overall well-being as well as symptom alleviation. Unlike more conventional medical practices that center mostly on disease treatment, palliative care places emphasis on enhancing the quality of life for afflicted patients with serious conditions. This supportive care is particularly germane to individuals with chronic pain because it not only encompasses pain relief interventions but also psychological, social, and spiritual dimensions of care. Caring for these multifaceted aspects, palliative care ensures patients receive comprehensive support according to their respective needs to enjoy a more enduring experience with their disease. This multidisciplinary approach not only decreases physical discomfort but also optimizes emotional and psychological resilience, significantly affecting global patient satisfaction and participation in their own care. Interdisciplinary collaboration among palliative care providers and primary healthcare providers is essential in effectively managing chronic pain. Interdisciplinary care teams consist of an assembly of varied professionals, including nurses, social workers, and pain management professionals, to create an entire treatment plan that addresses the complex needs of patients. This setting facilitates the sharing of varied expertise, which can lead to innovative solutions and a deeper knowledge of individual pain processes. Moreover, via open lines of communication, palliative care experts can inform primary caregivers on effective measures of pain management so that practice can continually improve. This kind of collaboration is critical, particularly in the treatment of chronic pain conditions since patients may require management over a long period. Through teamwork, medical practitioners can help ensure not only that patients are managed effectively but also that they walk them through the emotional and psychological components of chronic pain. The applicability of palliative care additionally grows with reference to the recently developed health concerns, i.e., the chronic symptoms that follow COVID-19, also referred to as long COVID. With studies identifying various chronic symptoms like tiredness and breathlessness, the necessity of professional palliative care also becomes vital to address the complexity of these issues. Patients are going to endure not just physical discomfort but also anxiety and emotional distress regarding their health ambiguity. Palliative care offers a framework for responding to these interconnected complications through tailored interventions and empathic communication strategies. By creating a supportive system, palliative care can validate patients' concerns, reinforce their coping mechanisms, and ultimately maximize their quality of life during and after such medical emergencies (Nehmeet al., 2020; Vahanian et al., 2021). This strategy spotlights the significance of integrating palliative care values into broader health systems to improve care to meet the evolving needs of patients (Figure 11.7).

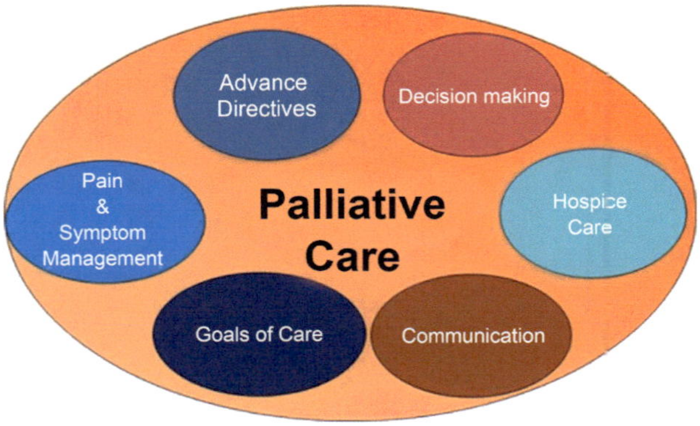

Figure 11.7. The palliative care assumes a pivotal role by prioritizing holistic patient well-being alongside symptom control.

Source: https://external-content.duckduckgo.com/iu/?u=https%3A%2F%2Fuchealth-wp-uploads.s3.amazonaws.com%2Fwp-content%2Fuploads%2Fsites%2F6%2F1970%2F01%2F28144624%2Fpalliative20care20components.jpg&f=1&nofb=1&ipt=1924ea1ecd0a2e124fdfd059b62f690c34f4f6fd7cd3bc676d4bad4258fda0e1.

11.2.1. Definition and Goals of Palliative Care

Palliative medicine is an integral part of medicine that is intended to improve the quality of life for patients with severe illnesses. Palliative medicine not only seeks to alleviate physical symptoms, such as chronic pain, but also addresses the emotional, psychological, and spiritual problems that accompany a severe health status. The integrated aspect of palliative care is critical in the management of chronic pain since it deems chronic pain as an intricate phenomenon beyond mere physical agony. By comprehensive support including pain control interventions, psychological therapy, and spiritual guidance, palliative care aims to optimize the health of patients and, therefore, is a critical component of chronic pain treatment interventions (Roat et al., 2010). Thus, the palliative care definition highlights its commitment to the care of the person and not only on the disease's clinical presentation. Palliative care goals extend beyond symptom relief; they include maintaining dignity, autonomy, and quality of life in patients with chronic pain syndromes. A primary objective is to offer patients and families assistance along the course of illness so there can be informed decision-making about treatment. This is particularly relevant for patients who have chronic pain, who might be experiencing difficulty with how their condition affects daily living. By providing advice and support, palliative care teams help patients voice their values and preferences regarding treatment, which comes a long way in ensuring a sense of control and individualization in their care experience (García-Navarro & Teixeira da Costa, 2017). Feeling heard and understood by the healthcare team has a high ability to boost the emotional resilience of patients, ultimately leading to a better living experience with chronic pain. With interdisciplinary approaches, palliative care is based on collaboration between a wide variety of healthcare professionals, such as doctors, nurses, social workers, and chaplains. Collaboration is often necessary in the achievement of holistic care aimed at the complicated nature of long-term pain. Every stakeholder contributes his or her skill to ensure that patients are subjected to holistic therapies with their own circumstances and cultural backgrounds in mind. For instance, having an intercultural mediator as part of the team can be particularly beneficial in managing cultural differences and enhancing communication among health professionals and patients with diverse backgrounds (García-Navarro & Teixeira da Costa, 2017). This emphasis on teamwork not only assists in effective pain management but also inspires a working environment where patients and families can manage the problems of serious illness as a team. Lastly, the interdisciplinary nature of palliative care underscores the goal of rendering caring and individualized care to patients with chronic pain (Figure 11.8).

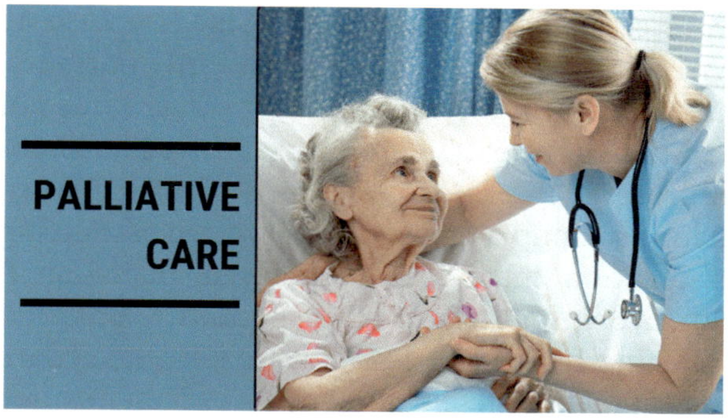

Figure 11.8. Palliative care is an essential component of healthcare.

Source: https://external-content.duckduckgo.com/iu/?u=https%3A%2F%2Fmeetcaregivers.com%2Fwp-content%2Fuploads%2F2020%2F10%2FPalliative-Care.png&f=1&nofb=1&ipt=738a2c33f7a1c00316e374214ec5d766cb9abe9dc5f7ff4a6945e3b3a9cb179c.

11.2.2. Differences Between Palliative Care and Hospice Care

The distinction between palliative care and hospice care is significant in addressing the needs of patients with chronic pain. Palliative care provides wide-ranging symptom management and psychosocial support throughout the course of the illness, from the moment of diagnosis. Such an approach may be utilized at any stage in a chronic illness so that curative treatments may be given alongside it. The primary goal is to enhance the quality of life by minimizing pain, helping with informed decisions, and providing care to patients as well as their relatives. Hospice care is, however, only end-of-life care, typically provided when a patient has a prognosis of six months or less to live. The objective of hospice is to administer comfort instead of curative care, with an emphasis on pain management and emotional support during the terminal stage of life. Understanding the differences among these two paradigms is particularly significant in managing patients with chronic, multifactorial pain disorders. For instance, palliative care can involve several therapies, including pain relief from cancer or other chronic disease, with or without disease terminability. The patients, therefore, undergo palliative therapies in addition to life-extending or disease-progression-addressing therapies. Hospice care, however, involves comfort measures only, often eschewing medication that would otherwise be taken if curative intent exists. Consequently, patients suffering from complex chronic pain disorders can transition from palliative care to hospice care, necessitating an individualized approach that respects the dynamic trajectory of their care needs as they approach death. Additionally, palliative care has shown a promising impact on patient outcomes in various settings, ranging from hospitalized patients with chronic diseases. Research determines that earlier palliative care involvement is correlated with lower in-hospital mortality, especially in cases of complications like infection in patients with multiple myeloma.

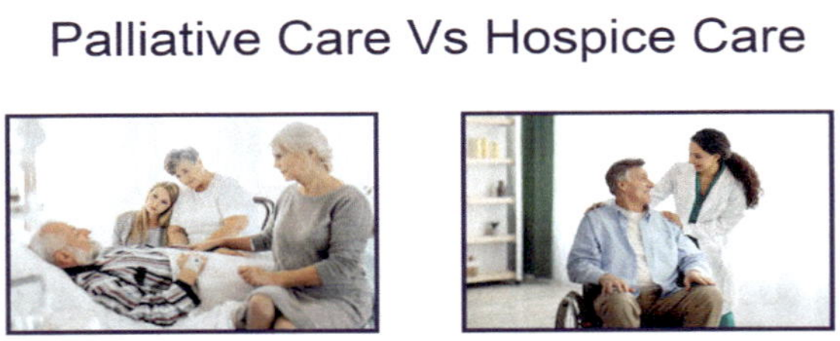

Figure 11.9. Differences between palliative care and hospice care.

Source: https://external-content.duckduckgo.com/iu/?u=https%3A%2F%2Fimedclaims.com%2Fwp-content%2Fuploads%2F2022%2F11%2FPalliative-Care-and-Hospice-Care-2.jpg&f=1&nofb=1&ipt=e035a3f624b979f68bf8f8828166461b9f38602abc71a1f74eb42cd89d9621b9.

It indicates that high-intensity, symptom-focused care during the course of the illness is able to enhance overall health outcomes and quality of life in patients with chronic pain. Conversely, hospice care, while adept at coping with end-of-life concerns, is not as flexible and broad in operation as palliative care, which can manage chronic pain at any stage of the disease process. It is important that doctors are aware of these distinctions in order to give their patients appropriate care tailored to their conditions as they advance through their chronic pain process (Figure 11.9).

11.2.3. Multidisciplinary Approach in Palliative Care

Multidisciplinary care is essential in the care of patients with complex needs in palliative care, as it involves a team of healthcare providers with various disciplines. It includes doctors, nurses, social workers, psychologists, and spiritual counselors who all contribute unique perspectives and qualifications to work with their patients. By bringing their diverse skills together, the multidisciplinary team can design individualized pain management plans that respect the biopsychosocial approach to health. For instance, while medical clinicians are busy eliminating physical symptoms, social workers have the liberty of targeting the psychosocial stressors that usually accompany chronic pain and result in increased overall well-being. This holistic model of care recognizes that pain is not merely a physiological occurrence but has profound emotional and social dimensions as well and, therefore, attempts to treat the patient holistically. By embracing a multidisciplinary approach to palliative care, not only is relief from chronic pain provided immediately, but the quality of both the patient's and their family members' lives is also improved. Team members' communication needs to be proper since it will ensure that all sections of care are coordinated and will reduce the likelihood of confused treatments or miscommunication. Open team sessions to discuss patients' progress and reconsider treatment plans give caregivers a sense of esprit de corps and a common purpose. In addition, this multidisciplinary strategy helps provide education and support to families, which equips them with the ability to cope with the complexity of managing chronic pain. With the extension of palliative care, there is a need for such multidisciplinary teams to be present in diverse populations across different settings, mirroring the belief that "palliative and end-of-life care must be available to all who require it" (Department of Anesthesia, University of Iowa, 2011). The outcome of a multidisciplinary model in palliative care is always good, as studies have shown that patients who have incorporated care are more satisfied and less uncomfortable. For individuals living with chronic pain, this model not only accommodates their acute medical care requirements but also facilitates empathy and psycho-emotional care, facilitation of their coping mechanisms. Moreover, educational training programs for healthcare professionals using this model of collaboration can strengthen healthcare professionals' ability to meet the multiple aspects of chronic pain. Through augmenting inter-disciplinary role understanding, these training programs create a culture of collaboration that culminates in better healthcare outcomes. As the providers strive to create equitable care systems, it is important to realize the importance of multidisciplinary input, so patients receive integrated care that is tailored to their unique experience (Inbadas et al., 2016).

Test Your Knowledge

1. What is the primary goal of palliative care for patients with serious illnesses?
2. Why is a multidisciplinary approach important in palliative care?

11.3. Assessment of Chronic Pain

Learning Outcome

1. Tools and methods for pain assessment
2. Importance of patient self-reporting
3. Challenges in assessing chronic pain

Chronic pain assessment is a central aspect of effective palliative care because it has a direct influence on treatments and patient quality of life. A holistic approach with both subjective and objective assessment methods is required in addressing the intricate nature of chronic pain. These instruments are instrumental in quantifying pain severity and symptom burden and allow healthcare providers to tailor interventions individually. In particular, the evidence indicates that symptoms like feeling bad, fatigue, and depression are typically mixed with chronic pain disorders, further complicating patients' overall clinical presentation (Angeli et al., 2024). Thus, an appropriate assessment not only establishes pain severity but also identifies associated dimensions that need to be addressed, resulting in an integrated and patient-centered approach in palliative care settings. Also, heterogeneity of patient experience necessitates tailored assessment techniques in the management of chronic pain. Chronic pain in patients with co-existing comorbidities, for instance, is characterized by unique challenges that can be addressed by targeted interventions. Non-drug therapies like acupuncture have been reported to be helpful in pain management among such populations, and it is important to consider the specialized profiles of individuals when creating care plans (Yan et al., 2024). Individualized care enables one to comprehend the complexity of chronic pain so that clinicians can apply diverse methods that are applicable to the needs and preferences of individual patients. By continuing to advance evaluation methods, clinicians will be capable of enhancing the effectiveness of palliative intervention, ultimately contributing to improving the outcome in patients. Lastly, the necessity of repeated evaluation cannot be overstated, in that chronic pain syndromes have a propensity for changing and varying in character over time. As patients undergo therapies, repeated evaluation of pain and associated symptoms will be necessary to measure the success of the intervention and implement changes. This practice not only enhances symptom care but also promotes a patient-centered conversation among healthcare practitioners and patients. Chronic evaluation can uncover changes in patient experiences that may signal new or aggravating conditions, necessitating immediate attention and changed treatment plans. Thus, it is vital to adopt a systematic evaluation model that gives centrality to patient feedback and symptom monitoring to maximize palliative care for those experiencing chronic pain, making sure that treatment is proactive in addressing their changing health status (Figure 11.10).

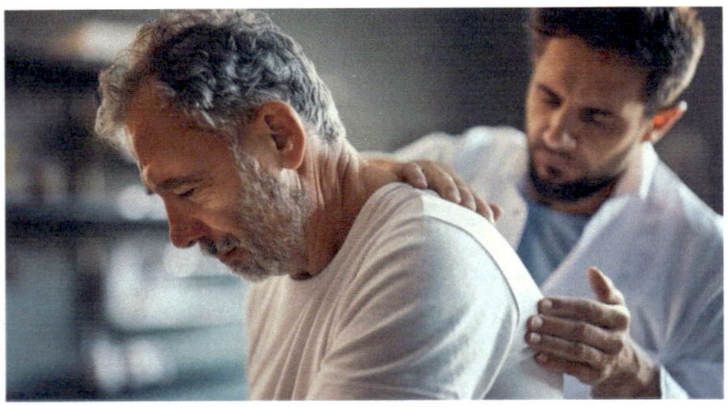

Figure 11.10. The assessment of chronic pain.

Source: https://external-content.duckduckgo.com/iu/?u=https%3A%2F%2Fimg.freepik.com%2Fpremium-photo%2Fcomprehensive-assessment-chronic-pain-conditions-use-diagnostic-tests-like-imaging-studies-nerve-blocks-development-personalized-treatment-plans-involving-medications-physical-therapy_10541-15113.jpg&f=1&nofb=1&ipt=84fa3e75959b237a5096af88c8f911522ac4987f6b671df04cd26e768a28d698.

11.3.1. Tools and Methods for Pain Assessment

Effective pain evaluation is critical in the treatment of chronic pain and in palliative medicine because pain is a subjective phenomenon and significantly impacts quality of life. Various instruments can be used to help healthcare professionals evaluate the severity of pain and its associated factors. Well-established instruments such as the numerical rating scale (NRS) and the visual analog scale (VAS) provide easy methods of quantifying pain intensity, allowing patients to tell others about their pain in an understandable, clear manner. They facilitate patient-provider communication by ensuring that there is an entire comprehension of the pain experience. Further, the use of multidimensional measures, like the Brief Pain Inventory, incorporates pain interference and emotional functioning measures, which promotes an interdisciplinary approach to palliative care pain management. Multidimensionality is particularly significant because it acknowledges that chronic pain is not merely a body-centered process but is highly intertwined with psychological and social dimensions of patient care. Aside from usual self-reporting devices, observational methods and clinical rating are integral parts of pain measurement, particularly in patients with communication impairments. Observation of behavior becomes crucial when it is necessary to measure pain in non-verbal or communication-impaired patients. Facial expression monitoring, body language, and physiological measures—such as heart rate and blood pressure—can provide invaluable information about a patient's level of pain. Second, the integration of both observation techniques with conventional pain assessment measures enhances accuracy in evaluations. For palliative care, the understanding of how chronic pain affects patients' quality of life is essential. The use of both self-report and observational tools thus promotes effective approaches to holistically managing pain based on individual patient needs, which is required for effective palliative care. The evolving landscape of digital health technology has also introduced new devices for pain measurement, adding variety to the choices available to healthcare professionals. Telehealth platforms and smartphone apps now enable remote monitoring and real-time reporting of pain from patients, enabling easier longitudinal tracking of changes in pain scores. All these technological advances enable proactive modification in pain management strategies, providing timely interventions crucial in palliative care. Further, the construction of pain assessment models based on artificial intelligence can analyze vast amounts of data and forecast pain trajectories so as to adopt customized treatment strategies. Nevertheless, such technologies also require thoughtful consideration of privacy, ethical protocols, and accessibility to provide universal care. Technology use in assessing pain is a promising path forward for managing chronic pain that could potentially enhance patient outcomes and align with the principles of palliative care in dealing with the complexity of suffering (Schofield et al., 2007; Kluger et al., 2017).

11.3.2. Importance of Patient Self-Reporting

Self-reporting by the patient is a wealth of information in chronic and palliative pain treatment, providing immediate access to how the patient perceives the illness. In its ability to make patients report their symptoms, response to treatment, and overall well-being, self-reporting provides the possibility for a more responsive and personalized type of treatment. It is particularly useful in settings where chronic disease exists because it enables the patient to be an active participant in his or her treatment. While objective assessments and clinical tests are important, they do not always gauge the complex realities of a patient's experience. Lastly, patient history validation through self-reporting again updates pain and symptom management to enable healthcare workers to make informed decisions based on patient options and needs, as seen in guidelines emphasizing the multidimensional nature of palliative care for certain illnesses, including chronic illnesses like cirrhosis (Shari et al., 2022). Secondly, self-reporting forms the backbone of facilitating communication among patients and healthcare providers. The process creates an environment of openness where patients feel their voice matters, which is important in palliative care centers. With continuous observation and documentation of patient-reported symptoms, clinicians are able to identify patterns of shifting symptoms and adjust care processes accordingly. This dynamic active engagement fosters trust and patient satisfaction since they are more actively engaged in planning care discussions. For instance, in chronic pain treatment, the effectiveness of therapies might be extremely variable across patients, which necessitates self-reporting as a critical method for tracking reactions to interventions by each patient. Management is effective on an open communication basis, and self-reporting not only offers sound treatment approaches but also aids in identifying psychosocial factors in the patient's experience. These have been realized as vital for holistic care, particularly emphasized in interdisciplinary palliative models (Nehme et al., 2020). In addition to facilitating individualized care, patient self-reporting maximizes the quality of life among patients with chronic pain. As patients are stimulated into discussing their feelings and symptoms, they should be likely to get appropriate and timely interventions that can alleviate distress and enhance functioning on an everyday level. This feedback cycle is significant, especially in chronic conditions where long-term management strategies have to be continuously optimized. Further, understanding a patient's subjective experience—like emotional impairment and functional distress—can help healthcare professionals offer individualized psychosocial care, which is an elementary aspect of palliative care. Encouraging self-reporting not only empowers patients but also advances healthcare practitioners' ability to implement care and caring plans, enabling the treatment to be tailored towards each patient's unique goals and values, a critical aspect in the integrated approach advocated in palliative care guidelines (Shari et al., 2022) (Figure 11.11).

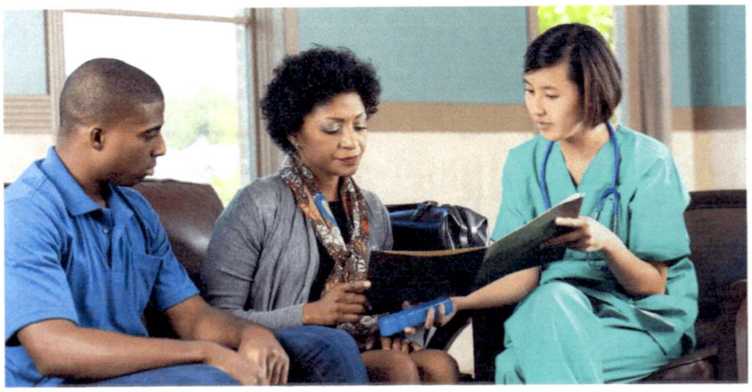

Figure 11.11. Patient self-reporting.

Source: https://external-content.duckduckgo.com/iu/?u=https%3A%2F%2Fthenerdynurse.com%2Fwp-content%2Fuploads%2F2021%2F08%2FWhy-Patient-Education-is-Important-FB.png.webp&f=1&nofb=1&ipt=0c03de81caa01ddf082689f3e70064561673c941de8968f81989784d3866323c.

11.3.3. Challenges in Assessing Chronic Pain

Chronic pain measurement is specific in challenges that limit useful management and treatment in the context of palliative care. Pain is by nature subjective, to the extent that every patient's experience is unique and influenced by unique psychological and situational variables. Subjective nature creates an obstacle to the proper use of standard assessment tools as valid, creating a difference between the perceptions of patients regarding pain and the knowledge of healthcare providers. Secondly, the multidimensional nature of chronic pain, often with physical, emotional, and social components, necessitates a multidisciplinary approach to evaluation. Traditional pain scales by themselves could miss the nuances of each case, the value of comprehensive evaluation instruments addressing psychological and socioeconomic issues as well as physical symptoms. These nuances necessitate innovative measures of assessment that better capture the diversity of individual experience and lead to tailored interventions for improving patient outcomes in palliative care. Additionally, barriers to communication between health professionals and patients further complicate the issues involved with evaluating chronic pain. Many patients may have trouble accurately explaining their pain, depending on fear of stigma, lack of assertiveness in discussing their experience, or inadequate knowledge of pain terminology. Such a discrepancy may result in an inadequate understanding of the patient's experience of pain, with potential suboptimal treatment choices. Involvement by caregivers can, in some cases, break this issue; however, reliance on caregivers introduces other variables like differences in perception of pain and priorities for treatment. In palliative care settings, where communication is critical to symptom control, these concerns require the use of supportive interventions that enhance patient-provider communication, such as trained facilitators or the use of visual pain assessment tools that engage patients in the process of their care. Furthermore, the psychological elements of chronic pain, such as depression and anxiety, render it particularly challenging to assess. Pain is also common to occur chronically along with psychological distress, which can further amplify the pain experience and create a spiral of increasing symptoms and tension. This interrelation necessitates a dual assessment approach that bridges pain and mental health issues. For instance, tools like the Edmonton symptom assessment scale (ESAS) can help to demarcate the burden of physical as well as psychological symptoms and lead clinicians to the right interventions. Incorporating tools like the integrated palliative care outcome scale (IPOS) can provide additional depth to the effectiveness of treatment programs in several areas of patient health. Therefore, understanding the multifactorial nature of chronic pain is essential in creating inclusive assessment models that enable maximum care outcomes in palliative care, directing therapy beyond the mere alleviation of pain (Sushma, 2024; Park et al., 2024).

Test Your Knowledge

1. What key factors are evaluated during the assessment of chronic pain?
2. Why is it important to assess both the intensity and impact of chronic pain on daily life?

11.4. Treatment Options for Chronic Pain

Learning Outcome

1. Pharmacological interventions
2. Non-pharmacological therapies
3. Integrative and complementary approaches

In the handling of the multifaceted issue of chronic pain, there are various treatment options available aimed at enhancing the quality of life of patients. Of considerable interest is that the World Health Organization (WHO) has come up with guidelines targeting chronic primary low back pain, which is a pervasive issue that affects millions of individuals worldwide. The guidelines summarize 37 potential interventions, of which 24 were given direct endorsement based on strong evidence. These policies encourage individualized care according to the patient's individual circumstances, setting an inclination for non-invasive intervention approaches within primary health centers. The emphasis on diverse interventions demonstrates the WHO's consideration of chronic pain's complex nature and the necessity for a comprehensive approach to management to minimize the condition's significant impact on daily living and health systems (Department of Anesthesia, University of Iowa, 2011). Pharmacologic interventions play a key role in managing chronic pain, and opioids are among the most commonly prescribed drugs. Opioid use for the treatment of chronic non-cancer pain is, however, increasingly criticized for risk and abuse potential. In response to this, the Korean Pain Society (KPS) developed new guidelines to act as a template for safe opioid prescribing. These guidelines stress starting with an adequate dose, ongoing monitoring of the treatment, and careful consideration of the risk-to-benefit ratio to prevent side effects. Although opioids do provide considerable relief, physicians are encouraged to be clinically astute and make patient-centered decisions when adding these medications to pain management protocols, such that the treatment is synchronized with the general intent of chronic pain management and palliative approaches (Kim et al., 2024). Alongside pharmacologic interventions, non-pharmacologic treatments also provide significant benefits in chronic pain management, particularly in a multidisciplinary setting. Interventions such as cognitive-behavioral therapy, exercise programs, acupuncture, and physical therapy have proven beneficial in reducing pain intensity along with improving functionality. Promoting whole-person care, such interventions effectively attend to the physical, psychological, and emotional aspects of chronic pain. Lifestyle modification, along with complementary therapies in customized treatment programs, can empower the patient, allowing them to feel a sense of control over their pain. This integrated model is essential in the application of palliative care, reaffirming that supportive treatments should follow the issue of comfort and overall welfare, ultimately enhancing the quality of life of patients experiencing chronic pain (Figure 11.12).

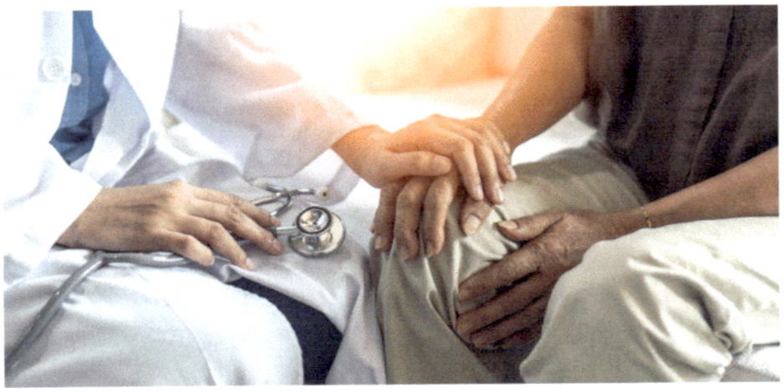

Figure 11.12. In addressing the multifaceted challenge of chronic pain.

Source: https://external-content.duckduckgo.com/iu/?u=https%3A%2F%2Fwestmichiganhospice.com%2Fwp-content%2Fuploads%2F2022%2F03%2Fchronic-pain-treatments-1024x512.jpg&f=1&nofb=1&ipt=e4a2b76748bec65d3d204d7df61b20e9fd8947a78ef20bdf7c198ecc2667f259.

11.4.1. Pharmacological Interventions

Pharmacological intervention plays a key role in palliative care, in which the treatment is employed to treat chronic pain. Pharmacological intervention is tailored to relieve pain and enhance the quality of life in patients suffering from life-threatening illnesses, which is justified by the nature of chronic diseases. Opioids, non-steroidal anti-inflammatory drugs (NSAIDs), and adjuvant drugs such as antidepressants and anticonvulsants typically form the basis of treatment regimes. In chronic obstructive pulmonary disease (COPD) patients and other advanced respiratory diseases, the evidence is that despite the administration of several therapies, the majority of them continue to experience uncontrolled pain and dyspnea (Boland et al., 2013). Thus, the inclusion of pharmacologic modalities in palliative care is indispensable not only for the management of physical symptomatology but also in addressing the broader psychosocial dimensions of suffering. The efficacy of pharmacological management of chronic pain is more than mere relief of symptoms; it is also a means of decreasing the social and affective burden generally endured by patients. Pain control by medication has the power to significantly transform patient's abilities in activities of daily living and to maintain their social support systems, which are generally under tension as a result of physical pain. Chronic problems in managing pain in chronic non-malignant lung disease patients have highlighted the necessity for adding specialist palliative care teams, regardless of patient prognosis (Boland et al., 2013). Innovative approaches such as enhanced delivery models and individualized medication plans are core to achieving maximum outcomes. As studies become more and more able to unlock the complex nature of pharmacological treatments, attention must also be given to how they are able to bring quality of life to patients, particularly those most at risk. While innovation has been seen with pharmacological treatments for chronic pain, there remains much to be learned about the full potential they hold, particularly in some conditions like COPD. There should be cooperation between palliative care teams and research institutions to determine the most effective use of medications. Continuous monitoring of pharmacological treatment is required, both to ascertain their safety and efficacy and to learn about the nitty-gritty of patient experience and response. Although healthcare professionals strive to maximize care delivery, funding for high-quality trials is required to determine the optimal management strategies. Underpinned by a strong evidence base for a variety of pharmacological options, increasingly patient-centered and complex mechanisms of pain management can be constructed in palliative care (Figure 11.13).

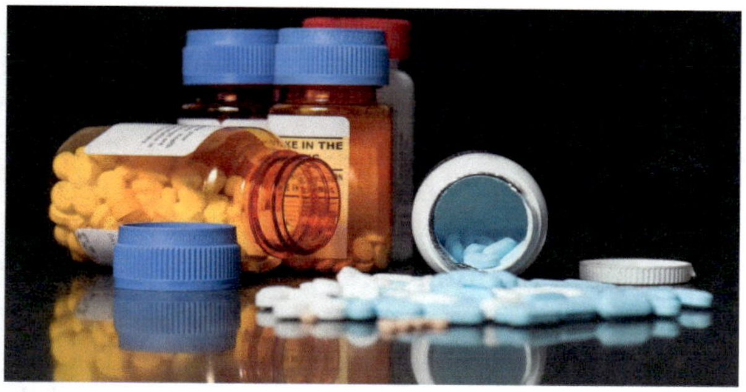

Figure 11.13. Pharmacological interventions possess a pivotal role in the management of chronic pain within palliative care settings.

Source: https://external-content.duckduckgo.com/iu/?u=https%3A%2F%2Fwww.findatopdoc.com%2Fvar%2Ffatd%2Fstorage%2Fimages%2F_aliases%2Ffb_thumb%2Fhealthy-living%2Fmedical-advancements-new-treatments-and-perspectives-on-fibromyalgia%2Fpharmacological-treatments%2F3584078-1-eng-US%2FPharmacological-treatments.jpg&f=1&nofb=1&ipt=9ee0fd8065ad9df3883698411f9d2dbc7fac18ed7cf38b0bc7053d4ef7acf1b5.

11.4.2. Non-Pharmacological Therapies

The increasing prevalence of chronic pain has necessitated the knowledge of therapeutic modalities other than pharmacology. The non-pharmacological interventions have come to signify a critical component in the management of chronic pain, particularly that of a palliative nature. The treatments incorporate a range of practices like cognitive behavioral therapy (CBT), mindfulness skills, and acceptance and commitment therapy (ACT), all for addressing the psychological and physical sides of pain. Adding these modalities to treatment can help healthcare providers offer patients more holistic care that can potentially reduce opioid medication dependency, typically associated with abuse and dependency behaviors in chronic pain patients. The success of the interventions suggests greater potential to improve patients' quality of life, especially since the comorbidities often associated with chronic pain, i.e., depression and anxiety (Samuel et al., 2024), may be treated. Apart from treating psychological aspects, non-pharmacological therapies also attach great importance to lifestyle modification and rehabilitation techniques in palliative care. For instance, regular exercise and stress management techniques have proven to alleviate some of the debilitating effects of chronic illness, thereby fostering emotional health and physical functioning. Integrating formal rehabilitation programs can also improve compliance with treatment and participation in one's own care management. The multi-faceted strategy, in addition to alleviating pain, also encourages the empowerment of patients by counteracting feelings of helplessness that are usual in chronic disease settings. Such strategies emphasize the need for healthcare workers to be multi-disciplinary in their approach, and how effective communication between patients, caregivers, and medical personnel is crucial (Shevcova et al., 2024). Besides that, the role of support systems cannot be overstated when applying non-pharmacological interventions for the management of chronic pain. Communication and coordination between healthcare providers, patients, and families create a supportive environment that facilitates compliance with such interventions. Education of patients on the potential advantage of non-pharmacological treatment fosters a higher appreciation and compliance with such interventions. For example, the integration of practitioners experienced with techniques such as mindfulness or relaxation therapy may improve patients' experiences and contribute to pain coping resources. With the healthcare landscape becoming increasingly patient-centered models of care, the integration of non-pharmacologic therapies will not only transform the treatment of chronic pain but also optimize quality of life as a whole, as much attention is being drawn to carrying out more research and validation of such practices within the framework of palliative care (Samuel et al., 2024) (Figure 11.14).

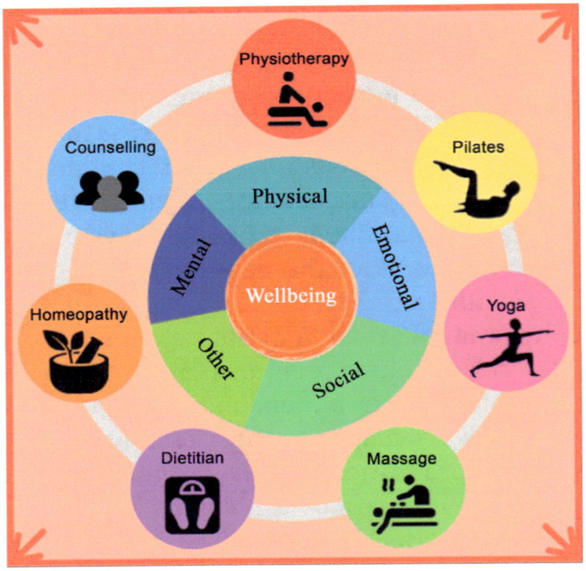

Figure 11.14. Non-pharmacological therapies.

Source: https://external-content.duckduckgo.com/iu/?u=https%3A%2F%2Fvicpainmanagement.com.au%2Fwp-content%2Fuploads%2F2020%2F06%2FPain-Management-550x550.png&f=1&nofb=1&ipt=8e99e8cabeb3a224f40b04fdf0ea4dc04145c0f237530fa096a32644f4664271.

11.4.3. Integrative and Complementary Approaches

Holistic and complementary approaches to the treatment of chronic pain have become increasingly prevalent in the practice of palliative care due to their promise of enhancing patient quality of life. Among these are a variety of non-pharmacological approaches, including acupuncture, mindfulness, yoga, and nutritional therapies. These approaches are intended to address not only the physical dimensions of suffering but also the emotional, psychological, and spiritual dimensions of pain. By integrating these approaches with conventional therapeutic medicine, clinicians can create an individualized care experience that caters to the unique desires and priorities of the patient. Such a patient-centered process is critical since it respects patients' preferences and values, thereby facilitating a respectful mutual partnership between healthcare professionals and chronic pain patients (Dowell et al., 2022). Moreover, research has demonstrated that integrative and complementary therapies can lead to better results in pain management. For instance, research has shown that acupuncture can bring significant pain relief for certain conditions, while mindfulness interventions can reduce perceived pain by changing cognitive as well as emotional processing of pain. In addition, exercise via such therapies as yoga not only relieves pain but also improves overall physical function and mental status. They are particularly appropriate in palliative care, in which the quality of life of patients suffering from chronic pain due to incapacitating diseases has to be improved. The integration of these complementary therapies can enhance conventional care modalities, and treatment regimens are more efficacious and comprehensive in enhancing the multifaceted symptoms of chronic pain (). Such an association between integrative treatment and routine medical therapy is further enhanced by guidelines developed by health organizations, which require an interdisciplinary model of pain management. In addition to this, the CDC Guidelines focus on evaluation of all treatment options, indicating a shift towards a wider reflection on care (Dowell et al., 2022). This model encourages reflection on risk and benefit across a spectrum of interventions, thereby allowing informed decision-making by both clinicians and patients. By combining pharmacologic treatment, such as opioids for terminal pain, with complementary measures, patients can rely on the strengths of both worlds leading to overall enhanced pain management and enhanced quality of life. Ongoing research into these combination methods highlights the necessity of an adaptable and responsive model of chronic pain treatment within palliative care settings that offers the proper support according to each patient's individual experience and need.

Test Your Knowledge

1. What are common pharmacological treatments for chronic pain?
2. Name one non-pharmacological approach used to manage chronic pain.

11.5. Psychological Aspects of Chronic Pain

Learning Outcome

1. Emotional and mental health implications
2. Coping strategies for patients
3. Role of mental health professionals in palliative care

Chronic pain is intrinsically interwoven with complex psychological processes that also have a substantial impact on the life and management of the illness of a patient. Psychological states such as stress, depression, and anxiety are most often aggravated by chronic pain, thus perpetuating a vicious cycle where each also contributes to aggravating the other. Patients will complain that their pain is not just a sensation, but an emotional and psychosocial one that disrupts their daily function and overall quality of life. What is most important to treat is these psychosocial issues, as it is imperative to intervention in palliative care, and once again indicative of the need for an integrated model to treat mind and body. This association emphasizes the importance of interdisciplinary care in the management of chronic pain, ensuring that psychological well-being takes precedence along with physical attention to reap greater therapeutic gain and patient satisfaction. Furthermore, a biopsychosocial model presents a powerful conceptualization of the nature of chronic pain. This model acknowledges that biological, psychological, and social factors are interconnected and contribute to the pain condition. Particularly, coping mechanisms and psychological resilience can have a great impact on whether or not a patient can effectively deal with his or her chronic pain, as well as treatment protocols. Self-management is key to this, whereby patients with sound coping skills can have improved outcomes regarding pain. For example, one study into COPD found that patients who exercised lifestyle coping responses had better emotional health and lower psychological distress levels, paralleling improved general health outcomes. This would mean that applying the same psychosocial interventions in the management of chronic pain could be of great benefit to patients in palliative care, with the importance of personalized psychological support arising from it. Lastly, the role of exercise as an approach to treatment in managing chronic pain demonstrates the intersection of physical and psychological well-being. The EPIC-Neck program is a well-established example of a co-produced exercise program aimed at optimizing patient adherence and outcomes by addressing the behavioral and psychological factors. With components that address the psychological barriers to participation, i.e., pain fear with activity, this new strategy aims to develop long-term treatment adherence. Moreover, it demonstrates that psychological preparation and support can contribute to improved physical functioning as well as pain reduction. The consequences of greater adherence and exercise participation are that management of chronic pain in palliative care would be greatly enhanced by addressing the psychological aspects within structured programs, thereby creating an integrative model of care that addresses each component of the patient's experience and encourages integrative healing (Figure 11.15).

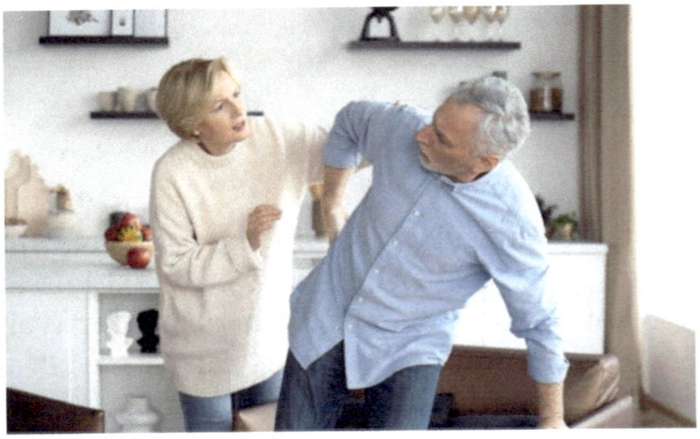

Figure 11.15. Psychological aspects of chronic pain.

Source: https://external-content.duckduckgo.com/iu/?u=https%3A%2F%2Fatlantichealthclinic.com%2Fwp-content%2Fuploads%2F2024%2F02%2FScreenshot-2024-02-07-at-2.10.58-PM.png&f=1&nofb=1&ipt=776cf552294b9631c3a43c2059d35ab0ef380d6408d7056c89e1f6c347ab29a7.

11.5.1. Emotional and Mental Health Implications

Chronic pain imposes a profound effect on mental and emotional health, and therefore requires an integral approach by palliative care. Psychological distress in pain coping may lead to profound emotional suffering through depression and anxiety. Furthermore, chronic pain exposes individuals to a reduced perception of well-being, which may manifest in terms of social isolation and hopelessness. This psychological landscape is further aggravated by the chronic pain stigma, whereby patients become belittled, overlooked, or not understood by medical professionals and society at large. Confronting the psychological impact of chronic pain is essential to creating effective palliative care strategies that not only alleviate physical symptoms but also convey psychological relief, affirming the interconnected role of mental and physical health in managing chronic conditions. Parenting in chronic pain exhibits a profound intersection of bodily suffering and affective burden, particularly as evidenced in vulnerable subgroups. Research indicates that parents' levels of pain severity and disability play a strong role in children's pain and psychological distress, such as anxiety and depression. The extension of parental pain beyond the self is profound, highly influencing the affective states of children. This is accentuated by the imperative of dealing with family dynamics within palliative care frameworks. Clarifying the impact of parental distress resulting from chronic pain on children enables healthcare workers to personalize support systems not only for the patient but also for the family, thereby providing a comprehensive treatment plan that addresses the needs of both generations and alleviates the broader emotional ramifications of chronic pain (Efua, 2024).

Furthermore, the effects of chronic pain have implications for specific circumstances, including post-childbirth recovery when women are destined to endure physical as well as psychological challenges. Evidence shows that there is a strong correlation between physical injuries like perineal tears and adverse mental health outcomes, including risks of postpartum depression and anxiety. These affective burdens are compounded by the physical pain endured during the recovery process and can be a vicious cycle on quality of life. Substitution with complete care in specialized perineal clinics that address both the physical and psychological elements of recovery is essential. Diversification ensures medical attention for physical injuries, alongside emotional healing that is vital for complete healing. Thus, detection and intervention for the psychological impact of chronic pain may facilitate an easier recovery process, significantly enhancing maternal and child well-being (Efua, 2024).

11.5.2. Coping Strategies for Patients

When it comes to palliative care and chronic pain, patients are likely to undergo multifaceted issues that need capable coping strategies. Pain is more than physical discomfort; it is also an emotional and psychological burden that has a powerful ability to dictate the quality of life. Becoming adaptive in coping strategies, therefore, becomes crucial. Evidence suggests that patients who are most actively engaged in problem-solving techniques, such as cognitive reframing and seeking social support, can best cope with their experiences of pain. Not only do these strategies promote resilience, but they also allow patients to take charge of their own care to a greater extent, feeling in control of their circumstances (Guziak et al., 2024). By addressing distinct coping styles, professionals can create interventions tailored to patients' particular needs and situation. Integrating technology into coping mechanisms of patients with chronic pain presents a potentially dynamic future for palliative care. In recent years, the creation of mobile app interventions has been promising in equipping patients with necessary self-management tools.

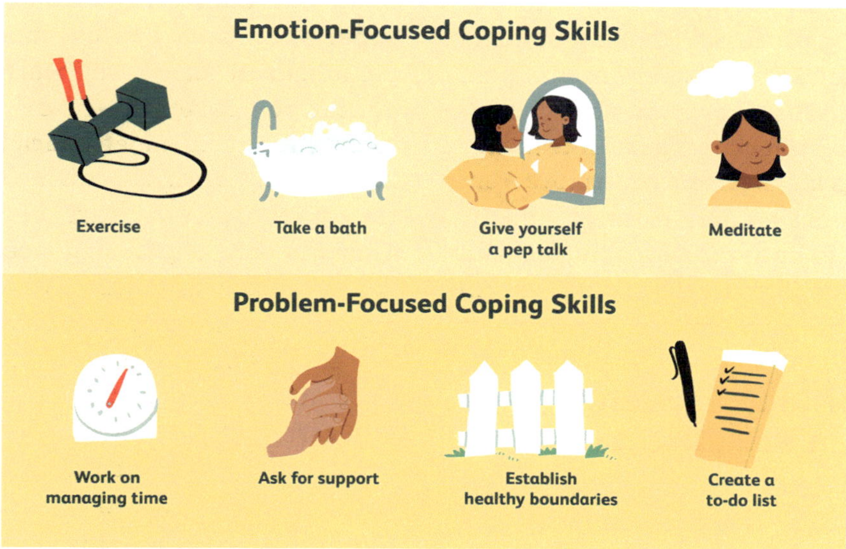
Emotion-Focused Coping Skills
Exercise
Take a bath
Give yourself a pep talk
Meditate
Problem-Focused Coping Skills
Work on managing time
Ask for support
Establish healthy boundaries
Create a to-do list

Figure 11.16. The context of chronic pain and palliative care.

Source: https://external-content.duckduckgo.com/iu/?u=https%3A%2F%2Fwww.verywellmind.com%2Fthmb%2FjLY9Yo-rud_N1-fH-xqTnYj9Hbw%3D%2F6000x4000%2Ffilters%3Ano_upscale()%3Amax_bytes(150000)%3Astrip_icc()%2Fforty-healthy-coping-skills-4586742_v61-4e1f6f67b5a14bf1abd0e3a472a069d2.png&f=1&nofb=1&ipt=e31114c304b8cd99d513ffb155a7630d354403940908dec4d3dc8f0b459a6c42.

These apps typically incorporate functionalities that allow patients to track pain severity, track medication, and offer access to educational material related to managing chronic pain. Evidence involving these web-based resources indicates that these resources can enhance the engagement of patients in their care plan, thereby enhancing adherence and outcomes (Guziak et al., 2024). Additionally, the fact that this technology is available to be continued beyond clinic attendance creates an environment where patients feel less lonely in their experience. As healthcare evolves, the use of technological advancements in coping strategies will be vital in addressing the complex needs of chronic pain patients. Moreover, the integration of psychological support among coping strategies for chronic pain patients has been found to significantly decrease symptoms and improve overall well-being. Research emphasizes the synergy between mental illness and chronic pain, with patients developing co-morbid illnesses such as depression and anxiety. Evidence-based interventions such as cognitive-behavioral therapy can empower patients with coping strategies to manage pain and stress better (Chandra et al., 2024). Moreover, establishing a healthy alliance between patients and healthcare professionals is essential for an adaptive coping process. Providing patients with opportunities to reveal experiences of pain and emotional consequences allows them to get validated in their suffering. These integrative approaches to pain management are a move from the more traditional models to more holistic care that attends to both the psychological and the physiological underpinnings of chronic pain in palliative care (Figure 11.16).

11.5.3. Role of Mental Health Professionals in Palliative Care

Application of mental health professionals in palliative care is essential, especially in the control of chronic pain. Mental health professionals provide essential psychological care to life-limited patients, navigating them through the emotional challenges of such conditions. Chronic pain is often associated with mental health conditions such as depression and anxiety, requiring interdisciplinary care. Mental health professionals can employ therapeutic interventions, such as cognitive-behavioral therapy, to assist patients in learning coping skills that minimize the psychological effects of chronic pain.

Additionally, their inclusion in multidisciplinary teams ensures that patients receive balanced evaluations that inform care plans that foster not only physical but also mental welfare within a palliative setting. Furthermore, integrating mental health services with palliative care can lead to improved outcomes for patients. Research has indicated that patients who receive psychological support adjust to their condition more effectively, and it significantly enhances the quality of their lives during the therapy. Emphasis on mental health enables practitioners to address issues of existential distress, which is often present in chronic pain patients. Incorporation of mental health professionals also facilitates personalized treatment, addressing each patient's personal experience and coping mechanisms. This personalized answer appeals to the present palliative care ethic of individualized interventions to meet special patient needs, in harmony with a growing appreciation of the psychosocial nature of serious illness. There is also a pressing need for increased access to mental health care as palliative care expands, particularly among older patients. As life expectancy increases, there is a greater need for palliative care services integrated into care, including mental health input. Older individuals have generally been lower on the list of priorities in palliative care systems, yet they often present with complicated clinical issues and considerable psychosocial challenges (Department of Anesthesia, University of Iowa, 2011). Providing equal access to mental health professionals for all patients is of utmost priority when creating palliative care programs that meet diversified needs, including chronic pain conditions. This aligns with the perception that all patients have a right to access palliative care irrespective of their location or resource status and that mental health is essential in the creation of a fully inclusive, humane, and effective palliative care system (Department of Anesthesia, University of Iowa, 2011).

Test Your Knowledge

1. How can chronic pain affect a patient's mental health?
2. Why is addressing psychological factors important in chronic pain management?

11.6. Ethical Considerations in Palliative Care

Learning Outcome

1. Informed consent and patient autonomy
2. Balancing pain management and potential side effects
3. Cultural sensitivity in treatment approaches

Ethics are fundamental in palliative care, particularly where the unique issues in patients suffering from chronic pain are concerned. Ethical dilemmas arise when there are thoughts about end-of-life possibilities for care and the extent to which patients should be included in decisions about their care. Autonomy is the virtue that argues in favor of patients being able to exercise autonomous choices regarding their treatment and life quality, such as being able to forego aggressive interventions. In cases where patients have declining conditions such as dementia, caregivers can be confronted with ethical challenges since there is little guidance on how to respect the wishes of those who may not be able to make their own. The disparity in care standards of individuals with chronic disease, identified in Robinson et al. (2006), further indicates the need for an equitable system that upholds patient autonomy, particularly as the number of elderly individuals with chronic disease continues to grow. Another important ethical concern is the disparities in various populations in obtaining palliative care. Ethnic minority patients go through a close network of barriers, such as the problem of communication and unfamiliarity with health systems, as noted in Green et al. (2018). These problems can silence their ability to take an active participation in their care choices and enjoy high-quality end-of-life care. Health professionals should achieve cultural competence in ethical practice to fully interact with patients from different backgrounds. By being aware of the specific needs and experiences of these groups, including their migration history and family roles, palliative care professionals can better tailor their response. Not only does this enhance patient comfort and safety, but it also allows care be delivered in line with the values and beliefs of the recipients, and supports a family-friendly and respectful setting for families and patients.

Lastly, the integration of ethical considerations in palliative care also involves a commitment to the provision of holistic and individualized care that addresses both physical and psychosocial issues. The decision-makers must balance the effects of treatment interventions not only according to medicine but also according to the effect these interventions have on patients' and their families' well-being. For example, responsiveness to attitudes of death and dying in culture can radically transform the patient's care experience, from ease with the use of pain management methods to family involvement preferences, as described in Green et al. (2018). As the demand for palliative care for pain continues to expand, it is increasingly vital to develop systems that are sensitive to ethical principles and offer efficient and empathetic care. By making communication, trust, and respect for patient autonomy priorities, the profession can adopt more equitable and effective end-of-life care practices (Figure 11.17).

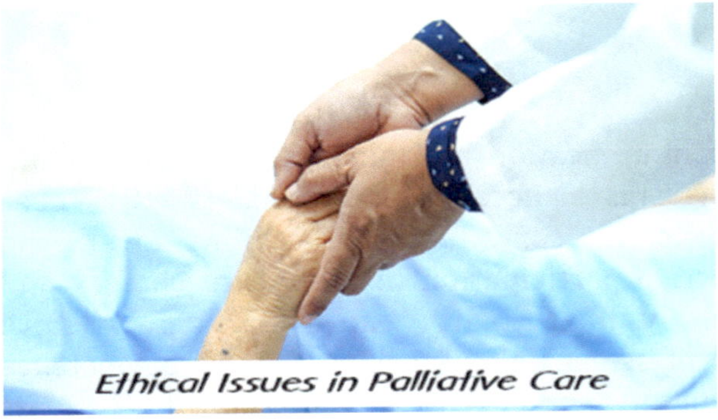

Figure 11.17. Ethical considerations in palliative care.

Source: https://www.rgcirc.org/wp-content/uploads/2024/07/ethical-issues-palliative-care.png.

11.6.1. Informed Consent and Patient Autonomy

In the instance of chronic pain and palliative care, patient autonomy and informed consent are the foundation on which effective treatment regimens are established. Patients must be provided with full disclosure regarding their condition, treatment alternatives, risks, benefits, and other alternatives. This process not only allows patients to make choices about their care but also encourages a therapeutic relationship between patients and healthcare professionals that is the foundation in chronic pain management.

Effective communication thus becomes pivotal to allowing patients understand their choices completely and to communicate their wishes. A robust informed consent system is essential as it enhances patient satisfaction and leads to compliance with the treatment plan, ultimately leading to improved health outcomes. Patient autonomy, which is also strongly linked with informed consent, emphasizes the liberty of individuals in making their own healthcare decisions.

Particularly in palliative care, where hard moral and ethical decisions are the standard, patient autonomy ensures that treatment is aligned with the values and desires of individuals suffering from chronic pain. Not only does such respect for this type of autonomy affirm the dignity of the patient, but it also honors their experiences and unique situation. Current studies, including those associated with the Hospice Friendly Hospitals Program, point to the necessity of proactively involving patients in discussions around their end-of-life care, valuing the paramount role of autonomy in developing a more nurturing healthcare environment (Green et al., 2018).

Amidst the intricacies of treatment options, patient opinions need to guide the course of their care. Moreover, end-of-life care is supported by ethical frameworks that stipulate the importance of informed consent and patient autonomy to be maintained in practice. The Ethical Framework for End-of-Life Care is used as a guide source for healthcare professionals, which stipulates how to approach problems related to chronic pain management and palliative care (McCarthy et al., 2010). With the integration of ethical principles such as respect for persons and legitimate informed decision-making, healthcare professionals can offer an environment that respects patient autonomy while at the same time ensuring that the patients are properly informed about their options. As healthcare systems continue to put more emphasis on person-centered care, the alignment of ethical principles with everyday practices will be crucial to enhance the quality of life of individuals living with chronic conditions and promote dignified strategies in their care journey (Figure 11.18).

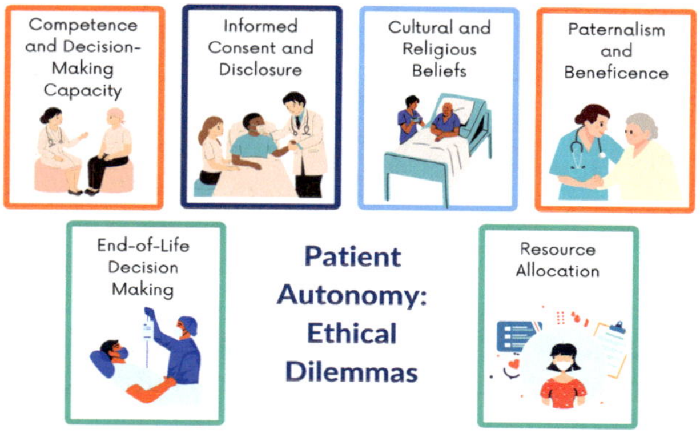
Competence and Decision-Making Capacity
Informed Consent and Disclosure
Cultural and Religious Beliefs
Paternalism and Beneficence
End-of-Life Decision Making
Patient Autonomy: Ethical Dilemmas
Resource Allocation

Figure 11.18. The principles of informed consent and patient autonomy.

Source: https://www.themedicportal.com/wp-content/uploads/2024/01/Social-Dilemma-Prompts-in-Education-Flashcards-in-Colorful-Bold-Style-.png.

11.6.2. Balancing Pain Management and Potential Side Effects

Successful pain management is a cornerstone of chronic pain treatment and palliative medicine, but it is fraught with pitfalls, primarily with the potential side effects of the intervention. Patients with chronic pain are typically in need of an interdisciplinary treatment with pharmacologic and non-pharmacologic interventions. Opioids, despite their efficacy in most situations, carry risks of addiction, sedation, and gastrointestinal upset. Therefore, clinicians encounter these risks to achieve the greatest pain relief and the least amount of side effects. Haloperidol, an antipsychotic, is one of the newer options to alleviate pain and has proven to be of potential analgesic application. Current literature indicates that haloperidol can successfully treat pain of conditions like gastroparesis and migraine without significant side effects like QT-related problems, thereby having a favorable profile in the array of drugs for pain relief in palliative care (Barnosky et al., 2025). Balance also needs to be achieved with postoperative care, as inadequate control of pain can lead to serious complications. Studies show that poorly controlled postoperative pain increases the risk for cardiopulmonary complications, prolonged hospital stay, and the development of chronic pain syndromes. Procedure-specific postoperative pain management has emerged as the solution concept to these issues. By tailoring analgesic measures to the specific procedure, clinicians can optimize relief of pain without the risks associated with pain drugs. This multimodal approach employs more than one analgesic and regional technique to offer effective pain relief without risking overwhelming patients with side effects such as opioid hyperalgesia or addiction (Barnosky et al., 2025). Monitoring of side effects is part of any pain management program, especially palliative care. With quality-of-life concerns for patients with chronic diseases increasingly in the limelight, measurement of relief of pain as well as side effects becomes of prime importance. Continuous monitoring of a patient's response to therapy allows clinicians to institute proper adjustments in therapy in good time such that pain is maximally controlled without compromising the patient's overall well-being. The haloperidol administration, for instance, provides an opportunity for pain relief while limiting excessive side effects conventionally caused by stronger opioids. Such strategies emphasize the importance of individualization in the management of chronic pain, where the goal is to achieve a balance between adequate analgesia and minimal adverse effects, ultimately enhancing the patient's experience during their illness (Barnosky et al., 2025).

11.6.3. Cultural Sensitivity in Treatment Approaches

Treatment of chronic pain in palliative care demands a solid understanding of cultural sensitivity in treatment plans. Acknowledgment of patients' diversity of background according to culture makes clinicians provide an intervention that is aligned with patients' beliefs and values. Such sensitivity not only enhances patients' trust but also enhances patients' engagement in their care plan. Cultural considerations may influence how individuals experience pain, report distress, and have expectations of curative response. Later, culturally competent health care practitioners have better capacities for negotiating discussions regarding accessible pain management, thereby increasing patients' general quality of life when they have chronic conditions. Thus, adding cultural sensitivity to the practice protocols becomes relevant in ensuring that patients are heard, understood, and fully participating in their treatment program, ultimately leading to more successful patient-care relationships. Treatment interventions can be most effective if cultural sensitivity is incorporated into the model of palliative care. For instance, palliative care values holistic management such that physical relief from symptoms is not the only aspect, but also emotional and social problems. This applies more so to terminally ill patients who may have unique cultural determinants of health attitudes and behavior. By promoting shared decision-making processes, medical professionals are able to explore culturally suitable options that resonate with patients and their families. Not only does such a participatory approach preserve respect for personal autonomy, but it also fortifies patient-provider therapeutic alliance, leading to more suitable and effective interventions in pain management. By reconciling treatment modalities into alignment with patients' cultures, care providers enhance the quality of the entire therapeutic process and potential outcomes in palliative care. In addition, the incorporation of cultural sensitivity in the management of pain requires close scrutiny of barriers and facilitators potentially present within different healthcare systems. According to studies, there has been evidence showing healthcare providers frequently face difficulty in identifying and addressing the specific cultural influences that impact pain experience and treatment compliance. For example, clinical interventions like intrathecal drug delivery systems (IDDS) may be very effective but must possess a sensitive awareness of the history of individual patients to be appropriately utilized and utilized. The findings of recent studies bring to light the necessity for cultural competency training and education of clinicians, which can be very useful in bridging pain service gaps among culturally diverse populations. With an emphasis on cultural sensitivity to palliative care, both the immediate physical concerns of patients are met and their emotional and psychological concerns as well, becoming a more comprehensive care philosophy. The outcome is the best, patient-tailored pain management strategies and improved patient satisfaction in the realm of chronic pain and palliative care (Jeff et al., 2025; Barnosky et al., 2025).

Test Your Knowledge

1. Why is patient autonomy important in palliative care decisions?
2. How does informed consent guide ethical practice in palliative care?

SUMMARY

The study of chronic pain in the palliative medicine setting demonstrates the major impact that individualized pain treatment regimens can have on patient quality of life. The creation of greater research, particularly the efforts brought together in comprehensive bibliographies on pain management, emphasizes the importance of a multidisciplinary approach. This methodology not only facilitates an improved understanding of pain mechanisms but also facilitates the development of targeted interventions. The meta-analysis by the University of Sheffield research team proves that an informed approach can bring about remarkable improvements in patient outcomes, thereby substantiating the hypothesis that effective pain relief is crucial in the enhancement of the overall experience of recipients of palliative care. The findings of these bibliographies call for continuous dedication to study and learning on approaches to pain management, affirming their position in guaranteeing proper treatment of chronic pain. The findings of current research, such as the trial of combination analgesics in cancer pain, also verify the tangible benefits of changing treatment strategies in palliative care. The use of extended-release oxycodone/naloxone combined with pregabalin is one of the newer strategies that can achieve significant pain relief and maximize patient satisfaction. The documented reduction in average pain severity, along with better quality-of-life measures, emphasizes the critical importance of physicians adopting evidence-based practice for treating chronic pain. As health care systems continue to evolve, the combination of these approaches will not only establish palliative care models but also improve patient experience, showcasing the interlacing of effective pain management and integrative care. Briefly, chronic pain management in palliative care is a multi-dimensional approach centered on patient outcomes and making use of a rich tapestry of clinical literature. The combination of traditional approaches with the development of novel treatments could lead to progress in individual and societal experiences of care. The need to establish comprehensive bibliographies of effective practice cannot be overstated because they constitute the single most valuable learning resource for the healthcare community. Lastly, maximizing pain experience for patients not only fulfils a fundamental ethical obligation but also maximizes the worldwide impact of palliative care. Such a strategy demands ongoing study and activism that uphold the principles of empathy and understanding in facing the complexities of chronic pain and improving the quality of life of the afflicted.

The complexity of managing chronic pain in palliative care necessitates a complex comprehension of patient requirements and treatment dynamics. A wide range of proactive intervention techniques, ranging from extensive primary care models, can substantially enhance functional outcomes in activity of daily living among older vulnerable adults suffering from chronic pain. One study highlighted that, at two-year follow-up, patients who had been actively cared for showed less decrease in functioning capacity compared to patients who received standard care protocols despite a lack of substantial differences in pain level. This suggests that while continued control of pain remains paramount, maintenance and enhancement of general functioning must also be crucial in the palliative care model, which points toward individually tailored interventions that prioritize both components of the patients' experience as being of utmost significance (Dong et al., 2024). Second, in addition to the challenges presented by cancer and other chronic diseases, the issues these diseases create highlight the need to make palliative care available everywhere across the world. Given the rise expected in Africa's cancer incidences, treatment access inequalities compromise patient survival and quality of life. There is a need to step up palliative care incorporation into health systems, particularly in resource-poor settings. Palliative care has proven to enhance patients' quality of life, providing evidence to support the assertion that pain management is a universal human right. Initiatives like the African Palliative Care Association advocate for the complete incorporation of palliative care practice into health policy at the national level, supporting evidence that such interventions are required to improve health outcomes (Rawlinson & Luyirika, 2014). In conclusion, education's role in increasing palliative care capability cannot be overemphasized. The ongoing educational activity, in this case through innovative digital media, is aimed at facilitating skill transfer within settings with limited resources as well as addressing training logistics challenges. For instance, adaptive education modules have been developed that address several aspects of symptom control, ethics, and patient communication, depending on context-dependent needs. Assisting local healthcare workers to undertake online and onsite training encourages practical implementation, hence the quality of patients' care in the clinical setting. Under the dynamic palliative care environment, maintaining a patient-centered approach in conjunction with this practice determines success in alleviating chronic pain and improving overall health outcomes (Rawlinson & Luyirika, 2014).

KEY TERMS FROM THIS CHAPTER

- Cannabis-based therapies
- Inequities
- Palliative care
- Psychological distress
- Public policy
- Chronic pain
- Numerous
- Patient-reported outcome measures (PROMs)
- Public health
- Symptom management

CRITICAL THINKING QUESTIONS

1. **What is the first-line pharmacological treatment for neuropathic pain?**
   a. NSAIDs
   b. Opioids
   c. Gabapentinoids
   d. Acetaminophen
2. **Which of the following is NOT a commonly used opioid for chronic pain management?**
   a. Morphine
   b. Fentanyl
   c. Ketorolac
   d. Oxycodone
3. **The World Health Organization (WHO) pain ladder recommends which first-line treatment for mild pain?**
   a. Strong opioids
   b. Non-opioid analgesics
   c. Adjuvant therapy
   d. Invasive procedures
4. **Which of the following is a key principle of palliative care?**
   a. Prolonging life at all costs
   b. Prevention and relief of suffering
   c. Focus exclusively on cancer patients
   d. Use of high-dose chemotherapy
5. **A patient with metastatic cancer experiences breakthrough pain. What is the best management?**
   a. Increase the dose of long-acting opioids
   b. Administer a short-acting opioid
   c. Add a non-opioid analgesic
   d. Switch to a different opioid

Short Answer Questions

1. What are the key differences between nociceptive pain and neuropathic pain, and how does this distinction influence treatment strategies?
2. Describe the principles of the World Health Organization (WHO) analgesic ladder and its application in managing chronic pain.
3. What are the primary indications for using adjuvant medications such as antidepressants or anticonvulsants in chronic pain management?
4. Discuss the role of bisphosphonates in managing bone pain associated with metastatic cancer.
5. What are the common side effects of long-term opioid therapy, and how can they be mitigated in patients with chronic pain?
6. Explain the concept of total pain in palliative care and how it guides the holistic management of patients.

Answer to Critical Thinking Questions

1. (c); 2. (c); 3. (c); 4.(b); 5. (b)

REFERENCES

1. Angeli, E., Zambelli, A., Corli, O., Bestetti, G., Landonio, S., Merli, S., Cheli, S., et al. (2024). High symptom burden in patients with advanced chronic or prolonged infectious diseases: Not only pain. *Cureus, 16*. https://www.semanticscholar.org/paper/2e8d0566b8c9a9295586c7a0aaf458e9366caf7d (accessed on 28th June 2025).
2. Schofield, P., Smith, P., and Aveyard, B. (2007) Developing annotated bibliographies : a tool for education, collaboration and research development. Journal of Orthopaedic Nursing. https://core.ac.uk/download/177011.pdf (accessed on 28th June 2025).
3. Robinson, L., Hughes, J., Daley, S., Keady, J., Ballard, C., & Volicer, L. (2005). End-of-life care and dementia. Reviews in Clinical Gerontology, 15(2), 135–148. doi:10.1017/S0959259806001833(accessed on 28th June 2025).
4. Barnosky, V., Brown, M., Bagchi, S., Blain, R., Husejnovic, D., Johnson, S., & Mackworth-Praed, M. (2025). Underutilized treatments for patients with refractory cancer pain: A qualitative study assessing the use of intrathecal drug delivery devices in the United Kingdom compared to alternative treatments in cancer pain management. *Frontiers in Pain Research, 6*. https://www.semanticscholar.org/paper/bea517649497fa8b825e4047604d9f0cf7039c6d (accessed on 28th June 2025).
5. Barton, L., Nisan, C., Burleigh, C., & Fredericks, S. (2021). Case presentation of safe and effective use of medical cannabis in the elderly. *Nurse Practitioner Open Journal*. https://www.semanticscholar.org/paper/6dd56bbcc4f39d5169da8ff490b03ca2ff0bb5ae (accessed on 28th June 2025).
6. Kluger, B. M., Fox, S., Timmons, S., Katz, M., Galifianakis, N. B., Subramanian, I., Carter, J. H., Johnson, M. J., Richfield, E. W., Bekelman, D., Kutner, J. S., & Miyasaki, J. (2017). Palliative care and Parkinson's disease: Meeting summary and recommendations for clinical research. *Parkinsonism & related disorders, 37*, 19–26. https://doi.org/10.1016/j.parkreldis.2017.01.008(accessed on 28th June 2025).
7. Boland, J., Martin, J., Wells, A. U., & Ross, J. R. (2013). Palliative care for people with non-malignant lung disease: summary of current evidence and future direction. *Palliative medicine, 27*(9), 811–816. https://doi.org/10.1177/0269216313493467(accessed on 28th June 2025).
8. De Santis S, Borghesi C, Ricciardi S, et al. Analgesic effectiveness and tolerability of oral oxycodone/naloxone and pregabalin in patients with lung cancer and neuropathic pain: an observational analysis. *Onco Targets Ther*. 2016;9:4043-4052. Published 2016 Jul 4. doi:10.2147/OTT.S108144(accessed on 28th June 2025).
9. Ščiupokas, A., Brogiene, L., & Skorupskienė, D. (2019). Cancer Pain. From Conventional to Innovative Approaches for Pain Treatment.https://core.ac.uk/download/322441459.pdf (accessed on 28th June 2025).
10. Juba, K. M., Khadem, T. M., Hutchinson, D. J., & Brown, J. E. (2017). Methadone and Corrected QT Prolongation in Pain and Palliative Care Patients: A Case-Control Study. *Journal of palliative medicine, 20*(7), 722–728. https://doi.org/10.1089/jpm.2016.0411(accessed on 28th June 2025).

11. McCarthy, Joan; Donnelly, Mary; Dooley, Dolores; Campbell, Louise; Smith, David; O'Neill, Catherine; et al. (2010). The Complete Ethical Framework for End-of-Life Care. Royal College of Surgeons in Ireland. Report. https://doi.org/10.25419/rcsi.10779956.v2(accessed on 28th June 2025).

12. Begoña García-Navarro, Emilia Martins Teixeira da Costa, (2017). Intercultural mediation at the end of life: Different perceptions of the same process. Procedia - Social and Behavioral Sciences, https://core.ac.uk/download/186632139.pdf (accessed on 28th June 2025).

13. Chandra, R., Kumar, B. J., Taj, D. M., Devaki, K., Shekhar, N. R., Kommireddy, S., Chittipolu, A. K., et al. (2024). Effect of coping strategies on pain intensity in patients with rheumatoid arthritis. *Journal of Pharmacology and Pharmacotherapeutics, 15*, 277–283. https://www.semanticscholar.org/paper/384d3c7985edf7f15abd2d2c1023da20c11a13f0 (accessed on 28th June 2025).

14. Cho, J., Goldfeld, K. S., Grudzen, C. R., Schmucker, A., et al. (2019). Emergency Medicine Palliative Care Access (EMPallA): Protocol for a multicenter randomized controlled trial comparing the effectiveness of specialty outpatient versus nurse-led telephonic palliative care of older adults with advanced illness. https://core.ac.uk/download/213444890.pdf (accessed on 28th June 2025).

15. Inbadas H, Zaman S, Whitelaw A, Clark D. Palliative Care Declarations: Mapping a New Form of Intervention. *J Pain Symptom Manage*. 2016;52(3):e7-e15. doi:10.1016/j.jpainsymman.2016.05.009(accessed on 28th June 2025).

16. Krawczyk, M., Sawatzky, R., Schick-Makaroff, K., Stajduhar, K., Öhlen, J., Reimer-Kirkham, S., Mercedes Laforest, E., & Cohen, R. (2019). Micro-Meso-Macro Practice Tensions in Using Patient-Reported Outcome and Experience Measures in Hospital Palliative Care. *Qualitative health research, 29*(4), 510–521. https://doi.org/10.1177/1049732318761366(accessed on 28th June 2025).

17. Dong, H. J., Peolsson, A., & Johansson, M. M. (2024). Effects of proactive healthcare on pain, physical and activities of daily living functioning in vulnerable older adults with chronic pain: A pragmatic clinical trial with one- and two-year follow-up. *European Geriatric Medicine, 15*, 709–718. https://www.semanticscholar.org/paper/697b6aa4a273b9e17957c00d612681d2fff266af (accessed on 28th June 2025).

18. Dowell, D., Ragan, K., Jones, C. M., Baldwin, G., & Chou, R. (2022). CDC clinical practice guideline for prescribing opioids for pain—United States, 2022. *MMWR Recommendations and Reports, 71*, 1–95. https://doi.org/10.15585/mmwr.rr7103a1 (accessed on 28th June 2025).

19. Duncan, B., Natuhwera, G., Nassuuna, D., Katusabe, R., Kasozi, H., & Acuda, W. (2025). Serious adverse drug reactions to long-term oral liquid morphine in patients with chronic pain: A cross-sectional survey in palliative care. *Journal of Pain Research, 18*, 2361–2371. https://www.semanticscholar.org/paper/2b1c6df9cb1a16a54e431285615a2f2105fe0c7d (accessed on 28th June 2025).

20. Efua, S. S. (2024). Perineal lacerations and postpartum well-being: Exploring mental health and chronic pain. *World Journal of Advanced Research and Reviews*. https://www.semanticscholar.org/paper/f296f18bb7b16aac170a1df0c147d6c5de188a2d (accessed on 28th June 2025).

21. Fallon, M., Giusti, R., Aielli, F., Hoskin, P., Rolke, R., Sharma, M., & Ripamonti, C. (2018). Management of cancer pain in adult patients: ESMO Clinical Practice Guidelines. *Annals of*

Oncology, 29, iv166–iv191. https://doi.org/10.1093/annonc/mdy152 (accessed on 28th June 2025).

22. Roat, C. Fernandez, A., & Kinderman, A. (2011). Interpreting in palliative care: A continuing education workshop. https://core.ac.uk/download/71358555.pdf (accessed on 28th June 2025).
23. Gold, M. (2018). An introduction to the Biennial Review of Pain. *Pain*. https://www.semanticscholar.org/paper/50c2ee9cf0b3ed85d21b6a77ac31abbacf9996ca (accessed on 28th June 2025).
24. Gonçalves, B., Lusher, J., Cund, A., Sime, C., & Harkess-Murphy, E. (2025). Understanding the psychosocial burden of living with advanced COPD in context of palliative care: A mixed methods study. *Journal of Health Psychology*. https://www.semanticscholar.org/paper/169338ad523520c50c0e1f206a0d1b1d993e95a7 (accessed on 28th June 2025).
25. Green, A., Green, M., Jerzmanowska, N., Lobb, C., et al. (2018). 'Death is difficult in any language': A qualitative study of palliative care professionals' experiences when providing end-of-life care to patients from culturally and linguistically diverse backgrounds. https://core.ac.uk/download/213607752.pdf (accessed on 28th June 2025).
26. Guziak, M., Szot, O., Bastrzyk, Z., & Sobocki, B. (2024). Pain management apps in palliative care: Landscape, challenges & possibilities. *Progress in Palliative Care, 33*, 20–23. https://www.semanticscholar.org/paper/d5a6d13c5838e1d19533e101912427ed7955efe6 (accessed on 28th June 2025).
27. Ibrahim, A. M., Abdel-Aziz, H., Zaghamir, D. E. F., Elneblawi, N., Elhoty, M. A. E. E., Sweelam, R. K. M., Mohamed, H. A. O., et al. (2025). Ethics and moral empathy in end-of-life palliative care. *Palliative and Supportive Care, 23*. https://www.semanticscholar.org/paper/9e267d46a544012ebdf969b0dfa4c53ee82c0a47 (accessed on 28th June 2025).
28. Inbadas, H. (2016). History, culture and traditions: The silent spaces in the study of spirituality at the end of life. https://core.ac.uk/download/42371436.pdf (accessed on 28th June 2025).
29. Ingle, P., Lian, W. K., Ting, S. J., Ngui, Y. U., Chong, C. W., Teoh, H. Q., & Hatware, K. (2025). Current developments in palliative care for patients with lung cancer. *Current Cancer Therapy Reviews*. https://www.semanticscholar.org/paper/8530046e0bcf7e3a4c6d9fa06e9d9cce370e4aea (accessed on 28th June 2025).
30. Jennings, B., D., C., Baily, M. A., & Ryndes, T. (2003). Access to hospice care: Expanding boundaries, overcoming barriers. https://core.ac.uk/download/71364924.pdf (accessed on 28th June 2025).
31. Kapke, T. L., Nehls, S., LiaBraaten, B. M., Zhang, J., Yan, K., Weisman, S., & Hainsworth, K. (2025). Pain and mental health variables for youth with chronic pain: The role of caregiver stress, pain, and resilience. *Families, Systems & Health: The Journal of Collaborative Family Healthcare*. https://www.semanticscholar.org/paper/1d7571c65fee0b0915ee12e41409813a4193708e (accessed on 28th June 2025).
32. Kim, M., Park, S. K., Kim, W. M., Kim, E., Kim, H., Park, J. M., Choi, S. S., et al. (2024). Updated guidelines for prescribing opioids to treat patients with chronic non-cancer pain in Korea: Developed by Committee on Hospice and Palliative Care of the Korean Pain Society. *The Korean Journal of Pain, 37*, 119–131. https://www.semanticscholar.org/paper/acc0d280d31a26c45ebcc38b1caf76faf788e1ed (accessed on 28th June 2025).

33. Lyon, A. R., López-Fernández, T., Couch, L. S., Asteggiano, R., Aznar, M. C., Bergler-Klein, J., Boriani, G., et al. (2022). 2022 ESC guidelines on cardio-oncology developed in collaboration with the European Hematology Association (EHA), the European Society for Therapeutic Radiology and Oncology (ESTRO) and the International Cardio-Oncology Society (IC-OS). *European Heart Journal, 43*, 4229–4361. https://doi.org/10.1093/eurheartj/ehac244 (accessed on 28th June 2025).

34. Majerić Kogler, V., Lončarić Katušin, M., & Kogler, J. (2023). Evidence-based strategies for multimodal postoperative pain management. *Acta Clinica Croatia, 62*, 107–114. https://www.semanticscholar.org/paper/c5406e0d6b6dced2b6f7abb452f038d1f56c3acc (accessed on 28th June 2025).

35. McCaffrey, N., Flint, T., Kaambwa, B., Fazekas, B., Rowett, D., Currow, D., Hardy, J., et al. (2018). Economic evaluation of the randomized, double-blind, placebo-controlled study of subcutaneous ketamine in the management of chronic cancer pain. *Palliative Medicine, 33*, 74–81. https://www.semanticscholar.org/paper/a04b3d1431931336e566059f370c0c2d51c9f97a (accessed on 28th June 2025).

36. Mendez Araque, S. J., Nguyen, L. T., & Nadal, C. N. (2024). Outcomes of psychotherapy for co-morbid pain and substance use disorders: A review of the literature. *Journal of Pain & Palliative Care Pharmacotherapy, 38*, 264–280. https://www.semanticscholar.org/paper/29e8aaa7a6fb5b4bd1158d4c1c583b5a1de2c91d (accessed on 28th June 2025).

37. Nehme, M., Braillard, O., Alcoba, G., Aebischer Perone, S., Courvoisier, D. S., Chappuis, F., & Guessous, I. (2020). COVID-19 symptoms: Longitudinal evolution and persistence in outpatient settings. *Annals of Internal Medicine, 174*, 723–725. https://doi.org/10.7326/m20-5926 (accessed on 28th June 2025).

38. O'Boyle, C., & McCarthy, S. (2010). Family views of end-of-life care in acute and community hospitals. https://core.ac.uk/download/75777805.pdf (accessed on 28th June 2025).

39. Park, S. J., Park, Y., Han, M., Kim, S. H., Hwang, I. C., Woo, G., Lee, Y. J., et al. (2024). Validity and reliability of the Integrated Palliative Care Outcome Scale (IPOS) in Korea: A multicenter study of terminally ill cancer patients. *BMC Palliative Care, 23*. https://www.semanticscholar.org/paper/c8b273e3e83a15ed4903000eb2ad57b055883a00 (accessed on 28th June 2025).

40. Price, J., Rushton, A., Ives, N., Jolly, K., Parmar, P., & Greaves, C. (2025). Co-designed neck exercise (EPIC-Neck) vs usual exercise care for people with chronic non-specific neck pain: Protocol for a randomised feasibility study with process evaluation. *Pilot and Feasibility Studies, 11*. https://www.semanticscholar.org/paper/db1d905863e68d1e83fa8e22d753fde34394b4ac (accessed on 28th June 2025).

41. Rajadurai, J. W., Likhit, C. S., Kumar, S., & Purushothaman, K. (2025). Integrating palliative care principles in orthopedic management of end-stage musculoskeletal conditions: A path towards holistic patient-centered care. *International Journal of Science and Research Archive*. https://www.semanticscholar.org/paper/b860e14ccaf139889da3b7b8a34e747f034e4677 (accessed on 28th June 2025).

42. Rawlinson, F., & Luyirika, E. (2014). Collaboration across continents to produce e-learning for palliative care education in Sub Saharan Africa. *Ecancermedicalscience, 8*, ed36. https://doi.org/10.3332/ecancer.2014.ed36 (accessed on 28th June 2025).

43. Rogal, S. S., Hansen, L., Patel, A., Ufere, N. N., Verma, M., Woodrell, C. D., & Kanwal, F. (2022).

AASLD practice guidance: Palliative care and symptom-based management in decompensated cirrhosis. *Hepatology, 76*, 819–853. https://doi.org/10.1002/hep.32378 (accessed on 28th June 2025).

44. Roldan, C. J., Rowland, J. W., & Ye, A. L. (2024). Haloperidol for pain management: A narrative review. *Pharmaceuticals, 17*. https://www.semanticscholar.org/paper/4473627703fbc0d54bd1e0d1f843a1a4ee856e0e (accessed on 28th June 2025).

45. Department of Anesthesia. University of Iowa. Spring 2011. https://core.ac.uk/download/18608347.pdf

46. Shah, P., Eltaher, B., Mahmoud, A., & Herman, A. (2024). Association of palliative care involvement and infectious complications in hospitalized multiple myeloma patients–National inpatient database study. *Blood*. https://www.semanticscholar.org/paper/8efc7d9f1391798e803f80050b9b6983bc32a741 (accessed on 28th June 2025).

47. Shevcova, V. I., Pashkova, A. A., Kolpacheva, M. G., & Salamatova, V. N. (2024). Palliative care for chronic heart failure: Non-pharmacological methods of relieving the main symptoms. *Meditsinskiy Soviet = Medical Council*. https://www.semanticscholar.org/paper/855ea3b62a0755e588dcb2b36b0454a0d2c247bb (accessed on 28th June 2025).

48. Sushma, M. N. (2024). IJCM_200A: Symptom burden profile of individuals facing chronic life-limiting illnesses and barriers to effective management of symptoms in palliative care–Grounded theory qualitative study. *Indian Journal of Community Medicine, 49*, S58. https://www.semanticscholar.org/paper/2a36dd9593705a2e2eb09510783854d05a0ecaf6 (accessed on 28th June 2025).

49. Tikkanen, A. U., Buxton, K., Ullrich, C., Stone, S., & Nimec, D. (2019). The palliative use of intrathecal baclofen in Niemann-Pick disease type C. *Pediatrics, 144*. https://www.semanticscholar.org/paper/18ec8206a7d4fdc26caf644eca7682dc77858c65 (accessed on 28th June 2025).

50. Vahanian, A., Beyersdorf, F., Praz, F., Milojevic, M., Baldus, S., Bauersachs, J., Capodanno, D., et al. (2021). 2021 ESC/EACTS guidelines for the management of valvular heart disease. *European Heart Journal, 43*, 561–632. https://doi.org/10.1093/eurheartj/ehab395 (accessed on 28th June 2025).

51. Yan, C., Liu, H. R., Kong, Q., Gan, J. Y., Liu, K., Yao, W. G., & Yao, X. M. (2024). Effect of acupuncture intervention on chronic musculoskeletal pain in hemodialysis-dependent kidney failure patients: Study protocol for a randomized controlled clinical trial. *Journal of Pain Research, 17*, 4289–4300. https://www.semanticscholar.org/paper/b2f903ed62bd587d2ee00a3488b2008e7ab3aa16 (accessed on 28th June 2025).

RECENT ADVANCES AND EVIDENCE-BASED ANESTHESIA

12

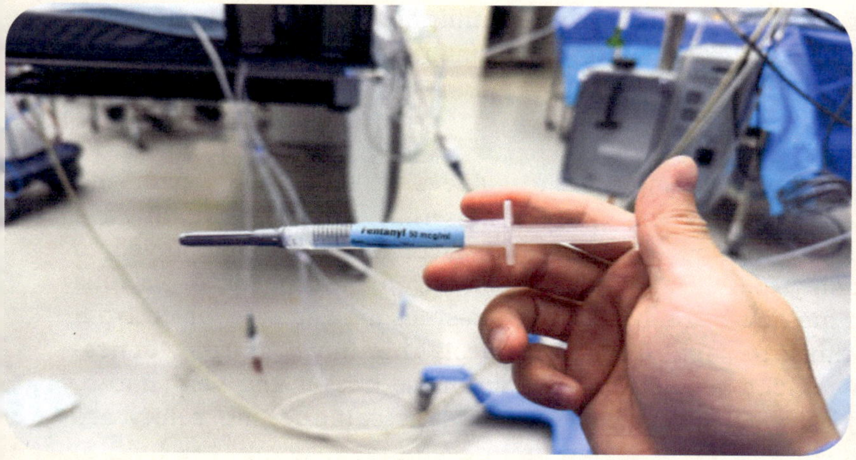

LEARNING OBJECTIVES

After studying this chapter, you will be able to:

1. Discuss the historical context of anesthesia
2. Focus on pharmacological innovations
3. Explain the technological advancements
4. Know evidence-based guidelines
5. Evaluate patient safety and quality improvement
6. Learn about future directions in anesthesia

Introduction

In the modern era of medicine, anesthesia also has an important role to play, providing access to a wide variety of surgical interventions while also maintaining patient safety and comfort. Recent advances in anesthetic strategies, drugs, and monitoring technology have immensely optimized the utility of anesthesia, besides minimizing complications. Progress has been primarily propelled by evidence-based policies putting high value on empirical evidence and clinical practice. As we delve into recent advances, it is essential to recognize the impactful role of anesthesia on operating outcomes and recovery in patients. The importance of personalized anesthetic care plans according to the individual needs of patients has become a spotlight in contemporary anesthesia practice, with potential directions to optimize perioperative care. Anesthesia evolution is marked by an incessant drift away from traditional practices towards new, evidence-driven practices. New technology and research methods enable practitioners to make decisions based on the latest findings and recommendations. For instance, multimodal analgesia studies emphasize the need to use more than one analgesic method in pain relief and avoid opioid dependence. These practices not only counteract short-term postoperative pain but also set the foundation for improved long-term results. Through the incorporation of results from high-quality clinical trials, anesthetists are able to enhance techniques more suited to the nuances of patient profiles so that the delivery of both effective and safe anesthesia is realized. Of equal concern to this debate is the role of ongoing education and training for anesthesia professionals in order to facilitate the integration of new developments into practice. Continuous professional education in anesthesia provides for the implementation of new findings to improve patient care. Further, inter-professional practice among practitioners remains essential in maintaining anesthesia practice to guarantee an interdisciplinary approach to patient management. Given the history of recent progress and evidence-based use of anesthesia, it is very clear that a robust platform supporting research as well as education is important. Such a commitment not only teaches best practices but also develops perioperative patient care safety and quality culture.

Definition of Anesthesia

Anesthesia can be defined as a medical method employed to achieve insensibility to pain and sensation while undergoing surgery, thereby allowing interventions that otherwise would have been extremely painful or distressful. It encompasses a wide array of techniques employed to cause reversible loss of awareness, analgesia, or paralysis, depending on the needs of various medical procedures. With advances in medicine, the practice of anesthesia has also evolved from the rudimentary methods of ancient times to sophisticated protocols that incorporate evidence-based practices to achieve maximum patient benefit. This evolution addresses the very nature of anesthesia's role in contemporary surgical practice, where patient comfort and safety are paramount, and addresses the continued need for research and development within the field to address the needs of diverse populations of patients and the complexity of surgery. Anesthesia's definition also transcends pain management alone; it is a multifaceted system for preserving a patient's physiological status during surgery. Improvements in anesthesia over recent years have led to enhanced monitoring techniques and anesthetic agents with better safety profiles, as well as improved recovery from surgery after the operation. Anesthesiologists today employ evidence-based practice regularly considering patients' medical status, the type of surgery, and potential complications. For instance, the addition of local anesthesia techniques has revolutionized pain control methods to make more directed efforts with reduced side effects but enhanced analgesia. Greater consciousness and application of customized anesthesia methods form the basis of the need for ongoing education and adaptation in the specialty, underlining the need for evidence-based medicine to enhance standards and techniques of anesthesia. Furthermore, an anesthetic definition must also account for global disparities in access to these basic services.

While advances in anesthesia have made safety and efficacy much greater in developed economies, low- and middle-income countries often face substantial hurdles to implementing these processes. Disease burdens amenable to access to effective neurosurgery and anesthesia remain under a great deal of undertreatment in much of the world, as Fezeu et al. (2018) find. In addition, the loads of surgical evaluation, particularly in the developing world, call for the need for robust structures that facilitate surgical research and innovation, as described in Ergina et al. (2009). In order to tackle these inequalities, not only is more technology needed, but also efforts aligned towards understanding local issues and developing context-based solutions for anesthetic practice. This global action on the definition of anesthesia fortifies the premise that safe and effective care should be accessible to patients where they reside, regardless of location (Figure 12.1).

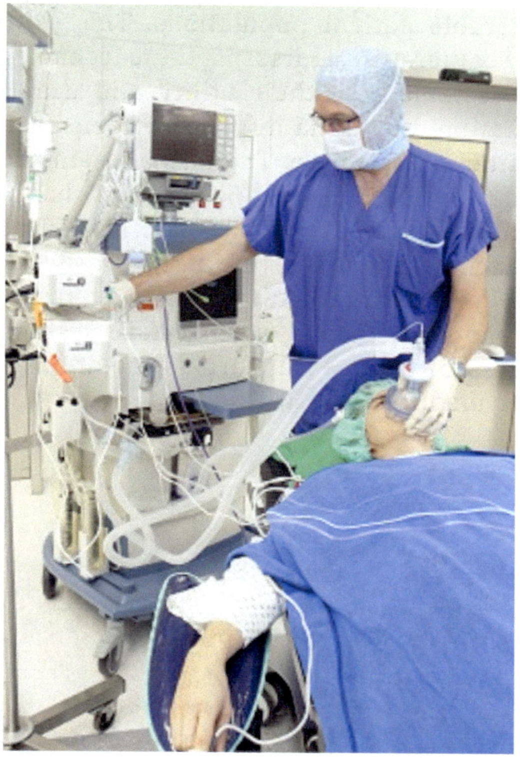

Figure 12.1. Anesthesia can be defined as a medical practice.

Source: https://study.com/cimages/multimages/16/aa61e4fb-a134-4634-b0d0-db11716eeced_anes4243.jpg.

Importance of Evidence-Based Practice

Evidence-based practice (EBP) is core to the enhancement of anesthesia interventions' safety and efficacy, particularly with the ever-evolving research work continuing to redefine the field. Through critically evaluating evidence from studies and integrating clinical experience, EBP prepares anesthesiologists to make informed decisions based on the best evidence available. This is particularly pertinent in the environment of surgical procedures, where complexity is the rule. As noted, "surgical evaluation is especially demanding because many of these challenges intersect," highlighting the necessity of grounding anesthetic practice in solid research. The imperative for stringent evidence-based recommendations ensures anesthetic choices not only reflect current knowledge but also ensure the patient's safety, finally leading to improved outcomes. By facilitating continuous education and examination of new techniques and medications, EBP positions professionals at the forefront of anesthesiology, poised to address evolving clinical circumstances efficiently. Furthermore, adopting EBP as a component of practice in anesthesia allows for a culture of accountability and quality in healthcare institutions. Informed decision-making, in the meantime, not only relies on scientific evidence but also entails patient values and choices, bridging clinical experience to individualized care. The more recent development of making evidence-based standards, as witnessed in many outpatient procedures, is a focus on optimizing patient safety without unnecessarily burdening providers. Procedure standards, including anesthesia standards, must be written through consensus by providers who have direct contact with the procedures so that relevant expertise shapes best practices. Such collaborative efforts emphasize the importance of EBP, as they lead to enhanced techniques in anesthesia that enhance not only effectiveness but also the general well-being of patients undergoing surgery. Moreover, overcoming obstacles to implementing evidence into clinical practice is essential in fostering anesthesia methodologies. Obstacles continue to emerge due to limited access to quality research, as well as political issues surrounding some procedures, particularly contentious ones like abortion care. It is critical to know that, as is true with the routine development process for other outpatient procedures, anesthesia guidelines need to be based on sound scientific research in order to efficiently avoid risks. In situations when definitive studies are lacking, clinicians must resort to their experience and established best practice based on collegial discussion and existing literature. The consideration that there is a reliance on clinical practice rather than expressed evidence, as seen with the challenge in developing facility standards for healthcare, emphasizes that while EBP is fundamental, expert practitioner experience and knowledge cannot be substituted in developing anesthesia protocol where patient safety and quality outcome are prioritized (Ergina et al., 2009; Berglas & Roberts, 2018).

Overview of Recent Advances

Recent innovations in anesthetics have significantly altered perioperative care by emphasizing a robust emphasis on evidence-based practice. Improved innovations in multimodal analgesia have developed means for clinicians to integrate analgesic modalities and agents to enhance comfort and maximize opioid-sparing strategies. This method not only minimizes the risk of opioid-related complications but also allows for faster recovery and higher overall patient satisfaction. Further, the use of enhanced recovery after surgery (ERAS) protocols has proven to be beneficial, allowing for a scientific attitude towards perioperative care that is patient-centered and outcome-based. Through the implementation of such protocols, patients benefit from reduced pain, shorter hospital stays, and reduced postoperative complications, reflecting a shift from the paradigm to a more inclusive and holistic perspective of care in surgery. Technological advancements have also played an important role in the development of anesthetic practice. The addition of sophisticated monitoring devices and algorithms has led to the capacity to better assess the condition of patients undergoing procedures. Technological innovations enable real-time examination of data so that anesthesiologists can make decisions based on evolving patient needs. The application of point-of-care ultrasound (POCUS) is a prime example of this direction, augmenting the ability to perform regional anesthesia in a better way. With these technologies being embraced by anesthesiologists, the potential of improved outcomes becomes a reality, particularly for vulnerable patient populations. The growing body of literature addressing these technologies is a testament to their utility and usability, facilitating the arena in which evidence-based anesthesia can thrive. The formal examination of anesthesia guidelines and standards has been in the spotlight during the past few decades, advancing the course of the discipline. Breaking away from traditional patterns of practice, current methods allow for a more systematic process of facility standard formulation from other medical specialties.

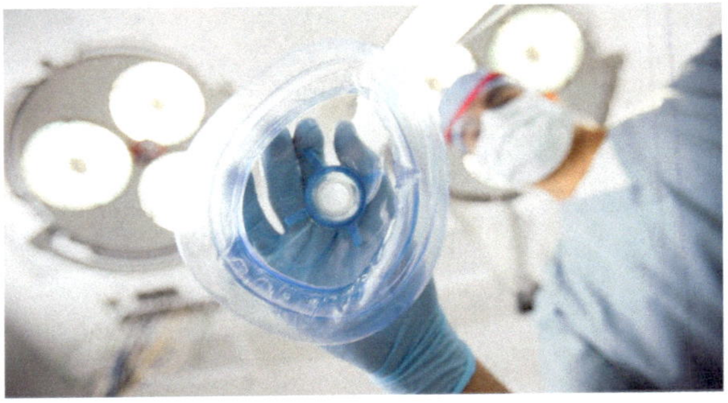

Figure 12.2. Recent advances in anesthesia.

Source: https://cdn.theatlantic.com/thumbor/K6xofLtaGoVjkIEaTcAFk8Wx6L4=/0x297:5616x3456/960x540/media/img/mt/2017/12/GettyImages_85501281/original.jpg.

By providing access to the collective knowledge of clinicians who are engaged in optimizing best practices through methods applied in outpatient processes, the anesthetic community can benefit. This process emphasizes a balance in guaranteeing patient safety while providing an effective care setting. However, there are still challenges concerning the inadequacy of research as well as practice differences in relation to standards across regions.

Consequently, as the practice of anesthesia evolves and transforms over time, more focus on collaborative approaches and evidence-based models must underpin consistency and quality in care for the patient, backed by evidence from recent research undertaken in this field (Berglas & Roberts, 2018; Fezeu et al., 2018) (Figure 12.2).

12.1. Historical Context of Anesthesia

Learning Outcome

1. Evolution of anesthetic techniques
2. Milestones in anesthesia research
3. Impact of historical advances on current practices

The history of anesthesia has moved dramatically since then, a revolution in the very nature of surgical medicine. Surgery was initially performed with no pain reduction whatsoever, which led to horrific pain and limited the kinds of surgery that could be performed. The early 19th century witnessed a gigantic revolution with the introduction of ether and chloroform, as these provided a means to guide patients to unconsciousness and dampen the sensation of pain in surgery. Pioneers like Crawford Long, who first employed ether in 1842, and James Simpson, who advocated for chloroform in obstetrics, played a key role in showing the promise of anesthetic drugs. This advancement not only made more widespread and invasive procedures possible but also revolutionized the patient experience, placing significant importance on humane treatment during medical procedures. With advancements in anesthesia skills, a more systematic methodology became the norm, placing greater importance on safety and efficacy. The late 19th and early 20th centuries saw significant technological advancements, including the development of inhalational anesthetics and the introduction of anesthetic machines, making the administration of these agents more efficient and standardized. The introduction of local anesthesia, pioneered by the use of novocaine in dentistry, offered an alternative to general anesthesia, enabling practitioners to perform procedures with reduced systemic effects. The historical development of anesthesia is closely associated with advancing knowledge regarding pharmacology and the body's reactions, which served as the basis for evidence-based practices that inform present-day anesthesia administration. Recent progress in the specialty reflects a broader understanding of the importance of multimodal analgesia as a cornerstone of contemporary anesthetic care. This approach, employing a combination of analgesic medications to target the various pathways of pain, is intended to minimize opioid addiction while maximizing pain control and minimizing side effects. According to recent literature, such treatments employing this integrated method must be tailored to the specific surgical case as well as the individual needs of the patient (Schwenk & Mariano, 2018). Besides, ongoing research into mechanisms of consciousness and anesthetic action draws on previous success, integrating older and more recent data to refine clinical methods. Neuroimaging techniques, for instance, have become essential in quantifying levels of consciousness in patients and remain vital in elucidating the brain's response to anesthetics (Boly & Seth, 2012).

12.1.1. Evolution of Anesthetic Techniques

The history of anesthetic practice has been marked by a dramatic movement towards evidence-based practice, ensuring patient safety and better outcomes. Traditionally, anesthetic delivery was hazardous, dependent on primitive methods and the primitive knowledge of pharmacological agents. But advances in drug development, monitoring equipment, and education have made anesthesia a more predictable and controlled specialty. The advent of regional anesthetics, in combination with general anesthesia, has permitted site-specific pain control techniques that reduce systemic impact and increase recovery times. These advances are themselves part of a greater development toward increased understanding of the need for individualized anesthesia protocols based on patient and procedural variables, opening the way for the multimodal analgesia techniques that are now commonplace practice. Against the background of recent progress, the incorporation of dexmedetomidine into anesthetic protocols is the epitome of the shift towards opioid-sparing strategies. Recent data have demonstrated the effectiveness of dexmedetomidine in blunting surgical stress responses, with consequent improved recovery profiles and opioid decreases. An influential project evaluated the educational initiatives aimed at anesthesia practitioners regarding the advantages of this drug before induction, encouraging its implementation in clinical settings. With focused education interventions, the knowledge and practice of dexmedetomidine were notably increased among the practitioners, reflecting a cultural change in anesthesia toward embracing innovations based on solid evidence. Through the use of such innovation, anesthesia professionals are more able to provide efficient and safe care, which ultimately benefits the patient experience. In addition, as the field of anesthesiology advances, focus on postoperative complications, including nausea and vomiting, is crucial. According to the protocols that were adopted for the prevention of postoperative nausea and vomiting, outpatients undergoing surgery are content since such implantation was evidence-based. According to this fact, this contributes to the benefit of patient recovery since evidence-based guidance attributed to the minimization of postoperative complications results in rapid recovery. The continuous development of anesthetic methods demonstrates a universal focus on incorporating scientific data into practice to enhance patient outcomes and general safety. The development of anesthetic methods is thus a test of the dynamic nature of the discipline, consistently keeping up with new evidence and patient-centered care models such as those advocated through (Betts, 2015; Nilsson, 2024) (Figure 12.3).

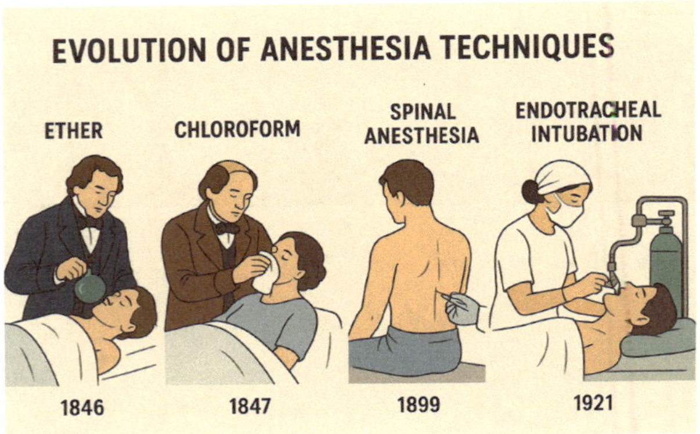

Figure 12.3. The evolution of anesthetic techniques.

Source: https://drmanjushah.in/wp-content/uploads/2025/05/ChatGPT-Image-May-4-2025-12_31_26-AM.png.

12.1.2. Milestones in Anesthesia Research

The history of research in anesthesia has witnessed many revolutionary milestones that have significantly impacted contemporary practice. One of the first breakthroughs occurred in the 19th century when ether and chloroform were discovered, transforming surgical procedures by making it possible for patients to be exposed to operations without experiencing pain. This discovery was a turning point, as it led to future developments in modern anesthetics and future scientific studies. Advances in the anesthetic field were fueled by research into the pharmacodynamics and pharmacokinetics of anesthetic agents. Such discoveries provided information regarding the action and process of various agents within the body, making anesthesia administration safer and more effective in various patient populations. These early achievements only serve to emphasize the importance of ongoing research in the evolution of anesthesia techniques and improving patient outcomes in the operating room. In the future, the development of regional anesthesia represented a defining milestone in the specialty with the advent of new modalities that were added to the arsenal of techniques available to anesthesiologists. The technique provides for selective blockade of chosen nerve pathways, thus providing effective pain relief with fewer systemic side effects. Methods such as spinal and epidural anesthesia became inseparable tools for clinical anesthesia practice, especially in obstetrics and pain management. Regional anesthesia development with ultrasonography also made it easier to perform blocks and ensured tighter accuracy of the needle placement. This shift to more evidence-based techniques continues to involve the ongoing action between research and practice in anesthesia as practitioners upgrade and upgrade their strategies with empirical data and technological developments. Recently, the hybridization of anesthesiology and molecular biology has unveiled the possibilities for thrilling developments in anesthesiology and pain control. This multidisciplinary field is unveiling research into the mechanisms of pain and how anesthetics can act on these mechanisms at the cellular level. The quest for new anesthetic medications, spurred by developing genetic knowledge and directed therapy, is beginning to offer increasingly customized approaches to patient care. Further, the emphasis on evidence-based practice within anesthesiology is allowing a culture of vigorous critique and quality improvement in the field. As scientists continue to understand more about the intricacies of anesthesia and its impact on human physiology, the future possibilities for advancements are promising for enhancing patient safety and optimizing clinical results in various surgical populations.

12.1.3. Impact of Historical Advances on Current Practices

The evolution of history in developments has had a significant influence on the development of anesthesia practices to form the basis of today's evidence-based practice. The use of several agents of analgesia to achieve optimal pain coverage with minimal opioids is one of the largest breakthroughs in multimodal analgesia. The opioid drugs dominated the plan of pain management for long periods and were succeeded by a myriad of complications arising from their use. But with appreciation for the reality that different pharmacological classes target unique pathways for pain modulation, clinicians can now individualize pain management regimens for their patients. This shift not only enhances perioperative patient comfort but also attempts to minimize opioid-related side effects, a valuable concern that has gained prominence in the last few years as opioid dependency has increased throughout the healthcare continuum (Schwenk & Mariano, 2018). The translation of historical advances into current practice has also been a component of the development of integrated analgesic protocols for different surgical procedures. These protocols are more of a checklist than a rigid recipe and reflect a less standardized, more individualized strategy for patient care that acknowledges variability. Through the use of multiple analgesic modalities—non-steroidal anti-inflammatory drugs, acetaminophen, and regional anesthetic techniques—anesthesiologists are better able to manage heterogeneity in postoperative pain management. This practice both illustrates compliance with evidence-based medicine and facilitates an integrative model of patient care, which emphasizes the importance of investigating and responding to each patient's unique needs. Historical data on the effectiveness and safety of these diverse analgesics form the basis for these modern practices, thus enhancing the quality of care provided during operation (Schwenk & Mariano, 2018). Despite these favorable developments in anesthesia care, concurrent problems such as shortages of drugs overshadow the advent of evidence-based practice. Balancing the requirement for multimodal analgesia against the reality that some essential drugs are absent when they are needed most complicates treatment plans. It is up to the anesthesiologists and pain medicine physicians not only to optimize the use of whatever resources exist but also to facilitate a safe supply of analgesic drugs at the local and national levels. Trends from the past that shape current practice underscore the need for adaptability in the face of such hardship in ensuring preservation of the legacy of effective pain control. By recognizing the complementarity of past progress and current challenges, medical professionals can set their sights on the future with a focus on patient-centered care in the evolving practice of anesthesia (Schwenk & Mariano, 2018).

Test Your Knowledge

1. Who is credited with demonstrating the first successful use of surgical anesthesia?
2. How has anesthesia evolved from early techniques to modern practice?

12.2. Pharmacological Innovations

Learning Outcome

1. Development of new anesthetic agents
2. Advances in opioid-sparing techniques
3. Role of adjuvant medications in anesthesia

The anesthetic practice environment has been significantly enhanced by developments in the field of pharmacology that are aimed at improving patient outcomes and procedural effectiveness. Developments in recent years have resulted in novel anesthetic drugs with improved pharmacokinetic properties that facilitate more rapid onset and recovery of action. This is especially relevant in environments like outpatient surgery, where shorter recovery is desirable to both patients and the medical system. Additionally, the integration of technology, such as artificial intelligence, has been pivotal in the optimization of drug options and delivery, enabling anesthesiologists to personalize anesthetic regimens according to individual patients' needs. The technologies not only enhance safety profiles but also reduce patients' physical and emotional burdens, resulting in more effective healthcare consistent with evidence-based anesthesia practice. Moreover, the introduction of new adjuncts and modalities, e.g., multimodal analgesia, is also a great milestone in pharmacologic pain management during and after surgery. With the administration of multiple classes of drugs, anesthesiologists can target several pathways of pain to achieve better analgesia with a lesser intake of opioids.

This is particularly relevant given that there has been a constant opioid crisis, which necessitates the use of other safer alternatives to pain control. Empirical data in support of these multimodal strategies validate their applicability in modern anesthetic practice, as not only do they reduce unnecessary drug-related complications but also maximize patient recovery outcomes. Pharmacological innovations and techniques are thus the key to modifying anesthetic practices with regard to both efficacy and patient safety according to current evidence-based guidelines. Finally, ongoing research into the pharmacologic developments relevant to anesthesia is not just in terms of new drug development but redesigning already existing agents to maximize their properties. The newer local anesthetics with greater duration and reduced toxicity levels are being researched, which may revolutionize the management of postoperative pain. In addition, studies of adjunctive therapies such as dexmedetomidine and gabapentinoids augment traditional anesthetics, providing anesthesiologists with more individualized options. The move towards precision medicine, which will be fueled by a better understanding of how patients respond to anesthetics, will further accelerate these advancements. Thus, the continuous evolution of pharmacologic drugs is a milestone in anesthesia practice, and it reflects commitment to improving patient care through scientific inquiry and application (Stecca et al., 2023; Karalis, 2024) (Figure 12.4).

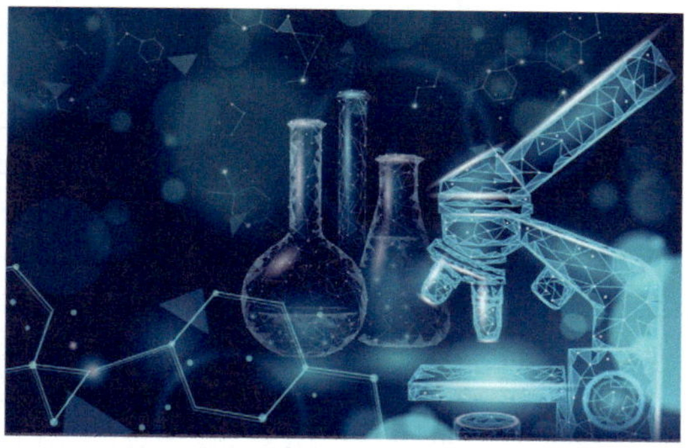

Figure 12.4. The landscape of anesthetic practice has been significantly enhanced through pharmacological innovations.

Source: https://media.licdn.com/dms/image/v2/C4D12AQHne1z4FwFpmA/article-cover_image-shrink_720_1280/article-cover_image-shrink_720_1280/0/1614849388421?e=2147483647&v=beta&t=K_W7rVPk5eNUFrZhfWbAWkG9SOIk1haBFx63cjLcCio.

12.2.1. Development of New Anesthetic Agents

The development of new anesthetic agents is a landmark achievement in the science of anesthesia, a demonstration of ongoing effort towards better surgery safety and patient recovery. Developments are aimed at overcoming limitations of traditional anesthetics, including side effects, time to induce, and action duration. Recent advances have witnessed the creation of agents with faster induction and recovery times, thereby enabling outpatient procedures and reduced hospital stays. For instance, newer intravenous and inhalational anesthetics have been impressive in improving hemodynamic stability and reducing postoperative nausea, long problematic for patients. Moreover, these drugs are increasingly being formulated with consideration of their pharmacokinetics and pharmacodynamics that can be designed to suit patient-specific needs, varying anesthetic plans for optimal efficacy and safety. Volatile anesthetics are, in particular, becoming increasingly popular for their unexpected cardioprotective properties, which may have a profound impact on perioperative care. Studies have demonstrated that these agents can induce a protective state known as anesthetic-induced preconditioning (APC) that protects the myocardium from damage during surgery, especially among at-risk cardiology patients. Substantial experimental evidence demonstrates that volatile anesthetics enhance recovery from cardiac ischemia and reduce myocardial infarct size, supporting their use as therapeutic drugs as opposed to mere sedatives and analgesics (Ludwig et al., 2003). Such new insight opens the door to the use of these anesthetics in cardiac surgery, with the hope of lowering morbidity and mortality that accompany perioperative myocardial ischemia. This paradigm change emphasizes the need for continued investigation of anesthetics not just as sedatives but also as central components of total surgical management strategies. In addition to the advancement of volatile anesthetics, advancement in neuromonitoring techniques in surgery, particularly in sophisticated procedures such as endoscopic, endonasal access to the skull base, has been groundbreaking. Recent literature favors the efficacy of multimodal intraoperative neurophysiological monitoring, in which a mix of test procedures is used to safeguard sensitive neurological structures. Application of electroencephalography, somatosensory evoked potentials, and motor evoked potentials improves the practice through the potential of real-time assessment of nervous system integrity in sensitive operations (Singh et al., 2016). This comprehensive monitoring plan enhances operative safety as well as enables aggressive therapy of skull base tumors, ultimately leading to improved outcomes. With ongoing anesthetic innovation embracing sophisticated monitoring techniques, the synergy between them reflects the evolution of anesthesia toward a more precise and patient-centered discipline.

12.2.2. Advances in Opioid-Sparing Techniques

The development of opioid-sparing techniques in clinical practice is an outstanding evolution of anesthetic care strategies that attempt to offset the opioid epidemic without sacrificing the control of pain. Evidence-based enhanced recovery after surgery (ERAS) guidelines are a prime example of this methodology, using multimodal analgesia to minimize postoperative use of opioids. This holds particular significance in orthopedic surgery, where opioid dependence was a hallmark of pain control. Through combining non-opioid analgesics, local anesthetics, and adjunct treatments, the recovery of patients and complications resulting from opioids can be optimized by surgeons. Specifically, ERAS protocols have produced excellent results in the surgery of lumbar fusion, decreasing the length of hospital stay and enhancing patient outcomes. Thus, the incorporation of these evidence-based treatments will help benefit healthcare systems as well as patients in terms of lowering the risks and costs involved with opioid use (Debono et al., 2021). Physical therapy has also been shown to be an important aspect of opioid-sparing interventions, particularly for the management of illnesses such as knee osteoarthritis. Research has shown that involvement in individually tailored physical therapy interventions results in reduced pain and functional improvement, with decreased opioid medication use. Supervised physical therapy and home exercise programs have proven effective in achieving better functional outcomes compared to medical management alone. For instance, clinical trials indicate that patients treated by individually tailored physical therapy demonstrate significant improvement in pain status and strength. This emphasizes the importance of patient management in a combined holistic approach, whereby opioid-sparing techniques are part of care plans that center on non-operative strategies, bound to lead to a change of paradigm in managing chronic pain syndromes (Michael, 2019). The role of new pharmacological agents and techniques in achieving success in pain relief without the risk of exacerbating opioid use cannot be overstated. Drugs such as regional anesthesia techniques, peripheral nerve blocks, and liposomal bupivacaine application have been questioned in terms of efficacy in delivering focused pain management. Regional anesthesia is particularly capable of yielding significant advantages with decreased systemic opioid requirements and accelerated recovery. Additionally, trial data in support of liposomal bupivacaine indicate that it can prolong analgesia and reduce postoperative opioid requirements. By embracing these evidence-based practices in clinical practice, anesthesiologists are able to advance patient care at large, supporting effective pain relief that is safety-focused and minimizes opioid dependence within contemporary surgical settings (Debono et al., 2021) (Figure 12.5).

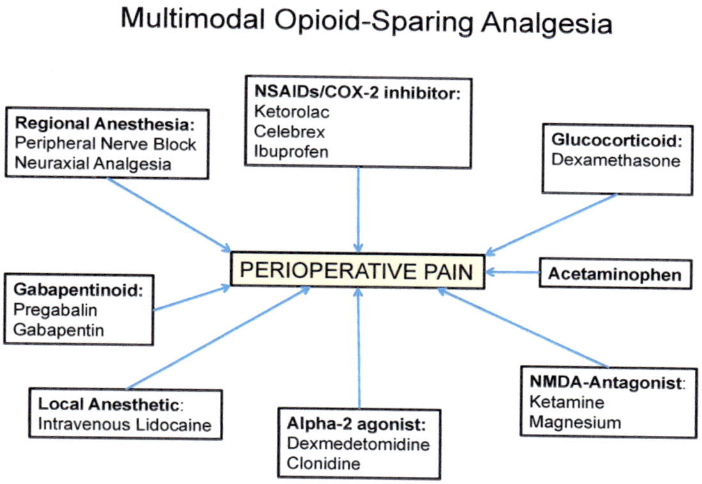

Figure 12.5. The emergence of opioid-sparing techniques.

Source: https://www.tandfonline.com/cms/asset/9d03b946-20d2-4847-8fc9-c59aa88ff1b9/ieop_a_1583743_f0001_oc.jpg.

12.2.3. Role of Adjuvant Medications in Anesthesia

Adjuvant medications play a vital role in anesthesia by amplifying the effect of primary anesthetic agents with a diminishment of side effects. A combination of drugs can have synergistic action, leading to improved patient outcomes, particularly sedation and pain relief. For instance, adjuvants such as non-steroidal anti-inflammatory drugs (NSAIDs), corticosteroids, and certain anticonvulsants have been employed to reduce required dosages of opioids, thereby reducing the risks associated with opioid therapy, such as respiratory depression and postoperative nausea. The systematic administration of these drugs not only optimizes intraoperative anesthesia but also optimizes postoperative recovery by favoring superior pain control and avoiding opioid-induced complications, ultimately culminating in patient satisfaction and comfort in the perioperative period. Of the promising adjuvant medications, dexmedetomidine is exceptional due to its wide-ranging pharmacological effects. As a selective α2-adrenoceptor agonist, dexmedetomidine exhibits anxiolytic, analgesic, and sedative effects without the adverse respiratory effects of other sedatives. With this medication, changes between wakefulness and sedation are smoother and patients are more cooperative in postoperative assessment. Moreover, its extended duration of analgesia has been reported in varying surgical environments because it not only inhibits the incidence of postoperative pain but also reduces opioid usage. Its clinical applications across different settings emphasize the need for integrating emerging pharmacological advancements, particularly with the anesthetic setting being diversified in the wake of a multicultural patient population (Liu et al., 2021). When discussing the role of adjuvant drugs in anesthesia, there is a need to analyze the evolving setting of evidence-based practice. While a majority of the current research emphasizes the effectiveness of these adjuncts, research quality is typically unbalanced, and there is a need for more rigorous, large-scale trials. While there has been some progress made, such as research on varying administration modes and utility of dexmedetomidines in specific situations, many studies are being limited by sample size and issues of generalizability of findings. As emphasized in recent literature, bridging these gaps through high-quality research is imperative to maximize anesthetic protocols through emphasizing patient safety and comfort. Last but not least, to achieve the full potential of adjuvant medications, there is a continuous need to explore and innovate to remain updated with the challenges of individual patient needs (Harden et al., 2022).

Test Your Knowledge

1. What is the purpose of adjuvant medications in anesthesia?
2. Name one class of adjuvant drugs commonly used to enhance anesthetic effects.

12.3. Technological Advancements

Learning Outcome

1. Introduction of monitoring technologies
2. Use of simulation in anesthesia training
3. Impact of telemedicine on anesthesia practice

The integration of innovative technologies in anesthesia has greatly transformed clinical practice, both enhancing patient safety and procedure efficacy. One of the most impactful innovations is the application of ultrasound in regional anesthesia. Imaging technology allows anesthetists to visualize anatomical structures in real-time, facilitating the accuracy of needle placement and reducing complications. The use of ultrasound-guided regional anesthesia (UGRA) has revolutionized pain management procedures and improved the success rates of nerve blocks. Existing literature identifies that the incorporation of advanced imaging technologies in curriculum programs improves the competency of healthcare practitioners to perform intricate procedures, therefore highlighting the need for modern learning aids in the practice of anesthesiology (Jacobs et al., 2023). These advancements not only enhance procedural self-assurance in the practitioner but also enhance patient outcomes, a paradigm shift in the administration of anesthesia. Artificial intelligence (AI) is rapidly emerging as another pillar of technological advancement in anesthesiology, streamlining clinical processes and optimizing decision-making protocols. AI has been visionary in a number of medical areas, such as anesthesia, where it helps with image analysis in real-time and predictive modeling. For example, machine learning models trained on large sets of ultrasound images can assist anesthetists in the automatic identification and classification of anatomical structures with high precision. Software like ScanNav Anatomy PNB applies convolutional neural networks to superimpose instructive color marks upon ultrasound images, thus facilitating improved identification of important structures during UGRA. This not only enhances educational results for trainees but also the accuracy of expert professionals, ultimately leading to safer and more effective anesthetic interventions (Pennazio et al., 2022). As these AI-based technologies become more integrated into clinical practice, they are likely to change the educational environment of anesthesia. Furthermore, the introduction of new simulation technologies is remodeling educational approaches to anesthesia training. High-fidelity simulators allow students and residents to practice critical skills in a controlled environment where patient safety is never at risk and iterative learning is possible. The use of virtual reality (VR) technology for anesthesia education also become more popular, with immersive simulations that model real-life clinical scenarios. This not only enhances the competence of anesthetists but also encourages critical decision-making when under simulated stress conditions. By leveraging these technologies, schools can better prepare future anesthesia professionals to address complex clinical situations. The use of advanced imaging, AI technology, and simulation technologies is a forward-looking approach that emphasizes evidence-based practice in anesthesia for improved patient safety and quality of care (Jacobs et al., 2023) (Figure 12.6).

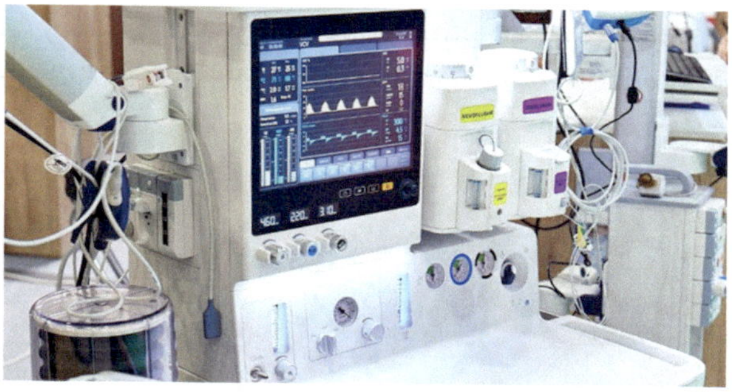

Figure 12.6. The integration of technological advancements in anesthesia.

Source: https://medicalbuyer.co.in/wp-content/uploads/2023/02/Anestatia.jpg.

12.3.1. Introduction of Monitoring Technologies

Inclusion of high-tech monitoring technologies in anesthesia has introduced an age of increased patient safety and surgical efficacy. With shifts in anesthesia practice, implementation of multimodal monitoring platforms allows continuous assessment of key functions and thus enhances real-time intraoperative decision-making. These technologies include electroencephalography (EEG), which provides data on the depth of anesthesia, and various somatosensory evoked potentials that monitor neurological integrity. Through the use of these advanced tools, anesthesiologists are better able to customize anesthetic depth and deal with complications that may arise, ultimately producing better patient outcomes. This insistence on utilizing leading-edge monitoring systems is part of a larger movement within the medical community toward data-based practices and evidence-based decision-making aimed primarily at ensuring that patient safety is paramount. Besides, the application of multimodal neuromonitoring in surgery, particularly that of critical neurological structures, has been extremely promising in intraoperative brain function detection and preservation. For instance, during performing endoscopic, endonasal skull base procedures, many neuro-monitoring tests have been shown to be feasible and safe, hence verifying their value in real-time studies. A number of modalities are employed, including free-running electromyography and transcranial electric motor evoked potentials, which together provide an overall impression of nervous system functional integrity. Multimodal examination has been shown to greatly improve the surgeon's ability to manage advanced procedures with greater confidence, hence minimizing the risks of cranial nerve and brainstem trauma during operations (Singh et al., 2016). With the increasing complexity of surgical practices, the challenges in evaluating monitoring technology and its impact on practice cannot be overstated. Surgical trials generally face idiosyncratic methodological challenges like the intricacy of randomization in trials of live procedures and heterogeneity of outcomes by surgeon experience. However, seeking good evidence for the use of these advanced monitoring technologies is crucial. Evidence-based practice, as it has been contended through argument over surgical innovation, is needed to assess the safety and efficacy of such interventions within everyday practice. With continued advances in technology, overcoming such obstacles will be important to ensure that monitoring technologies are not only being introduced into practice but properly evaluated for their safety and efficacy (Ergina et al., 2009).

12.3.2. Use of Simulation in Anesthesia Training

The use of simulation in training for anesthesia is a significant step in the practice of medicine, making trainees more ready for real practice. Simulation education allows for simulating complex clinical situations without risking patient health, hence providing practical experience in a simulated setup. The approach favors in developing technical skills and decision-making necessary for anesthesiologists. Recent studies have pointed to the fact that concentrated practice through simulation promotes improved competence in anesthesia management, leading to improved clinical outcomes for patients. Through interactive simulation scenarios and high-fidelity mannequins, students are able to experience multiple crises and develop their ability to successfully manage challenging situations. Also, built-in feedback mechanisms within simulation exercises enhance learning objectives even further so that practitioners can refresh their skills continuously. Additionally, teaching methods, like simulation training, complete what appeared to be the gaps in traditional anesthesia education. Targeted and brief teaching intervention with simulation has been shown in current studies to significantly enhance anesthesiologists' interpretation skills, like EEG monitoring skills, now increasingly appreciated for its role in optimal anesthesia depth (Berger-Estilita et al., 2025). By incorporating simulation into curricular design, anesthesiology residency programs are innovatively redesigning curricula. This enables the transition from conventional didactic methods to more active learning experiences that encourage critical thinking and in-the-moment problem-solving abilities, which better prepare trainees to manage the complexity of perioperative care. Furthermore, the benefits of simulation extend beyond the technical skill set; they lie at the heart of building non-technical skills such as communication and teamwork within the operating environment. Anesthesia may necessitate the coordination of various medical professionals, and therefore, teamwork is paramount for good outcomes. Simulation training enables these all-important interpersonal skills to be developed by placing trainees in real-world conditions where effective communication and cooperative strategies are paramount. Evidence suggests that such simulated situations not just reinforce individual capability but also team dynamics as a whole (Mokin & Kan, 2022). Emphasizing these traits is vital in creating mature anesthesiologists skilled not just in technical competence but in building a supporting environment that ultimately ends up centering on patient security and quality of care in challenging clinical situations (Figure 12.7).

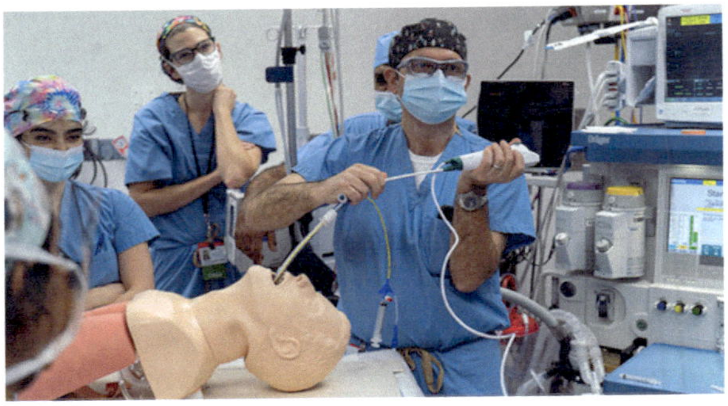

Figure 12.7. The integration of simulation in anesthesia training represents a significant advancement in medical education.

Source: https://www.bumc.bu.edu/anesthesiology/files/2022/06/SimCenterTraining1.png.

12.3.3. Impact of Telemedicine on Anesthesia Practice

The integration of telemedicine into the practice of anesthesia is a massive shift in the way preoperative evaluation is carried out. Traditionally face-to-face reliant, anesthesia care has begun utilizing the strength of virtual consult to facilitate more efficiency and patient accessibility. This trend is most beneficial in tackling logistical challenges since patients may struggle to arrive for appointments due to distances between locations, mobility, or the need for transport. Telemedicine allows anesthesiologists to perform complete assessments remotely, allowing for timely decision-making and potentially improving patient outcomes as well as decreasing delays associated with in-office visits. These advances resonate with the larger goals of advancing patient-centered care among anesthesia practices and thus paving the way for further research on how these virtual visits impact clinical guidelines and patient satisfaction levels (Department of Anesthesia, University of Iowa, 2011). A large study at the University of California, Los Angeles, evaluated the impact of telemedicine on preoperative consultation for anesthesia. The researchers found that patients who were seen through telehealth reported higher appointment completion and lower cancellation rates than their counterparts who underwent in-person consultations. Specifically, the completion rate for appointments was 81.38% for telemedicine and 76.60% for in-person evaluation, demonstrating the efficiency of virtual consultations in reducing barriers to care (Le et al., 2024). These findings look to the potential of telemedicine to optimize the scheduling processes inherent to anesthesia practice, allowing more patients to access preoperative evaluations without the limitations previously present in physical appointments. Yet, as telemedicine presents its myriad benefits, its execution shows limitations that deserve close scrutiny. The patient demographics for using telehealth platforms typically reveal a younger population that has more access to technology, perhaps screening out elderly patients or patients who need interpreter services. These inequalities give rise to significant ethical concerns about fairness in access to care. Moreover, during the study, it was discovered that telemedicine patients were more likely to have private insurance than Medicare, and this may reflect a potential socioeconomic gap which is able to perpetuate disparities in anesthesia care (Le et al., 2024). These constraints must be tackled to avoid the development of telemedicine inadvertently increasing existing inequality in healthcare, causing a shift in telehealth strategies to effectively support different patient populations in anesthesia practice.

Test Your Knowledge

1. How does simulation technology improve anesthesia training?
2. Why is practicing emergency scenarios in simulation important for anesthesia providers?

12.4. Evidence-Based Guidelines

Learning Outcome

1. Importance of clinical trials in anesthesia
2. Development of practice guidelines
3. Role of professional organizations in guideline dissemination

The establishment and implementation of evidence-based guidelines for anesthetic practice are a significant step towards improving patient outcomes and safety. The process of creating these guidelines is teamwork-based, considering the most recent research, clinical experience, and patient preferences and therefore resulting in an inclusive practice of anesthesia care. One of the most distinguishing aspects of these guidelines is that they rely on sound data analysis in supporting best practices, particularly in determining adequate anesthesia approaches to certain surgical procedures. By aligning clinical practice with such evidence-based measures, anesthesia providers can better deliver care that prevents risk and promotes recovery. In addition, continually evolving studies and systematic reviews continually fine-tune such guidelines, instilling an environment of ongoing development in the anesthesia protocols. Of particular importance, evidence-based guideline utilization is not uniformly spread throughout all aspects of anesthesia practice because of variations in accessing studies and clinical tools. For instance, while high-income countries may be able to have extensive information available for the formulation of such guidelines, low- and middle-income countries lack similar access, which hinders their implementation. This disparity raises red flags regarding inequalities in the quality of anesthetic care worldwide. The process by which guidelines are formulated within high-income environments is more dependent on scientific evidence, with limited data to consult, necessitating a recourse to clinical experience and established best practices that have been proven. In order to this extent, increasing the consolidation of evidence-based guidelines within every environment becomes a priority in order to ensure even access to good quality anesthesia care, regardless of geographical limitations. Besides, collaboration among clinicians, researchers, and professional organizations is necessary to drive the production and application of evidence-based guidelines in anesthesia.

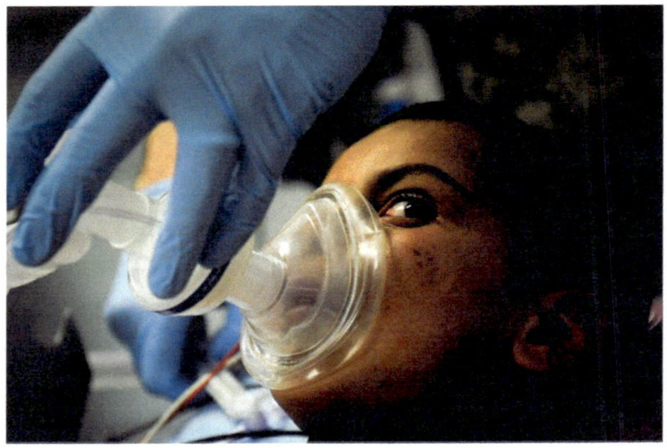

Figure 12.8. The creation and implementation of evidence-based guidelines in anesthesia practice.

Source: https://upload.wikimedia.org/wikipedia/commons/thumb/3/3d/Preoxygenation_before_anesthetic_induction.jpg/1200px-Preoxygenation_before_anesthetic_induction.jpg.

It has the potential to facilitate knowledge and resource sharing, particularly in low- and middle-income countries where guidelines are likely in the initial stages. Recent studies have demonstrated growing awareness of the need for region-specific recommendations that consider specific regional health care challenges, such as resource constraints and disease incidence variability. Through the facilitation of international collaboration and knowledge sharing between high-income and low-income countries, the anesthetic community can better address these challenges and deliver evidence-based care that is flexible and applicable to a broad spectrum of health care environments. This cooperative approach is a critical element towards enhancing the efficacy and usability of evidence-based guidelines for anesthesia, finally resulting in improved patient care globally (Figure 12.8).

12.4.1. Importance of Clinical Trials in Anesthesia

Clinical trials are crucial to the future advancement of the practice of anesthesia because they provide precious information that drives evidence-based practices. In an era in which the complexities of anesthetic care are amplified by patient diversity and evolving surgical techniques, the findings derived from clinical trials are invaluable. These trials are designed to evaluate the efficacy and safety of various anesthetic drugs for use, as well as methods to inform us about their pharmacokinetics and potential side effects. This is critical information not only to optimize patient care but also in creating guidelines that maximize perioperative outcomes. Therefore, incorporation of robust clinical trial strategies becomes imperative in establishing a scientific foundation for anesthesia practices, so that practitioners can be apprised of current best practices as determined by new research findings. Clinical trials offer more than mere efficacy data; they also account for the variability of patient-specific factors, i.e., comorbidities and surgery types, that directly affect anesthetic management. Emerging research design developments, such as stratified randomization and adaptive trial methodology, have allowed for a greater understanding of how different populations respond under anesthesia. Crucially, clinical trials in diverse groups facilitate generalizability of findings and facilitate inclusivity while assuring that new anesthetic regimens prove effective in diverse patient populations. This is particularly relevant to anesthetic procedures that may be influenced by genetic, age-related, or ethnic factors, as a recent article in the University of Iowa Department of Anesthesia newsletter (Department of Anesthesia, University of Iowa, 2011) highlighted. In the end, these trials empower anesthesiologists to tailor their approach to suit individual cases based on evidence accumulated from rigorous science. Moreover, the ethical aspects of clinical trials in anesthesia need to be stressed since they play a pivotal role in the safety of patients while advancing therapeutic techniques. Not every trial is an attempt at knowledge, but rather a pledge to uphold the highest standards of ethics in the treatment of patients. Conducting trials according to pre-specified techniques serves as a contribution towards an equipoise system that minimizes risk and maximizes benefits for patients. Clinical trials also create useful knowledge about possible side effects and complications that are uncommon, thus empowering practitioners with the right kind of information in order to make appropriate decisions. An example is how the results of trials that impact the use of preoperative testing and postoperative observation procedures can significantly guide patient safety measures. As in the studies of stroke management, adding high-quality evidence from clinical trials has enhanced the treatment methods, stamping its impact on universal patient outcomes in anesthesia (Campbell & Macrae, 2015). Continued commitment to conducting clinical trials will ensure the field evolves in evidence with both technological advancements and the overall ethical obligation to provide the best care.

12.4.2. Development of Practice Guidelines

Development of practice guidelines in the field of anesthesia is a critical process aimed at enhancing patient safety and improving outcomes through evidence-based recommendations. To this end, various stakeholder groups like clinical practitioners and professional associations play a vital role. Development of guidelines in anesthesia tends to be done by specialist committees that incorporate existing research evidence, clinical expertise, and patient safety considerations. Such committees are often confronted with issues of the availability of robust evidence, particularly where practice contexts are confounded by variability in the populations of patients and resources within an area. In this regard, some guidelines may be derived from the collective clinical judgment of practitioners where there is minimal empirical evidence, to emphasize the value of ongoing research and collaboration in this evolving discipline (Berglas & Roberts, 2018). There is also added complexity in the guidelines being practiced in different clinical settings, especially between resource-rich centers and low- and middle-income countries (LMIC). While high-income countries might have access to ample funding for research and infrastructure to support guideline development, LMICs pose unique challenges in the form of a scarcity of surgical services and a higher rate of anesthesia-related morbidity and mortality. Therefore, the policy guidelines in such regions have to be adaptable to fit local conditions and contain feasible interventions that reflect both accessibility and safety. This requires an acknowledgment of asymmetry in anesthesia practice worldwide and the need for evidence-based but context-adjusted guidelines that also facilitate interaction between institutions operating out of different economic environments (Fezeu et al., 2018). Since these dynamics are present, it is of utmost importance that clinicians participate in the process of developing guidelines. The engagement of front-line practitioners ensures that the ensuing guidelines are not just scientific but also practical and actionable in actual clinical practice. Care must be taken to frequently revise guidelines to reflect emerging evidence and changing clinical environments. A balance between investigation activities, clinician input, and ongoing tracking of guideline use will be necessary to guide and enhance evidence-based practice in anesthesia. As the profession matures, robust mechanisms for measuring the impact of practice guidelines on patient outcomes will be critical to sustaining ongoing relevance and usefulness for safe anesthesia care (Berglas & Roberts, 2018) (Figure 12.9).

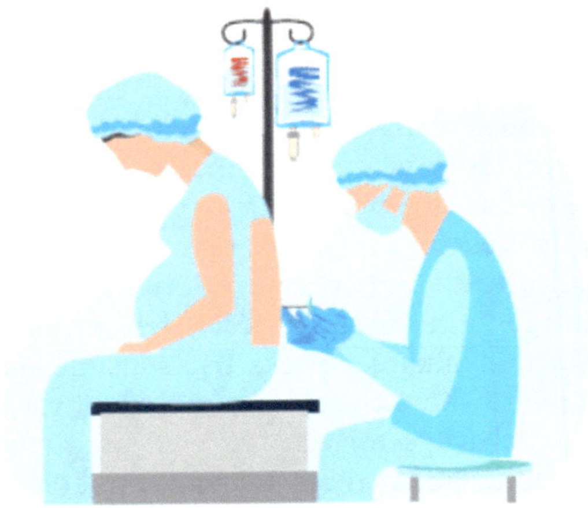

Figure 12.9. The development of practice guidelines in the field of anesthesia.

Source: https://asa.org.au/wp-content/uploads/2024/04/Anaesthesia_Epidural.png.

12.4.3. Role of Professional Organizations in Guideline Dissemination

Professional organizations play a key role in the communication of clinical guidelines for numerous medical specialties, such as anesthesia. These organizations usually possess the authority and expertise necessary to examine, develop, and communicate guidelines based on the available evidence. With the help of their established networks, they help spread practices that aim to improve patient outcomes.

For example, they can turn around the barriers to evidence-based recommendations usage, such as provider defensiveness and service overuse. Through targeted education programs and collaborations, such organizations provide clinicians with the skills needed in order to put new practices in place effectively, opening a door for evidence-based care to reach front-line providers (Bovbjerg & Berenson, 2012). Thus, the proactive role of professional groups not only guarantees the establishment of clinical guidelines but also translates the guidelines into daily practice to maintain the standards of care. Postoperative pain control in anesthesiology is a prime example of the necessity of professional groups in guideline translation. Professional groups that specialize in anesthesiology have launched programs intended to educate providers in pain control, particularly in the post-anesthesia care unit (PACU). They are significant because ineffective management of pain can affect patient satisfaction and hospital stay, thus resulting in extra health care expenditure. Professional associations address gaps in clinicians' knowledge through the development of integrated educational interventions, which enhance interprofessional communication skills. Studies demonstrate that systematic educational interventions can lead to measurable enhancement of the competence of nurses to manage pain in PACU settings (Madenski, 2014). By such dissemination of guidelines, such organizations encourage both the quality improvement of patient care and the culture of continuous education of healthcare workers. Professional organization intervention in guideline dissemination also brings consistency of practice across different areas and institutions. By extensive dissemination of guidelines, they bring a framework of care standards that all can aspire to achieve. This standardization is particularly important in anesthesia, where variation in practice can lead to extreme variation in patient outcomes. By promoting adherence to evidence-based guidelines, professional organizations help decrease variability in the provision of care. Apart from that, they also tend to establish forums for feedback and continuous improvement, so that guidelines continue to evolve and are responsive to emerging evidence. Hence, the collective efforts of these associations, apart from supporting compliance with best practices, lead to community advancement in the field of anesthesia, finally contributing to enhanced patient safety and care efficiency.

Test Your Knowledge

1. Why are clinical trials important in developing anesthesia practices?
2. How do evidence-based guidelines improve patient safety in anesthesia?

12.5. Patient Safety and Quality Improvement

Learning Outcome

1. Strategies for reducing anesthesia-related complications
2. Implementation of checklists and protocols
3. Importance of reporting and analyzing adverse events

Both patient safety and quality improvement have been unprecedentedly emphasized in the last few years in healthcare systems generally, and particularly in the field of anesthesia. Improvements in these domains are grounded in evidence-based practices that aim to systematically decrease the risks of anesthetic administration. For instance, advanced preoperative evaluation procedures have been shown to significantly decrease complications during surgical procedures. In addition, technology integration such as electronic health records and anesthetic monitoring systems becomes critical in ensuring patient safety. Technology advancement gives real-time access to information so that clinicians can make decisions and react to any change in a patient's status immediately, which in turn highlights the importance of effective communication and teamwork among healthcare providers. Also, quality improvement initiatives are commonly motivated by case examples of effective innovations in patient safety. Reports from research show that the implementation of some quality improvement approaches in specific health care institutions has yielded significant improvements in patient outcomes. For example, learning collaborations aimed at addressing interdisciplinary teamwork may enhance processes and reduce the frequency of adverse events. These initiatives not only present concrete results but also indicate the importance of sharing lessons gained across the health care community. Through a reading of these working models, practitioners in the field of anesthesiology are able to undertake similar actions in their respective settings, thus instilling a culture of continuous improvement across health care settings, as proposed by McCarthy & Blumenthal (2006). Furthermore, direct involvement of medical students and other trainees in quality improvement research has become a key component in enhancing patient safety. Programs that promote engagement with initiatives such as the SCaLPEL (Surgery Collaborative and Long-term Practical Experience Learning) Program foster an environment where new ideas are generated and new solutions developed. Engaging future professionals in conversation about safety and quality empowers them to carry forward these elements in their professional lives. Through the establishment of an education system focused on the improvement of quality and patient-centered care, health facilities are creating a workforce in the future that is informed and committed to upholding the highest possible standards of safety. Thus, continued education and participation become integral to the plan for long-term improvement in anesthesia practice and overall patient safety, as written in the paper by the Department of Anesthesia, University of Iowa (2011) (Figure 12.10).

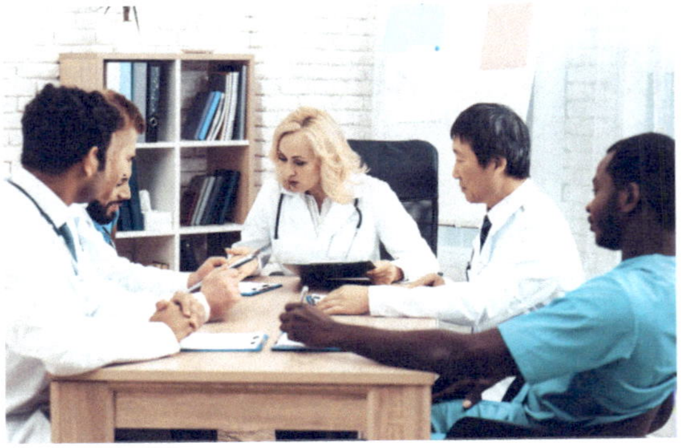

Figure 12.10. The domains of patient safety and quality improvement.

Source: https://www.ccianesthesia.com/wp-content/uploads/2022/12/AdobeStock_216718179-1-1024x684.jpeg.

12.5.1. Strategies for Reducing Anesthesia-Related Complications

Anesthesia-related complications are serious issues in perioperative care, and thus there is a search for effective measures to reduce them. One of the leading strategies is based on the enforcement of multimodal analgesia protocols. This technique entails the use of multiple diverse pharmacological agents that have actions on multiple receptors in the pain pathway, thus improving pain control with a reduced incidence of side effects of any single drug. Evidence supports the application of multimodal analgesia, particularly to reduce opioid use, which is related to a range of side effects, including respiratory depression and extended recovery. Further, a protocol specific to the surgery allows for tailored management of the patient, as different procedures may require tailored analgesic management. The challenge of drug shortage highlights the role of anesthesiologists and pain specialists in advocating for the use of both analgesics and appropriate alternatives to optimize perioperative pain relief and reduce complications (Schwenk & Mariano, 2018). Another possible way to reduce anesthesia-related complications is through the implementation of enhanced recovery after surgery (ERAS) protocols. These evidence-based multidisciplinary protocols are designed to ease the patient pathway and eliminate the physiological stress response to surgery. Enhancing such aspects of perioperative care as pain, fluid status, and early mobilization, ERAS has been proven to improve measurable outcomes from procedures like colorectal surgery. Of particular interest, studies have demonstrated lower markers of systemic inflammatory response with the utilization of components of ERAS protocols. For instance, laparoscopic techniques, a cornerstone of ERAS, have been implicated in lower postoperative C-reactive protein levels, hinting at lower inflammation and better recovery. By laying stress on the evidence-based practices that allow quick recovery, ERAS protocols are a vital component in minimizing the risks of anesthesia (Watt et al., 2015). Moreover, technological advancements and monitoring techniques have also been instrumental in minimizing the complications due to anesthesia. With innovations like real-time intraoperative monitoring, more advanced blood pressure and oxygen saturation monitoring, anesthesiologists have been able to react instantaneously in case of any instability. In addition, the use of targeted temperature management devices has also been shown to avoid complications like perioperative hypothermia, which might lead to greater morbidity. Such incorporation of technology requires intensive training of anesthesia practitioners along with dedication to strictly applying evidence-based practices within a broad variety of clinical settings. The interaction of these technological advances with established methods like multimodal analgesia and ERAS also indicates an interlinked solution to enhancing patient safety and minimizing complications in anesthesia, further solidifying the importance of ongoing research and education in this critical area.

12.5.2. Implementation of Checklists and Protocols

The application of checklists and protocols in the course of anesthesia is now a vital evolution intended to enhance patient protection in operating rooms. A good example is the roll-out of standardized readbacks, an idea conceived in aviation safety and now applied in perioperative services. Studies have shown that these readbacks reduce communication failures between healthcare professionals and consequently adverse outcomes in procedures. To give an example, a survey of providers within a level-one trauma center received near-unanimity in favor of readbacks' role in improving patient safety. Providers signaled assurance that these practices would improve handoffs, validate surgical instruments, and elucidate critical results, reporting their capacity to reengineer existing practice in anesthetic care. Hence, applying scripted communication methods in checklists can aid in bridging coordination gaps and promote safety culture in anesthesia, which is instrumental in providing optimal surgical results (Prabhakar et al., 2012). Also, the complexity of today's healthcare necessitates a more robust system for executing checklists and protocols. It has been suggested that the use of a standard training methodology, incorporated into educational curricula, will go a long way in strengthening the comprehension and efficacy of these tools among anesthesia professionals. Simulation-based education programs not only enhance technical skills but also strengthen non-technical abilities that are essential to patient safety. Through the exploitation of controlled and tested processes within training systems, professionals are more equipped to handle high-risk cases. The application of checklists within the same training makes every team member familiar with protocols that direct patient interaction in critical care. Through this, education and practice using simulation reinforce the necessity of checklists as a part of safe anesthetic practice with direct effects on team function and patient care (Escudero et al., 2019). Furthermore, despite the obvious advantage of checklists and protocols in anesthesia, there are still barriers to their widespread use. One of the significant barriers identified in recent literature is resistance to these standardized procedures by providers. For instance, it was demonstrated through studies that resident physicians were less inclined to participate in readback training than more experienced physicians. This difference highlights the necessity of tailored education plans for specific generational attitudes toward checklists. In addition, there is a pressing requirement to recognize clinical contexts where these protocols yield the greatest benefits. As healthcare systems strive to continuously improve, standardization of best practices must be accompanied by general evaluation to optimize and calibrate checklists for varied environments. With the overcoming of these obstacles, the application of checklists and protocols can revolutionize anesthesia practice and significantly enhance patient safety (Prabhakar et al., 2012) (Figure 12.11).

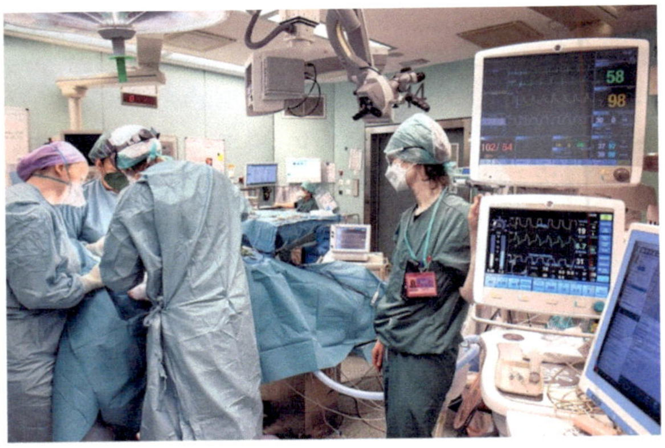

Figure 12.11. The implementation of checklists and protocols in anesthesia.

Source: https://nextlevelcme.com/storage/app/public/photos/54/WhatsApp%20Image%202021-05-04%20at%2009.47.05.jpeg.

12.5.3. Importance of Reporting and Analyzing Adverse Events

The significance of reporting and investigating adverse events in the practice of anesthesiology cannot be emphasized strongly enough, since these are a determining factor for improving the quality of patient care and safety. Adverse events, from minor issues to life-threatening consequences like death, provide useful information that can be carefully scrutinized by medical professionals collectively. In documenting such occurrences, institutions develop an atmosphere of transparency, where staff members are free to report cases of near-miss and error without any fear of retaliation. Transparency is crucial in establishing baseline levels of safety as well as enhancing the application of evidence-based practices. Systematic reporting is a process that allows anesthesia professionals to document trends and choose areas of work to be improved, ultimately leading to improved patient care competency as well as a reduction in the number of adverse events, thus highlighting the importance of strategic data collection in the clinical setting. Analysis of adverse events not only assists the immediate objective of enhancing patient safety but also assists in developing evidence-based guidelines with the potential to revolutionize anesthesia practice. By analyzing successful healthcare organizations that have experienced enhanced levels of safety through case studies, the field is able to acquire effective strategies and methods. For instance, programs focused on root-cause analysis are informative because it identifies essential problems that result in adverse events. Reporting systems combined with critical evaluation allow health care teams to engage in continuous learning and improvement. As different organizations come together to evaluate incidents collectively, they can formulate recommendations on short- and long-term improvements in the practice of anesthesia, solidifying a quality improvement system (McCarthy & Blumenthal, 2006). Also, the implementation of structured reporting systems along with careful analysis aligns with overall systemic reforms aimed at enhancing higher degrees of organizational safety cultures. Organizations such as the Veterans Affairs (VA) health system are exemplars through their establishment of the National Center for Patient Safety, highlighting organizational accountability and safety at all levels. Innovations associated with effective education and communication between surgical teams have yielded actual dividends, including reduced surgical mortality rates and improved care quality. Further, programs stimulating immediate root-cause analyses ensure an active approach towards prevention of future accidents—a model that can be replicated in other healthcare sectors. The interaction of reporting, analysis, and organizational commitment produces a strong safety culture, ultimately leading to improved outcomes for patients undergoing anesthesia (McCarthy & Chase, 2011).

Test Your Knowledge

1. What is one key strategy to minimize anesthesia-related complications?
2. How does continuous monitoring contribute to patient safety during anesthesia?

12.6. Future Directions in Anesthesia

Learning Outcome

1. Personalized anesthesia approaches
2. Integration of artificial intelligence in anesthesia
3. Potential for global health initiatives in anesthesia

Evolution of anesthesia is on the verge of significant advances, primarily with the deployment of evidence-based practice interventions aimed at patient outcomes and safety. Currently, there is a move towards multimodal analgesia modalities that provide improved pain control without limiting opioid consumption. One such instance includes pre-induction infusion of dexmedetomidine, which has gained attention for its opioid-sparing effect. Current studies show that education of anesthesia practitioners on the efficacy of dexmedetomidine not only enhances their knowledge but also encourages the drug's use in the clinical setting. It is the action that is crucial as it aims to reduce surgical stress responses and improve perioperative care, and that aligns with the general objective of reducing surgical patients' reliance on opioids (Nilsson, 2024). Such integration approaches herald the beginning of a new age in anesthesia wherein caregivers use modern-age methods to optimize patient experiences and surgical outcomes. In addition to this, future directions in anesthesia are centered on leveraging technology to facilitate tailored patient treatment. Advanced monitoring equipment and artificial intelligence are increasingly used to tailor anesthetic plans to specific patients according to their own needs. Through data analysis, the profession of anesthesiology can analyze enormous amounts of patient information, and this enables them to make well-informed decisions during the period of surgery. Implementation of these technologies not only improves the accuracy of anesthetic drug delivery but also assists in the forecasting of potential complications and improving overall patient safety. As health organizations implement such technological innovation, they become lifesavers in case studies that demonstrate effective innovation towards improving anesthesia practice. These case studies offer practical lessons that can be disseminated across the entire medical community, further driving the trend toward evidence-based, individualized anesthesia care (McCarthy & Blumenthal, 2006). Incorporating educational programs into anesthesiology procedures remains a vital area to target in the future for continued improvement. Ongoing professional development is needed to ensure that anesthesia professionals are up to date on new techniques and evidence-based practices. Training and educational programs for healthcare workers on the effects of multimodal analgesia and the benefits of adjunct agent use, like dexmedetomidine, have been shown to contribute towards a paradigm shift in clinical practice. Evidence shows that there are significant changes in prescribing patterns following enhanced education and training, with significant reductions in perioperative opioid dependence (Nilsson, 2024). The ongoing emphasis on education not only generates a culture of safety in operating rooms but also builds a culture of collaboration in which providers can share information and experiences. Such collaborative efforts will definitely shape the future of anesthesia, pushing it towards evidence-based practices and quality patient-centered care overall (Figure 12.12).

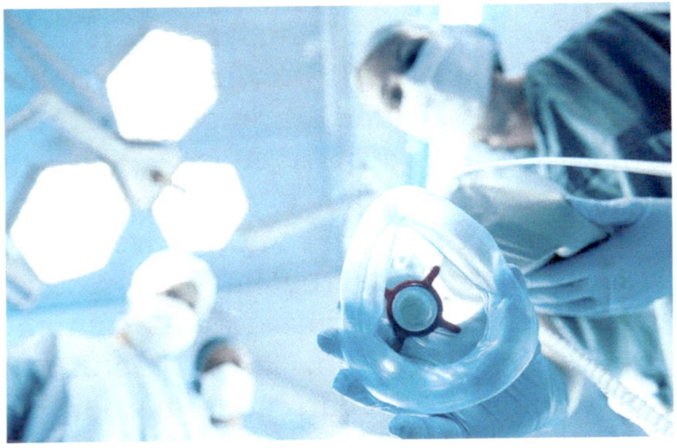

Figure 12.12. The evolution of anesthesia is poised for significant advancements.

Source: https://media.licdn.com/dms/image/v2/D4E12AQE8WvuHOJ9-lg/article-cover_image-shrink_720_1280/article-cover_image-shrink_720_1280/0/1691597874480?e=2147483647&v=beta&t=kxWZVQ6ID5hapmekeyM8TWMgOkMdrjfjjXvAa2a1meA.

12.6.1. Personalized Anesthesia Approaches

The field of anesthesia is revolutionizing itself with a trend towards individualized approaches that are based on patient-specific characteristics like genetic profile, comorbidities, and special surgical requirements. Individualized anesthesia is applicable for maximizing patient benefits with minimal adverse effects. Individualized anesthesia aims at modifying anesthetic techniques and drug choice based on a thorough understanding of a patient's individual physiology and drug response. For example, drug metabolism gene polymorphisms can have a significant impact on the efficacy and safety of anesthetic medications. So, pharmacogenomics is also emerging as a crucial factor in the formulation of personalized anesthesia plans, which enable anesthesiologists to select drugs better adapted to a person's metabolic capabilities, ultimately leading to improved procedural outcomes and recovery, along with reduced complications. Furthermore, individualized anesthesia relies on the use of advanced monitoring technologies. Real-time data collection and analysis, in turn, allow anesthesiologists to make dynamic adjustments to drug delivery and fluid management, thereby providing a more customized anesthetic experience. For instance, the use of multivariate monitoring systems can provide information regarding patient responses to anesthesia, allowing clinicians to make on-the-fly adjustments to doses or anesthetic techniques to prevent hypotension or hypoxia. This movement towards more interactive and responsive care is particularly beneficial in complex cases, such as those with geriatric patients or with high comorbidities. Additionally, employing a customized method can enhance a patient-centered care model with emphasis on safety, comfort, and satisfaction, enhancing general surgical outcome further. Emerging evidence-based strategies are also refining personalized anesthesia methods, particularly by employing artificial intelligence and machine learning algorithms. These technologies have the potential to review immense data sets to make individualized predictions regarding response to anesthesia based on hundreds of preoperative factors, such as age, weight, and comorbidities. Artificial intelligence -developed risk models, for instance, have revolutionized perioperative assessment by enabling the identification of patients with higher complication risk and thus more aggressive anesthetic monitoring and individualized care pathways. Through the incorporation of data from other clinical settings, such as the addition of ERAS protocols, customized anesthesia practices can ultimately bridge the gap between clinic practice and research development. This direction towards a data-driven practice is a significant step forward, embodying both precision medicine and an ethos of ongoing improvement in patient outcomes within the discipline of anesthesia care, as mandated in more recent developments set forth in the literature, e.g., (Malik et al., 2023; Singh et al., 2025) (Figure 12.13).

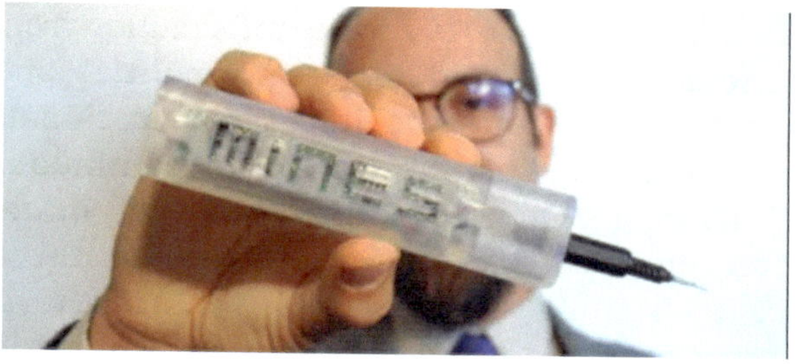

Figure 12.13. Personalized anesthesia approaches.

Source: https://res.cloudinary.com/tbmg/c_scale,w_400,f_auto,q_auto/v1625672982/sites/mdb/articles/2021/briefs/MDB-0721-p30_fig1.jpg.

12.6.2. Integration of Artificial Intelligence in Anesthesia

The use of AI in the field of anesthesiology is a paradigm shift that enhances accuracy as well as efficiency in clinical practice. Through the means of advanced machine learning techniques, anesthesiologists can currently use predictive analytics to forecast potential complications during surgery, and hence enhance anesthesia protocols to the specifications of individual patients. With the advancement of AI technologies in processing high volumes of data that encompass patient populations, medical histories, and intraoperative factors, AI provides real-time feedback and decision support to healthcare professionals. Not only do these technological innovations result in improved patient outcomes, but they also decrease the incidence of adverse events related to anesthesia administration, as AI facilitates a proactive rather than reactive approach in the management of patients. The transformation enabled by AI therefore constitutes a significant step forward in the safe delivery of anesthesia care within evidence-based frameworks. Furthermore, the newly emerging potential of AI in anesthesia practice is not limited to intraoperative care but extends to postoperative recovery as well. AI systems have the capacity to constantly monitor vital signs, leveraging information from various sources to detect abnormalities and appropriately notify healthcare professionals about evolving complications. This continuous monitoring enhances patient safety as initial interventions can be initiated when there are variations from expected parameters. Furthermore, the integration of AI-driven predictive models enables the identification of those patients at high risk for postoperative pain or complications, such that analgesic plans can be suitably readapted proactively. These advancements form a critical role in the era of personalized medicine, where individualized care pathways are optimized to achieve peak recovery, pain minimization, and peak resource utilization in clinical settings. Such application justifies the use of AI as a primary agent to improve the quality and effectiveness of anesthesia care. Finally, while the potential for AI in anesthesia is vast, one must consider the ethical implications of applying it to clinical practice. With emerging AI systems come challenges relating to data privacy, security, and the risk of algorithms being biased in their judgments. Reliance on large datasets necessitates consideration of the quality of the data in use, particularly because inaccuracy in the data may lead to incorrect clinical predictions. Besides, the challenge of the emotional aspect of patient care also comes forth as a central theme; while AI can be valuable in optimizing logistical features of anesthesia, it cannot substitute for the human touch that is the essence of patient-provider relationships. The argument for balance between embracing AIs strengths and holding on to the empathetic features that are an integral of healthcare is central to ensuring patient care remains rooted in compassion and empathy. As more of AI gets integrated, it will be necessary to cross these ethical borders to achieve optimal gains while ensuring patient rights and well-being (Figure 12.14).

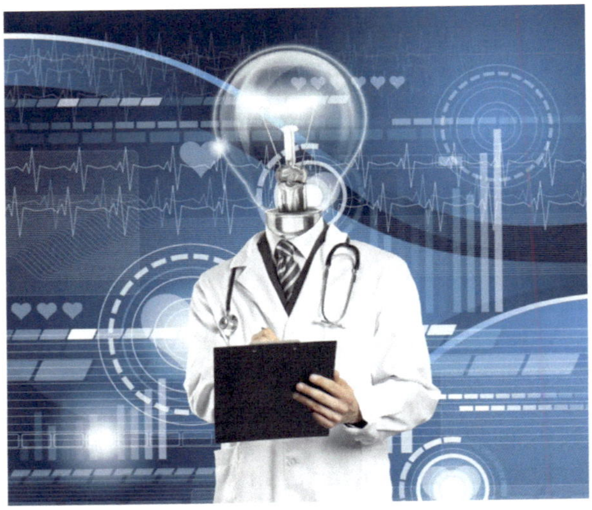

Figure 12.14. The integration of artificial intelligence (AI) within the field of anesthesia.

Source: https://i0.wp.com/theanesthesiaconsultant.com/wp-content/uploads/2017/08/ai-medical-1-orig.jpg?resize=788%2C677&ssl=1.

12.6.3. Potential for Global Health Initiatives in Anesthesia

The potential for global health opportunities in anesthesia is underscored by the growing recognition of access to safe and effective anesthetic care as a vital support for surgical success. With the lower-income nations struggling with high surgical mortality, the role of anesthesia in improved health outcomes becomes increasingly significant. Improving surgical infrastructure and training programs are emphasized by present global health efforts, most critically in resource-constrained settings. Through the promotion of standardized procedures and evidence-based practice, the global community of health professionals aims to improve the delivery of quality anesthesia interventions, ultimately leading to better postoperative recovery and reduced healthcare disparities. Cross-fertilization in the form of collaboration between international and national health governments is required for the creation of sustainable models for the dissemination of innovative anesthesia practice in different healthcare environments. Further, the introduction of new technologies is a key advancement in world health programs within the area of anesthesia. The development of nanotechnology, as revealed by recent research, signifies possible uses in drug delivery systems, target therapeutics for pain management, and enhancing anesthesia security measures. These advances are also able to give additional assistance to infrastructure that supports adequate anesthetic practice in underdeveloped countries and supplement efforts for the training and education of medical personnel in modern anesthesiology practice. As researchers increasingly push the boundaries of what is possible in the field of anesthetic care, clinicians' collaboration with technologists will be key to developing scalable solutions that are adaptive to local conditions and thereby establishing a more distributive model of global health. Finally, the emergence of data science and machine learning for anesthesia is indicative of the ways in which evidence-based medicine can be used to guide inclusive health initiatives. Surgical data science (SDS) facilitates the acquisition, organization, and analysis of large clinical data sets with value that can improve anesthetic decision-making and patient care. Through SDS, health systems can optimize resource utilization, identify high-risk populations, and implement tailored interventions. Most importantly, emphasis is placed on enhancing the translational effects of such innovations in the operating room globally so that advances in anesthesia are made accessible and impactful. As the technologies continue to evolve, they can assist in advancing the global health priorities focused on improved anesthetic care, ultimately as part of the bigger picture of enhancing health equity across the globe (Maier-Hein et al., 2021; Malik et al., 2023) (Figure 12.15).

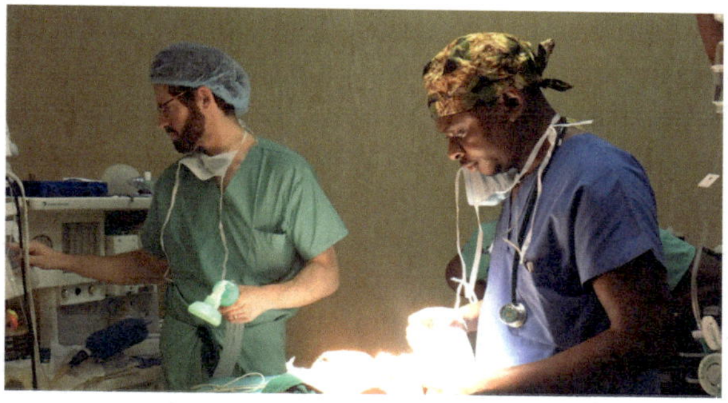

Figure 12.15. The potential for global health initiatives in anesthesia.

Source: https://anesthesiology.weill.cornell.edu/sites/default/files/styles/panopoly_image_original/public/media_uploads/img_0056_web.jpg?itok=12pzJY6m.

Test Your Knowledge

1. How can artificial intelligence improve decision-making in anesthesia management?
2. What is one potential benefit of using AI for patient monitoring during surgery?

SUMMARY

It is worth mentioning the significant progress within the field that has enhanced patient safety and results. Evidence-based practice has revolutionized anesthesia protocols, ensuring that clinicians utilize the latest and relevant scientific evidence when making clinical decisions. This guarantees that maximum possible attention is placed on eliminating the application of outmoded standards and addressing the necessity to follow new research and technology. Though problems still prevail with the pervasive use of evidence-based guidelines in most medical centers, the possible scope of improved patient care cannot be overlooked. The need for ongoing education and involvement on the part of anesthesia providers is pertinent in these contexts, culminating in enhanced levels of practice standards and improved patient safety. Beyond that, examining the development of anesthesia practices under the lens of proven standards in other ambulatory procedures offers lessons of monumental value. For instance, in setting facility standards, it was observed that anesthesia practice would benefit from the same rigorous development processes applied to other outpatient services. By encouraging professionalism among professionals working in anesthesia, for instance, those on surgical facility standard-setting committees, the profession can move towards more collaborative and established standards. As evidenced in literature, the absence of clear-cut research guidelines has a tendency to create reliance on clinician experience. This allows for continued professional development and more contact with health policy as it aligns with best practice, hence maximizing anesthesia delivery and patient care in various clinical settings (Berglas & Roberts, 2018). Finally, not only individual practitioners but also learning schools have an obligation to incorporate current practices within their learning curricula. Recent studies show that nursing education has been late to adopt evidence-based knowledge that would be applicable to current surgical practice and has impacted the preparedness of healthcare professionals in anesthetic settings (Mitchell, 2005). By bridging these gaps and fostering interdisciplinarity, the medical community can thus come together to equip all healthcare workers with the resources necessary for the introduction of sophisticated and evidence-based anesthetic practice. Therefore, with continued emphasis on education, adherence to evidence-based practice guidelines, and the strengthening of interprofessional ties will ultimately result in continued refinement of anesthesia so that patient well-being and safety are put at the top, so that advances made in the practice are effectively translated into practice.

Later advances in evidence-based anesthesiology have led to the door opening for optimizing clinical practice, mainly through the development and implementation of guidelines that achieve the best possible patient outcomes and safety. The implementation of evidence-based recommendations into practice has encouraged a more uniform process of care, reducing variability among providers. These guidelines not only help minimize the risk for surgical complications but also enhance the overall success of anesthetic approaches used. Studies highlight that compliance with evidence-based practice significantly reduces provider defensiveness and overuse, a trend that can have detrimental effects on healthcare provision. This trend toward standardization underscores the necessity of regular revision of these guidelines with new research becoming known to direct best practices in anesthesia management (Bovbjergm & Berenson, 2012). In addition, competency-based education for anesthesia professionals has also been pivotal in ensuring a higher quality of care. Highlighting the process of building competence, education programs now are designed to list the knowledge, skills, and attitudes to be acquired by practitioners in anesthesiology at various stages of their career. It encourages the culture of continuous learning and growth, allowing anesthesiologists to keep up with the fast-changing platform of medical advancements. By also reconciling clinical competencies with educational outcomes, the efforts ensure that anesthesiologists are capable of providing safe and effective care in varying settings. This symbiotic balance between practice and education ultimately enhances the quality of anesthesia services provided to patients, highlighting the importance of tailored educational frameworks in shaping competent clinicians (Hodges et al., 2013). Generally, the greatest progress in evidence-based anesthesia is both the creation of clinical guidelines and competency-based training, which collectively enhance patient care. Emphasizing evidence-based practice resolves not only current problems in anesthesia but also equips practitioners to continually enhance their abilities as new evidence is crafted. This dual-pronged approach is most important for building a health milieu that is both responsive and adaptive to patient requirements. Inclusion of guidelines and competency development is crucial, as it will help ensure that anesthesia professionals are trained to handle the complexities of modern medicine in an environment where patient outcomes are still the top priority. As the specialty continues to mature, ongoing innovation and collaboration will be necessary to preserve these advancements and shape the course of future safe anesthesia care (Taunton, 2019).

KEY TERMS FROM THIS CHAPTER

- Anesthesia protocols
- Bolster anesthesia
- Complexity
- Healthcare professionals
- Mitigate risks
- Patient safety
- Anesthetic community
- Clinical experiences
- Evidence-based practice (EBP)
- Innovation
- Neurosurgery
- Patients physiological

CRITICAL THINKING QUESTIONS

1. **What is the primary advantage of Sugammadex over neostigmine for reversal of neuromuscular blockade?**
   a. Rapid reversal of non-depolarizing block
   b. Reversal of depolarizing block
   c. No effect on hemodynamics
   d. Effective for all types of neuromuscular blockers
2. **Which opioid-sparing strategy has shown significant benefit in enhanced recovery after surgery (ERAS) protocols?**
   a. Patient-controlled analgesia (PCA)
   b. Regional anesthesia and multimodal analgesia
   c. Continuous intravenous morphine infusion
   d. Use of high-dose ketamine
3. **What is the mechanism of action of Dexmedetomidine, a sedative increasingly used in anesthesia?**
   a. GABA receptor agonist
   b. NMDA receptor antagonist
   c. Alpha-2 adrenergic receptor agonist
   d. Sodium channel blocker
4. **In patients with obstructive sleep apnea (OSA), what is the recommended anesthetic management strategy?**
   a. Avoid regional anesthesia
   b. Use of short-acting opioids and non-opioid analgesics
   c. Prolonged postoperative intubation
   d. Liberal use of benzodiazepines
5. **Which of the following is an advantage of total intravenous anesthesia (TIVA) with propofol over inhalational anesthesia?**
   a. Faster induction time
   b. Reduced risk of postoperative nausea and vomiting (PONV)
   c. Lower cost
   d. Universal applicability for all surgical procedures

Short Answer Questions

1. Explain the role of ERAS protocols in improving perioperative outcomes. How do these protocols incorporate evidence-based practices?
2. Discuss the benefits of Dexmedetomidine for sedation compared to traditional sedatives like midazolam or propofol.
3. How has video laryngoscopy improved the safety and success rates of airway management in difficult intubation scenarios?
4. What is the significance of capnography in monitoring procedural sedation, especially outside the operating room?
5. Describe the concept of goal-directed fluid therapy (GDFT) and its role in perioperative hemodynamic optimization.

Answer to Critical Thinking Questions

1. (a); 2. (b); 3. (b); 4. (b); 5.(d)

REFERENCES

1. Al-Ariki, M. K., Sidik, A., Ghosh, D., Hossain, M. L., Asadi, R., Mishra, R., Abuirayyeh, A. M. A., et al. (2025). Perioperative advances in repair of abdominal aortic aneurysm: A narrative review of strategies to enhance outcomes and reduce complications. *Cureus, 17*. https://www.semanticscholar.org/paper/bcf9906fef0f2cfd540b5c4a2f0b476830a783f4 (accessed on 28th June 2025).
2. Berger-Estilita, J., Saxena, S., & Gisselbaek, M. (2025). Advancing electroencephalography education in anesthesiology. *Current opinion in anaesthesiology, 38*(5), 576–583. https://doi.org/10.1097/ACO.0000000000001521(accessed on 28th June 2025).
3. Berglas, N. F., & Roberts, S. C. M. (2018). The development of facility standards for common outpatient procedures and implications for the context of abortion. *BMC health services research, 18*(1), 212. https://doi.org/10.1186/s12913-018-3048-3(accessed on 28th June 2025).
4. Betts, M. (2015). Utilization of an outpatient nausea prevention protocol. https://core.ac.uk/download/159581235.pdf (accessed on 28th June 2025).
5. Ergina, P. L., Cook, J. A., Blazeby, J. M., Boutron, I., Clavien, P. A., Reeves, B. C., Seiler, C. M., Balliol Collaboration, Altman, D. G., Aronson, J. K., Barkun, J. S., Campbell, W. B., Cook, J. A., Feldman, L. S., Flum, D. R., Glasziou, P., Maddern, G. J., Marshall, J. C., McCulloch, P., Nicholl, J., ... Vandenbroucke, J. (2009). Challenges in evaluating surgical innovation. *Lancet (London, England), 374*(9695), 1097–1104. https://doi.org/10.1016/S0140-6736(09)61086-2 (accessed on 28th June 2025).
6. Bloom, D. E., River Path Associates, & Fang, K. (2025). Social technology and human health. https://core.ac.uk/download/pdf/6248694.pdf (accessed on 28th June 2025).
7. McCarthy, D., & Blumenthal, D. (2006). Committed to safety: Ten case studies on reducing harm to patients. https://core.ac.uk/download/71350251.pdf (accessed on 28th June 2025).
8. Boly, M., & Seth, A.K. (2012). Modes and models in disorders of consciousness science. Archives italiennes de biologie, 150 2-3, 172-84 .(accessed on 28th June 2025).
9. Bovbjerg, R. R., & Berenson, R. A. (2012). The value of clinical practice guidelines as malpractice "safe harbors." https://core.ac.uk/download/71357531.pdf (accessed on 28th June 2025).
10. Le, D. Q., Burton, B. N., Tejeda, C. J., Jalilian, L., & Kamdar, N. (2024). Improvement in Adherance to Anesthesia Preoperative Appointment With Telemedicine: A Retrospective Analysis. *Cureus, 16*(5), e60805. https://doi.org/10.7759/cureus.60805(accessed on 28th June 2025).
11. Campbell, B. C., & Macrae, I. M. (2015). Translational perspectives on perfusion-diffusion mismatch in ischemic stroke. *International journal of stroke : official journal of the International Stroke Society, 10*(2), 153–162. https://doi.org/10.1111/ijs.12186 (accessed on 28th June 2025).
12. D. McCarthy and D. Chase, Advancing Patient Safety in the U.S. Department of Veterans Affairs, The Commonwealth Fund, March 2011.(accessed on 28th June 2025).
13. Prabhakar, H., Cooper, J. B., Sabel, A., Weckbach, S., Mehler, P. S., & Stahel, P. F. (2012). Introducing standardized "readbacks" to improve patient safety in surgery: a prospective survey in 92 providers at a public safety-net hospital. *BMC surgery, 12*, 8. https://doi.org/10.1186/1471-2482-12-8(accessed on 28th June 2025).

14. Escudero, E., ., Silva, M., & Corvetto, M(2019). Simulation: A training resource for quality care and improving patient safety. in: Serpil Celik Durmus (ed.), Nursing - New Perspectives, IntechOpen.

15. https://core.ac.uk/download/322444304.pdf (accessed on 28th June 2025).

16. Debono, B., Wainwright, T. W., Wang, M. Y., Sigmundsson, F., Yang, M., Smid-Nanninga, H., Bonnal, A., et al. (2021). Consensus statement for perioperative care in lumbar spinal fusion: Enhanced Recovery After Surgery (ERAS®) Society recommendations. *The Spine Journal, 21*, 729–752. https://doi.org/10.1016/j.spinee.2021.01.001 (accessed on 28th June 2025).

17. Singh, H., Vogel, R. W., Lober, R. M., Doan, A. T., Matsumoto, C. I., Kenning, T. J., & Evans, J. J. (2016). Intraoperative Neurophysiological Monitoring for Endoscopic Endonasal Approaches to the Skull Base: A Technical Guide. *Scientifica, 2016*, 1751245. https://doi.org/10.1155/2016/1751245(accessed on 28th June 2025).

18. Iqbal, R., Doctor, F., More, B., Mahmud, S., & Yousuf, U. (2020). Big data analytics: Computational intelligence techniques and application areas. Technological Forecasting and Social Change.. https://core.ac.uk/download/228156656.pdf (accessed on 28th June 2025).

19. Fezeu F, Ramesh A, Melmer PD, Moosa S, Larson PS, Henderson F Jr. Challenges and Solutions for Functional Neurosurgery in Developing Countries. *Cureus*. 2018;10(9):e3314. Published 2018 Sep 17. doi:10.7759/cureus.3314(accessed on 28th June 2025).

20. Ludwig, Lynda M.; Kersten, Judy R.; Tanaka, Katsuya; Gu, Weidong; LaDisa, John F.; Warltier, David C.; and Pagel, Paul S., "Mechanisms of Volatile Anesthetic-Induced Myocardial Protection" (2003). Biomedical Engineering Faculty Research and Publications. 233. https://epublications.marquette.edu/bioengin_fac/233(accessed on 28th June 2025).

21. Haladjian, H. H., & Montemayor, C. (2016). Artificial consciousness and the consciousness-attention dissociation. *Consciousness and cognition, 45*, 210–225. https://doi.org/10.1016/j.concog.2016.08.011(accessed on 28th June 2025).

22. Harden, R. N., McCabe, C., Göebel, A., Massey, M., Suvar, T., Grieve, S., & Bruehl, S. (2022). Complex Regional Pain Syndrome: Practical diagnostic and treatment guidelines, 5th edition. *Pain Medicine, 23*, S1–S53. https://doi.org/10.1093/pm/pnac046 (accessed on 28th June 2025).

23. Hodges, B. D., & Lingard, L. (2013). *The Question of Competence: Reconsidering Medical Education in The Twenty-First Century*. https://core.ac.uk/download/19958654.pdf (accessed on 28th June 2025).

24. Watt, D. G., McSorley, S. T., Horgan, P. G., & McMillan, D. C. (2015). Enhanced Recovery After Surgery: Which Components, If Any, Impact on The Systemic Inflammatory Response Following Colorectal Surgery?: A Systematic Review. *Medicine, 94*(36), e1286. https://doi.org/10.1097/MD.0000000000001286(accessed on 28th June 2025).

25. Jacobs, E., Wainman, B., & Bowness, J. (2023). Applying artificial intelligence to the use of ultrasound as an educational tool: A focus on ultrasound-guided regional anesthesia. *Anatomical Sciences Education, 17*, 919–925. https://doi.org/10.1002/ase.2266 (accessed on 28th June 2025).

26. Karalis, V. (2024). The integration of artificial intelligence into clinical practice. *Applied Biosciences, 3*, 14–44. https://doi.org/10.3390/applbiosci3010002 (accessed on 28th June 2025).

27. Liu, X., Li, Y., Kang, L., & Wang, Q. (2021). Recent advances in the clinical value and potential of dexmedetomidine. *Journal of Inflammation Research, 14*, 7507–7527. https://doi.org/10.2147/jir.s346089 (accessed on 28th June 2025).

28. Madenski, A. D. (2014). Improving nurses' pain management in the Post Anesthesia Care Unit (PACU). https://core.ac.uk/download/20252157.pdf (accessed on 28th June 2025).

29. Maier-Hein, L., Eisenmann, M., Sarıkaya, D., März, K., Collins, T., Malpani, A., Fallert, J., et al. (2021). Surgical data science–From concepts toward clinical translation. *Medical Image Analysis, 76*, 102306. https://doi.org/10.1016/j.media.2021.102306 (accessed on 28th June 2025).

30. Malik, S., Muhammad, K., & Waheed, Y. (2023). Emerging applications of nanotechnology in healthcare and medicine. *Molecules, 28*, 6624. https://doi.org/10.3390/molecules28186624 (accessed on 28th June 2025).

31. Schwenk, E. S., & Mariano, E. R. (2018). Designing the ideal perioperative pain management plan starts with multimodal analgesia. *Korean journal of anesthesiology, 71*(5), 345–352. https://doi.org/10.4097/kja.d.18.00217 (accessed on 28th June 2025).

32. Mitchell, M. J. (2005). Nursing knowledge and the expansion of day surgery in the United Kingdom. https://core.ac.uk/download/104292.pdf (accessed on 28th June 2025).

33. Mokin, M., & Kan, P. T. (2022). Balancing technical innovation and competence in the age of evidence-based medicine. *Journal of Neurointerventional Surgery, 14*, 949–950. https://www.semanticscholar.org/paper/6dda6ea49b0cd7f9dcff3664146903e79b48d493 (accessed on 28th June 2025).

34. Nilsson, A. (2024). Reducing perioperative opioid use through utilization of dexmedetomidine prior to induction: Provider education. https://core.ac.uk/download/604145967.pdf (accessed on 28th June 2025).

35. Pennazio, M., Rondonotti, E., Despott, E. J., Dray, X., Keuchel, M., Moreels, T. G., Sanders, D. S., et al. (2022). Small-bowel capsule endoscopy and device-assisted enterostomy for diagnosis and treatment of small-bowel disorders: ESGE Guideline–Update 2022. *Endoscopy, 55*, 58–95. https://doi.org/10.1055/a-1973-3796 (accessed on 28th June 2025).

36. Singh, A., Kanda, A., & Kanda, J. (2025). Recent approaches on oncolytic viruses, aptamers, TTFields and personalized treatment used for the management of glioblastoma: A comprehensive review. *Anti-Cancer Agents in Medicinal Chemistry*. https://www.semanticscholar.org/paper/17ad38becf67f54e05c0e60da1417329441fdfcb (accessed on 28th June 2025).

37. Stecca, T., Nistri, C., Pauletti, B., Di Giacomo, A., Colaut, F., Ruperto, M., Caratozzolo, E., et al. (2023). *Management of Acute and Chronic Pancreatitis*. Intech Open eBooks. https://doi.org/10.5772/intechopen.109115 (accessed on 28th June 2025).

38. Taunton, M. J. (2019). What's new in adult reconstructive knee surgery. *Journal of Bone and Joint Surgery, 102*, 91–100. https://doi.org/10.2106/jbjs.19.01063 (accessed on 28th June 2025).

39. Department of Anesthesia. University of Iowa. Spring 2011. https://core.ac.uk/download/18608347.pdf

INDEX

D

E

F

G

H

I

L

M

N

O

P

Q

R

S

T

U

V

W